Veterinary Science and Medicine: An Integrated Study

Veterinary Science and Medicine: An Integrated Study

Editor: Gerardo Bailey

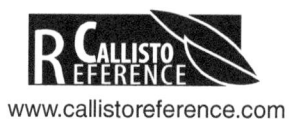

www.callistoreference.com

Callisto Reference,
118-35 Queens Blvd., Suite 400,
Forest Hills, NY 11375, USA

Visit us on the World Wide Web at:
www.callistoreference.com

ISBN: 978-1-64116-094-0 (Hardback)

Trademark Notice: Registered trademark of products or corporate names are used only for explanation and identification without intent to infringe.

Cataloging-in-Publication Data

Veterinary science and medicine : an integrated study / edited by Gerardo Bailey.
    p. cm.
Includes bibliographical references and index.
ISBN 978-1-64116-094-0
1. Veterinary medicine. 2. Animals--Diseases. 3. Animal health. I. Bailey, Gerardo.
SF745 .V48 2019
636.089--dc23

Table of Contents

Preface

Veterinary medicine is a branch of medicine that is concerned with the diagnosis, treatment, control and prevention of diseases in animals. It also deals with the treatment of injuries and disorders that animals are prone to. This field extends medical interventions to all domesticated and wild species of animals. Studies in zoonotic disease monitoring and control, food safety, livestock health management, mental well-being of pets, etc. are also explored in veterinary science. This book is compiled to provide detailed information about this field while also exploring modern perspectives towards the same. Different approaches, evaluations, methodologies and advanced studies on veterinary science have also been included herein. It aims to serve as a resource guide to students, researchers, experts and practicing veterinarians.

The information shared in this book is based on empirical researches made by veterans in this field of study. The elaborative information provided in this book will help the readers further their scope of knowledge leading to advancements in this field.

Finally, I would like to thank my fellow researchers who gave constructive feedback and my family members who supported me at every step of my research.

Editor

Comparative Study on Newcastle Disease and Infectious Bursal Disease in Chicken Submitted to Upazilla Veterinary Hospital, Bogra Sadar, Bangladesh

Arup Sen[1]*, Abu Torab[1], Abdus Salam SM[2], Bhubon Halder[2] and Alauddin MD[2]

[1]Department of Microbiology and Veterinary Public Health, Chittagong Veterinary and Animal Sciences University, Chittagong, Khulshi, Bangladesh
[2]Faculty of Veterinary Medicine (FVM), Chittagong Veterinary and Animal Sciences University, Chittagong, Khulshi, Bangladesh

Abstract

The study was conducted on 123 chickens submitted to Upazila Veterinary Hospital, Bogra Sadar for the detection of Newcastle disease (ND) and Infectious Bursal disease (IBD) during the period of 9th February to 8th April 2017. On the basis of history and postmortem examination findings, the prevalence of ND and IBD was 8.13% and 23.58%, respectively. The morbidity was 6.19% and 3.69% in ND and IBD, respectively. The mortality of ND and IBD was 4.00% and 2.009%, respectively. The main pathological lesions observed in this study were pinpointed hemorrhage in the proventricular gland, thickness of proventriculus wall, hemorrhage in the duodenum in case of ND and hemorrhages on thigh and breast muscles; inflamed, edematous, hyperemic and hemorrhagic bursa of Fabricious in IBD. The study also showed that the chickens of more than 30 days old and chickens within 15-30 days old were highly susceptible to ND (27%) and IBD (44%), respectively.

Keywords: Chicken; Newcastle disease; Infectious bursal disease; Prevalence; Bogra Sadar

Introduction

The economy of Bangladesh is agro based. About 21.77% of Gross Domestic products (GDP) come from agriculture sector of which livestock alone shares 7.23% [1]. Within the livestock sector poultry has the highest contribution to GDP. The poultry industry is an important part of agriculture in our country. Poultry farming is gradually taking the shape of a large industry, and it is now one of the intensive forms of agri-business in our country. In order to achieve the Millennium Development Goal (MDG), Bangladesh is committed to developing the poultry sector. The total poultry population, both backyard, and commercial accounts to approximately 246 million, providing 5400 million pieces of eggs annually and nearly 15% of total animal protein. This sector employs about 5 million people of the country and has experienced a long-term growth rate of about 4.5%, which is one of the highest in the economy and is believed to have accomplished a silent revolution in Bangladesh [2]. Some diseases create problems to run poultry farming profitably, such as Newcastle disease, Infectious bursal disease, Colibacillosis, Salmonellosis, Mycoplasmosis, Coccidiosis, Necrotic enteritis etc. Among these, Newcastle disease and Infectious Bursal disease are the threat for both commercial poultry and backyard poultry farming.

Newcastle disease (ND) is indicated as the most significant viral disease of poultry in the world together with developing countries [3]. In Africa and Asia ND is a major constraint to the development of both industrial and village poultry production. NDV infections of poultry range from latent to rapidly fatal depending upon the pathotype of virus involved [4]. Chicks from immunized parents possess a high level of maternally derived antibodies (MDA) which protect them against virulent and vaccine viruses [5,6]. The outbreak of diseases in Bangladesh causes about 30% mortality of chickens [7]. Among them, infectious bursal disease (IBD) is one of the major viral diseases which cause 80% mortality in field outbreak [8].

The etiological agent of IBD, infectious bursal disease virus (IBDV), is a non-enveloped virus, belonging to the family Birnaviridae, with a bisegmented double-stranded RNA genome [9]. Since 1992, the poultry farms of Bangladesh have been experiencing the outbreaks of a disease resembling acute IBD. Swollen bursa and sometimes atrophied bursa, edematous and hyperemic bursa, gelatinous yellowish transudate covering the serosal surface and swollen kidney were observed in post-mortem examinations. Hemorrhage and areas of necrosis may be present in more severe cases of IBD. Hemorrhage may be seen in the thigh and pectoral muscles [10-14]. IBD causes significant mortality in chickens in Bangladesh. The disease is in both private and government farms in the country. IBD is frequently reported even from vaccinated flocks. Sometimes farmers are confused and cannot suspect clinically on their own the occurrences of ND and IBD and the prevalence estimates of these diseases at a particular upazilla level are not clearly known to them as well.

Materials and Methods

The study was conducted at Upazilla Veterinary Hospital, Bogra (UVH, B) Sadar, Bogra district, Bangladesh. The duration of the study was the period of 8 weeks, starting from 9th February 2017 to 8th April 2017. A total of 123 birds were examined which were submitted to UVH, B from different commercial farms. Birds were examined postmortem at the UVH, B. ND and IBD on the reported farms were suspected based on the farmers' perceptions on clinical histories of diseases as received by taking direct interviews with them which were recorded on

*Corresponding author: Dr. Arup Sen, DVM, MS, Department of Microbiology and Veterinary Public Health, Chittagong Veterinary and Animal Sciences University, Chittagong, Khulshi-4225, Bangladesh
E-mail: arup09dvm@gmail.com

questionnaires. Some epidemiological information, such as bio-security management of a farm, vaccination, mortality and feed/water source were also recorded on it.

Case definition

Most of the time sick birds or dead birds brought to the Veterinary Hospital, examined first, history was taken from the farmers and finally postmortem examination was done. The bird which represent swollen or atrophied Bursa, hemorrhage /edematous fluid in bursa, hemorrhage on thigh muscles and breast muscles etc found on the postmortem examination were considered as case of IBD and ND is considered if pinpoint hemorrhage at the tip of the proventicular glands, hemorrhagic/diptheric ulcers on the intestine and caecal tonsils were found on post-mortem. The clinical signs and post-mortem findings of other concomitant infections with ND and IBD were recorded. Post-mortems examinations were carried out and the different disease conditions of the birds were examined and tentative diagnoses were made as described by Calnek [15]. The clinical signs as seen or described by the owners and postmortem examination findings based on which ND and IBD and other diseases were diagnosed. The prevalence (%) of ND or IBD in the birds examined was calculated on the following formula:

$$Prevalence = \frac{Total\ number\ of\ infected\ birds}{Total\ number\ of\ birds} \times 100$$

Data analysis

All data were entered into a spreadsheet program. Data management and analysis were performed using ANOVA Test: Single Factor using Microsoft Excel 2007. ANOVA Test: Single Factor done for the explanatory variables (Flock size, Age groups, Vaccination) and those having P-value ≤ 0.05 were considered significant.

Results

In the UVH, B during study period 123 chicken was investigated of which 10 were found positive ND and 29 for IBD. The cardinal post mortem examination findings, especially lesions located into the proventriculus and Bursa of Fabricious based on which ND and IBD were diagnosed. The prevalence estimates of ND by type of birds, age groups, flock sizes and status of ND-vaccination are summarized in Table 1.

Of the total chickens investigated in the study, 8% were positive for ND. The prevalence (%) of ND in Sonali chickens was 14%, significantly higher in Sonali chickens compared to broiler ones (P<0.05). Compared with young ones the prevalence of ND was higher in chickens belonging to the age group >30 days (P<0.05). Surprisingly, ND was evenly distributed in ND-vaccinated and non-vaccinated chickens.

The prevalence estimates of IBD in chickens by type of birds, age, flock size and IBD-vaccination are presented in Table 2. The prevalence of IBD in chicks of 15-30 days' group was 44%, significantly higher than other age groups (p<0.05). Surprisingly, IBD was 29% in vaccinated chicks which are significantly higher than non-vaccinated ones (P<0.05). Table 3 is presented with the overall farm-based morbidity and mortality in chickens based on the available data. The overall farm-based mortality attributable to ND and IBD were 4% and 2%, respectively.

Discussion

About 8% of the chickens investigated were diagnosed positive

with ND which was similar to the findings of Beach, Banerjee et al. and Alexander [16-18]. Most commonly observed postmortem lesions were pinpoint hemorrhages at the tip of proventricular glands, hemorrhagic ulcers in the intestinal wall and caecal tonsils, petechial hemorrhage in the colon, hemorrhagic lungs, tracheitis with congestion and catarrhal exudates. These findings corroborate with the findings of Kotani et al., Crespo et al., Talha et al. and Pazhanivel et al. [19-22]. The prevalence of ND observed in the study is, however, lower than the reports of Biswas et al. on chickens including Sonali reared under backyard system in Bangladesh [23,24]. A higher prevalence of ND in Sonali chickens, as observed in the study might be relating to weaker biosecurity for them compared to a better system of rearing for broiler chicks. The even distribution of ND in vaccinated and non-vaccinated birds should raise a question on the quality of vaccine used or its preservation and time of vaccination. This high prevalence of IBD found in this study is in accordance with the observation of Islam et al. who reported the proportion to be 24% in broiler chickens in Sylhet region [25]. However, there are reports in the other parts of the country which demonstrated the occurrence of this disease is lower than the present findings [21,26]. The highest prevalence (44%) of IBD was found in the group of 15-30 days birds and lowest (0%) in the group of 0-15 days birds. Lukert and Saif reported that clinically infectious bursal disease mostly occurs in the young chicken between 3-6 weeks of age, but the disease has also been reported to occur between 9 days to 20 weeks of age [27]. Rahman et al. found that the broilers of four weeks of age were highly susceptible to IBD (55%), whereas in third week 12.5% and in the fifth week 32.5% chicks were infected with IBDV and the broilers of two weeks of age were not affected with the virus [28]. Khan et al. reported that IBD affected birds were four weeks old conclusively [29]. Rajaonarison et al. showed that the birds of three to five weeks of old were most susceptible to IBD [30]. Wyeth et al. carried out studies IBDV in Great Britain and reported that IBDV can infect some chicks as young as fifteen days old [31]. No bird was found affected up to fifteen days. In this study, the outbreak of IBD in vaccinated flocks was significantly higher (P<0.05) which has also been described previously by Anku in Southern Ghana, Islam and Samad in Bangladesh and Jindal et al. in India [11,25,32]. They opined that factors like improper vaccination, poor biosecurity measures and the existence of very virulent strains of IBD virus contributed to the occurrence of IBD in the vaccinated flocks. The mortality rate of IBD (2%) in this study was similar to a previous report of Jindal et al. [32]. Age of the bird had a significant relationship on the prevalence and mortality of the disease. Mortality due to IBD in

Variable	N	Prevalence% (No. positive)	95% CI	P value
Type of bird	Sonali (63)	14% (9)	6-25	0.0258
	Broiler (60)	2% (1)	0.04-8	
Age	<15 days (35)	0% (0)	0-10	0.0008
	15-30 days (66)	6% (4)	32-57	
	>30 days (22)	27% (6)	0-15	
Flock size	<1000 birds (36)	0% (0)	0-9	0.0738
	1000-<2000 birds (45)	16% (7)	6-29	
	2000-<4000 birds (34)	6% (2)	0.72-19	
	≥ 4000 birds (8)	12% (1)	0.32-52	
ND vaccinated	Yes (107)	8% (9)	3-15	0.8451
	No (16)	6% (1)	15-64	
Total	123	8.13%	3-14	

Table 1: Prevalence estimates of ND by type of birds, age, flock size and ND-vaccination in the investigated chickens.

Variable	N	Prevalence% (No. positive)	95% CI	P value
Type of bird	Sonali (63)	22% (14)	12-34	0.8805
	Broiler (60)	25% (15)	15-38	
Age	<15 days (35)	0% (0)	0-10	0.0001
	15-30 days (66)	44% (29)	32-57	
	> 30 days (22)	0% (0)	0-15	
Flock size	<1000 birds (36)	22% (8)	10-39	0.0655
	1000-<2000 birds (45)	13% (6)	5-27	
	2000-<4000 birds (34)	32% (11)	17-50	
	≥ 4000 birds (8)	50% (4)	15-84	
IBD vaccination	Yes (86)	29% (25)	20-40	0.0504
	No (37)	11% (4)	3-25	
Total	123	23.58%	16-32	

Table 2: Prevalence estimates of IBD in chickens by type of birds, age, flock size and IBD-vaccination in the investigated chickens.

Farm No.	Morbidity (%)		Mortality (%)	
	ND	IBD	ND	IBD
1		0.84		0.24
2		2		1
3		3.2		0.2
4		0.05		0.05
5		0.5		0
6	3.1		0.1	
7		1.55		0.67
8		3.18		2.92
9		1.37		1.25
10		6.4		0.4
11		4.16		1.67
12		0.72		0.73
13	17.5		16.66	
14		8		6
15		8		7.5
16		1.6		0.8
17		0.85		0.14
18	1.63		1.17	
19	17.14		14.28	
20	0.46		0.2	
21	1.1		0.5	
22	4		2.5	
23		6.25		3.13
24		7.5		2.5
25		1.2		0.8
26		5.9		4.09
27		1		0.6
28		15.22		10.87
29		1.37		0.13
30	10.27		1.18	
31	4		1	
32		4.09		1.82
33	2.72		2.27	
34		12		8
35		4.8		0.35
36		2.25		1.5
37		1.2		0.4
38		0.33		0.2
39		1.33		0.33
Average	6.19	3.69	4.00	2.00

Table 3: Comparison of morbidity and mortality in case of ND and IBD, on the basis of farms where the birds were from.

chicks was significantly higher in vaccinated chicks, an agreement with the findings of Shil et al. [33]. The prevalence, mortality, and morbidity of IBD were 7.75%, 6.38%, and 1.35%, respectively. Khan et al.; Sami and Baruah recorded 55 outbreaks of IBD in broiler flocks from 1993-95 with mortality ranging from 0.9-25.7% [30,34].

Conclusion

The important postmortem findings in ND and IBD cases during postmortem examinations might be observed in the proventriculus and the Bursa of Fabricious, respectively. The prevalence of ND in the UVH, B might be 8%. The prevalence (%) of ND in Sonali chickens was 14%, which is significantly higher than broiler chicks. ND was also higher in chickens more than one month of age than younger birds. The distribution of ND was even in ND-vaccinated and non-vaccinated chickens. The prevalence of IBD in chicks of 15-30 days' group was much higher than the younger chicks. IBD was also much higher in vaccinated chicks. Farm-based mortality attributable to ND and IBD appears to be 4% and 2%, respectively.

Conflicts of Interest

The authors declare no conflicts of interest.

Acknowledgements

The author expresses his deepest sense of gratitude, and respect to his honorable teacher and internship supervisor, Professor Dr. Paritosh Kumar Biswas, Department of Microbiology and Veterinary Public Health, Chittagong Veterinary and Animal Sciences University for his scholastic guidance, sympathetic supervision, valuable advice, continuous inspiration, radical investigation and constructive criticism in all phases of study.

References

1. Bangladesh Bureau of Statistics. Livestock Survey in 2005-2006.

2. BLRI (2008) A Study on Highly Pathogenic Avian Influenza in Bangladesh. Bangladesh Livestock Research Institute, Savar, Dhaka.

3. Spradbrow PB (1997) Policy framework for smallholder rural poultry development. In: Proceedings of International Workshop on Sustainable Poultry Production in Africa held in Addis Ababa, Ethiopia. pp: 30-39.

4. Alexander DJ (2003) Newcastle disease, other Paramyxoviruses and Pneumovirus Infections. In: Saif YM, Barnes HJ, Glossons GR, Fadly MA, McDougald DJ, Swayne DE (eds.), Diseases of Poultry, Iowa State Press, AMES, pp: 63-100.

5. Allan WH, Lancaster JA, Toth B (1978) Newcastle disease vaccines: their production and use. FAO Animal Production and Health Series. FAO, Rome.

6. Rahman MM, Bari ASM, Giusuddin M, Islam MR, Alam J, et al. (2002) Evaluation of maternal and humoral immunity against Newcastle disease virus in chicken. Int J Poult Sci 1: 161-163.

7. Ali MJ (1994) Current status of veterinary biologics production in Bangladesh and their quality control proceeding of BSVER symposium held on July 28, 1994 at NIPSOM auditorium, Mohakhali, Dhaka, Bangladesh.

8. Chowdhury EH, Rahman IA (1996) Observation of outbreaks and subsequent control of infectious bursal disease in the central poultry farm in Bangladesh. Bangladesh Vet J 30: 13-17.

9. Kibenge FSB, Dhillon AS, Russel RG (1988) Biochemistry and immunology of infectious bursal disease virus. J Gen Virol 69: 1757-1775.

10. Butcher GD, Miles RD (2001) Infectious bursal disease (Gumboro) in commercial broilers. University of Florida.

11. Anku GG (2003) Gumboro hampers efforts to improve nutrition of Ghana's growing population. Poult Int 12: 32-36.

12. Rodriguez-Chavez R, Issac WS, Cloud S, Sandra MD (2002) Characterization of antigenic, immunogenic and pathogenic variant of infectious bursal disease virus due to propagation in different host systems (Bursa, embryo and cell culture). Avian Pathol 31: 475-492.

13. Saif YM, Abdel-Amin GA (2001) Pathogenecity of cell culture derived and bursa derived infectious bursal disease viruses in specific pathogen free chickens. Avian Dis 45: 844-852.

14. Dybing K, Jackwood DJ (1998) Antigenic and Immunogenic properties of baculovirus-expressed infectious bursal disease viral proteins. Avian Dis 42: 80-91.

15. Calnek BW (1997) Infectious bursal disease. In: Lukert PD, Saif YM (eds.), 10th edn. International Publishers Limited, pp: 721-733.

16. Beach JR (1942) Avian Pneumoencephalitis. Proceeding of annual meeting in US livestock sanitary association, Springer, Milan, Berlin, Heidelberg, New York.

17. Banerjee M, Reed W, Fitzgerald SD, Paniger B (1994) Neurotropic, Velogenic Newcastle disease incormorants in Michigan: Pathology and virus characterization. Avian Dis 38: 873-878.

18. Alexnader DJ (1997) Newcastle disease and other avian paramyxoviridae infections. In: Calnek BW, et al. (eds.), Diseases of Poultry. 10th edn. Ames. Iowa State University Press, pp: 541-569.

19. Kotani T, Ddagiri Y, Nakamura J, Horiuchi T (1987) Pathological changes of tracheal mucosa in chickens infected with lentogenic NDV. Avian Dis 31: 491-497.

20. Crespo R, Shivaprasad HL, Woolcock PR, Chin RP, Davidson-York D, et al. (1999) Exotic Newcastle disease in a game chicken flock. Avian Dis 43: 349-355.

21. Talha AFSM, Hossain MM, Chowdury EH, Bari ASM, Islam MR, et al. (2010) Poultry Diseases Occurring in Mymensingh District of Bangladesh. Bangladesh Vet J 18: 20-23.

22. Pazhanivel N, Balsubramaniam GA, George VT, Mohan B (2002) Study of natural outbreak of Newcastle disease in and around Namakkal. Indian Vet J 79: 293-294.

23. Biswas PK, Biswas D, Ahmed S, Rahman A, Debnath NC (2005) A longitudinal study of the incidence of major endemic and epidemic diseases affecting semi-scavenging chickens reared under the Participatory Livestock Development Project areas in Bangladesh. Avian Pathol 34: 303-312.

24. Biswas PK, Uddin GM, Barua H, Roy K, Biswas D, et al. (2006) Causes of loss of Sonali chickens on smallholder households in Bangladesh. Prev Vet Med 76: 185-195.

25. Islam MT, Samad MA (2003) Outbreak of infectious bursal diseases in vaccinated and unvaccinated commercial cockerel farms in Bangladesh. Bangladesh J Vet Med 1: 21-24.

26. Giasuddin M, Sil BK, Alam J, Koike I, Islam MR, et al. (2002) Prevalence of Poultry Diseases in Bangladesh. Indian J Poult Sci 40: 99-101.

27. Lukert PD, Saif YM (1997) Infectious bursal disease: Disease of poultry. 9th edn. Wolfe Publishing Limited, pp: 684-663.

28. Rahman MS, Islam MS, Rahman MT, Parvez NH, Rahman MM (2010) Analysis of prevalence of infectious Bursal disease in broiler flocks in Dinajpur. Int J Sustain Crop Prod 5: 15-18.

29. Khan RW, Khan FA, Farid K, Khan I, Tariq M (2009) Prevalence of Infectious Bursal Disease in Broiler in District Peshawar. ARPN J Agric Biologic Sci 4: 1-5.

30. Rajaonarison JJ, Rakotonindrina E, Rakotondramary SM, Razafimanjary S (2006) Gumboro Disease (Infectious bursitis) in Madagascar. Rev Elev Med Vet Pays Trop 47: 15-17.

31. Wyeth PJ, Chettle NJ, Mohepat AR (2003) Infectious bursal disease in Great Britain. Vet Rec 130: 30-32.

32. Jindal N, Mahajan NK, Mittal D, Gupta SL, Khokhar RS (2004) Some epidemiological studies on infectious bursal disease in broiler chickens in parts of Haryana, India. Int J Poult Sci 3: 478-482.

33. Shil GC, Ehsam MA, Rahmn MS, Anower AKMM, Ismal MR (2003) Diseases associated with mortality and pathological changes in cockerel birds. Bangladesh J Vet Med 1: 33-38.

34. Sami W, Baruah GK (1997) Incidence of infectious bursal disease in broilers in Assam. Indian J Vet Pathol 21: 67-68.

Status of Helminthes Parasites of Cattle in Dairy Farms of Holleta Agricultural Research Center, Central Ethiopia

Chala Bedasa[1], Mekdes Getachow[1], Ararsa Duguma[2]* and Shubisa Abera[3]

[1]College of Agriculture and Veterinary Medicine, Jimma University, Jimma, Ethiopia
[2]College of Veterinary Medicine, Haramaya University, PO Box 138, Diredawa, Ethiopia
[3]Yabello Regional Veterinary Laboratory, Yabello, Ethiopia

Abstract

A cross-sectional study was under taken at dairy farms of Holleta Agricultural Research Center, Central Ethiopia, which was located at central highland of Oromia special zone surrounding Finfinne, to determine the prevalence of gastrointestinal helminthes parasites of cattle from October 2009 to June 2010. A total of 283 cattle were examined using standard coprological examination on 147 Boran × Fresia and 136 Jersey breed cattle from both farms. The over all prevalence of GI helminthes parasites was found to be 68.2% (193/283) with the predominant eggs of *paramphistomum* (18.0%) followed by *ascaris* (9.5%), *fasciola* (8.5%), *strongylus* (7.1%), *nematodirus* (6.7%) and *trichuris* (1.8%) obtained from the study. There was statistical significant difference between age, breed and body condition with prevalence of parasites (P<0.05). The higher prevalence was recorded from adult animals than in young group. A cross breed of Boran × Fresia had higher prevalence of 57% than that of pure Jersey (43.0%). The level of infections determined by using Mc Master Eggs counting indicated that mild infections accounted for 55.5%, sever 1.1% and 11.7% for sub clinical light infections. Based on the results obtained further study on determinant factors for the occurrence of helminthes parasites and implementation of appropriate control and prevention methods should be applied in study area.

Keywords: Gastrointestinal helminthes parasites; Dairy cattle; Prevalence; Holetta; Ethiopia

Introduction

In Ethiopia Livestock playing an important role in the livelihood of poor farmers and provide a vast range of products and services such as meat, milk, skin, hair, horns, bones, manure and urine, security, gifts, religious rituals and medicine [1]. Livestock diseases are one of the main production constraints in which helminthes parasites are among the biggest causes of production losses and are responsible for both direct and indirect losses [2]. Helminthiasis of domestic animals is of major importance in many agro-ecological zones in Africa, but their impact is greater in Sub-Saharan Africa in general and Ethiopia in particular [3].

The most important helminthes parasites in cattle include nematodes (round worms), trematodes (flukes) and cestodes (tape worms). These parasitic infections are problem for both small- and large-scale farmers worldwide, but their impact is greater in sub-Saharan Africa in general and Ethiopia in particular due to the availability of a wide range of agro-ecological factors suitable for diversified hosts and parasite species [4].

Gastrointestinal helminthes are one of the main problems to cause economic losses and disease in animals. The effect of infection is determined by a combination of factors of which the varying susceptibility of the host species, the pathogenicity of the parasite species, the host/parasites interaction and the infective dose are the most important. The direct losses caused by these parasites are attributed to acute illness and death, premature slaughter and rejection of some parts during meat inspection. Indirect losses include the diminution of productive potential such as milk production reduce in dairy cow, decrease growth rate, weight loss in young growing calves and late maturity of slaughter stock [5].

The pathogenic effect of gastro-intestinal parasites may be sub-clinical or clinical. Young animals are most susceptible. The effect of these parasites is strongly dependent on the number of parasites and the nutritional status of the animals they are infecting. The major clinical signs are weight loss, reduced feed intake, diarrhea, and mortality reduced carcass quality and reduced wool production/quality [6]. Young animals do not have a great deal of immunity to parasites during their first year at pasture. The second year, they have partial immunity and, although they may appear healthy, they eliminate many eggs. Adult animals are much less susceptible to most parasites, unless they are in poor living conditions [5].

Animals are sometimes kept in conditions that make them highly susceptible to parasites. In the case of a recently dewormed animal, internal parasites no longer exist. There is thus no equilibrium and such an animal put into a contaminated pasture may be seriously affected. Animals in poor condition (e.g., recent illness, food shortages) are also highly susceptible [7].

Previous reports on prevalence of helminthes parasites of cattle in different areas of Ethiopia showed that 71%, 82.8%, 50.2%, 54.4%, 47.1% and 77.6% which is reported by Manaye [8] from highlands of Asela and its surrounding, Estehewot [9] in dairy cows in and around Holleta, Fikru et al. [10] in Western region of Oromia, Berhanu [11] in West Shoa zone, Ephrem [11] in Addis Ababa dairy farms and Cherinet [12] in small holder dairy farms of Jimma town respectively. Continuous investigation of parasitism in specific area is important to

*Corresponding author: Ararsa Duguma, College of Veterinary Medicine, Haramaya University P.O.box 138, Diredawa, Ethiopia
E-mail: tararsad@yahoo.com

know its status for implementation of control and prevention strategies based on its determinant factors. Therefore the aim of the present study was to determine the status of helminthes parasites of cattle and its associated risk factors and to identify major GI helminthes affecting dairy cattle of Holleta agricultural research center, central Ethiopia.

Materials and Methods

Study area

The study was conducted at Holetta and Adea Berga dairy farms of Holleta Agricultural Research center (HARC), which is located about 29 km from Addis Ababa on the highway of Ambo road. Holetta is located in central highland of Oromia special zone surrounding - 9°15' N and longitude of 38°25'- 38°45' E, at altitude of 2060-3380 m above sea level. The area got annual rain fall in between 834-1300 mm and the annual temperature of 11-22°C. Rainy season occurs with bimodal distribution 70% of which occurs during the main rainy season (June to September) and 30% during the small rainy season (February to April) and relative humidity of 50.4%.

Study animals

The Study animals were cross-breed of the number of Boran × Friesian cattle and Jersey breed which were kept under semi-intensive management system by Holleta Agricultural Research center in two separate places. The farm of cross-breed were located in Holleta town where the main office of the center found and Jersey breed farm at about 20 km from the center in Adea berga District. A total of 283 cattle with different age groups were included in this study. The age and other related factors of individual animals were collected from record of the center. Body condition score was determined as described by Morgan [13] and further classified into poor, medium and good. The purposes of these farms were for breed improvement and increasing of milk production requirement by the country.

Sample size determination

The sample size was determined at 95% confidence interval, 5% precision and with an expected prevalence of 50%. Thus, the sample size value was read from Thrusfield [14] and calculated to be 384 animals; however for this particular study we have used 283 animals based on facilities and animal management during the study period. Simple random sampling was considered to select the animals from the two farms of the study area where there was small herd size of animals existed in the farms.

Study design

A cross sectional study type was carried out from October 2009 to June 2010 to determine the prevalence of gastrointestinal helminthes of cattle in dairy farms of Holetta Agricultural research center using different coprologic techniques like flotation, sedimentation and Modified Mc master egg counting. The study cattle were selected by simple random sampling method and fecal sample was collected from the selected animals. Each selected animals for study was identified by their code.

Sampling method

The fecal samples were collected directly from rectum of the selected animals or from the top layers of fresh voided feces with a labeled disposable container by the animals' identification code number. Then the sample transported to HARC Parasitology laboratory immediately after collection and stored in a refrigerator at 4°C at maximum for 24

hours only. During the sample collection the breeds of animals, age and code given for individual animals as well as sample collection date were recorded for each sampled animals. Also their body conditions were registered. The sample was collected from the dairy farm cattle with use of simple random methods.

Fecal examination/coprology

To investigate the eggs of the helminthes each fecal sample collected were processed by using standard flotation and sedimentation techniques [15]. Identifications of eggs also made on the basis of their morphology according to keys given by Soulsby [15]. Modified Mc master egg count techniques (used for fecal samples that were positive to the parasite; to identify the degree of infestation) and levels of the worm infection were extrapolated from severity index defined by Urquhart et al. and Smith et al. [16,17], where cattle was said to have low, moderate and severe infestations if their fecal egg counts were from 100-250, 250-400 and more than 400 respectively.

Statistical analysis

The data collected from the study area was coded and recorded in Microsoft excel spread sheet and then analyzed by using SPSS version 16. The prevalence was calculated by dividing the number of animals harboring a given parasite by the total number of animals examined. Percentage to measure the prevalence of helminthes and chi-square (χ^2) to measure association between prevalence of the helminthes and the breeds, age, and body conditions of animals were the statistical tools applied. In all the analyses, confidence level was held at 95% confidence level and P<0.05 were set for significance value.

Results

Of the total 283 cattle (Boran × Fresian and Jersey) examined, 68.2% were found to harbor one or more gastrointestinal parasites. The prevalence of gastrointestinal parasites was higher in Borena × Fresian 57% (110/193) than Jersey 43% (83/193) (Table 1).

The predominant helminthes, eggs identified were nematodes eggs (52.3%), trematodes (37.8%) and mixed infections were found to be rare in occurrence (9.8%) as shown in Table 2.

The major species of helminthes parasites identified in this study were *Paramphistomum* at rate of 18% (51/193), followed by *Ascaris* 9.5% (27/193), *Fasciola* spp.8.5% (24/193) and the least percentage were *Trichuris* spp. which accounted for 1.8% (5/193) even mixed infection of those others occurred (Table 3).

The prevalence study in the different age groups was also conducted and it was observed to be 7.8%, 13.0%, 42.5% and 36.8% in age categories of less than 6 months, 6 months to 1 year, Heifers and bulls and milking cows respectively. There was statistically significant difference among the age groups (χ^2=69.278, P=0.002) as shown in Table 3. Higher prevalence rate was shown in adult animals than young.

There were a significant difference in prevalence of parasites with body condition of the animals observed (χ^2=7.950, p=0.019). A higher prevalence rate was encountered in animals with poor body condition 62.7%, while 16.1% and 21.2% were in animals with medium and good body condition respectively (Table 3). The statistical analysis in between breeds of animals showed that there was significance difference (χ^2=8.830, P=0.032) with the prevalence of helminthes parasites (Table 4).

The greater proportion of the study cattle (55.5%) were with moderate EPG, while (11.7%) and were with severe EPG infection rates (1.1%). Statistically significant (P<0.05%) association was also revealed

Type of parasites	Breed		
	Borana × Friesian N (%)	Jersey N (%)	Total N (%)
Nematodes	42 (21.8)	59 (30.6)	101 (52.3)
Trematodes	53 (27.5)	20 (10.4)	73 (37.8)
Mixed infection	15 (7.8)	4 (2.1)	19 (9.8)
Over all	110 (57)	83 (43)	193 (100)

N=Number of positive

Table 1: Prevalence of major helminthes parasites among breeds of Cattle in the study area.

Species of parasites identified	No. Positive	Percent (%)	Boran × Fresia (%)	Jersey (%)
Strongylus	20	7.1	9(6.1)	11(8.1)
Ascaris	27	9.5	11(7.5)	16(11.8)
Nematodirus	19	6.7	2(1.4)	17(12.5)
Trichuris	5	1.8	2(1.4)	3(2.2)
Paramphistomum	51	18	47(32.0)	4(2.9)
Fasciola	24	8.5	7(4.8)	17(12.5)
Nematodirus & ascaris	23	8.1	14(9.5)	9(6.6)
Strongylus & ascaris	2	0.7	2(1.4)	0
Fasciola & ascaris	7	2.2	3(2.0)	4(2.9)
Trichuris & ascaris	2	0.7	0	2(1.5)
Paramphistomum and ascaris	9	3.2	9(6.1)	0
Paramphistomum and fasciola	2	0.7	2(1.4)	0
Paramphistomum, fasciola & ascaris	2	0.7	2(1.4)	0
Overall	193	68.2	110(57%)	83(43%)

Table 2: Species of helminthes parasites identified from different cattle breeds.

Factors	No. of animals examined	No. Positive (%)	χ^2	P-Value
Age				
<6 months	25	15(7.8)		
6 months to1year	42	25(13.0)	69.278	0.002
Heifers and bulls	110	82(42.5)		
Milking cow	106	71(36.8)		
Body condition				
Poor	164	121(62.7)		
Medium	45	31(16.1)	7.950	0.019
Good	74	41(21.2)		
Breed				
Boran × Fresia	147	110(57)	8.830	0.032
Jersey	136	83(43)		

Table 3: Prevalence of GI helminthes Parasites within different risk factors.

in parasite prevalence between the different cattle breeds as shown in Table 4.

Discussion

Gastrointestinal parasites are highly prevalent in cattle where grazing pastures are dominant feed resources. Moreover, the study indicated a high prevalence and wide distribution of trematodes and moderate prevalence of gastrointestinal nematodes. The overall prevalence of helminthes infection of cattle in the present study was (68.2%) which almost in line with prevalence reported by Manaye [8] in highlands of Asela and its surrounding (71%) and also by Tesfaye [4] in dairy cattle of south Wello who reported 60%. The present study was lower as compared to the prevalence of GI helminthes obtained in dairy cows by Cherinet [12] and Estehewot [9] who indicated 77.6% in small holder dairy farms of Jimma town and 82.8% in dairy cows in and around Holleta respectively. The preset study was higher as compared

to the prevalence of GI helminthes obtained by Ephrem [18] in Addis Ababa dairy farms; Dejene [19] in Tulo district, Western hararghe zone; Mohammed [20] in Jimma areas; Berhanu [11] in West Shoa zone who reported as 47.1%, 50.8%, 53.9%, 54.4% respectively. Differences in the prevalence of GI parasite between the different studies could be due to variations in deworming practices, sample sizes, the parasitological techniques utilized, management conditions and climate between the studies areas including breed of cattle considered.

The predominant GI helminthes parasites identified in this study indicated higher prevalence of nematode parasites at 52.3% than trematodes 37.8%, whereas 9.8% were mixed infections of the two. This is consistent with findings of [21] in Burkina Faso, but disagreed with the reports of [9,22]. The major parasites species identified were *paramphistomum* (18.0%) followed by *Ascaris* (9.5%), *Fasciola* (8.5%), *Strongylus* (7.1%), *nematodirus* (6.7%), and *Trichuris* (1.8%) in which Infection with more than one helminthes occurred as well. Among the

Breed	No. of examined	Positive animals (%)	EPG Category (%)		
			Light	Moderate	Heavy
Boran × Fresian	147	110 (57%)	17(11.6%)	90(61.2%)	3 (2.0%)
Jersey	136	83(43%)	16(11.8%)	67(49.3%)	0%
Total	283	193(100%)	33(11.7%)	157(55.5%)	3(1.1%)

EPG=Egg per Gram

Table 4: Degree of nematode parasites infection among cattle breeds.

species highest prevalence of *paramphistomum* recorded by Manaye [8] had similar reports with the present study. The prevalence difference among the genera and species of helminths in different study area indicates that the topography and climatic condition of each study area vary from one another in supporting infectivity of different parasite and development of their intermediate hosts.

The prevalence study in different age group was conducted and it was observed to be the significantly higher prevalence rate was recorded in adult animals. This finding is in agreement with most literatures [7,23]. The age at which young animals are weaned is an important factor as regard to parasite resistance. For example, it has been observed that milk-fed calves are distinctly less contaminated than weaned calves [24]. The present report may oppose the idea of young animals do not have a great deal of immunity to parasites during their first year at pasture. The second year, they have partial immunity and, although they may appear healthy, they eliminate many eggs. Adult animals are much less susceptible to most parasites, unless they are in poor living conditions [5]. The present study concludes that less chance of exposure to infective stage of parasites by calves made less frequency of its occurrence than in adult animals.

The significant difference (χ^2=7.950, P=0.019) was observed in body condition of the animal and the prevalence of the parasites. The higher prevalence that observed in poor body conditioned animals was similar with the report of [7,10,25] could be due to GI nematodes and immunological responses of the animals against parasitic infections. This idea is in consistent with FAO [26] that started ruminants that are on a higher plane of nutrition mount a better immune response to internal parasites than whose nutritional status is compromised.

The study further revealed that breed of the animals showed significant association (χ^2=8.830, P=0.032) with the prevalence of the parasites; in which cross breed Boran × Fresian highly infected at rate of 51.9% than pure breed Jersey 48.1%. This association between different groups of breed and prevalence of parasites agrees with the study reported by Etsehiwot [9] and Berhanu [11] that stated there is a significant difference between the breed of the animals with prevalence of parasites.

The egg count per gram of feces for nematode infection in the current study indicated mostly with low to moderate intensity of infection. This result agrees with observation made by Berhanu, Dejene and Mohammed [11,19,20], who indicated the sub clinical cases of GI helminthes parasites with subsequent subsistent low pasture contamination.

Conclusion and Recommendations

Gastrointestinal helminthes parasites were one of the main problems in animals in dairy farms of Holleta agricultural research center. The most predominant GI helminthes parasites identified in this study was *paramphistomum* followed with *Ascaris* and *Fasciola*. Some of the cattle were affected with two or more parasites at a time. However, different ages, breeds and body conditions of animals had different chance to harbor the GI parasites. Generally the prevalence

of parasites was depending upon variations in deworming practices, sample sizes, climate conditions, and presence of intermediate host, feeding system, breeds and ages. Most of the animals examined during the present study relatively harbor low to moderate parasites eggs suggesting that the infection were usually sub clinical. However, sub clinical infections may be very important economically leading to retarded growth; reduced productivity and animals were more susceptible to other infections and infected animals also contaminate pastures. Therefore strategic parasitic control programs should be designed, so there should be further study on epidemiology and determinant factors for the occurrence of helminthes parasites and implementation of appropriate control and prevention methods for GI parasites identified that cause economic losses and diseases of animals in this study.

Acknowledgements

The authors would like to acknowledge Jimma University, College of Agriculture and Veterinary Medicine for financial support and staff members of Holleta Agricultural research center for technical and material support during the study period. We would like to express our heartfelt gratitude to Dr. Abebaw Gashaw for his high standard guidance, valuable comments and all round assistance in this research.

References

1. Yami A, Merkel RC (2008) Sheep and Goat Production Hand Book for Ethiopia. Ethiopia Sheep and Goat Productivity Improvement Program (ESGPIP).

2. Hoste H, Torres-Acosta JF, Aguilar-Caballero AJ (2008) Nutrition-parasite interactions in goats: is immunoregulation involved in the control of gastrointestinal nematodes? Parasite Immunol 30: 79-88.

3. Kumsa B, Wossene A (2006) Efficacy of Albendazole and Tetramisole Anthelmintics against *Haemonchus contortus* in experimentally infected Lambs. Intern J Appl Res Vet Med 4: 94-99.

4. Tesfaye H (2006) Ovine and bovine helminthiasis in Kelela, South Wollo. In: proceedings of EVA conference, Addis Ababa, Ethiopia, pp: 30-34.

5. Hansen J, Perry B (1994) The Epidemiology, Diagnosis and Control of Helminthes Parasites of Ruminants. A handbook, ILRAD, Nairobi, Kenya.

6. Radiostits OM, Blood DC, Gay CC (2000) Text book of the disease of cattle, sheep, pigs, goats, and horses. 9th edn. Bailler Tindall, London, pp: 563-613.

7. Keyyu JD, Kassuku AA, Kyvsgaard NC, Willingham AL 3rd (2003) Gastrointestinal nematodes in indigenous Zebu cattle under pastoral and nomadic management systems in the lower plain of the southern highlands of Tanzania. Vet Res Commun 27: 371-380.

8. Manaye M (2002) Study on bovine gastrointestinal helminthes in Asella and its surrounding highland areas in the Oromia regional state. DVM Thesis, Debre Zeit, Ethiopia.

9. Etsehiwot W (2004) Study on bovine gastrointestinal helminthes in dairy cows in and around Holetta. DVM Thesis, Debre Zeit, Ethiopia.

10. Regassa F, Sori T, Dhuguma R, Kiros Y (2006) Epidemiology of Gastrointestinal Parasites of Ruminants in Western Oromia, Ethiopia. Intern J Appl Res Vet Med 4: 51-57.

11. Berhanu G (2008) A cross sectional study of major gastrointestinal parasites of cattle in Bako District of West Shoa. DVM Thesis, JUCAVM, Jimma, Ethiopia.

12. Cherinat A (2009) Prevalence of bovine gastrointestinal helminthes parasites and socio economic survey in small holder dairy farms of Jimma town. DVM Thesis, JUCAVM, Jimma, Ethiopia.

13. Morgan ER, Torgerson PR, Shaikenov BS, Usenbayev AE, Moore ABM, et al. (2006) Agricultural restructuring and gastrointestinal parasitism in domestic ruminants on the rangelands of Kazakhstan. Vet Parasitol 139: 180-191.

14. Thrusfield M (2013) Veterinary Epidemiology. 3rd edn. Black Well Science Ltd., London, UK, pp: 178-236.

15. Soulsby EJW (1982) Helminthes, Arthropods and Protozoa of Domesticated Animals. 7th edn. Bailliere Tindall, London: Lea and Febiger, Philadelphia, USA, pp: 212-258.

16. Urquhart GM, Duncan JL, Armour J, Dunn AM, Jenning (1998) Veterinary Parasitology. 2nd edn. Blackwell Science, UK, pp: 103-113.

17. Smith WD, Jackson F, Jackson E, Williams J (1985) Age immunity to Ostertagia circumcincta: comparison of the local immune responses of 412 and 10 month old lambs. J Comp Pathol 95: 235-245.

18. Epherem W (2007) Prevalence of Bovine GI helminths in selected Dairy farms of Addis Ababa. DVM Thesis, JUCAVM, Jimma, Ethiopia.

19. Dejene T (2009) A study on major gastrointestinal helminthes parasites of cattle in two district Hararghe zone. DVM Thesis, JUCAVM, Jimma, Ethiopia.

20. Mohammed B (2008) Prevalence of bovine gastrointestinal helminthes in Jimma area. DVM Thesis. JUCAVM, Jimma, Ethiopia.

21. Belem AMG, Ouédraogo OP, Bessin R (2001) Gastro-intestinal nematodes and cestodes of cattle in Burkina Faso. Biotechnol Agron Soc Environ 5: 17-21.

22. Derb Y (2005) Study on Endoparasites of Dairy Cattle in Bahir Dar and Its Surrounding. DVM Thesis, Faculty of Veterinary Medicine, Addis Ababa University, Debre Zeit, Ethiopia.

23. Nwosu CO, Ogunrinade AF, Fagbemi BO (1996) Prevalence and seasonal changes in the gastro-intestinal helminths of Nigerian goats. J Helminthol 70: 329-333.

24. Pandey VS, Ndao M, Kumar V (1994) Seasonal prevalence of gastrointestinal nematodes in communal land goats from the highveld of Zimbabwe. Vet Parasitol 51: 241-248.

25. Abebe R, Gebreyohannes M, Mekuria S, Abunna F, Regassa A (2010) Gastrointestinal nematode infections in small ruminants under the traditional husbandry system during the dry season in southern Ethiopia. Trop Anim Health Prod 42: 1111-1117.

26. FAO (2004) Guide lines resistances management and integrated parasites control in ruminants, Animal production and Health Division Agriculture Department. Food and Agriculture organization of the United Nations, Rome.

3

Prevalence of Intestinal Parasites in the Intestine of Dogs (Sheep-Keeper, Owned, Pet and Stray) in Duhok Province, Kurdistan Region

Teroj Abdulrehman Muhamed[1] and Lokman T Omer Al-barwary[2]*

[1]*Department of Medicine and Surgery, College of Veterinary Medicine, University of Duhok, Iraq*
[2]*Department of Pathology and Microbiology, College of Veterinary Medicine, University of Duhok, Iraq*

Abstract

This survey was done to investigate the prevalence of internal parasites in the intestine of dogs in Duhok province from February to October 2015. A total of 270 sheep-keepers, owned, pet and stray dogs' fecal samples from most areas in Duhok province were collected and examined by flotation technique, sedimentation technique and direct smear. During this study *Spirocerca lupi* (0.7%) and *Uncernia stenocephala* (2%) were recorded for the first time in Kurdistan region; while *Diplydium caninum* (16.7%), *Strongyloides* spp. (1.9%), *Ancylostoma caninum* (2.2%), *Isosporaspp* (9.3%), cyst of *Giardia* (5.2%), *Hymenolepis nana* (1.9%), *Eimeria oocyst* (3.7%), *Taenia* spp. (13.7%) and trematode eggs (1.9%) were recorded for the first time in dogs of Duhok province. The overall percentage of intestinal parasites in dogs was 65.9%.

Keywords: Internal parasite; Dogs; Duhok province; Kurdistan region

Introduction

There have been no recent surveys to determine the prevalence of intestinal parasites in dogs in Duhok province, Kurdistan region. Dogs are frequently infected by internal parasites. However, several of these parasites are zoonotic and are considered important to human health. Although dogs are often considered family members by their owners, it is important to seriously note that they may be transmitter of intestinal parasites. Most of these intestinal parasites have an oral-fecal transmission cycle; and a major component for the spread of these parasites is the shedding of eggs or oocysts into the environment [1]. The transmission of zoonotic agents could be through direct and indirect contact with animal and animal secretions and excretion [2]. Dogs are the main zoonotic disease source through which parasites, in particular helminthosis, can raise serious public health concerns worldwide [3].

Many canine gastrointestinal parasites eliminate their scuttle elements (egg, larvae and oocyst) through the faecal route [3]. Several intestinal helminths of dogs including *Toxocara canis, Ancylostoma braziliense* and *Ancylostoma caninum* are important causes of zoonotic diseases, including cutaneous, visceral, ocular larva migrans and eosinophilic enteritis [4,5].

The aim of this investigation was to determine the prevalence of internal parasites infections in stray, owned, sheep-keeper and pet dogs in Duhok province, Kurdistan region.

Materials and Methods

Faecal samples

In this study, 270 fecal samples were collected from dogs of both sexes and different ages from three months to 13 years old, as shown in Table 1.

Collection of fecal samples

The practical work was carried out from the beginning of September 2014 to end of June 2015 in different rural and urban areas of Duhok governorate in Kurdistan region to determine the prevalence of intestinal helminths. Faecal sample was collected directly from the rectum of each dogs by using plastic lop spatula in small dogs, plastic gloves in adult dogs [6], or collection from the ground after defecation directly or some days old feces, but not more than 5 to 7 days [7]. Samples were then put in plastic containers and labeled; after that they were kept in a cool box and brought to the research laboratory at the College of Veterinary Medicine for coprological examination.

Study area

The area studied in this research is Duhok governorate, Kurdistan region in the north of Iraq, and five districts around it, namely Duhok, Summel, Zakho, Amedi and Shikhan/Qesrok, as shown in Figure 1. The animal population in this area is more than 750,000, including sheep, goats and cattle, and each year more than 650,000 animals are vaccinated.

Macroscopic examination

The fresh fecal sample was examined by naked eyes for consistency, texture, color and for the presence of any helminths, mucus and blood.

Coprological examination

All fecal samples were examined microscopically by flotation concentration method and formalin-ether sedimentation.

Flotation concentration method (modified Sheathers solution): The flotation solution must have a higher specific gravity than oocysts or parasite egg. The modified Sheather solution was prepared by using the methods of Dryden et al. [8] and Dryden et al. [9] (Figure 2).

Formalin-ether sedimentation: Faecal samples were concentrated by formal-ether concentration technique. The formalin-ether sedimentation

***Corresponding author:** Lokman T Omer Al-Barwary, Department of Pathology and Microbiology, College of Veterinary Medicine, University of Duhok, Duhok 00964, Iraq
E-mail: luqman_ommar@uod.ac

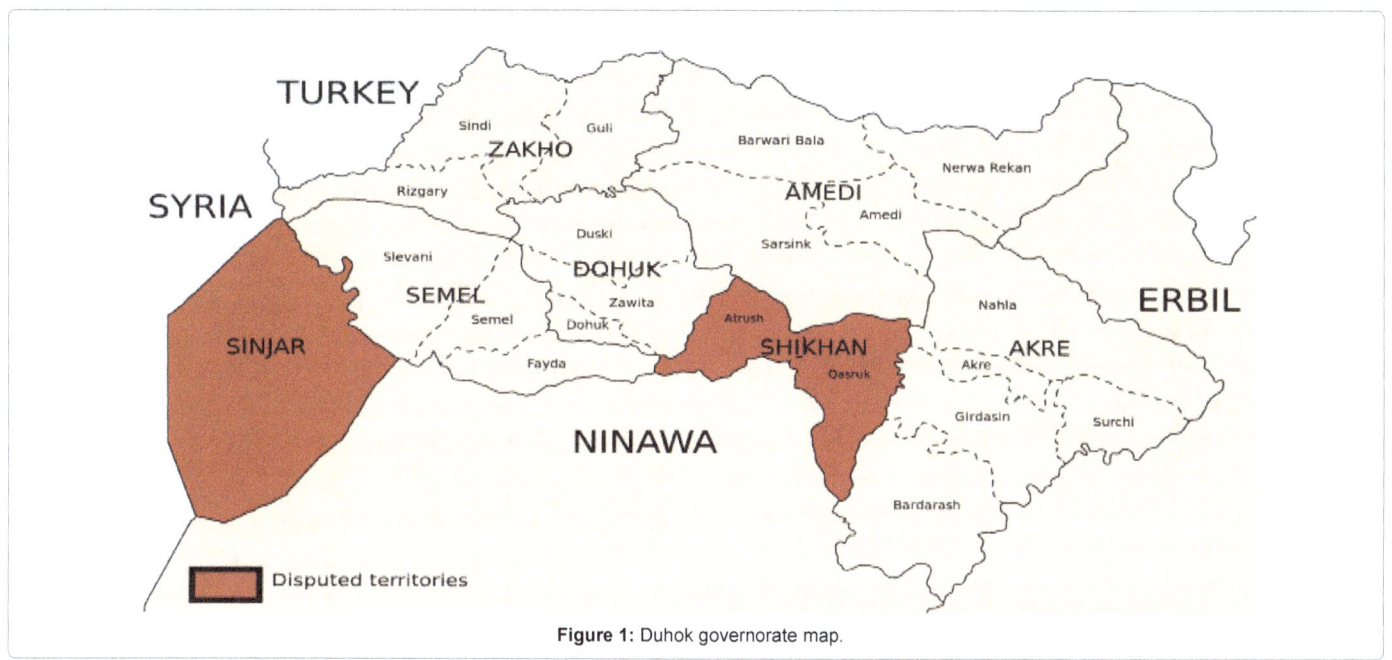

Figure 1: Duhok governorate map.

Faecal examination	Sex		Age		Type of dogs				Faecal collection	
	Female	Male	Young	Adult	Pet	Owned	Sheep keeper	Stary	Rectum	Ground
270	38	232	64	206	21	24	180	45	172	98

Table 1: Details of samples which were collected from dogs.

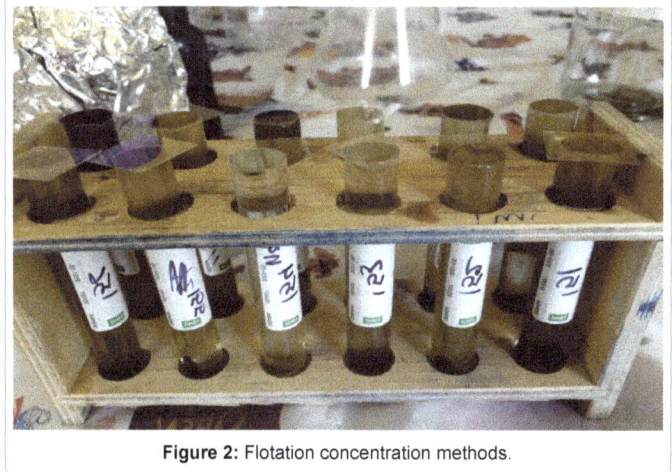

Figure 2: Flotation concentration methods.

was prepared by using the method of Allen and Ridley [10] and Zajac and Conboy [11]. Formalin 10% (1 volume of 40% formaldehyde diluted with 9 volume distilled water) and ether 99% (Figure 3).

Results

The following results were obtained from examination of fecal samples with methods of examination and each fecal sample was examined two times by Sheather concentration method and three times by formalin-ether sedimentation; and different ova of intestinal parasites were detected by these methods.

Out a total of 270 fecal samples examined, 65.9% were infected with ova of different intestinal parasites, while only 34.1% were free from ova of parasites, as shown in Table 2.

Table 3 shows ova of different intestinal parasites recorded by copro-parasitolgical examination methods. Ova of two parasites were detected for the first time in Kurdistan region, and these parasites were *Uncinaria stenocephala* and *Spicocera lupi* (Table 4).

Prevalence of intestinal parasites among 232 males examined recorded high infection rate of *T. canis* (22.84%) and low infection rate of *S. lupi* (0.86%); while the prevalence of intestinal parasites among 38 female dogs examined recorded high infection rate of *T. canis* (26.31%) and low infection rate of *H. nana* (2.63%).

Table 5 shows the percentages of single and mixed infection. Single infection had high frequency. As shown in Table 6, high prevalence of infection were found in stray and sheep keeper dogs with percentages of 73.3 and 70.5 respectively; while the lowest infection rate was in pet dogs (19.04%).

Discussion

Dog (*Canis familiaris*) is a domestic animal that has contact with man and other animals, any lack in the diagnosis or treatment of a certain disease may lead to the transmission of a zoonotic disease.

A total of 270 fecal samples were obtained for copro-parasitological examination, 178/270 (65.9%) were found to harbor at least one species of parasites, some had two to three species of parasites but only two samples harbored four species of parasites. The high prevalence of these helminthes in dogs is an indication of the degree of environmental contamination and poor hygienic level; also it indicates the lack of knowledge of dog owners in the role of dog in disease transmission and the importance of veterinary care.

Toxocariasis is one of the zoonotic diseases distributed worldwide by dogs. It is caused by *Toxocara canis*. Humans act as accidental host

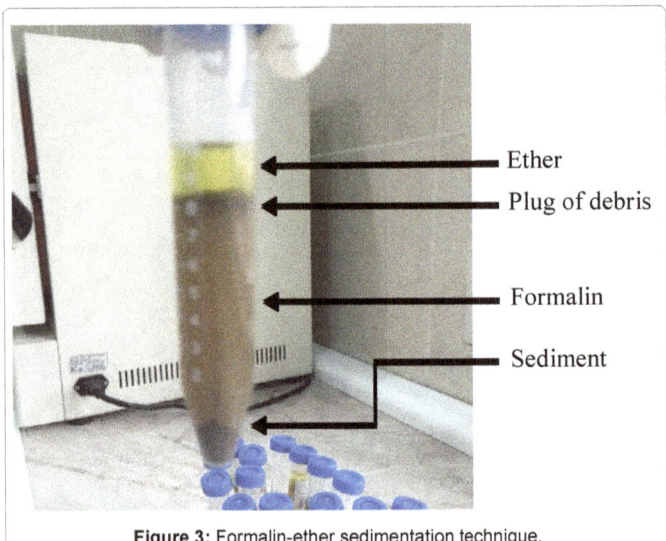

Figure 3: Formalin-ether sedimentation technique.

No. of dogs examined	Free from parasite microscopically		Infected with the parasite	
270	**Negative**	**%**	**Positive**	**%**
	92	34.1	178	65.9

Table 2: Overall percentage of intestinal parasites in dogs.

Name of parasite	No. of positive	%
Tremaode	5	1.9
Ancylostoma caninum	6	2.2
Ascaris spp.	11	4.1
Dipylidium caninum	45	16.7
Eimeria spp.	10	3.7
Cyst of Giardia	14	5.2
Hymenolepis nana	5	1.9
Isospora canis	25	9.3
Larvae of Toxocara canis	1	0.4
Rhabditiform larvae	6	2.2
Sarcocyst spp.	13	4.8
Strongyloides spp.	5	1.9
Spicocerca lupi	2	0.7
Taenia spp.	37	13.7
Toxocara canis	63	23.3
Toxascaris leonina	14	5.2
Uncinaria stenocephala	5	1.9

Table 3: Types of parasite ova, oocyst, cyst and larvae present in faecal samples examined by concentration technique with their infection rate.

and are infected accidentally through ingestion of the thick-shelled embryonated eggs, causing serious health problems [12,13]. The highest prevalence rate was found in *T. canis* eggs at 63/270 (23.3%) of the examined samples. This high prevalence rate of the infection is close to other results recorded in Iraq and Kurdistan region. Prevalence of 36% of 50 stray dogs examined in Sulaimani province, Kalar city was recorded by Bajalan [14]; the prevalence in cats was 30% in Mosul as obtained by Al-Obaidi [15] and 26.5% in Basrah according to Awad and Al-Aziz [16]. Dog sex had no effect on the copro-prevalence of the family Ascaridioidea and the same result was recorded by Dishow [17].

Diplidiasis is another zoonotic disease caused by dog tapeworm *Diplyidium caninum*. Human diplidiasis reported by Narasimham et al. [18] showed a prevalence of 45 (16.7%); this prevalence was

less than recorded in Diyala and Sulaimani provinces at 28 and 26%, respectively [14,19].

The prevalence of *Taenia* spp. in our work was 37/270 (13.7%); and the same result was recorded by Hasson [19] as 14.2%.

Hookworm was also observed in this work and the prevalence recorded was 2.2% (6/270) and 1.9% (5/270) for *Ancylostoma caninum* and *Uncinaria stenocephala*, respectively. The prevalence of *A. caninum* in Sulaimani is the same as in Duhok province, which was 2%. *U. stenocephala* had not been reported before this time in Kurdistan region and the prevalence was less than recorded in Albania which was 64.9% from a total of 111 dogs examined by Xhaxhiu et al. [20]; it was also less than recorded in Argentina by Dopchiz et al. [21] at 14.29%.

Trematode egg recovered from the fecal sample had prevalence of 1.9% (5/270); but in Basrah it was 67.1% from a total of 70 dogs examined by Awad et al. [22]. Low prevalence of trematode in Duhok province was due to little contact of the dog with water and the characteristic dry hot weather of this area.

As in the present work, for the first time *Spirocera lupi* was recorded in Kurdistan region, Duhok province and the prevalence was 0.7%

Parasite species	Male dog		Female dog	
	No. of infected dogs	Infection rate %	No. of infected dogs	Infection rate %
T. canis	53	22.84	10	26.31
D. caninum	37	15.94	2	5.26
Taenia spp.	32	13.79	5	13.15
Isospora spp.	20	8.62	5	13.15
T. leonina	12	5.17	2	5.26
Ascaris spp.	11	4.74		
Sarcocystis	9	3.87	4	10.52
Giardia spp.	8	3.44	6	15.78
Eimeria spp.	7	3.01	3	7.89
A. caninum	6	2.5		
Strongyloides spp.	5	2.15		
U. stenocephala	5	2.15		
H. nana	4	1.72	1	2.63
Rhabditiform larvae	4	1.72	2	5.26
Trematode	3	1.29	2	5.26
S. lupi	2	0.86		
Larvae of T. canis	1	0.43		

Table 4: Prevalence of intestinal parasites ova among 232 male and 38 female dogs examined.

No. of infection	No. of dogs infected	Infection rate (%)
0	92	34.07
1	113	41.85
2	49	18.14
3	14	5.18
4	2	0.74

Table 5: Frequency of single and mixed intestinal parasites infection in dogs.

Dog categories	No. of dog examined	No. of dog infected	Infection rate (%)
Stray dog	45	33	73.3
Owned dog	24	14	58.3
Sheep keeper	180	127	70.5
Pet dog	21	4	19.04
Total	270	178	65.9

Table 6: Prevalence of intestinal parasites in dogs of different functional categories.

(2/270); unfortunately, there is no available result in Iraq to compare the prevalence with. However, in neighbouring countries like Iran, the parasite was recorded and prevalence was 19.04% from a total of 105 dogs examined by Oryan et al. [23].

Other parasites were also recorded, but with low prevalence rate. Those parasites include *Strongyloides* spp. with prevalence of 1.9% (5/270) in fecal samples and this rate was less than recorded in Diyala province 7.1% by Hasson [19]; and *Hymenolepis nana* with observed prevalence rate of 1.9% (5/270).

Beside the presence of intestinal helminths in dogs of Duhok province, dog intestinal protozoa was present and the prevalence of cyst of *Giardia* was 5.2% (14/270), while the prevalence of *Eimeria* spp. and *Isospora* spp. were 3.7% (10/270) and 9.3% (25/70), respectively. Most of the infection rates were shown by dogs less than six months and this may be due to contact of puppies with feces of infected mother. High prevalence rate was also recorded in Baghdad and Diyala by Khalaf et al. [24] and Hasson [19] and the prevalence were 14.7 and 21.4%, respectively.

Sarcocystis spp. is one of the intestinal protozoa widely spread among sheep and goats in Duhok province and high prevalence of microcytic *Sarcocystis* spp. was recorded in sheep and goats; and the infection rate was 96.5% (220/228) of sheep and goats inspected in Duhok slaughter house by Hussein [25]. In the current study, it was found that the prevalence of the *Sarcocystis* spp. in the final host was 4.8% (13/270). This rate was more than recorded by Katagiri in Brazil with prevalence of 2.7% of a total of 254 dogs examined [26,27].

References

1. Claerebout E, Casaert S, Dalemans AC, De Wilde N, Levecke B, et al. (2009) Giardia and other intestinal parasites in different dog's populations in Northern Belgium. Vet Parasitol 161: 41-46.

2. Bugg RJ, Robertson ID, Eliot AD, Thompson RCA (1999) Gastrointestinal parasites of urban dogs in Perth, Western Australia. Vet J 157: 295-801.

3. Khante GS, Khan LA, Bodkhe AM, Suryawanshi PR, Majed MA, et al. (2009) Epidemiological survey of Gastro-intestinal parasites of Non-descript dogs in Nagpur city. Vet World 2: 22-23.

4. Krauss H (2003) Zoonoses: Infectious Diseases Transmissible from Animals to Humans. 3rd edn. Washington, DC: Am Soc Microbiol Press, pp: 369-371.

5. Prociv P, Croese J (1996) Human enteric infection with *Ancylostoma caninum*: Hookworms reappraised in light of a "new" zoonosis. Acta Tropica 62: 23-44.

6. Craig PS (1997) Immunodiagnosis of *Echinococcus granulosus*. In: Compendium on echinococcosis in Africa and in Middle Eastern Countries with special reference to Morocco. Andersen FL, Ouhelli H, Kachani M (eds.). Brigham Young University Print Services, Provo, Utah, pp: 85-118.

7. Guarnera EA, Santillan G, Botinelli R, Franco A (2000) Canine echinococcosis: an alternative for surveillance epidemiology. Vet Parasitol 88: 131-134.

8. Dryden MW, Payne PA, Ridley R, Smith V (2005) Comparison of common fecal flotation techniques for the recovery of parasite eggs and oocysts. Vet Therapeutics 6: 14-28.

9. Dryden MW, Payne PA, Ridley R, Smith V (2006) Gastrointestinal Parasites, the practice guide to accurate diagnosis and treatment. Compendium on continuing education for the practicing veterinarian 28: 3-3.

10. Allen AV, Ridley DS (1970) Further observations on the formol-ether concentration technique for faecal parasites. J Clin Pathol 23: 545-546.

11. Zajac AM, Conboy GA (2012) Veterinary Clinical Parasitology. 8th edn. John & Wiley Sons, Inc., pp: 40-88.

12. Despommier D (2003) Toxocariasis: clinical aspects, epidemiology, medical ecology, and molecular aspects. Clin Microbiol Rev 16: 265-272.

13. Marx JL, Masruha MR, Rodrigues MG, da Rocha AJ, Vilanova LC, et al. (2007) Toxocariasis of the CNS simulating acute disseminated encephalomyelitis. Neurology 69: 806-807.

14. Bajalan MMM (2010) Prevalence of intestinal helminths in stray dogs of Kalar city/Sulaimani province. Iraqi J Vet Med 34: 151-157.

15. Al-Obaidi QT (2012) Prevalence of Internal Helminthes in Stray Cats (*Felis catus*) in Mosul City, Mosul-Iraq. J Anim Vet Adv 11: 2732-2736.

16. Awad AHH, Al-Azizz SAAA (2004) Epidemiological study of *Toxocara canis* in Basrah (Cited: by Meerkhan Azad, 2007). Biochemical studies on hydatid cysts of *Echinococcus granulosus* isolated from different intermediate host (sheep, goat, cow and Human) tissues. MSc Thesis College of Education, University of Duhok.

17. Dishow MH (2014) Prevalence of Toxocariasis in dogs, cats and experimental infection in paratenic hosts and cats in Duhok province. A thesis submitted for the partial requirement of the degree of Master (MSc). College of Education, University of Duhok.

18. Narasimham MV, Panda P, Mohanty I, Sahu S, Padhi S, et al. (2013) *Dipylidium caninum* infection in a child: A rare case report. Indian J Med Microbiol 31: 82-84.

19. Hasson RH (2014) Stray dogs internal parasites from Baquba City, Diyala Province, Iraq. J Nat Sci Res 4: 30-38.

20. Xhaxhiu D, Ilir K, Dhimiter R, Elisabeta K, Rezart PLR, et al. (2011) Principal intestinal parasites of dogs in Tirana, Albania. Parasitol Res 108: 341-353.

21. Dopchiz MC, Carla ML, Roberto B, Patricia VG, Celina E, et al. (2013) Endoparasitic infections in dogs from rural areas in the Lobos District, Buenos Aires province, Argentina. Rev Bras Parasitol Vet 22: 92-97.

22. Awad AHH, Thamir M, Al-Azizz SAAA (2008) Intestinal trematoda of stray dogs as zoonoses agents in Basrah province. Journal of Thi-qar University 4: 34-38.

23. Oryan V, Sadjjadi SM, Mehrabani D, Kargar M (2008) Spirocercosis and its complications in stray dogs in Shiraz, southern Iran. Vet Med (Praha) 53: 617-624.

24. Khalaf JM, Shaimaa A, Majeed NK (2015) Epidemiological study of zoonotic gastrointestinal parasites in police and house dogs in Baghdad governorate, Iraq. MRVSA 4: 18-26.

25. Hussein SN (2015) Prevalence of *Sarcocystis* Infection in Small Ruminants (Sheep and Goats) and Experimental Infection in Dogs and Cats in Duhok Province. MSc thesis Submitted to Faculty of Veterinary Medicine, University of Duhok.

26. http://www.duhokgov.org

27. Parasitology Manual (2004) Microbiology Service Policy and Procedure Manual.

4

Whole Body Computed Tomography for Tumor Staging in Dogs: Review of 16 Cases

Bonaparte A[1]*, Dhaliwal RS[2], Heo J[1] and Murtaugh RJ[1]

[1]VCA All Care Animal Referral Center, 18440 Amistad Street, Fountain Valley, CA 92708, USA
[2]Silicon Valley Veterinary Specialists, 7160 Santa Teresa Boulevard, San Jose, CA 95139, USA

Abstract

Precise tumor staging encompassing the patient's entire body is essential in cancer management. While more advanced imaging modalities for tumor staging are available, in veterinary medicine, three-view thoracic radiography and abdominal ultrasonography are conventionally performed to screen for pulmonary and abdominal metastases. The objective of this retrospective study was to describe the use of whole-body computed tomography as an alternative in detecting lesions likely to be associated with primary or metastatic neoplasia in dogs. Sixteen dogs that underwent whole-body computed tomography were identified. Fifteen dogs had a histopathologic diagnosis of cancer. One dog had a cytologic diagnosis of thyroid carcinoma. The most common tumor types in this population included mast cell tumors [4; hind limbs (2), sternum (1), prepuce (1)], oral malignant melanomas (2), and spindle cell sarcomas [2; flank (1), cecum (1)]. The most commonly detected thoracic computed tomographic lesions were positional atelectasis (68.8%) and pulmonary nodules (12.5%). The most commonly detected abdominal computed tomographic lesions were splenomegaly (43.8%) and lymphadenomegaly (18.8%). The most commonly detected extra-thoracic/extra-abdominal computed tomographic lesions were cervical and retropharyngeal lymphadenomegaly (31.3%) and thyroid tumors (18.8%). No complications associated with anesthesia or contrast agents given during the procedure were observed and all dogs recovered uneventfully. Median scan time was 37.5 minutes. This study demonstrates that whole-body computed tomography is a safe and time-efficient imaging modality that is effective in identifying a range of pathologic changes important to tumor staging. Further prospective studies are needed to correlate the sensitivity and specificity of whole-body computed tomography with those of a combination of three-view thoracic radiography and abdominal ultrasonography.

Keywords: Computed tomography; Malignancy; Metastasis; Neoplasia; Tumor staging

Abbreviations: WBCT: Whole-Body Computed Tomography; CT: Computed Tomography.

Introduction

Accurate clinical staging is essential to pre-treatment evaluation of cancer patients to determine optimal therapeutic options and accurate prognosis. Therefore, precise tumor staging encompassing the entire body is critical to cancer management. Thirty to 40 years ago, the introduction of instruments capable of Whole-Body Computed Tomography (WBCT) scanning heralded the use of this technology for the detection of intra-abdominal and intra-thoracic disease in human patients [1]. Since then, numerous reports in medical journals emphasize the value of WBCT in the diagnosis, staging, and management of malignancies [2]. While more advanced imaging modalities for tumor staging are available in veterinary medicine, three-view thoracic radiography and abdominal ultrasonography are still conventionally performed to detect pulmonary and visceral metastases, respectively [3-6].

This report details our cumulative clinical experience with the use of WBCT in detecting and defining either primary or metastatic cancer in veterinary patients. The case material was drawn from patients with documented neoplasia, and it was not our intention to statistically compare the efficacy of WBCT versus other diagnostic modalities. Rather, our goal was to assess the feasibility of using WBCT in a clinical setting to demonstrate the range of lesions which can be visualized by WBCT and to underscore the potential diagnostic benefits that WBCT may yield.

Materials and Methods

Medical records of dogs that underwent WBCT at VCA All Care Animal Referral Center (VCA-ACARC) between January 2010 and December 2012 were reviewed. Dogs with confirmed histological or cytological diagnosis for malignancy were included. Clinical information obtained included signalment, laboratory findings, results of histologic or cytologic examination, WBCT scan findings, results of pertinent ancillary diagnostics (thoracic radiography, abdominal ultrasonography) and patient clinical outcome.

All the patients had CT scans of the thorax and abdomen; additional body parts were scanned at the attending clinician's discretion. The CT images were acquired using a HiSpeed NX/I dual-slice unit (General Electric, United States). With this unit, lung scans can be performed in a single breath hold. Multi-phase studies of abdominal organs such as the liver and pancreas also benefit from its increased speed. All scans were performed within one month of confirmed cancer diagnosis. All dogs were scanned while under general anesthesia, having been induced with propofol, and maintained on isoflurane and 100% oxygen. Dogs were positioned in sternal recumbency and head first within the CT gantry. The CT protocol consisted of a whole body scan, from the nose to the ischii. In general, 3-5 mm thick slices were obtained in transverse plane with the majority of the thoracic scans having 3 mm slices and abdominal scans 5 mm slices. Prior to thoracic CT acquisition, the dogs were hyperventilated with 4-5 breaths followed

*Corresponding author: Ashtri Bonaparte, VCA All Care Animal Referral Center, 18440 Amistad Street, Fountain Valley, CA 92708, USA
E-mail: ashtri.bonaparte@vca.com

by breath holding at 20 cm H_2O for the length of the thoracic scan. No additional manipulation was performed for the abdominal CT scan or to scan any other additional body part. Thirteen of the 16 cases had pre- and post-contrast CT scans carried out after intravenous administration of iodine-containing contrast material (Isovue', Bracco Imaging, Italy).

All CT studies were evaluated by a single board-certified radiologist who was blind to the clinical diagnosis and from the original imaging reports at the time of retrospective analysis. The radiologist reviewed the location, size, margins, internal architecture, and density of lesions detected. Sternal lymph node height was measured when sternal lymphadenomegaly was observed.

Results

Signalment

Medical records of 31 dogs that underwent WBCT during the study period were reviewed and 16 cases met the criteria for inclusion in the study. For dogs included in the study, median age at time of CT scans was 9.5 years (range, 5-14 years). There were eight castrated males, two sexually intact males, and six spayed females. Three were mixed-breed dogs, and 13 were purebred, representing 11 breeds. The most common purebred breeds were Labrador Retrievers (2) and American pit bull terriers (2). One dog represented each of the following breeds: boxer,

dachshund, golden retriever, Great Dane, Rottweiler, Shar-Pei, Siberian husky, standard poodle, and toy poodle.

Laboratory findings

Eleven of the 16 hemograms available had complete blood counts with no abnormalities. The remaining five had mild changes: lymphocytosis (1), lymphopenia (1), non-regenerative anemia (1), regenerative anemia (1), and thrombocytosis (1). Seven dogs out of 16 had normal serum chemistry panels. The most common serum chemistry abnormality was elevated liver enzyme activity in seven of the remaining nine dogs. Additional chemistry abnormalities in these nine dogs included: hyperamylasemia (2), hypercholesterolemia (2), hypocalcemia (2), hypercalcemia (1), hypoalbuminemia (1), and hypoglobulinemia (1). Urinalyses available in nine of the 16 dogs were acellular and sediment-free. Five out of nine dogs had isosthenuria and three dogs had proteinuria. Thyroid function was normal for nine of 11 dogs and the two other dogs that were tested had a low free T4.

Results of tumor types evaluated

One out of the 16 dogs had a cytological diagnosis of thyroid carcinoma. Histopathological diagnosis of neoplasia was confirmed in 15 out of the 16 dogs (Table 1). The neoplasias included: four mast cell tumors [hindlimb area (2), sternal area (1) and left peripreputial

Case	Diagnosis	Thoracic CT findings	Abdominal CT findings	Additional CT findings	Additional imaging diagnostics	Sternal LN height (mm)
1	Right thoracic wall spindle cell sarcoma	NSFa	NSF	n/ab	n/a	7Lc, 10Rd
2	Lingual malignant melanoma	Atelectasis	-Left adrenomegaly -Prostatomegaly	Bilateral retropharyngeal lymph node enlargement	AUSe – prostatomegaly	n/a
3	Left metatarsal Mast cell tumor	Contrast enhancing sternal soft tissue subcutaneous nodule	NSF	n/a	n/a	4L, 5R
4	Thyroid carcinoma	Atelectasis	Caudate liver nodules	Left thyroid mass	n/a	10L, 9R
5	Left stifle Mast cell tumor	Atelectasis	Splenomegaly	n/a	n/a	4L, 6R
6	Left radial osteosarcoma	Atelectasis	Splenomegaly	-Aggressive bony lesion distal aspect left radius - Left superficial cervical lymph node enlargement	CXRf – unremarkable	n/a, 5R
7	Sternal Mast cell tumor	NSF	Splenomegaly	n/a	n/a	n/a, 3R
8	Right anal sac adenocarcinoma	NSF	-Right anal sac inflammation -Splenomegaly	n/a	CXR – unremarkable	n/a, 2R
9	Salivary gland malignant mixed tumor	-Atelectasis	Splenomegaly	-Left ventral cervical mass -Left retropharyngeal lymph node enlargement	n/a	n/a
10	Mediastinal lymphoma	-Large soft tissue mediastinal mass -Atelectasis	-Splenomegaly -Hepatic lymph node enlargement	n/a	CXR – unremarkable	n/a
11	Pulmonary adenocarcinoma	-right and left caudal lung lobe nodules -Atelectasis	-Splenomegaly	n/a	n/a	3L, 4R
12	Hepatocellular carcinoma	NSF	-Multiple liver lobe masses -Hepatic lymph node enlargement	n/a	-CXR – unremarkable -AUS – liver lobe masses	8L, 6R
13	Right ear ceruminous adenocarcinoma	Atelectasis	NSF	-Right ear mass -Right retropharyngeal lymph node enlargement -Left thyroid nodule	n/a	2L, 6R
14	-Left nasal bridge soft tissue sarcoma -Left peripreputial mast cell tumor	-left cranial lung lobe nodule -Atelectasis	NSF	Soft tissue swelling left nose	n/a	7L, 4R
15	Maxillary malignant melanoma	Atelectasis	NSF	-left maxillary mass with bone lysis -Cervical lymph node enlargement -Right thyroid nodule	n/a	5L, 5R
16	Cecal spindle cell tumor with omental metastasis	Atelectasis	-Multiple abdominal lymph node enlargement -Right adrenal mass invading caudal vena cava	n/a	-CXR – unremarkable -AXRg – cranial abdominal mass effect	6L, n/a

aNSF: No Significant Findings; bn/a: Not Applicable; cL: Left; dR: Right; eAUS: Abdominal Ultrasonography; fCXR: Thoracic Radiography; gAXR: Abdominal Radiography

Table 1: Summary of description of imaging findings for 16 dogs with confirmed diagnosis of neoplasia.

area (1)], two oral malignant melanomas, two spindle cell sarcomas [cecum (1) and flank area (1)], and one each of apocrine gland anal sac adenocarcinoma, ceruminous adenocarcinoma, hepatocellular carcinoma, malignant mixed tumor of the salivary gland, mediastinal lymphoma, osteosarcoma, pulmonary adenocarcinoma, and left nasal bridge soft tissue sarcoma. One out of the 15 dogs (case 14) was evaluated for two concurrent neoplasias (left preprepuotial mast cell tumor and left nasal bridge soft tissue sarcoma).

Radiographic and/or abdominal ultrasonographic findings

Five of the 16 dogs (cases 6, 8, 10, 12, and 16) had three-view thoracic radiographs available at the time of the CT scan; no radiographic abnormalities were detected. Only one dog (case 16) had abdominal radiographs available, which showed evidence of abdominal masses. Two dogs (cases 2 and 12) had abdominal ultrasonography performed, which showed prostatomegaly and liver lobar masses, respectively.

Computed tomography scan findings

The scan time for all dogs ranged from 12-90 minutes; the median scan time was 37.5 minutes for dogs undergoing WBCT. Twelve of 16 dogs had lesions detected on thoracic CT scans. The most common CT abnormality was positional atelectasis, which was detected in 10 of 12 dogs. Two of 12 dogs had lung nodules detected on thoracic CT scans, and three dogs had additional single lesions: large mediastinal mass (1), right lateral thoracic wall subcutaneous nodule (1), and a contrast-enhancing soft tissue sternal subcutaneous nodule (1). Sternal lymph nodes were visible in 13 dogs and were measured accordingly (Table 1). The median left sternal lymph node height was 6.6 mm in 10 dogs and right sternal lymph node height was 5.3 mm in 12 dogs.

Abdominal lesions were detected in 11 of 16 dogs, with splenomegaly being the most common finding (7), followed by abdominal lymphadenomegaly (3), liver nodules (2), left adrenomegaly (1), right adrenal mass invading the caudal vena cava (1), prostatomegaly (1), and right anal sac inflammation (1).

Additional body parts evaluated by CT scan included the head, neck, and extremities; these scans were performed on seven of the 16 dogs. All seven dogs had detectable extra-thoracic/extra-abdominal CT lesions which included retropharyngeal lymphadenomegaly in three dogs (cases 2, 9, and 13), thyroid mass or nodule in three dogs (cases 4, 13, and 15), cervical lymphadenomegaly in two dogs (cases 6 and 15). One dog each was observed to have each of the following lesions: ventral cervical mass, left nasal soft tissue swelling, left maxillary mass with bone lysis, right ear canal mass, and an aggressive lesion located at the distal aspect of the left radius.

Discussion

The results of our current study show that WBCT can play a primary or complementary role in staging canine patients with known or suspected malignancy via lesion localization. Since CT allows visualization of normal anatomic structures as well as pathologic processes, this imaging modality provides information regarding the texture and internal architecture of lesions under investigation. In the assessment of the primary tumor, CT is particularly helpful for identifying tumor spread into adjacent tissues. In this study, we assessed primary tumors of the skull and oral cavity, thorax (primary lung tumors, mediastinal tumors), abdomen, and of the integument and extremities. CT imaging can readily define the presence of compression and/or invasion of surrounding structures, as was seen in case 16 (Figure 1). Whole body CT identified this right adrenal mass invasion

of the caudal vena cava. Although histopathology was not performed to confirm malignancy, this invasion may be correlated with extension of malignancy, which in turn could impact treatment approach and prognosis for the patient [7-9].

Contrast agents are applied in CT protocols to aid differentiation of anatomic structures, improve lesion localization, and support lesion characterization. With the aid of injected contrast, solid lesions can be further categorized into hypovascular or hypervascular masses [10]. An example is demonstrated in case 4 (Figure 2). Studies of human patients comparing contrast-enhanced with non-enhanced CT protocols in the experimental setting, as well as in standard radiology practice, demonstrate a substantial benefit of the contrast-enhanced approach [9,11]. Violante and Dean show an increase in accuracy for detection of liver lesions, from 63% to 90%, when applying intravenous contrast agents [11]. Schultz et al. reports the sensitivity and specificity of contrast-enhanced CT for vascular invasion, compared with observation at surgery or necropsy, to be 92% and 100%, respectively [9].

Lymphadenomegaly was a lesion most commonly detected on CT in our patients. This finding may alert the clinician to potential tumor

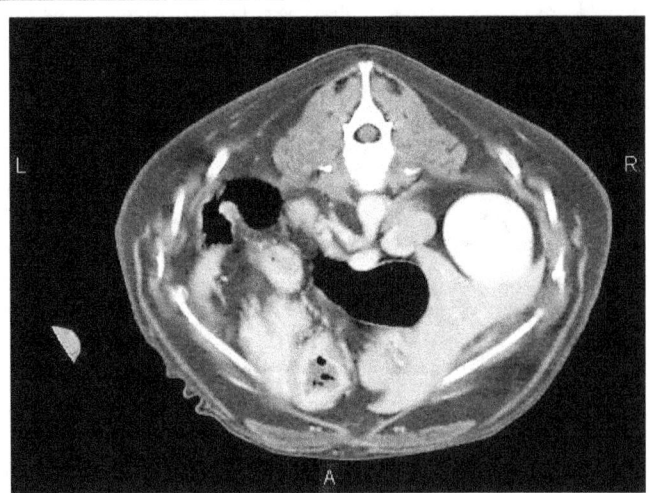

Figure 1: Case 16 - right adrenal tumor with caudal vena cava invasion; contrast-enhancement.

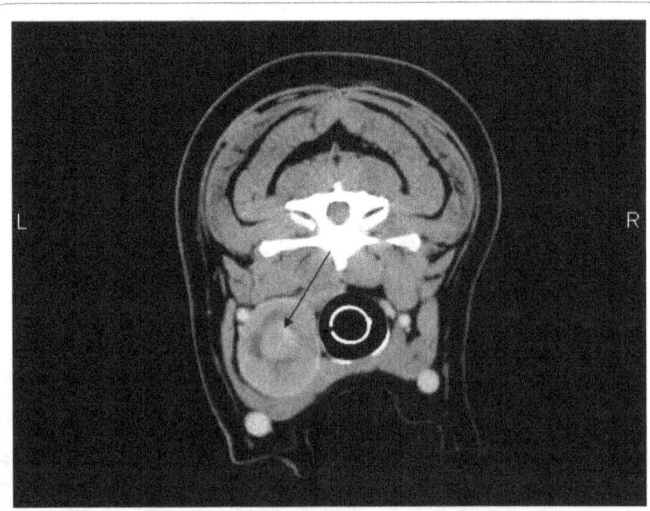

Figure 2: Case 4 - left thyroid carcinoma; contrast enhancement.

spread. The pattern of tumor spread to regional and distant lymph nodes depends on the tumor type and the use of CT examination must be tailored to include the appropriate areas. Enlarged lymph nodes often appear as soft tissue masses of homogenous density. A recent study evaluated CT characteristics of canine tracheobronchial lymph node metastasis for thoracic neoplasia and identified that lymph node enlargement, as well as contrast enhancement, was associated with metastatic disease [12]. Moreover, tracheobronchial lymph node enlargement is a prognostic factor for dogs with primary lung tumors [13]. In our study, the one dog with pulmonary adenocarcinoma (case 11) did not have associated lymph node enlargement, and this information was helpful in staging and formulating treatment planning.

The sternal lymph node chain may drain either the thorax or cranial abdomen. These lymph nodes are located in the intercostal spaces and may drain organs from the liver, to the diaphragm, to the thoracic wall, including mammary tissue. These lymph nodes may also drain dermal structures in this region. In human medicine, (para)sternal lymph nodes are staged in women with breast carcinoma, and when enlarged, are found to represent metastasis to the internal mammary lymphatic chain, which confers a poor prognosis for survival [14]. A recent veterinary study described radiographic findings of sternal lymphadenomegaly in cats and dogs. Neoplastic disease is the most prevalent condition associated with sternal lymphadenomegaly [15]. In that study, the median height of the left and right sternal lymph nodes in dogs with neoplastic, inflammatory, and hematologic diseases was 18 mm and 20 mm, respectively.

We measured sternal lymph nodes to assess for potential metastatic disease. To the authors' knowledge, there are no studies that measure sternal lymph nodes via CT in veterinary cancer patients. In our study, sternal lymph nodes were visible in 13 dogs; the median left sternal lymph node height was 6.6 mm in 10 dogs, and right sternal lymph node height was 5.3 mm in 12 dogs. Although the imaging modalities are different, one can conclude that sternal lymph nodes in our dogs were not enlarged compared to those observed in the dogs in the Smith and O'Brien study [15]. The results of our study appear to describe normal sternal lymph node size in dogs by CT scan, and thus could serve as a potential reference; however, cytological or histopathological confirmation is needed. Prospective studies are needed to further investigate this finding.

Splenomegaly was the most commonly detected abdominal CT finding. One possible cause for splenomegaly in our dogs is neoplasia. The most common neoplastic diseases of the spleen include hemangiosarcoma, lymphoma, and mast cell tumors [16]. No dogs included in this study had diagnosed hemangiosarcoma, but one dog had mediastinal lymphoma (case 10), and four dogs had mast cell tumors (cases 3, 5, 7 and 14). Three of these five dogs had splenomegaly on CT scan. While biopsy of the spleen would have been optimal for staging purposes, two of the three dogs with splenomegaly (cases 5 and 7) had fine needle aspiration performed. Normal splenic cytology, as interpreted by a board-certified cytopathologist at a reference laboratory, make it less likely that splenomegaly was attributable to metastatic round cell tumor in those two dogs.

Another cause for splenomegaly is use of anesthetic drugs. The concern for the effect of drugs on spleen size has been recognized, and drug-induced (propofol) splenomegaly may be misdiagnosed as splenic disease, such as diffuse neoplastic infiltrates of the spleen [17]. In the present study, all dogs were anesthetized with propofol, and 11/16 dogs had splenomegaly. Despite this finding, one cannot exclude the possibility that splenomegaly detected on CT may be caused by

neoplasia, which then warrants confirmatory needle aspiration or biopsy. Whenever possible, anesthetic protocols that minimize the potential for splenomegaly should be employed for WBCT procedures on patients being evaluated for metastatic neoplasia.

With WBCT, identification of a lesion depends on the difference in Hounsfield units between the lesion and its surroundings; therefore, smaller lesions can be detected by CT scans compared to conventional radiographic studies [18]. This is particularly important in the pulmonary parenchyma, where pulmonary metastases can be identified at sizes as small as one millimeter in diameter by CT scanning, compared to 7-9 mm by conventional radiography [19]. In recent veterinary studies that compared thoracic radiographs to CT scanning for detection of pulmonary nodules, CT was found to be more sensitive [5,19,20]. In our study, two cases (11 and 14) had evidence of pulmonary nodules on WBCT. Case 11 had two nodules: right caudal lung nodule (50 mm) and left caudal lung nodule (28 mm). Case 14 had one left cranial lung nodule (7 mm). These dogs did not have thoracic radiographs available for comparison, but one can infer that while the dog in case 11 had nodules that would be readily detectable on radiographs, the nodule in case 14, perhaps, would have been less obvious.

The same theory holds true for abdominal CT, in that abdominal CT may prove to be a better screening test for abdominal disease in veterinary patients when compared to abdominal radiographs and/or abdominal ultrasound findings [21]. Three of our dogs had abdominal ultrasonography (cases 2 and 12) or abdominal radiography performed (case 16). In case 2, abdominal CT and ultrasound detected prostatomegaly. The dog in case 12 had an abdominal ultrasound that detected liver masses, but CT was able to definitively identify the location and extent of the liver masses in the left and right medial liver lobe. Finally, case 16 had a cranial abdominal mass effect detected on abdominal radiographs, but CT was able to further characterize this mass effect as a right adrenal mass with multiple lymph node (mesenteric and medial iliac) rim enhancement lesions. A prospective study specifically comparing WBCT with thoracic radiography and abdominal radiography and/or abdominal ultrasound is warranted in the future.

Despite WBCT being an important, safe, and time-efficient diagnostic tool, there are some concerns associated with its use. Perhaps the most common concern for routine use of WBCT is the current necessity of employing general anesthesia in immune-compromised and often older cancer patients. Physiologic changes impede the body's ability to maintain homeostasis during times of physiological stress, with a subsequent decrease in physiological reserve. This can lead to physiological dysfunction, resulting in peri-anesthetic complications [22]. None of our patients had anesthetic complications; this was aided by a thorough pre-anesthetic patient evaluation to assess patient suitability for the procedure.

A critical component of the pre-anesthetic patient evaluation is laboratory analysis. There is no evidence to indicate the minimum time frame before anesthesia within which laboratory analysis should be performed. However, the timing should be reasonable to detect changes that impact anesthetic risk [23]. There was no clear association evident between the clinical pathological abnormalities in our patients and the results of their WBCT scans. Mildly elevated serum alkaline phosphatase activity was the most common serum chemistry abnormality in patients in our study. This elevation could represent a paraneoplastic elevation of serum alkaline phosphatase. Garzotto et al. describes the relationship between serum alkaline phosphatase and appendicular osteosarcoma and survival times [24]. The one dog in this study with appendicular osteosarcoma (case 6) did not have elevated alkaline phosphatase activity, however. The relatively minor clinical pathological abnormalities noted in our patients did not complicate or contraindicate pursuing WBCT, and all similar patients should have pre-anesthetic testing in order to properly evaluate the patient's status and adjust anesthetic agents or protocols as needed. Fortunately, with the advance of CT scanning equipment, newer multi-slice models (16, 32, or 40-slice) will allow for shorter anesthesia time, and even allow some studies to be performed using sedation only. Faster scanning also helps to eliminate artifacts from patient motion such as breathing or peristalsis. The increased slice count is useful for cancer diagnosis because it offers better resolution, making it possible to diagnose and assess the extent of the disease. A higher-slice count CT should more accurately measure the margins of a mass and allow for a greater precision in surgery and radiation therapy.

Another concern for the routine use of WBCT in veterinary patients is adverse reactions to contrast media. There are reports of reactions to iodinated contrast media in the human and veterinary literature [25-27]. These reactions are reported to include allergic reactions, cardiovascular reactions, gastrointestinal disturbances, nephrotoxicity, shock, and even sudden death. No dogs in this study developed any adverse reactions. Furthermore, the adverse reactions in the two anesthetized dogs described in the case report by Pollard and Pascoe were secondary to an ionic iodinated contrast media, whereas the dogs in our study received nonionic iodinated contrast media. Minor acute reactions occur in only three percent of people given nonionic iodinated contrast media [26]. These results, combined with prior clinical experience, suggest that veterinary patients undergoing WBCT with nonionic contrast media are highly unlikely to develop an adverse reaction.

An additional concern to both the clinician and client related to CT evaluation is cost. At our facility, the average cost of WBCT is $800-$1,200, whereas the cost of thoracic radiographs and abdominal ultrasound together average a cost of $700-$900. The apparent utility of WBCT to detect and more completely evaluate primary or metastatic lesions, along with the relatively short time to perform the study, offer good clinical and financial value when compared to a combination of abdominal ultrasound and thoracic radiographs.

CT has been more readily available in the recent years to clinicians and clients. Results of a 1999 survey of the American College of Veterinary Radiology members on the availability of CT scanners reported that in-house CT scanners accounted for 56% of the CT scanning instruments available to veterinary radiologists; off-site transport to local imaging centers, 26%; and regularly scheduled mobile units on site, 5%. However, the availability of CT scanners is likely to be considerably greater at the time of this writing.

Conclusions

WBCT is safe and provides valuable information for clinical staging in cancer patients. In this study, we highlighted tissue findings that may not have been detected through more commonly used imaging modalities. We also described sternal lymph node size in a variety of veterinary cancer patients, which could provide an objective reference for future studies. The potential advantages of WBCT in comparison to radiography and ultrasonography for staging cancer patients will likely become more evident with the increased availability of more advanced equipment. Newer multi-slice CT scanning instruments will dramatically reduce scan times, further limiting anesthetic risk while simultaneously improving spatial resolution and facilitating

multiplanar reconstruction. The results of our retrospective study support further work evaluating WBCT compared to radiographic and ultrasonographic evaluations for staging veterinary cancer patients.

Acknowledgements

The authors wish to thank Terry Rhodes, Jill Rodriguez, and Moises Sanchez for their technical assistance.

References

1. Husband JE (1985) Whole body computed tomography in cancer management. Br J Hosp Med 34: 25-31.

2. Riegger C, Herrmann J, Nagarajah J, Hecktor J, Kuemmel S, et al. (2012) Whole-body FDG PET/CT is more accurate than conventional imaging for staging primary breast cancer patients. Eur J Nucl Med Mol Imaging 39: 852-863.

3. Armbrust LJ, Biller DS, Hoskinson JJ (2000) Case examples demonstrating the clinical utility of obtaining both right and left lateral abdominal radiographs in small animals. J Am Anim Hosp Assoc 36: 531-536.

4. Mattoon JS, Bryan JN (2013) The future of imaging in veterinary oncology: learning from human medicine. Vet J 197: 541-552.

5. Oblak ML, Boston SE, Woods JP, Nykamp S (2015) Comparison of concurrent imaging modalities for staging of dogs with appendicular primary bone tumours. Vet Comp Oncol 13: 28-39.

6. Vignoli M, Terragni R, Rossi F, Frühauf L, Bacci B, et al. (2013) Whole body computed tomographic characteristics of skeletal and cardiac muscular metastatic neoplasia in dogs and cats. Vet Radiol Ultrasound 54: 223-230.

7. Barrera JS, Bernard F, Ehrhart EJ, Withrow SJ, Monnet E (2013) Evaluation of risk factors for outcome associated with adrenal gland tumors with or without invasion of the caudal vena cava and treated via adrenalectomy in dogs: 86 cases (1993-2009). J Am Vet Med Assoc 242: 1715-1721.

8. Gregori T, Mantis P, Benigni L, Priestnall SL, Lamb CR (2015) Comparison of computed tomographic and pathologic findings in 17 dogs with primary adrenal neoplasia. Vet Radiol Ultrasound 56: 153-159.

9. Schultz RM, Wisner ER, Johnson EG, MacLeod JS (2009) Contrast-enhanced computed tomography as a preoperative indicator of vascular invasion from adrenal masses in dogs. Vet Radiol Ultrasound 50: 625-629.

10. LeBlanc AK, Daniel GB (2007) Advanced imaging for veterinary cancer patients. Vet Clin North Am Small Anim Pract 37: 1059-1077.

11. Violante MR, Dean PB (1980) Improved detectability of VX2 carcinoma in the rabbit liver with contrast enhancement in computed tomography. Radiology 134: 237-239.

12. Ballegeer EA, Adams WM, Dubielzig RR, Paoloni MC, Klauer JM, et al. (2010) Computed tomography characteristics of canine tracheobronchial lymph node metastasis. Vet Radiol Ultrasound 51: 397-403.

13. Paoloni MC, Adams WM, Dubielzig RR, Kurzman I, Vail DM, et al. (2006) Comparison of results of computed tomography and radiography with histopathologic findings in tracheobronchial lymph nodes in dogs with primary lung tumors: 14 cases (1999-2002). J Am Vet Med Assoc 228: 1718-1722.

14. Maalej M, Hentati D, Afrit M, Boudabous H, Nasr C, et al. (2013) Sternal or parasternal involvement from breast cancer: a misleading clinical sign. Tunis Med 91: 54-58.

15. Smith K, O'Brien R (2012) Radiographic characterization of enlarged sternal lymph nodes in 71 dogs and 13 cats. J Am Anim Hosp Assoc 48: 176-181.

16. Johnson KA, Powers BE, Withrow SJ, Sheetz MJ, Curtis CR, et al. (1989) Splenomegaly in dogs. Predictors of neoplasia and survival after splenectomy. J Vet Intern Med 3: 160-166.

17. Baldo CF, Garcia-Pereira FL, Nelson NC, Hauptman JG, Shih AC (2012) Effects of anesthetic drugs on canine splenic volume determined via computed tomography. Am J Vet Res 73: 1715-1719.

18. Schurawitzki H, Stiglbauer R, Graninger W, Herold C, Pölzleitner D, et al. (1990) Interstitial lung disease in progressive systemic sclerosis: high-resolution CT versus radiography. Radiology 176: 755-759.

19. Nemanic S, London CA, Wisner ER (2006) Comparison of thoracic radiographs and single breath-hold helical CT for detection of pulmonary nodules in dogs with metastatic neoplasia. J Vet Intern Med 20: 508-515.

20. Armbrust LJ, Biller DS, Bamford A, Chun R, Garrett LD, et al. (2012) Comparison of three-view thoracic radiography and computed tomography for detection of pulmonary nodules in dogs with neoplasia. J Am Vet Med Assoc 240: 1088-1094.

21. Fields EL, Robertson ID, Osborne JA, Brown JC Jr (2012) Comparison of abdominal computed tomography and abdominal ultrasound in sedated dogs. Vet Radiol Ultrasound 53: 513-517.

22. Brodbelt DC, Pfeiffer DU, Young LE, Wood JL (2008) Results of the confidential enquiry into perioperative small animal fatalities regarding risk factors for anesthetic-related death in dogs. J Am Vet Med Assoc 233: 1096-1104.

23. Bednarski R, Grimm K, Harvey R, Lukasik VM, Penn WS, et al. (2011) AAHA anesthesia guidelines for dogs and cats. J Am Anim Hosp Assoc 47: 377-385.

24. Garzotto CK, Berg J, Hoffmann WE, Rand WM (2000) Prognostic significance of serum alkaline phosphatase activity in canine appendicular osteosarcoma. J Vet Intern Med 14: 587-592.

25. Morcos SK, Thomsen HS (2001) Adverse reactions to iodinated contrast media. Eur Radiol 11: 1267-1275.

26. Pollard RE, Pascoe PJ (2008) Severe reaction to intravenous administration of an ionic iodinated contrast agent in two anesthetized dogs. J Am Vet Med Assoc 233: 274-278.

27. Pollard RE, Puchalski SM, Pascoe PJ (2008) Hemodynamic and serum biochemical alterations associated with intravenous administration of three types of contrast media in anesthetized dogs. Am J Vet Res 69: 1268-1273.

Efficacy of Feed Coated Newcastle Disease I$_2$ Vaccine in Village Chickens in Gombe State, Nigeria

Lawal JR[1]*, El-Yuguda AD[2] and Ibrahim UI[1]

[1]*Department of Veterinary Medicine, University of Maiduguri, Nigeria*
[2]*Animal Virus Research Laboratory, Department of Veterinary Microbiology and Parasitology, University of Maiduguri, Nigeria*

Abstract

A study of response of village chickens to vaccination with ND I$_2$ vaccine coated on maize grit as vaccine carrier was carried out in some selected LGAs of Gombe State, using haemagglutination inhibition (HI) test. Vaccination efficacy of maize grit coated with Newcastles Disease I$_2$ vaccine has been compared between adult and young, village chickens. The study showed that 94.3% of the vaccinated village chickens (adults and chicks) seroconverted with protective levels of antibodies against ND virus. Those vaccinated with the maize grit coated vaccine exhibited antibody titres of between 1:16 to 1:8192 with GMT values of 109 to 245. There was a significant difference (P<0.05) in the response of the vaccinated adult village chickens as compared to the younger birds (chicks). It is concluded from the study that maize grit is a very suitable vaccine carrier for the delivery of ND I$_2$ vaccine to village chickens.

Keywords: Newcastle disease I$_2$ vaccine; Maize grit; Village chickens; Seroconversion; Gombe State; Nigeria

Introduction

Newcastle disease (ND) is an acute, contagious and highly pathogenic viral disease of both domestic and wild birds worldwide [1-4]. This disease is caused by a diverse group of viruses with the highly virulent strains endemic in Nigeria [5,6]. It is considered the most economically important avian viral disease in the world especially in developed countries due to its devastating effect on the industry [7-9]. It can produce mortality of up to 100% among infected populations of birds [10,11], and unfortunately the prognosis is poor [12,13]. Vaccination is currently the most effective method of controlling endemic Newcastle disease in both commercial and village chickens, but is rarely given priority in rural communities in Nigeria where majority of poultry are kept [14-16]. The administration of vaccines is by far the most humane and cost effective method of combating the spread of diseases [15,17]. The protection afforded by an efficacious vaccine not only removes the need for the administration of treatments, but also guards against the economically damaging consequences of disease [15,18]. Avirulent NDV$_4$ and ND I$_2$ strains of ND vaccines have been reported to give varying degrees of successes in both laboratory and field trials [19-22]. This study is therefore aimed at studying the responses of village chickens to Newcastle disease I$_2$ vaccine coated on maize grit as vaccine vehicle.

Materials and Methods

Study area

This study was carried out in some selected LGAs of Gombe State, Nigeria. Gombe State located between latitude 9°30' and 12° 3' N and longitude 8° 45' and 11° 45' E, has an estimated population of 2.4 million people based on the 2006 population census by the National Population commission [23]. The state is situated in the North Eastern zone of Nigeria and shares boundaries with Bauchi, Taraba, Adamawa, Yobe and Borno States. The state has Eleven Local Government Areas that are populated by ethnic groups including Hausa, Fulani, Tera, Waja, Tangale and Bolawa among others. The climatic and edaphic factors favour crop and livestock agriculture. The total poultry population in Gombe State is approximately 508,305 comprising 462,000 backyard poultry and 46,305 exotic poultry [24].

Source of Newcastle disease (ND) I$_2$ vaccine

The Newcastle disease I$_2$ vaccine that was used in this study was obtained from Viral Research Department, National Veterinary Research Institute (NVRI), Vom, Plateau State, Nigeria. The vials of the vaccines were 50 dose vials meant to be reconstituted in 50 ml of chlorine free water and to be giving orally at 1 ml/ bird. The batch number of the vaccines and expiration dates were 4 / 2011 and Oct / 2012 respectively.

Selection of villages for the Newcastle disease I$_2$ vaccination

Five (5) out of the eleven (11) Local Government Areas (LGAs) of Gombe State were selected for the study. In each LGA, four villages were selected, and from each village four (4) households that owns moderate number of village chickens and that were willing to volunteer, cooperate and give full support for the success of the study were randomly selected. The Local Government Areas that were used for this study were Gombe, Akko, Kwami, Funakaye and Yamaltu Deba Local Government Areas.

Processing and coating of vaccine carrier with the Newcastle disease I$_2$ vaccine

Maize grit that was used as the vaccine carrier in this study was maize that was per boiled for 15 minutes, washed and spread immediately to dry under the sun. The dried per boiled maize was then polished ('*surfe*') to remove the maize husk and then crushed into a gritty mash. The maize grit was soaked in hot water and allowed to stand until the water cools, washed thoroughly and sieved to reduce the starch content and was again sun dried. Using a weighing scale, the

*Corresponding author: Jallailudeen Rabana Lawal, Department of Veterinary Medicine, University of Maiduguri, PMB 1069, Maiduguri, Borno State, Nigeria
E-mail: rabanajallailudeen@yahoo.com

maize grit was weighed and packaged in polythene bags of 1 kg/package and stored at room temperature. Two vials of the 50 doses of ND I_2 vaccines were reconstituted in 100 ml of chlorine free water and used to mix each 1 kg of the maize grit (at a ratio of 1 ml to 10 g of the dried maize grit) using a hand sprayer. The maize grit coated ND I_2 vaccine was administering to the village chickens as previously described by Alders and Spradbrow [17].

Vaccination procedure

The village chickens from the selected households in the five LGAs were locked up in cages, raffia baskets and empty rooms when they returned to their owners' houses to roost in the evening from the scavenging of the day. They were denied access to any source of feed throughout the night before administering the ND I_2 vaccine coated feed to them the following morning. Some village chickens from a different village were used for the normal oral vaccination in water. Each of the birds used in the study were labeled using small number tags tied to their wings and were bled through the wing web vein prior to vaccination.

Blood sample collection

The vaccinated village chickens were bled twice on days zero and 28 post vaccination. Blood samples was collected from the live experimental village chickens through the brachial vein (wing vein) or jugular vein of adult and grower village chickens of both sexes using sterile 2 ml syringes and 21G needles. Each blood was carefully dispensed into plain vacutainer tubes, labeled appropriately and kept at a slanting position at room temperature to allow blood samples to clot. For chicks with tiny brachial veins through which a syringe and needle could not be used to collect blood directly, their veins were punctured using sterile 23G needles and then labeled strips of filter paper (Whatman' filter paper 1, Cat No 1001 125) were used to tap blood samples from the punctured veins and allowed to saturate up to a distance of 1-2 cm of the length of the strip as previously described [25,26]. Samples were air dried, labeled on both sides and stored in plastic bags and stored at 4°C for onward transport to the laboratory. In the laboratory, serum samples were eluted from the strips by punching 2 disks (6 mm in diameter) using a file punch and placed in a well of a microtitre plate and 100 μl of normal saline was added and the plate incubated at 4°C overnight.

Serology

Serum samples were tested for Newcastle disease virus specific antibodies using a modification of the Hemagglutination Inhibition (HI) test previously described by Baba et al. [27].

Data analysis

Hemagglutination inhibition titres obtained were expressed as geometric mean titre (GMT) values according to the method described by Garner et al. [28] using the formula $X_{geo}=antilog_{10}\{1/n\ (\Sigma f_i log_{10} X_i)\}$ where n=number tested, X_i=the reciprocal of dilution and f_i=frequency. The data generated from the study was entered to excel spreadsheet. All categorical data were entered into contingency tables and analyzed using chi square test, while the geometric means of all numeric data were compared using t-statistic or analysis of variance (ANOVA) for paired or multiple data columns respectively using Statgraphic plus Version 5.0, November 2000 (Statistical Graphics Corp.). The level of statistical significance was set a p-value less than or equal to 0.05.

Results

Tables 1 and 2 shows the distribution of ND HI antibodies at pre and post vaccination of village chickens in some selected areas of Gombe state. The distribution of the pre-vaccinal (baseline titre) ND HI antibodies among the different Local Government Areas of Gombe state showed no statistical difference (P>0.05) in prevalence rates and GMT values (Tables 1-3). The adult vaccines in all the 5 LGAs exhibited high seroconversion from 37.5% at day zero to 94.3% at day 28 post vaccination (Tables 1 and 2). The pre-vaccinal baseline titres of the adult vaccines varied from 1:2 to 1:128 and GMT of 14.1 as against the day 28 PV titres of 1:16 to 1:8192 and GMT of 190.1 (Tables 1 and 2). The vaccinated chicks exhibited a baseline titre of 1:2 to 1:64 with GMT of 3.1 and 1:2 to 1:64 with GMT of 12.3 on day 28 PV (Tables 3 and 4). The direct oral drench group showed a baseline titre of 1:2 to 1:64 with GMT of 3.6 and 1:512 to 1:2048 with GMT of 861 (Table 5). There was no statistical difference (P>0.05) noted among the vaccines from the different LGAs.

Discussion

The use of maize grit as the vaccine vehicle to deliver the ND I_2

LGA	No. tested	No. (%) positive	Distribution of HI antibody titres							
			2	4	8	16	32	64	128	GMT
Gombe	160	56 (35.0)	2	6	22	4	10	12	0	2.6
Akko	160	66 (41.3)	10	26	17	2	5	3	3	2.2
Kwami	160	45 (28.1)	1	6	12	4	6	16	0	2.3
Yamaltu Deba	160	70 (43.8)	1	9	18	5	4	33	0	3.8
Funakaye	160	63 (39.4)	1	12	16	10	5	18	1	3.0
Total	800	300 (37.5)	15	53	85	25	30	82	4	14.1

Table 1: Distribution of Newcastle disease HI antibody titres in sera of adult village chickens collected prior to vaccination with Newcastle disease I_2 vaccine coated on maize grit in some Local Government Areas of Gombe State.

LGA	No. tested	No.(%) positive	Distribution of the reciprocal of HI antibody titres													GMT values
			2	4	8	16	32	64	128	256	512	1024	2048	4096	8192	
Gombe	80	73(91.3)	0	0	0	2	0	4	18	6	24	6	4	8	1	245.1
Akko	80	71 (88.8)	0	0	0	1	2	10	23	10	13	7	3	1	0	114.4
Kwami	80	75 (93.8)	0	0	0	1	6	12	27	11	14	3	0	0	1	119.4
Yamaltu Deba	80	80 (100)	0	0	0	6	3	12	27	18	7	6	1	0	0	149.6
Funakaye	80	78 (97.5)	0	0	0	3	8	15	30	14	4	2	2	0	0	109.5
Total	400	377(94.3)	0	0	0	13	19	53	125	59	62	24	10	9	2	190.1

Table 2: Distribution of ND HI antibody titres in sera of adult village chickens 28 days post-vaccination with ND I_2 vaccine coated on maize grit in some Local Government Areas of Gombe State.

LGA	No. tested	No. (%) positive	Distribution of reciprocal of ND HI antibody titres							GMT values
			2	4	8	16	32	64	128	
Gombe	40	9 (22.5)	5	4	0	0	0	0	0	1.5
Akko	40	12 (30.0)	8	3	1	0	0	0	0	1.3
Kwami	40	7 (17.5)	3	4	0	0	0	0	0	1.2
Yamaltu Deba	40	10 (25.0)	7	3	0	0	0	0	0	1.3
Funakaye	40	16 (40.0)	5	8	1	0	1	1	0	1.8
Total	200	54 (27.0)	28	22	2	0	1	1	0	3.1

Table 3: Distribution of Newcastle disease HI antibody titres in sera collected prior to vaccination with Newcastle disease I_2 vaccine coated on maize grit in young village chickens (chicks) in some Local Government Areas of Gombe State.

LGA	No. tested	No.(%) positive	Distribution of reciprocal of ND HI antibody titres							GMT values
			2	4	8	16	32	64	128	
Gombe	32	31 (96.9)	5	4	11	6	3	2	0	8.2
Akko	32	32 (100)	0	1	17	9	3	2	0	12.3
Kwami	32	30 (93.8)	1	0	9	8	5	7	0	15.7
Yamaltu Deba	32	32 (100)	2	5	15	2	6	2	0	10.2
Funakaye	32	32 (100)	0	6	15	4	2	5	0	11.6
Total	160	157(98.1)	8	16	69	29	19	18	0	12.3

Table 4: Distribution of Newcastle disease HI antibody titres in chick sera collected 28 days post vaccination with ND I_2 vaccine coated on maize grit in some Local Government Areas of Gombe State.

Sampling period	Number tested	No. (%) positive samples	Distribution of reciprocal of ND HI antibody titres											GMT
			2	4	8	16	32	64	128	256	512	1024	2048	
Pre- vaccination	24	11 (45.8%)	1	2	2	0	3	3	0	0	0	0	0	3.6
Post- vaccination	24	24 (100%)	0	0	0	0	0	0	0	0	10	10	4	861

Table 5: Distribution of ND HI antibody titres of village chickens pre- vaccination and post-vaccination with oral drenches of ND I_2 vaccine.

vaccine in this study was meant to obviate the problem of chasing, catching and vaccinating individual bird which is difficult in the natural habitat of the village chickens. The choice of maize in this study to be used as vaccine carrier is in accordance to similar research by Ibrahim et al. [29] that reported maize to be a reliable vaccine carrier. The findings of this study showed that the ND I_2 vaccine coated on maize grit has led the vaccinated village chickens to seroconvert with high antibody titres in all the study areas. This finding concurs with field records in Mozambique which indicates that ND I_2 vaccine provided approximately 80% protection in the field in the face of an outbreak when coated on suitable carrier food [17] and also confirmed the findings of Echeonwu et al. [22] who reported the efficacy of the same vaccine under laboratory trials using maize meal waste (maize offal) as the vaccine carrier. The efficacy of any vaccine is determined mainly by assessment of the level of antibody produced in the target birds and the ability of the vaccinated bird to resist exposure to the virulent infectious agent when compared to the unvaccinated birds [30]. The advantage of the feed coated ND I_2 vaccine over the use of drinking water in the village chicken is that most village chickens are used to early morning feeding in the study area and this makes it easy for the vaccine coated feeds to be consumed early before the vaccine virus gets inactivated by environmental conditions. Whereas if the vaccine was to be given in drinking water, only a small percentage of the chickens may take the water within the required time, due to the availability of surface water in the environment. The study showed that significantly larger proportion of vaccinated adult village chickens seroconverted to higher antibodies levels than the chicks. This finding may not be unconnected to the possible repeated exposure and/or well developed immune system in the adult chickens leading to an adequate response. The high NDV HI antibody titres recorded in the vaccinated chickens in this study must have resulted from anamnestic response in the birds due to previous natural expose to NDV.

Although all the village chickens vaccinated with both the feed coated and direct oral drench vaccine demonstrated high antibody titres, the later demonstrated a more uniform response and hence higher GMT values. This could be because it was not possible to ensure that all the village chickens in the mass application of the ND I_2 vaccine coated on the maize grit receive the same and exact dose of the vaccine. This difference in the feed in take also appears to have been the primary cause for the difference in titres between the adult chickens and chicks in this present study. The adult chickens consumed much of the feed while the chicks just picked tiny grains. This resulted in higher immune response in the adult chickens when compared to the chicks. Similarly, Erick et al. [31] found that a significantly large proportion of vaccinated adult chickens attaining protective immunity against NDV as compared to growers and chicks which were attributed to repeated exposure and/or well developed immune system in adult chickens leading to an adequate response to vaccination. Other factors to consider include the prevalence of other infectious diseases like IBD capable of immunosuppressing the village chickens. El-Yuguda et al. [32] have reported significant depression of primary antibody of chickens to ND vaccine when administered one week after IBD infection or vaccination. It is therefore fundamental to monitor the prevalence of other infectious diseases capable of immunosuppression and to implement specific vaccination programme for their control. Also the rearing of ducks, guinea fowls, pigeons and doves (which are natural fliers) together with village chickens further compounds the difficulty in ND control strategies among the village poultry population. But vaccination in these classes of birds may be attempted using the feed coated ND I_2 vaccine by spraying over the locations where these birds usually scavenge for food. Since guinea fowl vaccination using different feeds as vaccine vehicles have been reported by Baba et al. [21] using thermostable NDV-V_4 vaccine. It is therefore suggestive that thermostable ND I_2 vaccine coated on feed such as maize grit be used to vaccinate free-living and scavenging birds.

Acknowledgements

The authors wish to thank the Technologists of the Animal Virus Research Laboratory, Department of Veterinary Microbiology and Parasitology, University of Maiduguri and those of the Department of Veterinary Medicine Research Laboratory, University of Maiduguri for their technical assistance.

References

1. Health BC, Lindsey MS, McManus KP, Claxon PD (1991) Newcastle disease vaccine for village chicken, Spradbrow PD (ed). Australian Centre for International Agriculture Research, Canberra, Australia, p: 103.

2. Seal BS, King DJ, Sellers HS (2000) The avian response to Newcastle disease virus. Dev Comp Immunol 24: 257-268.

3. Alexander DJ (2003) Newcastle disease and other avian Paramyxoviruses infections. In: Diseases of Poultry. 11th edn. Saif YM, Barnes HJ, Glisson JR, Fadly AM, McDougald LR, et al. (eds.). Iowa State University Press, Ames 1A, USA, pp: 63-99.

4. Okwor EC, Eze DC (2010) The Annual Prevalence of Newcastle disease in commercial chickens reared in South Eastern Savannah zone of Nigeria. Res J Poult Sci 3: 23-26.

5. Falcon M (2004) Newcastle disease. Semin Avian and Exot Pet Med 13: 79-85.

6. Aldous EW, Alexander DJ (2008) Newcastle disease in pheasants (Phasianus colchicus): a review. Vet J 175: 181-185.

7. El-Yuguda AD, Baba SS (2002) Prevalence of selected viral infections in various age groups of village chicken in Borno state, Nigeria. Nigeria Journal Animal Production 29: 245-250.

8. Ngaji LW, Nyaga PN, Mbuthia PG, Bebora LC, Michieka JN, et al. (2010) Prevalence of Newcastle disease virus in village indigenous chickens in varied agro-ecological zones in Kenya. Livestock Research for Rural Development 22: 1-4.

9. Aziz AGT, Ahmed TA (2010) Serological Survey of Newcastle disease in Domestic chickens in Sulaimani Province. Journal of Zankay Sulaimani 13: 31-38.

10. Ananth R, Kirubaharam JJ, Priyadarshini MLM, Albert A (2008) Isolation of Newcastle disease viruses of high virulence in unvaccinated healthy village chickens in South India. Int J Poult Sci 7: 368-373.

11. Ibu OJ, Okoye JOA, Adulugba EP, Chah KF, Shoyinka SVO, et al. (2009) Prevalence of Newcastle disease viruses in wild and captive birds in Central Nigeria. Int J Poult Sci 8: 574-578.

12. Al-Garib SO, Gielkens ALJ, Gruys E, Kochi G (2003) Review of Newcastle disease virus with particular references to immunity and vaccination. World's Poult Sci J 59: 185-200.

13. Hassanzadeh M, Fard MHB (2004) A Serological Study of Newcastle Disease in Pre- and Post- vaccinated Village Chickens in North of Iran. Int J Poult Sci 3: 658-661.

14. Abdu PA, Sa'idu L, Bawa EK, Umoh JU (2005) Factors that contribute to Newcastle disease. Infectious bursal disease and Fowl pox Outbreaks in Chickens. Presented at the 42nd Annual congress of the Nigerian Veterinary Medical Association. Held at University of Maiduguri.

15. Marangon S, Busani L (2006) The use of vaccination in poultry production. Rev Sci Tech Off Int Epiz 26: 265-274.

16. Nwanta JA, Abdu PA, Ezema WS (2008) Epidemiology, Challenges and Prospects for control of Newcastle disease in village poultry in Nigeria. Worlds Poult Sci J 64: 119-127.

17. Alders R, Spradbrow PB (2001) Controlling of Newcastle disease in village chickens. A field manual, Australian Centre for International Agriculture Research (ACIAR), Research monograph No. 82: 1-112.

18. Woolock RF, Harun M, Alders RG (2004) The impact of Newcastle disease control in village chickens on the welfare of rural household in Mozambique. Paper presented at the 4th Co-ordination Meeting of the FAO / IAEA Co-ordination Research Programme.

19. Wambura PN (2010) Detection of antibody to Newcastle disease virus in semi-domesticated free-range birds (Numida meleagris and Columba livia domestica) and the risk of transmission of Newcastle disease to village chickens. Short communication. Veterinarski Arhiv 80: 129-134.

20. Msami HM, Young MP (2005) Newcastle disease control using I_2 vaccine in Tanzania. Country report. In: Village chicken Poverty alleviation and the sustainable control of Newcastle disease. Australian Centre for International Agricultural Research (ACIAR), Proceedings 131: 67-73.

21. Baba SS, Iheanacho CC, Idris JM, El-Yuguda AD (2006) Food-Based Newcastle disease V4 vaccine in guinea fowl (Numida meleagris Galeata pallas) in Nigeria. Trop Vet 22: 37-45.

22. Echeonwu BC, Ngele MB, Echeonwu GON, Joannis TM, Onovoh EM, et al. (2008) Response of chickens to oral vaccination with Newcastle disease virus vaccine strain I_2 coated on maize offal. Afr J Biotechnol 7: 1594-1599.

23. http://www.qtsnigeria.com/

24. Adene DF, Oguntade AE (2006) The structure and importance of the commercial and village based poultry industry in Nigeria. FAO (Rome) Study, p: 22.

25. Ambali AG, Jones RC (1991) Efficiency of filter paper for measurement of IBHI antibody to Avian Infectious Bronchitis. Bull Anim Health Prod Afr 39: 213-218.

26. Roy P, Nachimuthu K, Venugopalan AT (1992) A modified filter paper technique for serosurveillance of Newcastle disease. Short Communication. Vet Res Commun 16: 403-406.

27. Baba SS, El-Yuguda AD, Baba MM (1998) Serological evidence of mixed infection with Newcastle disease and Egg drop syndrome 1976 viruses in Village chicken in Borno state, Nigeria. Tropical Veterinarian 16: 137-141.

28. Garner JS, Jarvis WR, Emori TG, Horan TC, Hughes JM (1988) CDC definitions for nosocomial infections, 1988. Am J Infect Control 16: 128-140.

29. Ibrahim UI, El-Yuguda AD, Tambari PS (2000) Trial of Feed-Based Newcastle disease 'Lasota' Vaccine in Chickens using feeds as Vaccine Vehicle. Nig J Exptl Appl Biol 1: 83-86.

30. Alders R, Spradbrow PB (1994) Newcastle disease in Village chickens. Poultry Science Review 5: 57-96.

31. Erick VGK, Albano OM, Rutashobya CTM (2012) Adoption of I_2 Vaccine in Immunization of Village Chickens against Newcastle disease virus in Southern Tanzania: Immune Status of Farmer vaccinated birds. Journal of Agricultural Science 4: 23-28.

32. El-Yuguda AD, Wachida AD, Baba SS (2007) Interference of Infectious Bursal Disease (IBD) Virus and Vaccine with the immune Responses of Guinea Fowls to Newcastle Disease Lasota Vaccination. Afr J Biomed Res 10: 189-192.

6

Contact-Independent Antagonism of *Ophidiomyces ophiodiicola,* the Causative Agent of Snake Fungal Disease by *Rhodococcus rhodochrous* DAP 96253 and Select Volatile Organic Compounds

Christopher T Cornelison*, Blake Cherney, Kyle T Gabriel, Courtney K Barlament and Sidney A Crow Jr

Applied and Environmental Microbiology, Georgia State University, Atlanta, GA, USA

Abstract

Snake fungal disease (SFD), caused by the ascomycete *Ophidiomyces ophiodiicola*, has been associated with severe morbidity and mortality of numerous species of wild snakes in 15 US states. Accordingly, SFD was added to the horizon scan of global conservation issues in 2014. Due to the itinerant and secluded nature of many snake species, as well as the diversity of species impacted by SFD, estimating SFD-associated mortalities has been challenging. Regardless, the impacts have been shown to be significant in local and regional instances. Currently there is no known therapeutic or prophylactic for SFD. This study evaluated a potential biological treatment option for SFD that has shown promise in managing white-nose syndrome in bats, the bacterium *Rhodococcus rhodochrous* DAP 96253. *R. rhodochrous* was evaluated for *in vitro* contact-independent antagonism of *O. ophiodiicola*, with positive results. Additionally, synthetic volatile organic compounds (VOCs) associated with fungistatic soils were evaluated individually and in combinations to determine their potential for use as chemical control agents of SFD. In all cases an inhibitory effect was observed and statistically significant (p<0.05) radial growth inhibition was observed in several cases. The results presented in this study provide initial evidence for the *in vivo* evaluation of the potential of these agents to prevent or reduce the morbidity and mortality associated with SFD.

Keywords: *Rhodococcus*; *Ophidiomyces*; Snakes; VOCs; Antagonism

Introduction

Beginning in 2006, an increasing number of snakes infected with a fungal dermatitis has been reported [1]. Cases have been confirmed in Florida, Georgia, Illinois, Massachusetts, Michigan, Minnesota, New Jersey, New York, Ohio, Tennessee, Wisconsin, and Virginia [1,2]. This disease is commonly known as snake fungal disease (SFD), and is attributed to *Ophidiomyces ophiodiicola* as the causative agent [3,4]. Most snakes develop symptoms of brittle scales, subcutaneous nodules, severe swelling in the periocular tissues, and premature shedding [1,2,5,6]. Most case studies on SFD with vipers have reported lesions around the facial region, which negatively influence the snake's ability to forage and survive in the wild [1,2,5,6]. The specific mechanism(s) of virulence and pathogenicity is currently unknown.

In 2014, SFD was declared in the horizon scan of global conservation issues due to the similar characteristics it shares with another fungal pathogen, *Pseudogymnoascus destructans*, the causative agent of white-nose syndrome (WNS) in bats [7]. The transmission route of SFD remains unknown, however, it is hypothesized to be environmentally transmitted due to the broad host range and annual cycle of infection [1,2,5,6]. Tracking the spread of this disease is very challenging due to the snake's varied habitat and secretive lifestyle, indicating that cases likely exists outside the currently known range of SFD.

Population declines of venomous and nonvenomous snake species is of significant ecological concern as many species (e.g., eastern indigo snake, *Drymarchon couperi*) are considered keystone species in their respective ecosystems. Snakes play the fundamental role of middle predator in the environment, which keeps small mammal populations, such as rodents, under control [7,8]. Rodents are known vectors of human pathogens, which the Centers for Disease Control (CDC) states can cause over 35 diseases capable of being spread to humans through direct or indirect contact via bodily fluids [9]. Healthy and stable populations of middle predators, such as snakes, limit rodent populations, which decreases the likelihood of diseases transmission to humans. Additionally, research on snake venom is now used as a form

of natural product for antivenins, anticoagulants, treating hemophilia, and studying neural toxins, myotoxins and their structure and function [10,11]. Snakes also play an enormous role in the private pet trade, amounting to an estimated total expenditure of $264 million a year in the US, making the US one of the largest exporters in this global industry [12].

With annually increasing reports of SFD, there is a growing concern for the health of snakes and the industries that rely on them, as well as the ecosystem services they provide. Clark et al. documented populations of the timber rattlesnake decreasing by 50 percent from 2006 to 2007 in New Hampshire [13]. Other states, such as Illinois, observed 100 percent mortality of massasauga rattlesnakes when infected with *O. ophiodiicola* [5]. Current antifungal treatments, such as ketoconazole and the surgical removal of an infected area, are often ineffective and lead to mortality [2,6].

Recently, a naturally-occurring Gram-positive bacterium, *Rhodococcus rhodochrous* was evaluated as a potential biological control agent for SFD. Previous research with this bacteria has shown promising results for the management of pathogenic fungal infections caused by *P. destructans*, the fungus responsible for the recent decline in bat populations in North America [14]. Given the similarity of traits

*Corresponding author: Christopher T Cornelison, Senior Scientist, Applied and Environmental Microbiology, Georgia State University, 161 Dr. Jesse Hill Jr., Atlanta, Georgia 30303, United States of America
E-mail: ccornelison1@gsu.edu

between SFD and WNS, it was hypothesized that *R. rhodochrous* could have similar effects on *O. ophiodiicola*.

R. rhodochrous has a long history in industrial applications [15]. This bacterium has been used extensively in bioremediation due to its diverse metabolic activity, including the ability to breakdown complex hydrophobic pollutants as well as the bacterium's presence in pristine and contaminated environments [15]. *R. rhodochrous* is also being evaluated for the ability to delay the ripening of climacteric fruits and vegetables to lengthen the shelf-life of human food stocks [16].

An additional line on inquiry in this study was evaluating the potential of naturally-occurring bacterially-produced volatile organic compounds (VOCs), associated with fungistatic soils, to inhibit the growth of *O. ophiodiicola in vitro*. Fungistatic soils occur globally and their antifungal activities are attributed to the generation of antagonistic VOCs by microbial community members [17-23]. Synthetically-produced VOCs were selected and introduced into a shared airspace with mycelia plugs to evaluate the antifungal activity of select VOCs. The compounds that were selected for this study were N, N dimethyloctylamine, benzothiazole, benzaldehyde, 2-phenylethanol, 2-ethyl-1-hexanol, propionic acid, 2-nonanone, decanal, styrene, and nonanal [17,19,21-23]. All compounds were introduced to fungal plug assays at 4 μmols. The five least toxic (based on LD50 with rats, S1) and the five most inhibitive (Table 1) were selected for combination trials of two and three VOCS to determine whether or not they have synergistic activities at equimolar ratios. Most fungistatic VOCs are produced by soil-dwelling bacteria [17,20]. There have been extensive studies conducted on fungistatic activity and the microbes that are correlated to the particular VOCs released into the soil [17-23]. Surveys of soil bacteria have reported that 30-60% of isolated microbiota produce VOCs that can inhibit fungi [20], indicative of the vast number of candidates not screened in this study and the potential of mining these communities for control agents for emerging fungal pathogens.

Current research showing induced cells of *R. rhodochrous* strain DAP 96253 and bacterially-produced VOCs as a possible treatment for WNS, establishes a precedent for this approach in the control of other emerging wildlife mycoses [14,18]. Initial *in vitro* evaluations of this approach in the management of SFD has been favourable and is presented below.

Materials and Methods

Culture acquisition and maintenance

Isolates of *O. ophiodiicola* (isolate number 10-1197) were obtained

VOC	Total area of mycelia (mm²) 7 days post inoculation
Nonanal	150.61
2-Ethyl-1-hexanol	204.13
Benzaldehyde	345.13
Propionic acid	365.23
N,N-Dimethyloctylamine	373.87
Decanal	378.95
2-Phenylethanol	418.93
Benzothiazole	638.96
2-Nonanone	650.02
Styrene	753.60
Control	681.85

Table 1: Averaged radial growth of single VOC exposures and control (most to least inhibitive). Each trial was performed in triplicate and the average of all exposures is represented below.

from the University of California Davis, School of Veterinary Medicine Department of Pathology, Microbiology & Immunology. Cultures were lawn streaked and grown on Sabouraud Dextrose Agar (SDA, Difco) then incubated for 7 to 10 days at 30°C or until the entire agar surface was covered with mycelial growth. Conidia of *O. ophiodiicola* were harvested according to the methods of Cornelison et al. [18]. For storage, the conidia solution was centrifuged at 3,000 rpm and the supernatant was removed. 10 ml of 25% glycerol solution was added to the resulting pellet and this mixture was vortexed. The conidia concentration was determined via hemocytometer (Bright-Line, Pennsylvania). Conidia solutions were stored at -80°C until use. All *R. rhodochrous* glycerol stock aliquots were prepared according to the methods of Pierce et al. [16,24,25]. Fresh glycerol stocks were used as the source of cells at the onset of each assay. The induction process was performed using the addition of either urea or urea and cobalt as described by Pierce et al. [16,24,25].

Co-culture assays with *R. rhodochrous*

Co-culture assays were carried out according to the methods of Cornelison et al. [14] and modified as follows. A Petri plate (60 mm × 15 mm) containing SDA was inoculated with 50 μl of *O. ophiodiicola* conidia solution (1.4×10^6 conidia ml^{-1}) and placed in a shared airspace (150 mm × 15 mm) with cells of *R. rhodochrous* (treatment) or alone (control) and sealed with Parafilm M (Sigma-Aldrich, Missouri). All experimental setups remained sealed for 8 days or until the controls had formed a congruent mycelial lawn on the SDA (60 mm × 15 mm). All assays were performed in triplicate. In order to identify if *R. rhodochrous* has the ability to inhibit vegetative hyphae growth of *O. ophiodiicola*, mycelial plug assays were used to quantify the radial growth of *O. ophiodiicola*. A lawn of *O. ophiodiicola* was grown from conidia for 7-10 days and a 5 mm diameter transfer tube (Spectrum Medical, SC) was used to extract full depth mycelial plugs from the lawn of *O. ophiodiicola*. Each plug was then inserted into a fresh plate of SDA (60 mm × 15 mm). The resulting mycelial plug plates were placed into a shared airspace (150 mm × 15 mm) alone (control) or with two plates (60 mm × 15 mm) of induced *R. rhodochrous* (treatment) and sealed with Parafilm M.

Induced *R. rhodochrous* germule suppression assay

Germule suppression assays were conducted according to the methods of Cornelison et al. [14] and modified as follows. Slide agar overlays were inoculated with 50 μl of conidia suspension (1.4×10^6 conidia ml^{-1}). Plates of induced *R. rhodochrous* were removed after 24 and 48 hours of exposure. Slide agars were then observed at 21 days post inoculation. Microscopic observation of slide agar overlays utilized a Nikon Eclipse model E600 (Japan) in Differential Interference Contrast (DIC). The camera used to capture photos was a Nikon D7000. A germule is defined as a mycelial extension from a single conidia greater than the length of the intact conidia.

Preparation of fermentation cell-paste in non-growth conditions

The preparation of fermentation cell paste was produced according to the methods of Pierce et al. [16,24,25]. Fermentation cell paste is a high cell density aggregate from 30L fermentations of *R. rhodochrous* DAP96253 that has been centrifuged to remove spent media. The assessment of anti-fungal activity of *O. ophiodiicola* was observed by mycelial plugs assays, with 1 and 2 grams of fermentation paste per shared airspace in treatment samples and no cell paste in controls.

VOC combination assay for anti-*O. ophiodiicola* activity

VOCs were tested individually in exposure assays to determine if specific compounds were antifungal against *O. ophiodiicola*. Previous research has shown numerous naturally-occurring VOCs to have antifungal activity. The following compounds were selected for VOC exposure assays in this study: N,N-dimethyloctylamine, benzothiazole, benzaldehyde, 2-phenylethanol, 2-ethyl-1-hexanol, propionic acid, 2-nonanone, decanal, styrene, and nonanal [17,19,21-23]. All VOCs were procured as pure liquid research-grade chemical reagents (Sigma-Aldrich, Missouri) without any modification for exposure assays. Single VOC exposures were performed at a quantity of 4.0 μmol on each absorbent disc in a closed air space (150 mm × 15 mm). Fungal plugs from a fresh mycelial lawn were inserted into a SDA Petri plate (60 mm × 15 mm) and placed in the closed airspace with the specific VOC disc. All assays were sealed with Parafilm M and incubated for 7 days at 30°C. Plugs were photographed every 24 hours in order to measure radial mycelial expansion. Each VOC was ranked according to the level inhibition of *O. ophiodiicola* in single-dose exposures performed in triplicate and averaged. Compounds were also ranked based on toxicity, according to median lethal dose (LD50) reported in the literature (S1). From those rankings, five VOCs were selected and paired in all different combinations with 2 μmols of each compound (4 μmol total) in a closed airspace. Similarly, the same 5 compounds were combined in combinations of 3 with 1.3 μmols of each compound in a closed airspace. N, N-dimethyloctylamine was excluded from the combination trials because of its high toxicity (S1) and replaced with the next most inhibitory compound, decanal (47.6%). The goal was to select the most effective compounds with the lowest reported toxicity (S1). All trials were performed in triplicate and radial mycelial growth was quantified over 7 days and averaged.

Area measurement of radial growth with digital photography and open-source software

The area of radial mycelial growth was determined using the open-source photo editing software package GIMP (GNU Image Manipulation Program). Area quantification of mycelia plugs were obtained according to the methods of Cornelison et al. [18].

Results

Co-culture assays with *R. rhodochrous*

Plates of induced cells of *R. rhodochrous* were placed in a closed airspace along with conidia-inoculated SDA Petri plates of *O. ophiodiicola*. 7 days post-inoculation, the Petri plates in a shared airspace with *R. rhodochrous* had no visible growth (Figure 1a) whereas the controls had formed a congruent lawn over the entire agar surface (Figure 1b).

In the radial mycelial extension assays using vegetative mycelial plugs, *R. rhodochrous* produced statistically significant radial growth inhibition in days 3-6 post-inoculation (p<0.05, Figure 2). Radial area measurements on days 3, 5 and 6 showed a percent inhibition greater than 100%, due to the inhibited treatment plugs shrinking due to desiccation. Although the fungal plugs did show radial expansion in the first 24 hours post-inoculation, radial expansion was significantly inhibited in subsequent days (Figure 2).

Induced *R. rhodochrous* germule suppression assay

O. ophiodiicola conidia on slide agar overlays were exposed to cells of induced *R. rhodochrous* on media in a closed airspace at 30°C for 24

and 48 hours (Figures 3b-3d). After removal of *R. rhodochrous* from the shared airspace the slides were monitored for 21 days to determine if the exposed conidia were capable of generating germules. These exposed slides were compared to the unexposed control slides inoculated with *O. ophiodiicola* conidia, which had over-grown the slide agar overlays after 8 days (Figure 3a). No germules were identified on slides exposed to *R. rhodochrous* whereas control slides showed significant mycelial growth and sporulation. These results validate the hypothesis that *R. rhodochrous* can inhibit germination of *O. ophiodiicola* with as little as 24 hours of exposure (Figure 3b).

Anti-*O. ophiodiicola* activity of fermentation cell-paste

Non-growth cell-paste trials were conducted with 24 hour post-harvest cell-paste (fresh), and 44 day-old cell-paste stored at 4°C (stored), to evaluate the influence of cold storage on the antifungal activity of *R. rhodochrous* fermentation cell-paste. Both fresh and stored cell-paste demonstrated inhibitory activity against *O. ophiodiicola* (Figure 4), although fresh cell-paste was quantitatively more inhibitory.

Single VOC trials

O. ophiodiicola mycelial plugs were exposed to 4 μmol of ten different VOCs individually. The five most inhibitory VOCs were nonanal, 2-ethyl-1-hexanol, benzaldehyde, propionic acid, and N, N-dimethyloctylamine with averaged (n=3) percent inhibitions after 7 days of 80.6%, 80.5%, 52.9%, 59.0%, and 53.4% respectively (Figure 5).

Combinations of 2 VOCs

Overall combinations of 2 VOCs inhibited growth to a greater extent compared to the single VOC trials, supporting the hypothesis that select VOCs can work synergistically. The most effective combination was 2-ethyl-1-hexanol, and nonanal yielding an average of 94% inhibition over a period of 7 days (Figure 6). The second highest percent inhibition resulted from an equimolar combination of benzaldehyde, and 2-ethyl-1-hexanol, yielding an average of 93% inhibition over a period of 7 days (Figure 6).

Combinations of 3 VOCs

All combinations of VOCs were more effective at inhibiting radial mycelial extension of *O. ophiodiicola* compared to any VOC alone at equivalent moles (Figure 7). The two combinations of 3 VOCs that had the highest percent inhibition were benzaldehyde, propionic acid, and nonanal yielding an average of 88% inhibition over a period of 7 days, and nonanal, 2-ethyl-1-hexanol, and propionic acid yielding an average of 85.1% inhibition of radial growth compared to controls (Figure 7).

Discussion

Emerging fungal pathogens are threatening wildlife around the globe and have been reported to be increasing in incidence and severity over the past several decades [26]. Fungal pathogens present numerous challenges to disease management and microbial control efforts. This is primarily due to the ability of these fungi to thrive in host-free environmental reservoirs as well as their taxonomic similarity to their hosts (i.e., Eukarya/Eukarya). Consequently, antifungal agents used to treat human mycoses may have toxic effects on susceptible animals or be cost-prohibitive for large scale wildlife applications. Accordingly, the identification and evaluation of novel approaches to managing fungal pathogens of wildlife are needed to avert these potential ecological disasters.

Cases of SFD have increased significantly since 2006 [1]. Currently,

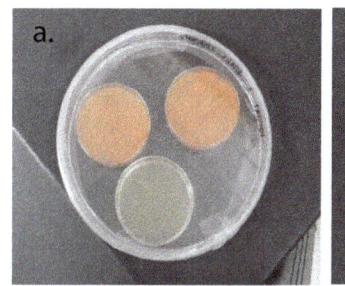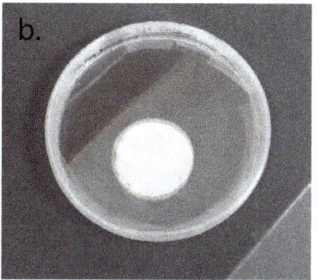

Figure 1: Co-culture assays with *R. rhodochrous*. 7 days post inoculation with 50 μl of 10^8 *O. ophiodiicola* conidia ml^{-1} in a closed airspace with induced *R. rhodochrous* **(a)** as well as in the absence of *R. rhodochrous* **(b)**.

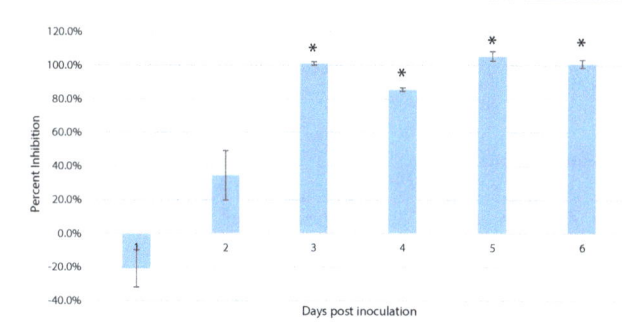

Figure 2: Average percent inhibition of *O. ophiodiicola* radial expansion in a shared airspace with *R. rhodochrous*. *indicates statistically significant ($p<0.05$) inhibition compared to unexposed controls.

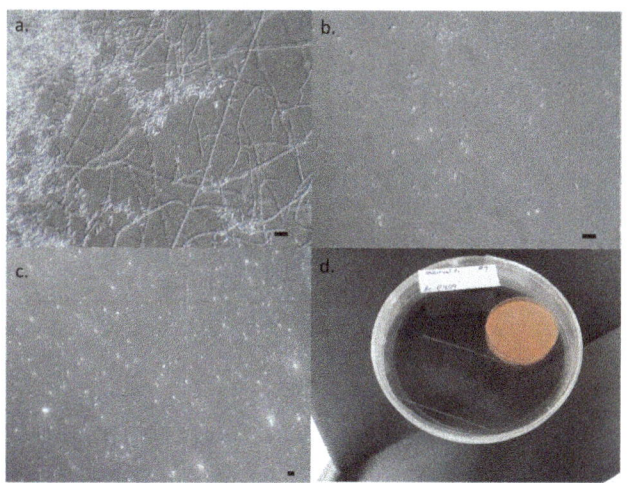

Figure 3: Germule suppression assay. 50 μl of 10^6 *O. ophiodiicola* conidia ml^{-1} were inoculated on slide agars overlays and stored at 30°C. Images were captured 8 days post inoculation. The control exhibits normal growth characteristics. **(a)** 24 hr. exposure of *R. rhodochrous* inhibits germination and germules are unable to recover after exposure. **(b)** 48 hr. exposure to *R. rhodochrous* inhibits germination. **(c)** Experimental setup **(d)** Images a and b are captured at 400X and c is captured at 200X. Scale bars are 10 μm.

SFD is confirmed in 15 states and continues to spread [1,2]. Disease management options for this mycosis are currently lacking, yet they may be vital to preventing regional extirpation of imperilled species such as the Eastern Massasauga Rattlesnake. The results presented in this study suggest that both *R. rhodochrous* and fungistatic soil-associated

VOCs may have utility in managing SFD, and warrant additional, *in vivo*, evaluation [27,28]. Specifically, evaluating the potential of these agents to address the deep tissue granulomas characteristic of advanced SFD will be critical for establishing these agents as clinical tools in the treatment of SFD [29].

Rhodococcus rhodochrous, a naturally-occurring soil bacterium, can irreversibly inhibit spore germination (Figure 3) and significantly inhibit radial mycelial elongation (Figure 2). Complete inhibition of conidia is beneficial for disease management purposes because it prevents any remnant conidia from germinating and growing after the treatment is complete. Additionally, as with many fungal pathogens, spores are likely the primary transmittable disease agent. Rendering these spores nonviable may reduce the spread of SFD in addition to potentially ameliorating the effects of SFD on individual hosts [30,31].

The ability to produce induced *R. rhodochrous* in large-scale fermentations, store at 4°C, and retain antifungal activity establishes the logistical feasibility of this organisms for disease management applications. Additionally, the well-established utility and safety of this organism for diverse industrial applications is supportive of the benign nature of large-scale applications and environmental release, although the evaluation of the potential for non-target effects will need to be conducted to ensure safety prior to any in situ applications being considered [32,33].

Mycelial plug assays using VOCs have also produced favourable results. Individual VOCs produced significant inhibition, but even greater inhibition was observed when VOCs were used in equimolar combinations, with select combinations demonstrating significant synergistic activities. In addition, snakes are not a traditional model for toxicity assessments; therefore, the toxicity, as LD50 with rats, was used only as general estimate for ranking individual VOC toxicity. Using a low dosage of less toxic compounds can be used as a way to achieve impactful efficacy in fungal control and limit the potential toxicity associated with antifungal agents [34]. The efficacy of antifungal VOCs for in situ application in the control of SFD is currently unknown. There are several key factors which play a role in natural examples of fungistasis that will also influence field performance in managing SFD (for example, physical barriers to diffusion, humidity, airflow and temperature). These factors will vary from site to site and must be considered when evaluating to the potential of VOCs for *in situ* applications.

As the incidence and prevalence of emerging fungal pathogens expands, novel tools must be developed to facilitate active management of these pathogens. Fungal pathogens, such as *O. ophiodiicola*, are capable of surviving and potentially amplifying in host-free environments requiring environmental mitigations to reduce disease incidence within a population. In these cases, agents capable of rendering conidia non-viable may have significant utility and should be the focus of efforts to develop mitigation plans for SFD in at-risk populations. However, *in vitro* activity, such as reported in this manuscript, does not serve as an ideal predictor of efficacy in the field. While in situ disease management for wild snakes will be the ultimate goal for managing SFD, developing disease mitigation tools for application in the natural environment presents numerous challenges and necessitates further investigation. The initial findings presented in this manuscript justify further *in vivo* evaluation of *R. rhodochrous* and select VOCs for the clinical management of SFD in captive recovery programs and in captive collections (e.g., zoos, pet trade) [35,36].

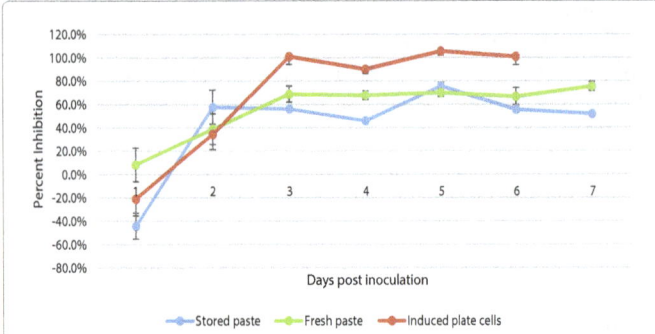

Figure 4: Biomass composition, age and media support influence efficacy against *O. ophiodiicola*. Percent inhibition of stored paste (44 days at 4°C), fresh paste (<24 hours after harvesting from fermentation vessel) and induced plate cells (used while on induction agar). Percent inhibition was determined by comparing growth to unexposed controls, and averaged from triplicate.

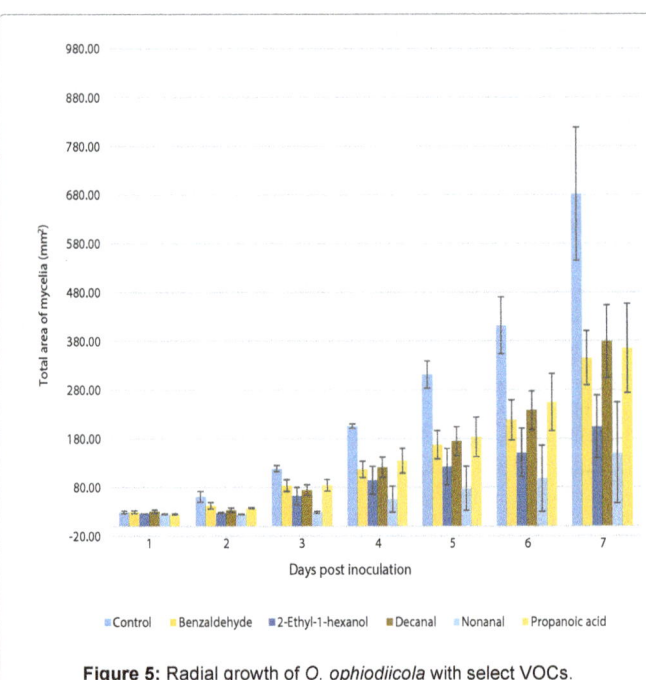

Figure 5: Radial growth of *O. ophiodiicola* with select VOCs.

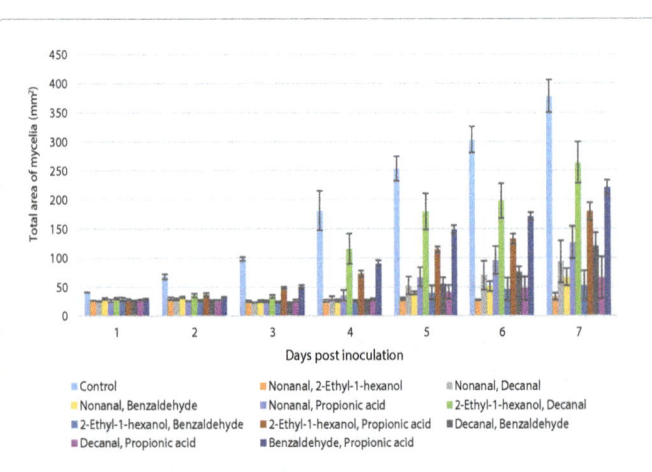

Figure 6: Radial growth of *O. ophiodiicola* with equimolar combinations of 2 VOCs.

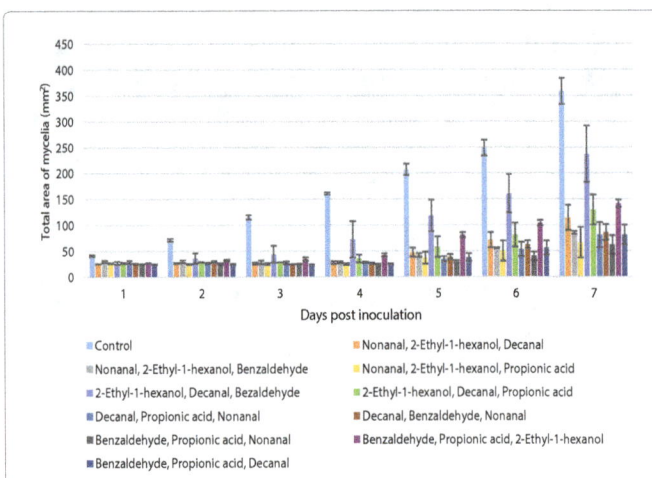

Figure 7: Radial growth of *O. ophiodiicola* with equimolar combinations of 3 VOCs.

Acknowledgments

This work was supported by the Environmental Research Center at Georgia State University as well as the Georgia State University Research Foundation.

Author Contributions

CTC, KTG, and SAC conceived and designed the experiments; BC performed the experiments; CTC, BC, and SAC analyzed the data; CKB and KTG contributed reagents/materials/analysis tools; CTC and BC wrote the paper.

Conflicts of Interest

SAC is an inventor on the seminal patents on *Rhodococcus rhodoochrous* DAP 96253 induction and application. CTC and KTG are the inventors on a patent submission regarding VOC formulations for treating fungal disease. All issued and submitted patents relating to this work are held by the Georgia State University Research Foundation.

References

1. Sleeman J (2013) Snake fungal disease in the United States. National Wildlife Health Center Wildlife Health Bulletin 2: 1-3.

2. Allender MC, Raudabaugh DB, Gleason FH, Miller AN (2015) The natural history, ecology, and epidemiology of *Ophidiomyces ophiodiicola* and its potential impact on free-ranging snake populations. Fungal Ecology 17: 187-196.

3. Allender MC, Baker S, Wylie D, Loper D, Dreslik MJ, et al. (2015) Development of snake fungal disease after experimental challenge with *Ophidiomyces ophiodiicola* in cottonmouths (*Agkistrodon piscivorous*). PLoS One 10: e0140193.

4. Lorch JM, Lankton J, Werner K, Falendysz EA, McCurley K, et al. (2015) Experimental infection of snakes with *Ophidiomyces ophiodiicola* causes pathological changes that typify snake fungal disease. mBio 6: e01534-15.

5. Allender MC, Dreslik M, Wylie S, Phillips C, Wylie DB, et al. (2011) *Chrysosporium* sp. infection in eastern massasauga rattlesnakes. Emerg Infect Dis 17: 2383-2385.

6. Rajeev S, Sutton DA, Wickes BL, Miller DL, Giri D, et al. (2009) Isolation and characterization of a new fungal species, *Chrysosporium ophiodiicola*, from a mycotic granuloma of a black rat snake (*Elaphe obsoleta obsoleta*). J Clin Microbiol 47: 1264-1268.

7. Sutherland WJ, Aveling R, Brooks TM, Clout M, Dicks LV, et al. (2014) A horizon scan of global conservation issues for 2014. Trends Ecol Evol 29: 15-22.

8. Linzey DW, Clifford MJ (2002) Snakes of Virginia. 1st edn. University Press of Virginia, Charlottesville, USA.

9. Center of Disease Control and Prevention (2010) Rodents.

10. Hahn G (2009) Target Animal Safety for Veterinary Pharmaceutical Products

(VICH GL 43). In Berichte zu Tierarzneimitteln, Birkhäuser Basel, pp: 58-69.

11. Koh DCI, Armugam A, Jeyaseelan K (2006) Snake venom components and their applications in biomedicine. Cell Mol Life Sci CMLS 63: 3030-3041.

12. Collis AH, Fenili RN (2011) The Modern US Reptile Industry. Economic Analysis Group.

13. Clark RW, Marchand MN, Clifford BJ, Stechert R, Stephens S (2011) Decline of an isolated timber rattlesnake (Crotalus horridus) population: interactions between climate change, disease, and loss of genetic diversity. Biological Conservation 144: 886-891.

14. Cornelison CT, Keel MK, Gabriel KT, Barlament CK, Tucker TA, et al. (2014) A preliminary report on the contact-independent antagonism of Pseudogymnoascus destructans by Rhodococcus rhodochrous strain DAP96253. BMC Microbiol 14: 246.

15. Bell KS, Philp JC, Aw DWJ, Christofi N (1998) The genus Rhodococcus. J Appl Microbiol 85: 195-210.

16. Pierce GE, Drago GK, Ganguly S, Tucker TA, Hooker JW, Jones S, et al. (2011) Preliminary report on a catalyst derived from induced cells of Rhodococcus rhodochrous strain DAP 96253 that delays the ripening of selected climacteric fruit: bananas, avocados, and peaches. J Ind Microbiol Biotechnol 38: 1567-1573.

17. Chuankun X, Minghe M, Leming Z, Keqin Z (2004) Soil volatile fungistasis and volatile fungistatic compounds. Soil Biol Biochem 36: 1997-2004.

18. Cornelison CT, Gabriel KT, Barlament C, Crow Jr. SA (2014) Inhibition of Pseudogymnoascus destructans growth from conidia and mycelial extension by bacterially produced volatile organic compounds. Mycopathologia 177: 1-10.

19. Fernando WD, Ramarathnam R, Krishnamoorthy AS, Savchuk SC (2005) Identification and use of potential bacterial organic antifungal volatiles in biocontrol. Soil Biol Biochem 37: 955-964.

20. Garbeva P, Hol WG, Termorshuizen AJ, Kowalchuk GA, De Boer W (2011) Fungistasis and general soil biostasis-a new synthesis. Soil Biol Biochem 43: 469-477.

21. Liu W, Mu W, Zhu B, Liu F (2008) Antifungal activities and components of VOCs produced by Bacillus subtilis G8. Curr Res Bacteriol 1: 28-34.

22. Strobel GA, Kluck K, Hess WM, Sears J, Ezra D, et al. (2007) Muscodor albus E-6, an endophyte of Guazuma ulmifolia making volatile antibiotics: isolation, characterization and experimental establishment in the host plant. Microbiol 153: 2613-2620.

23. Yuan J, Raza W, Shen Q, Huang Q (2012) Antifungal activity of Bacillus amyloliquefaciens NJN-6 volatile compounds against Fusarium oxysporum f. sp. cubense. Appl Environ Microbiol 78: 5942-5944.

24. Pierce GE, Drago G, Ganguly S (2009) Induction and stabilization of enzymatic activity in microorganisms. US 7531343 B2.

25. Pierce GE, Drago G, Ganguly S (2009) Induction and stabilization of enzymatic activity in microorganisms. US 7531344 B2.

26. Fisher MC, Henk DA, Briggs CJ, Brownstein JS, Madoff LC, et al. (2012) Emerging fungal threats to animal, plant and ecosystem health. Nature 484: 186-194.

27. Chem ID plus. Octyldimethylamine. ChemIDplus Datatbank Number 7378-99-6. National Library of Medicine Bethesda (MD), USA.

28. Chem ID plus. 2-Nonanone. ChemIDplus Datatbank Number 821-55-6. National Library of Medicine Bethesda (MD), USA.

29. Hazardous Substances Data Bank (2015) 2-Ethyl-1-Hexanol. Hazard Hazardous Substances Databank Number: 1118. National Library of Medicine, Bethesda (MD), USA.

30. Hazardous Substances Data Bank (2015) Nonanal. Hazard Hazardous Substances Databank Number: 7229. National Library of Medicine, Bethesda (MD), USA.

31. Hazardous Substances Data Bank (2015) Propionic Acid. Hazard Hazardous Substances Databank Number: 1192. National Library of Medicine, Bethesda (MD), USA.

32. Hazardous Substances Data Bank (2015) 1-Decanol. Hazard Hazardous Substances Databank Number: 1072. National Library of Medicine, Bethesda (MD), USA.

33. Hazardous Substances Data Bank (2005) Benzaldehyde. Hazard Hazardous Substances Databank Number: 388. National Library of Medicine, Bethesda (MD), USA.

34. Hazardous Substances Data Bank (2002) 2-Phenylethanol. Hazard Hazardous Substances Databank Number: 5002. National Library of Medicine, Bethesda (MD), USA.

35. Hazardous Substances Data Bank (2014) Styrene. Hazard Hazardous Substances Databank Number: 171. National Library of Medicine, Bethesda (MD), USA.

36. Reddy G, Mayhew DA (1992) Acute oral toxicity (LD50) study in rats with benzothiazole. Int J Toxicol 11: 666-666.

7

Sheep Mange Mites and Lice: Prevalence and Risk Factors in Asella and its Surroundings, South Eastern Ethiopia

Desalegn Deferes[1] and Minda Asfaw Geresu[2]*

[1]Lemu Bilbilo District Livestock and Fisheries Resource and Development Office, Arsi, Ethiopia
[2]School of Agriculture, Animal and Range Sciences Course Team, Madda Walabu University, Bale-Robe, Ethiopia

Abstract

A cross-sectional study was conducted to determine the prevalence and risk factors for sheep mange mites and lice infestation in Asella and its surroundings of south eastern Ethiopia, from November, 2009 to April, 2010. The study revealed that 212 (55.21%) of the 384 sheep examined were infested with mange mites or lice in the study area. A higher prevalence of pediculosis (49.5%) was observed compared to mange mite infestation which was rarely observed with prevalence rate of 5.72%. Mange mites genera identified in the present study were Sarcoptes (2.6%), Psoroptes (2.3%), Chorioptes (0.8%) while no Demodex was identified in the study settings of sheep. Pertaining to lice infestation, *Bovicola ovis* (36.7%) and *Linognathus ovillus* (16.9%) were the only identified species of lice. A negative association ($p>0.05$) of mange mites and lice infestation was observed among the sex groups while only lice infestation was positively associated ($p<0.05$) with the age groups of sheep in the study environs. Concerning to body condition scores, a chi-square analysis revealed that lice infestation was highly positively associated ($p=0.000$) with the covariates (different body condition score group) in which the highest prevalence of lice infestation was observed in sheep with poor body condition score (67.36%). Nevertheless, mange mite infestation was negatively associated ($p>0.05$) with different body condition scores as the statistical analysis revealed. The result of this study revealed that as an ever increasing threat of mange mite and lice infestation on overall sheep productivity and tanning industry in Ethiopia warrants urgent control intervention. Hence, to reduce mange mite and lice infestation prevalence and impact on the productivity and health status, planning of integrated control measures with sustainable veterinary services aiming at creating awareness about the importance and control of the ectoparasites for small ruminant's owners is recommended.

Keywords: Lice; Mange mites; Prevalence; Risk factors; Sheep; Asella

Introduction

Ethiopia with its greatest variation in climate and topography possesses one of the largest small ruminant populations in the world, which is kept extensively mostly by small holder farmers and adjacent to crop production [1-3]. The country is home to 23.6 million sheep [4], but the immense potential these numbers represent has yet to be realized due to a multitude of factors. Ectoparasites are very common and widely distributed in all agro-ecological zones in Ethiopia [5,6]. They are one of the major hindrances to the productivity of sheep in the country and infestation caused by the ectoparasites could lead to considerable economic losses to farmers due to loss of productivity, mortality, and skin diseases. Among the ectoparasites; lice, sheep keds, ticks, fleas and mange mites causes a great preslaughter defects responsible for downgrading and rejection of skins that confront the productivity of sheep [7]. About 35% of sheep and 56% of goat skin rejections in Ethiopia are attributed to ectoparasites [8] and all these established facts revealed that the ectoparasites pose serious economic losses to the farmer, the tanning industry and the country as a whole [7,9].

Mange mites are common in Ethiopia and therefore are reported from many regions and different agro climates. Based on the reports so far, mange mites are most prevalent in four national regional states of Ethiopia namely, the Amhara, Oromia, Tigray and Southern Nation and Nationalities regional states [10-12]. In all reports, three genera of mites namely, Sarcoptes, Psoroptes and Demodex were reported to affect small ruminants. In addition to this, lice infestation in the country is the most frequently reported and the most important skin disease of small ruminants this is because lice are found to be the cause of cockle [13].

Various studies have been conducted to determine the prevalence of mange mites and lice infestation in various regions of Ethiopia. Among the three genera of mites, *Sarcoptic scabiei var. caprae* and *Sarcoptic scabiei var. ovis* have a wide geographic distribution in many goat and sheep rearing in arid and semi-arid areas of Ethiopia, and it is more commonly seen in goats than sheep. In Ethiopia, they are widely distributed in lowland mainly [10-12], low and midlands [7] as well as central midland part of the country [14]. Studies conducted by Kedir [15] in Tigray (30.32%) and Fekadu et al. [12] in Southern Ethiopia (57.6%) disclosed the highest prevalence of sarcoptic mites in sheep and goats in the country.

Concerning, mites of the genus Psoroptes that cause psoroptic mange in sheep and goats, its prevalence is found greater than in goats therefore, it causes greater damage in sheep than in goats [13] and recent studies depicted that Psoroptic mange is most common among small ruminants in lowland areas of north [8,11] and South ecological zones in Ethiopia as reported by Yacob et al. [10] in central lowland of Oromia; by Sertse et al. [16] in midland and highlands of Amhara region, and [12] in lowland and midland areas in southern part of the

*Corresponding author: Minda Asfaw Geresu, School of Agriculture, Animal and Range Sciences Course Team, Madda Walabu University, Bale-Robe, Ethiopia
E-mail: minda.asfaw@gmail.com

country. Demodectic mange has also been reported different authors in sheep (*Demodex ovis*) and goats (*Demodex caprae*) and it is distributed in different agro ecological zones of the country as the works of [10] in central lowland of Oromia region, [16] in midland and highlands of Amhara region and [12] in lowland and midland areas in southern part of the country revealed.

Nowadays, in addition to mange mite infestation, pediculosis is a serious health problem of small ruminants in Ethiopia which is caused by lice infestation and it is the most frequently reported and important skin disease of small ruminants this is because lice are found to be the cause of cockle. Studies conducted by Yacob, Mulugeta, Sertse, Hailu et al. [10,11,17,18] reported different lice spp infestation in sheep from Wolaita Soddo, Tigray, Amhara regional state and Asella in the country respectively.

Nevertheless all the above study revealed that as mange mite and lice infestation seriously devastating sheep production system and tanning industry in Ethiopia, there is paucity of published data (information) about the prevalence of mange mites and lice infestation in sheep production system in Arsi Zone in general and in Asella and its surroundings as the potential it has in particular. This scarcity of information on the presence and prevalence of mange mites and lice infestation in sheep production system of the study area may reflect a lack of resources for the ectoparasite surveillance and control in sheep production system or most of the work done there may be left unpublished (left on shelf). In addition, most of mange mites and lice infestation, remain undiagnosed and only diazinon spray or Ivermectin injection has been applied without considering the efficacy and management system and the farmers consider skin losses as normal and natural. Therefore, information on the prevalence and risk factors exposing to mange mite and lice infestation has to be studied in detail in order to apply control measures based on mass treatment or effective movement control.

Hence, this study was conducted: to determine the prevalence of mange mite and lice infestation in sheep in Asella and its surroundings and to assess the putative risk factors exposing to mange mite and lice infestation in the selected study area. Therefore, our study could be a foil for the paucity of information about the prevalence of mange mites and lice infestation and presumed risk factors exposing to the ectoparasite infestation in the sheep production system of the study area.

Materials and Methods

Description of the study area

The study was conducted in Asella town and its surrounding, Arsi Zone, Oromia Regional State. It is located at 175 km in south east of Ethiopia within 6°59-8°49'N latitude and 38°41'-40°44'E longitude. Topographically, Asella is a high land area with altitude ranging from 1300 to 1350 meter above sea level and has annual rain fall of 2300 to 2400 mm [19]. Vegetation of the area changes with altitude and rainfall ranging from scattered trees and bushes to dense shrubs and bushes from the total land of 43% used for grazing, 35% for cultivation 8.6% forest land, 10.7% pastureland. It is one of the highly populated areas in Ethiopia with estimated human population of 2,521,349 and livestock population of bovine-82,190; ovine-51,292; caprine-8,11,479; poultry-5, 62,915 and equine-22,055 [20,21].

Study animals

In our study, a total of 384 sheep of different age groups, both sexes and of local breeds coming to the Asella town Veterinary Clinic for

veterinary services, were examined for the presence of mange mites and lice infestation. During sampling, history, age, sex, and body condition scores of each animal were recorded. The animals were grouped into two age categories, as young (up to one year) and adult (older than one year) as described by Steele and ESGPIP [22,23]. Age determination was made using owner's information and by dentition. Body condition scores were determined following the procedures documented by Steele and ESGPIP [22,23] for sampled animals as poor, medium and good classes following 1 up to 5 grading system.

Study design and sample size determination

A cross-sectional study design was conducted to determine the prevalence of mange mites and lice infestation in the selected study area and to identify the potential risk factors associated with the two ectoparasite infestations. A simple random sampling method was employed and the study animals were randomly selected and examination was conducted through visual inspection and palpation to detect the presence of skin lesion. The sample size was calculated according to Thrusfield [24] by considering 50% expected prevalence (P), 95% confidence interval (CI) (Z=1.96) with 5% desired absolute precision (d), using the formula $N=(Z)^2 P (1-P)/d^2$. Hence, the calculated required sample size (N) was 384.

Ectoparasites collection and identification

After proper restraining, representative specimens were collected from infested and diseased animals. Ectoparasites (sheep keds, ticks, lice and fleas) either encountered on the skin surface or attached to the hair were collected manually from their sites of attachment. A coat brushing technique was applied to collect lice from host skin. Then the collected samples were placed in labeled universal bottles containing 70% ethanol and taken to the Parasitology Section, Laboratory of the Asella Regional Animal Health Diagnostic and Investigation Centre located in Asella town. In the laboratory, the ectoparasites were identified with the basis of their morphological structure using the recommendations of Urquhart et al. [25] and Wall and Shearer [26]. Further identification at species level was conducted using a stereomicroscope according to their key morphological structures for lice. In addition, skin scrapings for mange mites were collected from clinically suspected animals. This was made by clipping the hair around affected areas using scissors, scraping the edges of the lesion with the scalpel blades [25] until capillary blood oozing was evident. The scraped materials were transferred to a container containing 10% formalin and were taken for laboratory examination. Then in the laboratory, a few drops of 10% potassium hydroxide were added to the specimen, allowed to stand for 30 minutes, and examined under a light microscope at 40x magnification [7,25]. The mange mites were identified with the morphological keys of Urquhart et al. [25] and Kumsa et al. [26].

Data analysis

Data generated from the questionnaire survey and laboratory investigations were recorded and coded using Microsoft Excel spreadsheet (Microsoft Corporation) and analyzed using STATA version 11.0 for Windows (Stata Corp. College Station, TX, USA). The prevalence of pig mange mites and lice infestation was calculated as the number of positive samples divided by the total number of samples tested. To identify association of prevalence with the risk factors (sex, age and body condition scores) were computed by percentages and Pearson's chi-square (χ^2) test. In all cases $p<0.05$ was considered as statistically significant.

Results

Overall prevalence of mange mite and lice infestation in sheep identified in this study

Ectoparasitological data analysis revealed that 212 of 384 total sheep flock examined harbored either single or mixed infection. The overall prevalence of lice and mange mite infestation in the flock was 55.21%. Of 384 total sheep examined, 22 sheep were infected by both mange and lice (mixed infection). The result signified that the higher prevalence of pediculosis (49.5%) was observed in sheep in the study area. Nevertheless, mange mite infestation was rarely observed with prevalence rate of 5.72% as depicted in Table 1.

Prevalence of species of mange mites and lice in the study area

The three major genera of mange mites identified from the sampled sheep were *Sarcoptes* spp (2.6%), *Psoroptes* spp (2.3%) and *Chorioptes* spp (0.8%) while no *Demodex* spp was found in the present study. Pertaining to the lice infestation, *Bovicola ovis* (*B. ovis*) (36.7%) and *Linognathus ovillus* (*L. ovillus*) (16.9%) were observed in this study. *Sarcoptes* spp (2.6%) were the most relatively higher in prevalence among the mange mite species identified while the prevalence of *B. ovis* was higher when compared to *L. ovillus* among the lice infestation observed in this study (Table 2).

A chi-square analysis of association of the putative risk factors with mange mite and lice infestation in sheep

Prevalence of mange mite and lice infestation in sheep in relation to sex group: The prevalence of lice infestation in male sheep (55.39%) was roughly the same with that of female sheep (54.95%).

Furthermore, the prevalence of mange mite infestation in male (5.75%) and female (6.06) sheep flocks was almost similar and the covariate (sex) was negatively associated with the prevalence of mange mite and lice infestation in flocks of sheep in the study area as illustrated in Tables 3-5.

Prevalence of mange mite and lice infestation with respect to the age group of the animal: A relatively higher prevalence of mange mites (6.56%) and lice (52.44%) infestations were found in adult animals in the study area when compared to young animals. Both young (43.90%) and adult (52.44%) sheep were highly infested by lice than mange mites. The prevalence of lice infestation was positively associated (χ^2 =6.330; $p<0.05$) with the putative covariate (age group) whereas the prevalence of mange mite infestation was not considerably associated ($p>0.05$) with the putative risk factor (age group).

Prevalence of mange mite and lice in sheep by body condition scores: A relatively higher prevalence of mange mite infestation was found in animals with poor body condition score (6.94%) than in animals with medium and good body condition score while the highest lice infestation was observed in animals with poor body condition score in relation to the animals with medium and good body condition score. The prevalence of lice infestation was highly significantly associated (χ^2=44.103; $p=0.000$) with the independent variable (body condition score) whereas the prevalence of mange mite infestation was negatively associated ($p>0.05$) with the putative exposing risk factor (body condition score).

Discussion

The present study ascertained an overall prevalence of 55.21% of

Ectoparasite	No. of sheep examined	No. of sheep found positive	Overall prevalence (%)
Mange	384	22	5.72
Lice	384	190	49.5
Total	384	212	55.21

Table 1: Total prevalence of lice and mange infection in sheep in Asella and its surroundings.

Ectoparasite species		No. of animals examined	No. of positive animals	Prevalence (%)
Mange	Sarcoptes	384	10	2.6
	Psoroptes		9	2.3
	Chorioptes		3	0.8
	Demodex		0	0
Lice	*Bovicola ovis*	384	141	36.7
	Linognathus ovillus		65	16.9

Table 2: Prevalence of genera of mange and lice in Asella and its surroundings.

Ectoparasite identified	Covariate (sex group)		χ^2 (*p*-value)
	Male (N=139)	Female (N=245)	
	Prevalence (%)	Prevalence (%)	
Mange	5.75	6.06	0.000 (0.987)
Lice	55.39	54.95	3.05 (0.081)

N: Number of animals examined

Table 3: Lice and mange infestation association with the sex groups in Asella and its surrounding.

Ectoparasite identified	Covariate (age group)		χ^2 (*p*-value)
	Young (N=125)	Adult (N=259)	
	Prevalence (%)	Prevalence (%)	
Mange	4.06	6.56	1.086 (0.581)
Lice	43.90	52.44	6.330 (0.042)

N: Number of animals examined

Table 4: Prevalence of lice and mange mite infestation in relation to age groups in the selected study area.

Ectoparasite	Covariate (body condition score)			χ² (p-value)
	Poor BCS N (%)	Medium BCS N (%)	Good BCS N (%)	
Mange	10 (6.94)	8 (4.659)	4 (3.88)	0.767 (0.682)
Lice	97 (67.36)	80 (46.51)	13 (19.12)	44.103 (0.000**)
Overall prevalence	107 (27.86)	88 (22.91)	17 (4.43)	

BCS: Body Condition Score; N: Number of positive animals sampled; **: Highly significantly associated

Table 5: Prevalence of lice and mange mite infestation by body condition score of animals in the study area.

mange mites and lice infestations revealing that the great importance and widespread occurrence of the two ectoparasites in sheep in Asella and its surroundings. This finding is in agreement with the previous reports of the ectoparasites prevalence in small ruminants from different parts of Ethiopia [7,16,27,28] and other countries of the world [29,30]. Nonetheless, the finding of the current study was higher than the prevalence reported in the Southern range land of Oromia as reported by Molu [31] and Takele [32], and Zeryehun and Tadesse [33] at Nekemte Veterinary Clinic, Northwest of Ethiopia. The higher infestation rate is most probably attributable to several important factors including conducive environment, malnutrition and poor husbandry systems, poor awareness of farmers and inadequate veterinary services in study settings [3,34,35].

The prevalence of sheep lice (49.5%) recorded in this study is higher than the reports of Kumsa et al. [7] in three agro-ecological zones in central Oromia (28.7%), Sertse and Wossene [16] in the eastern part of Amhara region (39.5%), Mulugeta [28] in south-eastern parts of Tigray (30.5%) and Haffize [36] in central Ethiopia (2%). Such variations in prevalence might arise from differences in agro-ecology, the season during which the study was conducted, the management and health care of sheep in the study areas and the sensitivity of the diagnostic techniques employed. Louse infestations may indicate some other underlying problems such as malnutrition and chronic diseases [7,37].

Meanwhile, the current study sheep mange mite infestation (5.72%) was relatively higher than the report of Tefera [38] in selected sites of Amhara regional state and Israel et al. [39] in Sodo Zuria district of southern Ethiopia. This study revealed that three genera of mange mites identified, namely, *sarcoptes* (2.6%), *chorioptes* (2.3%) and *psoroptes* (0.8%) in the study area. These genera of mange mites have been commonly reported from different parts of Ethiopia [36,39-41]. A bit higher prevalence of *Sarcoptes* was observed in the present work which is in agreement with the report of Zeryehun and Tadesse [33] in sheep at Nekemte Veterinary Clinic of Northwest Ethiopia (2.5%). The lesion of *Sarcoptes scabiei var ovis* in sheep was observed mostly around the ear, face and head areas and nodule formation was the characteristics lesion recorded. Kettle [42] observed that, sarcoptic mange if they occur in sheep in general they are frequently observed in sparsely haired parts.

Pertaining to lice infestation in Ethiopia, it is the most frequently reported and important skin disease of small ruminants this is because lice are found to be the cause of cockle. The present study established a higher prevalence of *B. ovis* (36.7%) and *L. ovillus* (16.9%). This finding is in agreement with the work of Asnake et al. [12] who reported 14.6% of *L. ovillus* and 36.1% of *B. ovis* of sheep in three agro-ecological districts of southern Ethiopia. However, the present finding is higher than the works of Yacob et al. [10] and Mulugeta et al. [11] in which 26.64% of *B. ovis* from Wolayta Sodo, and 15.3% of *B. ovis* and 27. 9% of *L. ovillus* from Tigray region was reported. In contrary to these authors work, Hailu [18] reported the highest prevalence of *Linognathus* spp (75.5%) and *B. ovis* (67.1%) in sheep from Asella even which disagrees with the present work. This difference in prevalence could be attributed to the

effects of climate change and other factor such as changes in animal management and husbandry system practices, usage of acaricides and increase in animal trafficking or movements may also contribute to the changes in the prevalence, or emergence, of lice infestation in certain localities [43].

The current study established that almost closer prevalence of mange mites in both sex groups of sheep, an overall prevalence of 6.06% was observed in female while 5.75% mange mite infestation was recorded in the male sheep, and the covariate (sex) was negatively associated (p>0.05) with the prevalence of mange mite infestation. This finding was in agreement with previous observation made by Yacob et al. [10], Zeryehun and Tadesse [33], and Kassaye and Kebede [44] that revealed as sex has no significant effect on the prevalence of mange mites infestation. In addition to this, almost closer prevalence of lice infestation in both male (55.39%) and female (54.95%) sheep was observed in this study though there is no significant association between the lice infestation and sexes of the animal.

This study revealed as age group was insignificantly associated with mange mite's infestation. Though there was a negative association between the covariate (age) and mange mite infestation, there was a relatively higher prevalence in adult than young sheep which contradicts the work of Sheferaw et al. [40], and Kassaye and Kebede [44] who reported higher prevalence of mange mite infestation in young age group. Furthermore, age was reported to have no significant effect on the prevalence of mange mites [10].

Like that of mange mite, adult age group of sheep (52.44%) had a risk of acquiring higher lice infestation than younger sheep (43.90%) and the covariate (age) was positively associated (p<0.05) with lice infestation in the present work. This finding is inconsistent with the study of Kassaye and Kebede [44] whom their report revealed that lice infestation was higher in young than in adult animals in Tigray region. The observation of significantly higher prevalence of lice in adult sheep attributed to maternal grooming and separate house that could be reducing exposure in younger animals [38].

The prevalence of lice in poor, medium and good body condition score was 67.36%, 46.5% and 19.12%, respectively in the present study. Significant association (p<0.05) between the prevalence of lice infestation were evidenced by body condition score, showing a greater susceptibility of animals with poor body condition. However, lower prevalence of lice infestation was reported by Israel et al. [39] whom their finding revealed that 6.5%, 5.7% and 8.3% in poor, medium and good body condition, respectively in Sodo Zuria district of Southern Ethiopia. Observations that animals with poor body condition score had higher ectoparasite infestation rate suggest negative effect on productivity. Ectoparasites induce itching or worry (reduce time on grazing) and suck blood (compete for nutrients), both of which compromise the nutritional status of host animals [45].

Conclusion

This study established mange mite and lice infestation in sheep in

Asella town and its surroundings. A higher prevalence of pediculosis was observed compared to mange mite infestation which was rarely observed with lower prevalence rate. Mange mites genera identified in this study were Sarcoptes, Psoroptes and Chorioptes while no Demodex was identified in the study settings of sheep. With regard to lice infestation, *B. ovis* and *L. ovillus* were the only identified species of lice. The study also revealed that lice infestation was positively associated with the two covariates (age and body condition score) while a negative association was observed between the sex groups. Nonetheless, mange mite infestation was negatively associated with all the risk factors considered in this study. This study disclosed that the poor quality of husbandry practices and/or inadequate veterinary care given to sheep by their owner's. Therefore, the growing threat of mange mite and lice infestation to sheep flock in the study settings requires a well-coordinated control intervention.

References

1. Tadesse H (2005) Pre-slaughter defects of hides/skin and intervention options in east Africa: Harnessing the leather industry to benefit the poor. In: Regional Workshop Proceedings, April, pp: 18-20.

2. MOA (2010) Ministry of Agriculture: Annual Report on Livestock Production, MOA, Addis Ababa, Ethiopia.

3. Seyoum Z, Tadesse T, Addisu A (2015) Ectoparasites Prevalence in Small Ruminants in and around Sekela, Amhara Regional State, Northwest Ethiopia. J Vet Med 2015: 216085.

4. CSA (2008) Agricultural sample survey. Volume II, Report on livestock and livestock characteristics. Volume II, 2007/08, Addis Ababa, Ethiopia.

5. Kumsa BE, Mekonnen S (2011) Ixodid ticks, fleas and lice infesting dogs and cats in Hawassa, southern Ethiopia. Onderstepoort J Vet Res 78: 1-8.

6. Kumsa B, Tamrat H, Tadesse G, Aklilu N, Cassini R (2012) Prevalence and species composition of ixodid ticks infesting horses in three agroecologies in central Oromia, Ethiopia. Trop Anim Health Prod 44: 119-124.

7. Kumsa B, Beyecha K, Geloye M (2012) Ectoparasites of sheep in three agro-ecological zones in central Oromia, Ethiopia. Onderstepoort J Vet Res 79: 1-7.

8. Kassa B (2006) Cockle, mange and pox: Major threats to the leather industry in Ethiopia. Ethiopian leather industry: Perseverance towards value addition. In: Proceedings of the National Workshop, Addis Ababa, Ethiopia, Pp: 71-92.

9. Berhanu W, Negussie H, Alemu S, Mazengia H (2011) Assessment on major factors that cause skin rejection at Modjo export tannery, Ethiopia. Trop Anim Health Production 43: 989-993.

10. Yacob HT, Nesanet B, Dinka A (2008) Part II: Prevalences of major skin diseases in cattle, sheep and goats at Adama Veterinary Clinic, Oromia regional state, Ethiopia. Rev Med Vet-Toulouse 159: 455-461.

11. Mulugeta Y, Yacob HT, Ashenafi H (2010) Ectoparasites of small ruminants in three selected agro-ecological sites of Tigray Region, Ethiopia. Trop Anim Health Prod 42: 1219-1224.

12. Fekadu A, Tolossa YH, Ashenafi H (2013) Ectoparasitesof Small Ruminants in Three Agro-Ecological Districts of Southern Ethiopia. Afr J Basic Appl Sci 5: 47-54.

13. Tolossa YH (2014) Ectoparasitism: Threat to Ethiopian small ruminant population and tanning industry. J Vet Med Anim Health 6: 25-33.

14. Yacob HT, Yalew TA, Dinka AA (2008) Part I: Ectoparasite prevalences in sheep and in goats in and around Wolaita Soddo, Southern Ethiopia. Revue de Méd Vét 159: 450-454.

15. Kedir M (2000) Study on mange mite infestations in small ruminants and camel in to selected Agro climatic zones in Tigray, Northern Ethiopia. DVM Thesis, Addis Ababa University, Faculty of Veterinary Medicine, Debre Zeit, Ethiopia.

16. Sertse T, Wossene A (2007) A study on ectoparasites of sheep and goats in eastern part of Amhara region, northeast Ethiopia. Small Ruminant Res 69: 62-67.

17. Sertse T, Wossene A (2007) Effect of ectoparasites on quality of pickled skins and their impact on the tanning industries in Amhara regional state, Ethiopia. Small Ruminant Res 69: 55-61.

18. Hailu W (2010) Study on the prevalence of major ectoparasites of sheep and assess the major risk factors in Arsi zone of Oromia regional state and evaluate the *in vitro* and *in vivo* acaricidal efficacy of seven medicinal plants against lice in naturally infested sheep (Doctoral dissertation, MSc thesis, Addis ababa University, FVM).

19. TDAO (2006) Tiyo District Agricultural Office, Asella.

20. Teklehaimanot D, Gangwar SK (2011) Seroprevalence study of bovine brucellosis in Assela government dairy farm of Oromia regional state, Ethiopia. Int J Sci Nature 2: 692-697.

21. Geresu MA, Ameni G, Tuli G, Arenas A, Kassa GM (2016) Seropositivity and risk factors for Brucella in dairy cows in Asella and Bishoftu towns, Oromia Regional State, Ethiopia. Afr J Microbiol Res 10: 203-213.

22. Steele M (1996) Goats, The Tropical Agriculturalist Series, Macmillan, London, UK; CTA Education, Wageningen, The Netherlands.

23. Sheep E (2009) Goat Productivity Improvement Program (ESGPIP) Common defects of sheep and goat skins in Ethiopia and their causes. ESGPIP: Technical Bulletin 19: 1-14.

24. Thrusfield M (2007) Sample size determination. In: Veterinary Epidemiology. 3rd edn. Blackwell Science Limited, Oxford, UK, Pp: 185-189.

25. Taylor MA, Coop RL, Wall RL (1996) Veterinary Parasitology. 4th edn. Blackwell Science, Glasgow, Scotland.

26. Wall R, Shearer D (2001) Veterinary Ectoparasites: Biology, Pathology and Control. 2nd edn. Blackwell Science Ltd., UK.

27. Teshome W (2002) Study on skin diseases of small ruminant in sidama zone, Southern Ethiopia. DVM Thesis, Addis Ababa University, Debre Zeit.

28. Mulugeta Y (2008) A study on ectoparasites of small ruminants in selected sites of Tigray regional state and their impact on the tanning industry. Doctoral dissertation, MSc thesis, Faculty of Veterinary Medicine, Addis Ababa University, Debre Zeit, Ethiopia.

29. Mohammed Y, Ali H (2006) Prevalence of ectoparasites of sheep and goat flock in Urmia Subrub, Iran. Vet Parasit 76: 431-442.

30. Rahbari S, Nabian S, Bahonar AR (2009) Some observations on sheep sarcoptic mange in Tehran province, Iran. Trop Anim Health Prod 41: 397-401.

31. Molu N (2002) Epidemiological study on skin disease of small ruminants. DVM Thesis, Faculty of Veterinary Medicine, Addis Ababa University, Debre Zeit, Ethiopia.

32. Takele G (1986) Epidemiological study of small ruminant mange mites in Harrarghe region. DVM Thesis, Faculty of Veterinary Medicine, Addis Ababa University, Debre Zeit, Ethiopia.

33. Zeryehun T, Tadesse M (2012) Prevalence of mange mite on small Ruminants at Nekemte veterinary clinic, East wollega zone, Northwest Ethiopia. Middle East J Sci Res 11: 1411-1416.

34. Mekonnen S, Hussein I, Bedane B (2001) The distribution of ixodid ticks (Acari: Ixodidae) in central Ethiopia. The Onderstepoort J Vet Res 68: 243-251.

35. Mekonnen S, Pegram RG, Gebre S, Mekonnen A, Jobre Y, et al. (2007) A synthesis of ixodid (Acari: Ixodidae) and argasid (Acari: Argasidae) ticks in Ethiopian and their possible roles in disease transmission. Ethiopian Vet J 11: 1-17.

36. Haffize M (2001) Study on skin diseases of small ruminants in central Ethiopia. DVM Thesis, Addis Ababa University, Debre Zeit, Ethiopia.

37. Chalachew N (2001) Study on the skin diseases in cattle, sheep and goats in and around Wolayta Soddo, Southern Ethiopia. DVM Thesis, Addis Ababa University, Facul. Vet. Med. Debre Zeit, Ethiopia.

38. Tefera S (2004) Investigation on ectoparasites in small ruminant in selected sites of Amhara regional state and their impact on the tanning industry. MSc Thesis, Faculty of Veterinary Medicine, Addis Ababa University, Debre Zeit, Ethiopia.

39. Israel Y, Abera T, Wakayo BU (2015) Epidemiological study on ectoparasite infestation of small ruminants in Sodo Zuria District, Southern Ethiopia. J Vet Med Anim Health 7: 140-144.

40. Sheferaw D, Degefu H, Banteyirgu D (2010) Epidemiological study of small

ruminant mange mites in three agro-ecological zones of Wolaita, Southern Ethiopia. Ethiopian Vet J 14: 31-38.

41. Numery A (2001) Prevalence and effect of ectoparasites in goats and fresh goat pelts and assessment of wet-blue skin defects at Kombolcha Tannery, South Wollo. DVM Thesis, Addis Ababa University, Debre Zeit.

42. Mullen GR, Durden LA (1995) Medical and Veterinary entomology. 2nd edn. CAB International, USA, Pp: 387-420.

43. Shibeshi B, Bogale B, Chanie M (2013) Ectoparasite of Small Ruminants in

Guto-Gidda District, East Wollega, Western Ethiopia. Acta Parasitologica Globalis 4: 86-91.

44. Kassayeq E, Kebede E (2010) Epidemiological study on manage mite, lice and sheep keds of small ruminants in tigray region, northern Ethiopia. Ethiopian Vet J 14: 51-66.

45. Radostits OM, Gay CC, Hinchcliff KW, Constable PD (2007) Veterinary Medicine: A text book of diseases of cattle, sheep, pigs, goats and horses. 10th edn. Saunders, Edinburgh, London. pp: 1585-1612.

8

Magnetic Resonance Imaging and Histological Findings of Paranasal Sinus Tumors and Surgical Outcomes in Dogs and Cats

Pinar Can[1], Sevil Atalay Vural[2], Murat Caliskan[1], Irem Gul Sancak[1]*, Arda Selin Coskan[2], Cisel Yazgan[3] and Omer Besalti[1]

[1]Department of Surgery, Faculty of Veterinary Medicine, Ankara University, Ankara, Turkey
[2]Department of Pathology, Faculty of Veterinary Medicine, Ankara University, Ankara, Turkey
[3]Department of Radiology, Faculty of Medicine, Hacettepe University, Ankara, Turkey

Abstract

Objective of this study was to report Magnetic resonance imaging (MRI) features of histologically confirmed paranasal sinus tumors and surgical outcomes. Totally 17 dogs and 3 cats were included in the study. Medical records of dogs and cats which were presented between January 2008 and November 2015 due to paranasal sinus tumors were reviewed. Dogs and cats were included if they have full clinical findings, diagnosed by MRI, confirmed histologically, and treated just surgically. Collected data for sex, breed, age, tumor stage, localisation, surgical outcomes, histological diagnosis, survival time and cause of death were included. Soft tissue mass within the nasal cavity replacing the nasal conchae and/or ethmoturbinates and mass invading to the frontal sinuses were determined in 80% (n=16) of the cases in MRI. Nasal and/or frontal bones were destructed in 65% (n=13) of the cases. In 7 dogs bone flap was created to expose and remove the tumor, and the flap was replaced wired after operation. In 10 dogs and 3 cats frontal and/or nasal bone was involved by the tumor, and closure of the defects was carried out with PMMA and wire. In this case series 50% of the tumors were sarcomas, and it was followed by adenocarcinoma (20%) and neuroesthesioblastoma (15%) in decreased rates. Dedicated MRI examination is crucial for diagnosis of paranasal sinus tumors, and surgical intervention as sole treatments looks acceptable for providing better quality of life for certain time.

Keywords: Cat; Dog; MRI; Paranasal sinus tumour

Introduction

Tumors of nasal cavity and paranasal sinuses in dogs comprise approximately 1-2% of all canine neoplasia and most of them are malignant, and have poor prognosis [1-3]. Also feline nasal and paranasal tumors are rare, approximately 1% of all feline tumors reported [4]. These tumors have a slow rate distant metastases, but they are locally invasive to bone and cartilage. Most of the nasal tumors in dogs occure in the caudal two-thirds of the nasal cavities and generally extend into frontal and paranasal sinuses. Epitelial tumors which are different type of carcinomas constitute 51 to 75% of nasal tumors. The remaining tumors mostly originate from connective tissue, cartilage or bone [5-8]. Dolichocephalic and mesocephalic breeds are more prone to nasal tumors [1].

Mucopurulent or hemorrhagic nasal discharge, epistaxis, nasal dyspnea, sneezing, epiphora, facial deformity and exophthalmos are the general symptoms of the nasal tumors. In addition to these sypmtoms if the tumor extends to the brain, neurologic signs may occur. Altered mentation, seizure and behavioral changes are the most common symptoms due to tumor invasion to the brain [9].

Diagnostic approach to paranasal tumors directed with history, physical and clinical examination, radiography, Computed Tomography (CT), MRI, rhinoscopy, cytology and histology [10-12]. CT is advantageous in detecting bone destruction and soft tissue involvement. MRI has advanced soft tissue contrast, multiplanar imaging capacity, and lack of radiation and bone beam-hardening artefact [13].

Therapy is based upon local disease control, and it involves surgery [14], chemotherapy [15], radiation therapy [3,16] and immunotherapy, or combination [9,17]. Although surgical approach to those tumors is not suggested by some authors, it still retains its place in selected cases [14]. The objective of this study is to report the clinical, MRI, histopathological findings and surgical outcomes of the paranasal sinus tumors of dogs and cats.

Materials and Methods

Animals

Medical records of dogs and cats which were presented to Ankara University Faculty of Veterinary Medicine Department of Surgery Clinic between January 2008 and December 2015 due to nasal and paranasal sinus tumors were reviewed. Dogs and cats were included if they have clinical examination findings, diagnosed by MRI, confirmed histologically, and treated with surgery as sole treatment, and the patients which were treated by combination of chemotherapy or radiotherapy with surgery were excluded. Records of the cases were reviewed for sex, breed, age, tumor stage, localisation, surgical outcomes histological diagnosis, survival time and cause of death.

Diagnostic imaging

MR scan was performed for each animal under general anesthesia which was achieved by medetomidine 80 µg/kg iv and ketamine HCl 5 mg/kg iv with a 1.5 Tesla MRI unit (Vision plus, Siemens, Erlangen, Germany). T1-weighted, T2-weighted and contrast-enhanced T1-weighted images of the nasal cavities and paranasal sinuses (Figure 1) were acquired in the dorsal, transverse and sagittal planes. Gadolinium diethylen-etriaminepentaacetic acid (Magnevist, Bayer, Germany) was

*Corresponding author: İrem Gul Sancak, Associate Professor, Department of Surgery, Faculty of Veterinary Medicine, Ankara University, Ankara, Turkey
E-mail: Iremgulsancak@gmail.com

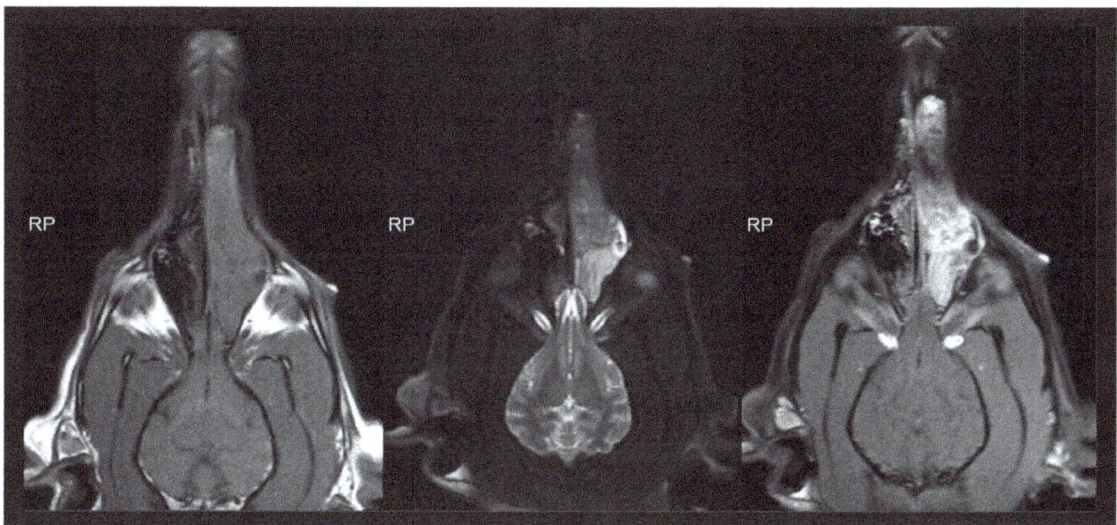

Figure 1: MRI features of the case 11. Dorsal T1-weighted and T2-weighted images of the nasal cavities show unilateral mass filling nasal cavity. T1-weighted postgadolinium images show extensive enhancement of tumor tissue. There is no any contrast enhancement in the brain suggesting with intracranial invasion.

used as the paramagnetic contrast medium, and was administered (dose: 0.2 mmol/kg) intravenously. All images were evaluated by board certified human radiologist and surgeons.

Tumor stage was determined based on the Modified World Health Organization Staging protocol by the evaluation of the MRI features. Dogs and cats were grouped into four clinical stages; T1-Confined to one nasal passage or paranasal sinus, with no bony involvement, T2 -Bony involvement, without evidence of orbital, subcutaneous, or submucosal mass, T3-Presence of orbital, subcutaneous, or submucosal mass, and T4-Tumor extension into nasopharynx or through cribriform plate. Tumors were also classified by location, on the basis of previously reported [13], into site 1 (unilateral nasal), 2 (unilateral nasal and sinus) and 3 (bilateral nasal). Staging and location of the tumors were based on the MRI images in three planes.

Clinical examination of the regional lenf nodes and chest X-ray were performed in order to assess metastasis before surgery. Surgery: Anesthesia was induced with propofol (Propofol, 10 mg/ml, Fresenius Kabi, Ltd., Sweden) and maintained with isoflurane-oxygen (Forane, Abbott Laboratories Ltd, Ireland). Perioperative analgesia was provided out using 0.5 mg/kg morphine-HCL (Morphine HCL, Galen, Turkey) in dogs and 0.1 mg/kg in cats. Tumor ablation was performed via dorsal approach under aseptic conditions. In the cases which frontal and nasal bones were involved by the tumor, the bone was removed totally and repaired by PMMA (polymetilmetacrilate) and wire (Figure 2). However in the cases which the frontal and nasal bone were not involved, a rectangle shaped frontonasal or nasal osteotomi was performed and tumor removed gross totally, then created nasal bone flap replaced and fixed with wire. Before replacing bone flap a gauze drain which rifampicine and bupivacain HCl-impregnated was placed into the nasal cavity. If the orbita was included in the tumor, it was extirpated. Postoperative analgesia was achieved with fentany patch (Duragesic® Janssen Pharmaceutica, Titusville, NJ; Cats and small dogs <10 kg: 25 µg/hr, Dogs 10-20 kg: 50 µg/hr, Dogs 20-30 kg: 75 µg/hr Dogs >30 kg: 100 µg/hr). Carprofen (Rimadyl, Pfizer, 3 mg/kg orally once daily) is used postoperatively for 7 days and antibiotherapy is maintained with amoxiciline (20 mg/kg orally twice daily) and metronidasole (20 mg/kg orally twice daily) for 10 days postoperatively.

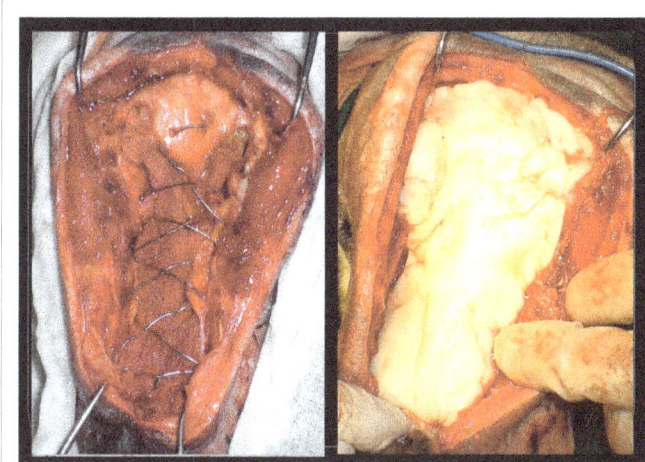

Figure 2: Repair of the bone defect with PMMA and wire (Case no. 1).

Collected samples of each mass were fixed 10% buffered formalin embedded in parafine and cut 5 µm-thick sections. All sections were stained according to Hematoxilen-Eosin (H&E).

Outcome assessment

The owner satisfaction and post operative survival time and cause of death (cardiac arrest during operation, euthanasia due to the tumor recurrence or infection and unrelated reasons) were recorded. Survival time was calculated due to the last day recieved report from the owner.

Statistical analysis

Mean survival time of the dogs was calculated due to Kaplan Meier Analysis, it wasn't calculated for cats because of the low case number. For data analysis, animals lost to followup and still alive were censored at their last known survival time. Dogs died during operation were not taken into account in estimating mean survival time.

Results

Twenty patients (17 dogs and 3 cats) have matched the inclusion criteria. Sex distribution was 14 males (12 intact, 2 castrated) and 3 females (1 intact, 2 spayed) for dogs, 2 males (intact) and 1 female (intact) for cats. The mean age of dogs was 8.67 (range 1.5 to 16 years) years. Mix breed dogs were most commonly represented 5/17 (% 29.41) and all the cats were domestic short hair (DSH). In cats mean age were 9.66 years. Distribution of sex, breed, age, tumor stage, localisation, MRI findings, histologic diaognosis, survival time and cause of death are listed in Table 1.

Most common clinical complaint was mucopurulent or nasal discharge (n=14), following with facial deformity (n=10), sneezing (n=7), epiphora (n=7), nasal dyspne (n=6), neurologic signs including circling and/or seizure (n=5), epistaxis (n=3) and exophtalmus (n=3) were observed. In three cases only chief complainment was neurologic signs (Case no 5, 6 and 7).

Imaging findings

On MR images, soft tissue mass within the nasal cavity replacing the nasal conchae and/or ethmoturbinates and mass invading to the frontal sinuses were determined in 80% (n=16) of the cases. Nasal and/

or frontal bones were destructed in 65% (n=13) of the cases. Retained secretions with or without mass lesion caudally in frontal sinuses were characteristic with a hyperintensity as like the fluids on T2-weighted images, and seen in 75% of the cases. Though meningeal hyperintensity on T2-weighted images around one or both olfactory bulbs was detected in 8 cases (40%), extension of mass into the cranial cavity affecting the brain was observed in 6 of these cases (30%). Both cases with meningeal hyperintensity and tumor extension to the brain were admitted obtundation, seizure, circling and some abnormal behavior. Detailed MRI findings were summarized on Table 2.

Frontal and nasal bones were intact in 7 dogs (Case no 2, 4, 6, 11, 14, 15, 16), in this context bone flap was created to expose and remove the tumor, and in these cases for the closure of the bone defect that occure due to the rhinotomy were closed by the replacing and wiring the flap. Rest of the cases (10 dogs and 3 cats) frontal and/or nasal bone was involved by the tumor, and closure of the defects were carried out with PMMA and wire. PMMA was well tolerated all the cases except for one case chondrosarcoma (Case no: 9) in which fistula was occured at 6th month, and tumor reoccured and displaced the PMMA. This case

	Case	Breed	Age (years)	Sex	Stage	MRI T1W	MRI T2W	MRI Gd	Site	Histopathology	Survival	Cause of death
Dogs	1	Siberian Husky	1.5	F	T4	iso	hyper	++ H	3	neuroesthesiablastoma	11 m	Euth.
	2	Mix	13	MC	T4	iso	hyper	++ H	2	neuroesthesiablastoma	7 m	Euth.
	3	Rottweiler	4	M	T2	Hyper mild	hyper	++ Ht	3	Squamous cell carcinoma	1 m	Euth.
	4	Kangal	4	M	T2	hypo	hyper	++ H	2	chondrosarcoma	9,5 m	unrelated
	5	English Setter	14	M	T4	Hyper mild	Hyper mild	++ H	2	Squamous cell carcinoma	-	Died during op.
	6	Kangal	6	M	T4	iso	hyper	++ H	2	Neuroestesiablastoma	2 m	Euth.
	7	Mix	11	M	T4	iso	Hyper mild	++ H	2	Meningioma	8 m	Loss of follow up
	8	Labrador	6	M	T3	hyper	hyper	++ H	3	osteosarcoma	-	Euthanasia during op.
	9	Mix	11	M	T2	hyper	hyper	+ H	3	Chondrosarcoma	19 m	Euth.
	10	Mix	11	M	T3	iso	hyper	+ H	2	osteosarcoma	4 m	Euth.
	11	Golden Retriever	10	M	T1	hyper	Hyper mild	++ H	3	chondrosarcoma	6 m	Euth.
	12	Maltese Terrier	16	M	T4	hyper	hyper	++ H	3	adenocarcinoma	1 m	Euth.
	13	Mix	6	M	T3	iso	hyper	+ H	3	Osteosarcoma	3 m	Euth.
	14	Rottweiler	12	MC	T2	hyper	Hyper mild	+ H	2	chondrosarcoma	9 m	unrelated
	15	English Setter	5	FS	T1	iso	hyper	++ H	3	adenocarcinoma	10 m	still living
	16	Cocker	7	FS	T1	iso	hyper	++ H	1	adenocarcinoma	5 m	Still living
	17	Golden Retriever	10	M	T4	iso	hyper	++ H	2	fibrosarcoma	2 m	Still living
Cats	18	Domestic short hair	11	F	T3	iso	hyper	++ Ht	2	Cystic ductal adenocarcinoma	1 m	Loss of folllow up
	19	Domestic short hair	9	M	T3	iso	hyper	++ H	2	osteosarcoma	2 m	Loss of follow up
	20	Domestic short hair	9	M	T2	iso	hyper	++ Ht	3	angiosarcoma and polip	2 y	unrelated

Table 1: Detailed information of the all cases.

MRI features of the cases	Number/Percent of all cases
Soft tissue mass within the nasal cavity replacing the nasal conchae and/or ethmoturbinates	16/80.0
Destruction of nasal septum (predominantly middle portion)	10/50.0
Mass invading the maxillary recesses (predominantly unilateral)	8/40.0
Mass extending into the nasal caudal recesses (predominantly unilateral)	9/45.0
Retained secretions with or without mass lesion caudally in frontal sinuses	15/75.0
Mass invading to the frontal sinuses	15/75.0
Destruction of the nasal/frontal bones	13/65.0
Destruction of the cribriform plate	7/35.0
Extension of mass into the cranial cavity (not necessarily through the cribriform plate) affecting the brain	6/30.0
Meningeal (dural) hyperintensity on T2-weighted around one or both olfactory bulbs (predominantly unilateral and on the side of the mass)	8/40.0

Table 2: MRI findings of all cases.

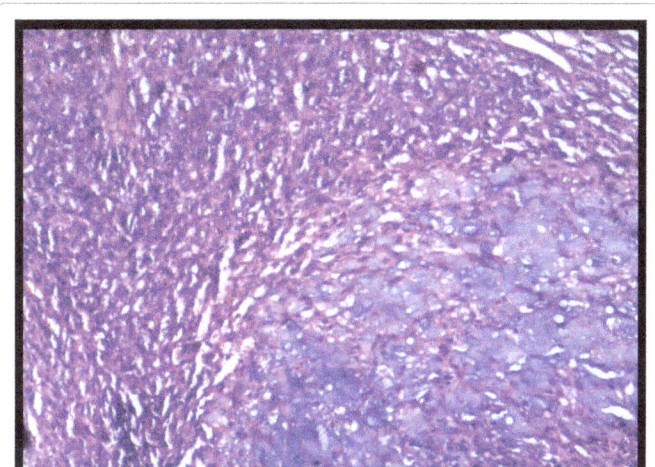

Figure 3: In differentiated round and/or spindle cartilage cells and condroid matrix, chondrosarcoma, HE, X100.

was reoperated, and survived for 19 months, and euthanaised due to owner request because of second time recurrence except 4 cases (Case no 3, 6, 12, 18) clinical complaints were roughly solved on 15 to 20 days after surgery. In four cases clinical complaints were not solved until one month postoperatively, which might be because of the tumor reoccurence, but further diagnostic workup was declined by the owner and animals were euthanaised.

Four chondrosarcoma (Figure 3), 4 osteosarcoma (3 dogs, 1 cat), 3 neuroesthesiablastoma, 1 cystic ductal adenocarcinoma (cat), 1 angiosarcoma and polip (cat), 2 squamous cell carcinoma, 1 meningioma, 1 fibrosarcoma and 3 adenocarcinoma were diagnosed histopathologically.

Mean survival time for dogs was found 7.95 ± 1.74 (95% confidence interval: 4.53-11.37). Estimated probabilty of survival was 78.6% at the 2nd month and it decreased to 38.6% at the 9th month postoperatively. Only 2 patients died spontaneously, rest of euthanized cases was performed over the request of owners.

Cause of death was euthanasia in 10 of the all cases due to tumor recurrence (n=8) and infection (n=1) and inability to remove tumor because of its more invasiveness (n=1). Three cases died with unrelated causes, and cardiac arrest was happened during operation in 1 cases. The cause of the death was unclear in 3 case because of lost to follow up (Case no: 7, 18, 19) and 3 of the cases are still alive.

Discussion

Characteristic MRI findings of paranasal sinus tumors and especially signs of affecting the frontal lobe of brain and histological findings according to WHO were represented in this case series. Surgical removal of paranasal tumor and repairement of created bone defect with PMMA and bone flap was found reliable and they were well tolerated by the dogs.

The mean age of the reported cases is similar with previous studies, which have reported a mean age of onset of nine to 10 years [5,8,14]. The prognosis for paranasal tumors without any treatment is poor and euthanasia is chosen in most animals as a result of progressive local invasion of tumor and related problems within three to six months of the onset of clinical signs [18]. The poor response of dogs with paranasal tumors to surgery is due to the advanced nature of most tumors at the time of diagnosis a propensity for this tumor to invade

bones that are inaccessible or that can not be surgically removed, and lack of appreciable encapsulation; each of which makes it impossible to completely remove tumors [19]. Even though surgery is not recommended as a sole therapy, but it can be an option in selected cases like mesenchymal tumors and collecting biopsy specimens, and it can be accepted as an option for increasing the quality of life, not just for increasing survival time [14]. Most of the patients suffer from sneezing, nasal discharge, epistaxis and nasal dyspne, after surgery clinical signs in some dogs paliated by alleviating obstruction and epistaxis. The clinical signs in the presented 16 cases were solved after operation and this can suggest the usefulness of surgery for a certain time. Restoration of bone defect with PMMA and wire are well tolerated in this case series. PMMA was found as a suitable material to repair the bone defect after nasal and/or frontal osteotomy which is necessary for radical removal of the diseased tissues in most of the cases presented in this study.

Mean survival time for the present study was counted 7.95 months and same as compared to the previous study [14]. The presented cases in this study had minimaly 3 to 5 months history of clinical complaining and were treated before presentation to our clinic medically, and also 60% of the dogs were stage 3-4. In addition, obscured time of beginning clinical signs may have caused the lower mean survival time.

Mucoprulent/haemoragic nasal discharge, facial deformity and sneezing were reported previously as most common clinical signs [1,20,21]. These signs were the main clinical complainments in the presented cases, but also in 5 patients neurological signs were recorded and extension of the mass into the cranial cavity is detected all these patients. Although extension of mass into the cranial cavity was identified in six cases by the MRI, five of these cases showed neurologic signs. Hyperintense lesions in the brain were also seen in cases the tumors were extended to the caudal nasal recess. Those findings represent the diagnostic power of MRI in paranasal sinus. MRI has an excellent soft tissue resolution, on the other hand CT is a valuable diagnostic tool for identifying bone destruction, and combined with rhinoscopy was reported as sensitive diagnostic approach [12,20]. In this study, nasal septum destruction and nasal and/or frontal bone destruction were identified in 10 and 13 patients respectively by MRI features; these findings were also confirmed by the operation. These findings represent that MRI is a very convenient diagnostic modality of choice in evaluating of nasal and paranasal sinus tumors even the bone structures involved in tumor and can lead the surgeon. However, in one with osteosarcoma, the margins and invasiveness of the tumor were worse than MRI findings, and he was euthenaised after the owner permision during the surgery. In addition to MRI, CT can be considered in cases with osteosarcoma for being sure about the tumor margins and it will provide valuable informations in deciding surgical treatments.

Conclusion

In conclusion, reconstruction of the bone defect with PMMA and wire in the cases which the nasal and/or frontal bone is invaded by the tumor and unrepairable after the opration can be suggested. However, if is it possible creating bone flap to expose the tumor to remove and nasal and/or frontal bone is repairable, reconstruction with bone flap should be the approach of choice. MRI is an ideal diagnostic tool in the evaluating of paranasal sinus tumors extending to cranial cavity, and even in the cases with bony involvment.

References

1. Confer AW, DePaoli A (1978) Primary neoplasms of the nasal cavity, paranasal sinuses and nasopharynx in the dog: A report of 16 cases from the files of the AFIP. Vet Pathol 15: 18-30.

2. Malinowski C (2006) Canine and feline nasal neoplasia. Clin Tech Small Anim Pract 21: 89-94.

3. Elliot KM, Mayer MN (2009) Radiation therapy for tumors of the nasal cavity and paranasal sinuses in dogs. Can Vet J 50: 309-312.

4. Mukaratirwa S, van der Linde-Sipman JS, Gruys E (2001) Feline nasal and paranasal sinus tumours: clinicopathological study, histomorphological description and diagnostic immunohistochemistry of 123 cases. J Feline Med Surg 3: 235-245.

5. Madewell BR, Priester WA, Gillette EL, Snyder SP (1976) Neoplasms of the nasal passages and paranasal sinuses in domesticated animals as reported by 13 veterinary colleges. Am J Vet Res 37: 851-856.

6. MacEwen EG, Withrow SJ, Patnaik AK (1977) Nasal tumors in the dog: retrospective evaluation of diagnosis, prognosis, and treatment. J Am Vet Med Assoc 170: 45-48.

7. Patnaik AK (1989) Canine sinonasal neoplasms: clinicopathological study of 285 cases. J Am Anim Hosp Assoc 25: 103-114.

8. Morris JS, Dunn KJ, Dobson JM, White RA (1996) Radiological assessment of severity of canine nasal tumours and relationship with survival. J Small Anim Pract 37: 1-6.

9. Forrest LJ (2009) Nasal tumors. Kirk's Current Veterinary Therapy XIV. 14th edn. Bonagura JD, Twedt DC (Editors). W.B Saunders Company, St. Louis, Missouri, USA.

10. Sullivan M, Lee R, Skae CA (1987) The radiological features of sixty cases of intra-nasal neoplasia in the dog. J Small Anim Pract 28: 575-586.

11. Ogilvie GK, LaRue SM (1992) Canine and feline nasal and paranasal sinus tumours. Vet Clin North Am Small Anim Pract 22: 1133-1144.

12. Auler Fde A, Torres LN, Pinto AC, Unruh SM, Matera JM, et al. (2015) Tomography, Radiography, and Rhinoscopy in Diagnosis of Benign and Malignant Lesions Affecting the Nasal Cavity and Paranasal Sinuses in Dogs: Comparative Study. Top Companion Anim Med 30: 39-42.

13. Ng SH, Chang TC, Ko SF, Yen PS, Wan YL, et al. (1997) Nasopharyngeal carcinoma: MRI and CT assessment. Neuroradiology 39: 741-746.

14. Laing EJ, Binnington AG (1988) Surgical therapy of canine nasal tumors: A retrospective study (1982-1986). Can Vet J 29: 809-813.

15. Hahn KA, Knapp DW, Richardson RC, Matlock CL (1992) Clinical response of nasal adenocarcinoma to cisplatin chemotherapy in 11 dogs. J Am Vet Med Assoc 200: 355-357.

16. Adams WM, Miller PE, Vail DM, Forrest LJ, MacEwen EG (1998) An accelerated technique for irradiation of malignant canine nasal and paranasal sinus tumors. Vet Radiol Ultrasound 39: 475-481.

17. Lana SE, Dernell WS, LaRue SM, Lafferty MJ, Douple EB, et al. (1997) Slow release cisplatin combined with radiation for the treatment of canine nasal tumors. Vet Radiol Ultrasound 38: 474-478.

18. Morris J, Dobson J (2001) Nasal cavity and paranasal sinuses. In: Small Animal Oncology. Blackwell Science Oxford, UK.

19. MacPhail CM (2012) Surgery of the upper respiratory system. In: Small Animal Surgery. 4th edn. Fossum TW (ed). Elsevier-Mosby Missouri, USA.

20. Avner A, Dobson JM, Sales JI, Herrtage ME (2008) Retrospective review of 50 canine nasal tumours evaluated by low-field magnetic resonance imaging. J Small Anim Pract 49: 233-239.

21. Kondo Y, Matsunaga S, Mochizuki M, Kadosawa T, Nakagawa T, et al. (2008) Prognosis of canine patients with nasal tumors according to modified clinical stages based on computed tomography: a retrospective study. J Vet Med Sci 70: 207-212.

9

Study on the Prevalance of Gastrointestinal Helminthes Infection in Equines in and around Kombolcha

Wondwossen Belay, Daniel Teshome* and Abebaw Abiye

School of Veterinary Medicine, Wollo University, Amhara, Ethiopia

Abstract

A cross sectional study was conducted from October 2013 to April 2014 in and around Kombolcha town to estimate the prevalence of gastro intestinal tract helminthes infection and to identify the common GIT helminthes parasites of equines. Gross examination, direct fecal smear, sedimentation and floatation techniques were utilized to identify the eggs of parasites in feces. A total of 384 horses, mules and donkeys were examined for gastrointestinal parasites. The overall prevalence of gastrointestinal parasites was 73.2% (281 from 384) with 57.0% (73 from 128), 82.5% (160 from 194) and 77.4% (48 from 62) in horses, donkeys and mules respectively. Prevalence of *Strongyle* spp, *Parascaris equorum, Oxyuris equi* and *Anoplocephala* spp was 44.5%, 3.1%, 2.3%, and 3.1% respectively in horses. Prevalence of gastrointestinal parasites was 63.4%, 8.6%, 2.1% and 3.1% for *Strongyle* spp, *Parascaris equorum, Oxyuris equi* and *Anoplocephala* spp in donkeys, respectively and the prevalence of GIT parasites was 48.4%, 12.9%, 3.2% and 6.5% for *Strongyle* spp, *Parascaris equorum, Oxyuris equi* and *Anoplocephala* spp in mules respectively. There was statistically significant difference between species, age, and body condition and among different management systems in prevalence of equine gastrointestinal parasites (p<0.05). However, there was no statistically significant difference in prevalence of gastrointestinal parasites based on sex. In conclusion, the present study revealed higher prevalence of gastrointestinal parasites in equines. Therefore, regular deworming, improvement of housing and feeding management were recommended.

Keywords: Mules; Donkeys; Kombolcha; Gastrointestinal parasites; Horse; Prevalence

Introduction

Ethiopia is a country with huge livestock population from Africa. The livestock population in the country is estimated to be 40.9 million head of cattle, 25.5 million head of sheep, 23.4 million head of goats, 2.7 million of horses, 5 million of donkeys, and 0.63 million mules [1]. There are an estimated 110 million equines (horses, donkeys and mules) in the developing world [2] where they provide an essential service. They are widely used as resource for traction and under saddle as a means of transport due to economic and /or topographical constraints on motorized alternatives [3].

In developing countries like Ethiopia, the contribution of equines in the energy scenario is of considerable significance as power source, for transportation, cultivation and post harvest activities in places where the road network is insufficiently developed [4]. Equines play a vital role both in economics as well as in social functions. They are kept and often used for land tillage, cultivation, and threshing as well as for pack purposes, riding, providing of manure for both energy and soil fertility [5]. In Ethiopia context especially in the marginal land of the country, equines are good vehicle and the main means of transport [6]. However, the contribution of equine power in the agriculture systems and the role in the production is not yet well organized and magnified [7].

Though equines play an indispensable role to the economy of nation, the treatment accorded to these species of animals has been far below that given to other species of animals. This can partly be due to the age- old erroneous concept that these species are hardly tolerant, and probably because they are not providers of meat and milk. The effective use of equine is moreover, constrained by absence of equine promotion program and policies practically in all developing countries [8].

As any other animal, equines are also vulnerable to a variety of diseases of biological origin, nutritional diseases or disorders and miscellaneous causes. Among the most common entities leading to ill-health, suffering and early demise and finally death are infectious diseases and parasitism, which resulted inconsiderably reduced animals work out put, reproductive performance and most of all their longevity [4].

Of the diseases that cause serious problems, parasitism represents a major impact on equine production in the tropics. Equine harbor a large quantity of parasites that prevail in the GIT which act up and damage the intestine depending on the age and natural defense of the individual equine [9].

Parasitic helminthes are one of the most common factors that constrain the health and working performance of donkeys, horses and mules worldwide. They cause various degrees of damage depending on the species and number present, nutritional and the immune status of equines [10].

Helminthosis is of considerable significance in the wide range of agro climatic zones in sub Saharan Africa and constitutes one of the most important constraints to working equines [11]. The most common internal parasites are small and large *Strongyle* spp, *Ascarids (Parascaris equorum)*, pin worms *(Oxyuris equi)*, and tape worms *(Anoplocephala* spp) [12].

The prevalence and type of internal parasites affecting equines, in general, have not been determined to great extent in Ethiopia. Available

*Corresponding author: Daniel Teshome, Lecturer and Researcher, Veterinary Medicine, Wollo University, Alimuhdine Street, Dessie, Amhara 1145, Ethiopia
E-mail: dteshome11@gmail.com

information however, indicated that gastro intestinal parasites are the major causes of every demises of working equines in Ethiopia [13].

Among the many disease problems affecting equines, Gastro Intestinal Tract (GIT) parasites are serious health hazards contributing to poor production performance and short life span. These parasites shares with equines digestible nutrients and cause inflammation and petechial hemorrhages as a result of adherence and penetration of mucus of GIT [14]. Gastrointestinal helminthes parasites infection is a major militating factor against profitable animal production over the world [15].

Despite the huge number of equine populations and their uncountable economic contribution, the attempt which has been made to improve the management aspect of these hard working animals is very much limited which is left to the mercy of nature particularly in the SWZARDO where there is huge equine population. Among the many problems, information regarding GIT parasites of equines is lacking. Therefore the study of equines GIT helminthes infection was carried out in the south wollo zone where there is large number of equine population with the following objectives:

- To estimate the prevalence of gastro intestinal tract helminthes infection in equine.

- To study risk factors involved in equine GIT helminthes infection in the south wollo zone of Amara national regional state

- To identify the common GIT helminthes parasites of equines

Literature Review

Major gastro intestinal helminthes parasites

Among the diseases affecting equines, helminthes infections are much extended. These parasites continue to be a significant threat to the health of equines. The nature or extent of damage varies with the parasites. They cause loss of nutrients, blood and serious economic losses [16].

Gastro intestinal helminthes are among the most important parasitic diseases in veterinary medicine, not only in livestock, but also in all mammals and in other cause of vertebrates. They are caused by varies species of nematodes, cestodes, or tremotodes at different stages of development (i.e., larvae and adult) [17].

Nematode contains worms of parasitic significant and they are commonly called round worms from their appearance in cross section [18]. The common nematode GIT parasites of equines are *Parascaris equorum*, *Strongyloides westeri*, *Oxyuris equi*, *Habronema muscae*, *Habronema majus* and *Draschia magastoma*, *Tricho strongylus axaie* and large and small *Strongyle* spp [19].

The cestode differs from the trematodes in having a tape like body with no alimentary canal. The body is segmented and each segmented containing one and sometimes two sets of male and female reproductive organs [20]. Trematodes are small helminthes having leaf shaped body and at its anterior end there is an oral sucker, at the ventral side there are ventral suckers which serves as organs attachment [21]. Equine GIT cestodes are *Anoplocephala magna*, *Anoplocephala perfoliata*, and *Paranoplocephala mamillana* [22].

Strongylosis

Etiology: Members of the genus *Strongylus* live in the large intestine of horses and donkeys and, with *Ttriodontophorous*, are commonly known as the large *Strongyles* [22].

Horses asses, and mules host a far greater variety of *Strongylid* parasites than ruminants and other domestic animals do. Even an apparently healthy horse may be infected with tens or even hundreds of thousands of small *Strongyle* worms (cyathostominae) [23]. The *Strongylus* species found in equines are *S. vulgaris*, *S. edentatus* and *S. equinus* [20].

Morphology and identification: *Strongylus* parasites are robust dark red worms which are easily seen against the intestinal mucosa. The well developed buccal capsule of the adult parasite is prominent, as is the bursa of the male. Male are 2.3-2.8 cm in size and females 3.3-4.4 cm and the head end is wider than the rest of the body. Male are 2.6-3.5 cm in size and females 3.8-4.7 cm and the head end is not marked off from the rest of the body and Male are 14-16 mm in size and females 20-24 mm and the head end is not marked off from the rest of the body are atypical features of *S. dentatus S. equinus* and *S. vulgaris* respectively [22]. Species identification is based on size and the presence and shape of the teeth in the base of bucal capsule. *S. vulgaris* has two ear shaped, rounded teeth and *S. equinus* posses three conical teeth, one is situated dorsally and is larger than the others. Whereas *S. edentatus* has no teeth [20] (Figure 1).

Life cycle: The life cycle of the equine *Strongylids* is direct and does not involve an intermediate host. It alternates between an exogeneous phase of free living stages present in the external environment and an endogenous phase of parasitic stages that develop in the host [17]. Eggs passed in faces are hatched in the environment and development to the infective larvae is take place. The larvae migrate up the blades of grass until ingested by horses. Infection is by ingestion of the L_3 and it migrates to the intestine then to mesenteric arteries and liver where they grow and molt to L_4 then migrates to the large intestine and molt to L_5 then the adult worm resides in the intestinal mucosa [18].

Epidemiology: Equine *Strongyle* spp infections occur specifically in domestic equines, i.e., horses, donkeys and their hybrids, but they are also frequently found in large numbers in zebras. The host is important terms of susceptibility to disease with the horse being the most susceptible to infection and disease especially through bred horses [17].

Strongylosis is a common disease of horses throughout the world and causes deaths when control measures are neglected. In areas with cold winters and mild summers, egg deposition peaks in spring and remains high over summer. At this time, temperatures are suitable for larval development and massive infective larvae may occur in late summer and early autumn, when young susceptible horses are present [24].

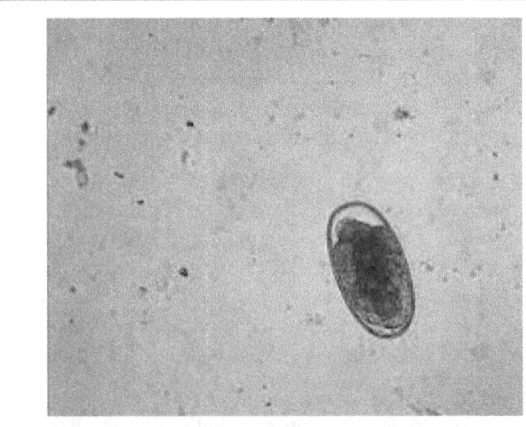

Figure 1: Morphology of strongyle egg.

Strongylosis is most frequently a problem of in young horse pastures, although cases of sever disease may occur in adult animals kept in sub urban paddocks and subjected to overcrowding and poor management [20].

Pathogenesis: The disease processes associated with the *Strongylus* can be divided in to those produced by migrating larvae, those provoked by the mass emergency of mucosal larvae and these associated adult worms. Heavy intestinal infection can alter intestinal motility, intestinal permeability and carbohydrate absorption [14]. The larvae of *S. vulgaris* are the most pathogenic, causing arthritis, thrombosis and thickening of the wall of the cranial mesenteric artery. Emboli may break away and lodge in smaller blood vessels, leading to partial or complete ischemia in part of the intestine, thus producing colic. The result of this depends on the length of the segment of the intestine affected and the ability of the collateral blood supply to become established before necrosis and gangrene occur [22]. The disease is due to migrating *S. vulgaris* larvae that are responsible for verminous arthritis. In case of massive infection, the clinical picture is severe with rapid weight loss; liquid diarrhea and frequent bouts of sever colic [17].

Clinical finding: The clinical picture varies in line with the intensity of parasite burden, the prevalence of certain parasitic species, and to the stage of development of the worms. Moderate infections due to larvae stages or adult worms result in sub clinical or chronic diseases with general clinical signs among which weight loss is the most common [17]. grazing horses usually carry a mixed burden of large and small *Strongyles* and the major signs associated with heavy infection in animals up to 2-3 years of age are unthriftness, anemia colic and sometimes diarrhea [18]. Marked clinical signs are less common in older animals although general performance may be impaired [20]. The effect of *Strongyle* spp in more chronic infestation results persistent low grade fever, poor appetite, intermittent colic and poor weight gain [14].

Diagnosis: Diagnosis of mixed *Strongyle* spp infection is based on demonstration of eggs in the feces. *Strongyle* spp eggs are oval, and thin shelled and are most of them observed during standared fecal flotation of faeces [18]. A specific diagnosis is difficult to achieve in every case. Few clinical observations or laboratory results are pathognomic for the disease syndromes associated with *Strongyle* spp infection. Often a judgment has to be made on an overall appraisal of clinical history, presenting signs and laboratory finding [14].

The presumptive diagnosis of *Strongylosis* due to adult worms are appropriate in young animals after weaning and in case of poor body condition, intermittent colic and irregular bots diarrhea [17].

Treatment: Treatment may be targeted against immature and adult large strongly worms in the lumen of intestine, against migrating *Stronglyl* spp larvae particularly *S. vulgaris* or against cyathostomins larvae, in the intestine mucosa [14]. Antihelmentic, ivermectin and moxidectin at a standard dosage are effective against the larval stages (L_4 and L_5) of effective against larval infection. A number of antihelmentics including the bezimidazoles, pyrantel, and ivermectin, are active against adult large *Strongyle* spp [25].

Control and prevention: The goal for control of horse strongly infection is to minimized the number of eggs and resultant infective L_3 larvae on the grazing areas and there by prevent clinical and sub clinical disease. Environmental contamination by infective larvae is the main determinant to the infective parasite control [26]. The concept of preventing parasite contamination of the environment can be accomplished by eliminating egg shedding back into the environment by strategically timed deworming [20].

Regular treatment of all animals in any group of horses, starting from the weaners, are typically used to eliminate adult *Strongyle* spp and these prevent heavy contamination of pastures with eggs and infective L_3 larvae [17].

Ascariosis

Etiology: *P. equorum* is the equine *ascarid* under the family of *Ascaridea* and it is found in the small intestine of young foals [18]. It is very large rigid, stout, whitish nematode, up to 40 cm in length, cannot be confused with any other intestinal parasites of equines. Males measure 15-25 cm and females up to 40 cm [22].

Epidemiology: Infection with *P. equorum* is common through out the world and is a major cause of unthriftness in young falls. There are two important factors in the epidemiology of infection, first is the high fecundity of the adult female parasites and secondly, the extreme resistance of the egg in the environment ensures its persistence for several years. The thick nature of the outer shell may also facilitate passive spread of eggs [22]. The main route of infection is by ingestion of larvae eggs. Because the eggs have very thick walls and the infective stage is protected from deleterious environmental influences. Few disinfectants will harm them and they are very resistant to cold but survive most readily in cool, moist surroundings. The period of survival of up to 5 years have been recorded [14] (Figure 2).

Life cycle: The life cycle is direct and migratory involving a hepato-pulmonary route [18]. The adult worms live in the small intestine and lay very large numbers of thick- shelled eggs. These are not infective until a larvae has developed inside. This process needs suitable warmth and humidity and takes place over a period of several weeks. When swallowed, infective eggs hatch quickly in the intestine of the host and larvae migrate through the intestinal wall, reach the portal vein and are transported to the liver [14]. They cross to hepatic venous systems and travel to the lungs, are passed up to the bronchi and trachea to the pharynx, are swallowed and come to rest in the intestine when the mature [27].

Pathogenesis and clinical findings: Migration of larvae through the liver results in hemorrhage and fibrosis appearing as white spots under the capsule. In heavy infection diffuse fibrosis may occur. The most serious damage occurs in the lungs where the larvae provoke alveolar injury with edema and consolidation. This damage can exacerbate pre-existing lung infections or provide a portal of entry into the body for pyogenic organisms [14]. In heavy infection coughing and circulating eosinonophilia are features of the prepatent period. Adult worm cause catarrhal enteritis which produce diarrhea which may be fetid in odor and pale in color [27]. Heavy infection with *Parascaris equorum* also

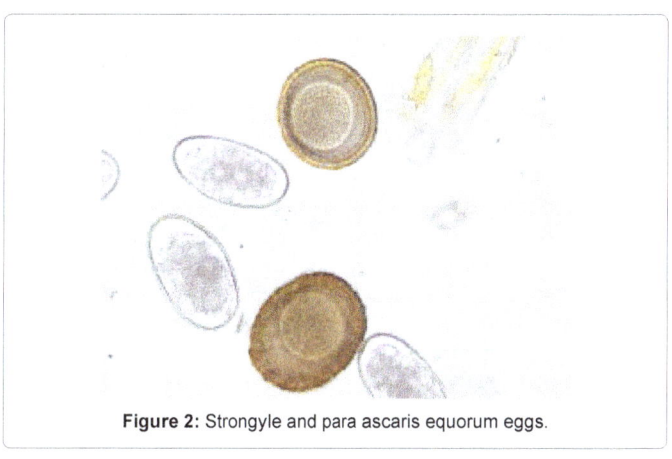

Figure 2: Strongyle and para ascaris equorum eggs.

results poor coat, diarrhea and occasionally colic. In addition in the foals, convulsions, intestinal obstruction and perforation may occur. Lung damage may give rise to fever, couphing and a muco-purulent nasal discharge and the migrating larvae may produce respiratory signs ("summer colds") as serious damage occurs to the lungs [25]. *Ascarid* infections may reduce rate of intestinal transit and heavy burdens can be associated with obstruction, intussusceptions or rarely perforation of the intestine [28].

Diagnosis: Diagnosis depends on clinical signs and the presence of spherical, thick, brownish rough shelled eggs on fecal examination. Sometimes atypical thick-walled eggs are seen that lack the dark outer shell [22]. *Ascarid* eggs are brown and have thick walls with appitted surface. These eggs measures 90-100 micrometers in diameter and the center of the eggs contain one or two cells and can be easily recovered on standard fecal flotation [18]. Migrating larvae are too small to be observed by the neck eye at post mortem examination. They can be recovered from macerated lung tissues by the barman's technique or seen microscopically in scraping of bronchial mucus [14].

Treatment: On farms where the infection is common, most foals become infected soon after birth. As a result, most of the worms are maturing when the foals are about 4-5 months old. Treatment should be started when foals are 8 weeks old and repeated at 6- to 8 week's intervals until they are yearlings. All broad-spectrum equine anthelmintics are effective against the adult and immature worms in the small intestine and, therefore, *Ascarids* are readily controlled by routine anthelmintic administration [25]. The most common anthelmintic administration includes benzimidazoles (such as fenbendazole, oxfendazole, oxibendazole), pyrantel, ivermectin and moxidectin are all effective against adult and larval stages when given orally [22].

Control and prevention: Important life cycle features which must be taken in to account when devising a control program for *Ascariosis* are the worms are prolific egg layers, the infective eggs are very resistant and long lived. Young animals are most susceptible; therefore emphasis must be place on preventing the environment from becoming contaminated. This is achieved by periodic treatment of animals likely to be shedding eggs-asymptomatic adult carriers as well as more vulnerable young stock. Exposure of foals to contaminated soil or bedding should be avoided [14]. Since transmission is largely on foal-to-foal basis it is good policy to avoid using the same paddocks for nursing mares and their foals in successive years [22].

Oxyuriodosis

Etiology: The cause of this disease is the nematodes of *O. equi* referred to *Oxyuidae* family. Adult's inhabitant large intestine and commonly called pinworms because of the pointed tail of the female parasite and the parasite has also a double bulb esophagus [29]. *Oxyuris equi* is a nematode that provokes irritation of the perianal region of horses, causing them to rub and bite their tails. This can result in the hair loss and sometimes physical damage to the tissue of the area. The parasite is ubiquitous but of greater prevalence in areas of high rainfall [14].

Morphology: *Oxyuris equi* occurs in the large intestine of equines in all parts of the world. The male is 9-12 mm long and the female up to 150 mm. The esophagus is narrow in the middle and the bulb is not distinctly marked off. The male has one pin shaped spicules which is 120-150 nm long and the tail bears two pairs of large and a few small papillae. The young females are almost grayish white in color, slightly curved and have relatively short -pointed tails [27]. *O. equi* L_4 are 5-10 mm in length, have tapering tails and are often attached orally to the intestinal mucosa [22] (Figure 3).

Life cycle: The male and young females inhabit the caecum and large colon. After fertilization the mature females wander down to the rectum and grawl out through the anal opening eggs are laid in the clusters on the skin on the perinea region. Development of the egg is rapid, reaching the infective stage in the 3-5 days [27]. Infection is by the ingestion of the infective stage on the fodder and bedding by the host. The infective eggs hatch in the intestine liberating the L_3, which reach large intestine where they penetrate the mucosa and molt in to the L_4 stage three to ten days after infection. L_4 larvae then emerge from the intestinal wall into the lumen and they attach to the intestinal mucosa where they feed from blood and tissue [17]. The prepatent period of *O. equi* is five months and the longevity of female worms is around 6 months [22].

Epidemiology: Although the infective stage may be reached on the skin, more often flakes of material containing eggs are dispersed in the environment by the animal rubbing on stable fittings, fencing posts or other solid objects. Heavy burdens may build up in horses in infected stables and there appears to be little immunity to reinfection [22]. Eggs of *O. equi* in the ground resist desiccation, may become air borne in the dust and remain viable in stables for long periods. Transmission then occurs via contaminated feed staffs. The parasite is ubiquitous but of greater prevalence in areas of high rain fall [14]. Pin worms are specific and are well adapted to their hosts, *O. equi* and *probstmaylia vivipara* are found in equids and *skrjabinema ovis* occurs in sheep and goats [17].

Pathogenesis: Severe infection with 3rd to fourth stage *Oxyuris equi* may produce significance inflammation of the cecal and colonic mucosa manifested by vague signs of abdominal discomfort [23]. The most important effects of *O. equi* are the perineal irritation and anal pruritis caused by the adult females during egg-laying. The resultant dull hair coat and loss of hair is known as rat-tail [22]. The fourth stage larva feeds on the intestinal mucosa of the host. The adult worms are, however, not found attached and probably feed on the intestinal contexts. The chive features of *Oxyuriasis* in equines are the anal pruritis produced by the egg-laying females [22].

Clinical signs: The presence of parasites in the intestine rarely causes any clinical signs, however, intestine pruritis around the anus causes solid objects, resulting in broken hairs, bare batches and inflammation and scaling of the skin over the rump and tail head [22]. The irritation caused by the anal pruritis produces restlessness and improper feeding, which results in the loss of condition and a dull coat. The animal rubs base of its tail against any suitable object, causing the hairs to break off and the tail to acquire ungroomed rat tail appearance [27].

Oxyurid infections are asymptomatic; however, clinical signs are sometimes present in equids. During the development of *O. equi* L_4, cases colic and softing of the faces may occur [17].

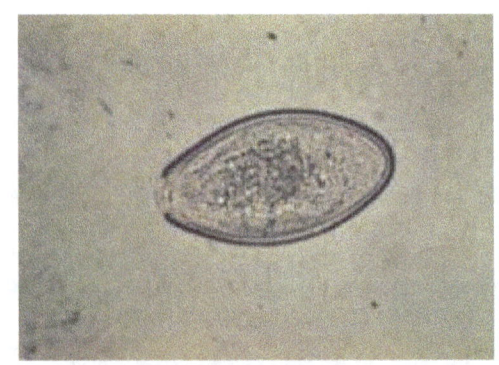

Figure 3: Morphology of oxyuris equi egg.

Diagnosis: The clinical signs should be adherence to an examination of the perinea region, where cream colored masses of eggs will be found [27]. Diagnosis is by the detection of operculated eggs, slightly flattened on one side, on transparent adhesive tape that has been pressed against the perineal skin and then passed on microscope slide for examination, or by the chance observation of an adult worm in the faeces [30]. Diagnosis is based on signs of anal pruritis and tail rubbing and the finding of grayish yellow egg masses on the perineal skin [22].

Treatment: *O. equi* is susceptible to many broad-spectrum anthelmentics and should be controlled by routine chemotherapy the more important horse parasites [18]. Treatment comprises the application of a mild disinfectant ointment to the perianal region and the administration of ivermectin, moxidectin, any of the newer broad spectrum benzimidizoles or pyrantel at the standard dose rate for horse piperazine salts are also effective [14].

Control and prevention: A high standard of stable hygiene should be observed, such as the frequent removal of bedding and the provision of feeding racks and water troughs than cannot easily be contaminated by bedding [22]. The control of *O. equi* depends on good hygiene in stables. Bedding should be removed frequently and feeding appliances constructed so that they are not contaminated by bedding. Clean supply of water should be available [27].

Equine tape worms

Etiology: Several tape worm species are found in horses, donkeys and other equines [22]. The most common encountered tape worms of equines fall under the family of *Anoplocephalidea* and the genus *Anoplocephala* [30]. The scolex of *Anoplocephala* species has neither rostellum nor hooks and the gravid segments are wider than they are long. Two species of this genus are parasitic in the intestine of equines and these are *A. perfoliata* and *A. magna*, *Paranoplocephala mamiallana* is also another tape worm of equines and it parasitize the small intestine occasionally stomach [20]. In horses, *A. magna*, *A. perfoliata*, *Anoplocephaloides* are cosmopolitan in their distribution [14].

Morphology: Tape worms Occur in the small intestines, particularly jejunum and rarely stomach, of horses and donkeys. It may reach 80 cm in length and 2.5 cm in breadth. The scolex is very large, 4-6 mm wide and without "lappets" eggs measure 50-60 nm in diameter [22] (Figure 4).

Life cycle: The life cycle of all the *Anoplocephalides* tape worms are very similar eggs, which are immediately infective and passé in the feces of the host, either singly or protected with in a tape worm segment. These are ingested by free living pasture (oribatids) mites and

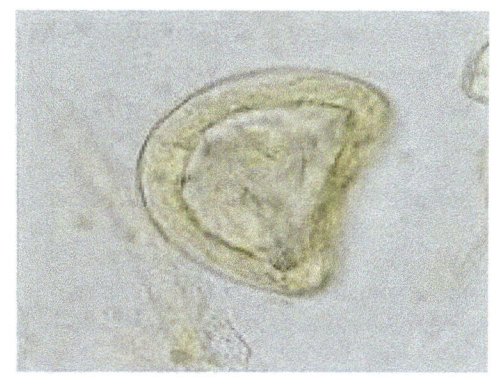

Figure 4: Morphology of Anoplocephala egg.

the intermediate stage (the metacestode) forms. Mature tape worms develop when the primary host accidentally swallows infected mites while grazing [14].

Epidemiology: Oribatid mites are ubiquitous but most numerous on permanent pastures in the summer months. All grazing animals are there for potentially at risk [14]. horses of all ages may be affected, but clinical cases have been reported mainly in animals up to 3-4 years of age [22].

Pathogenesis: Light infestation in horses produced no clinical signs, but very large numbers may cause ill health unthriftness and even death. *A. magna*, in very large numbers can cause catarrhal or hemorrhagic enteritis. Perforation of the intestine has been recorded in infestations with *A. perfoliata* and *A. magna* [27]. In horses the *Anoplocephala* species causes a mild local inflammatory response around its site of attachement, where 20 or more tape worms are clustered, ulcerations and other degenerative changes may occur. Heavy infestations may interfere with gut motility and increase the risk of ileo-cecal colic [14]. These worms are the cause of intestinal diseases such as caecal intussusceptions, caecal perforations, and peritonitis, but are rarely the cause of death [31].

Clinical finding: In horses, poor growth, unthriftness or mild colic may sometimes be seen in heavily infested animals [22]. Most infestations are as symptomatic but, on occasional, heavy burdens may result in unthrfitiness, poor coat, vague digestive disturbances including constipation, mild diarrhea, and dysentery and sometimes anemia. These signs are restricted chiefly to animals less than 6 months of on inadequate diet [14]. In most infections there are no clinical signs, however, when there are significance pathological changes in the intestine there may be unthriftness, enteritis and colic. Perforation of the intestine will prove rapidly fatal [22].

Diagnosis: Where clinical signs occur they may be difficult to differentiate from more common causes of unthriftness and digestive up sets, however, it may be possible to confirm the prevalence of *Anoplocephala* spp by the demonstration of the typical eggs on faecal examination or on post mortem [23]. Shed segments are very much wider than they are long. They can be seen to be full of charactestics eggs if broken in a drop of water on slide and examined microscopically. *Anoplocephalides* eggs are roughly D-shaped, thick shelled, and contain an embryo with a chitinous ring. They are not finding in feces. Centrifugation or flotation using a saturated solution is recommended for diagnostic in horses [14].

Treatment and control: Specific treatment for *Anoplocephala* spp infection is rarely but a number of compounds have been reported as effective, including pyrantel at increase dosage, including pyrantel at increase dosage rates(38 mg/kg), praziquantel at 1 mg/kg is also effective [22]. Control of mites which act as intermediate hosts is impractical. If a potential problem is perceived in for example valuable horses, consideration could be given to reduce the number of mites by plouphing permanent pasture and reseeding. Other ways stabling or tactical dosing at 6-10 weeks after turn out and in autumn are the only option [14]. Treatment with an effective anthelmentic before the animals enter new grazing may help to control *Anoplocephala* spp infections in areas where problems have arisen [22].

Materials and Methods

The study area

The study was conducted in Kombolcha town, south wollo administration zone of Amhara national regional state. Kombolcha is located in the north eastern parts of Ethiopia at a distance of about 375 km from Addis Ababa. The study area has an altitude range of 1500-1840 meters above sea level (masl). The topography of the zone generally is marked by the presence of numerous maintains, plateaus, hilly and sloppy areas with their topographic category including 14% of high altitude (dega), 34% of mild altitude (woynadega), and, 52% of low altitude (kola). The study area experiences abi modal rain fall, the short rain fall duration (half of march to may) with 39.63 mm and long rain fall time (September to November) with 1000 mm with the minimum and maximum annual rain fall of 750-900 mm. The recorded temperature in the area ranges from 23.3°C during short rain fall and 11.7°C during long rain fall. The relative humidity of the regions varies from 23.9% to 79% [32]. The vegetation in the area changes with an altitude ranging from scattered tree bushes to dense shrubs. The soil is vertisol, which is deep clay soil. The major crops grow in the area include teff, wheat, sorghgum, maize, barley, oats, and others. The farming system is mixed type (crop and livestock). According to Kombolcha and Kalu woreda agricultural and rural development office the livestock populations of the area comprises of 100386 cattle, 12975 sheep,31041 goats, 2540 horses,634 mules,7758 donkeys,1865 camels and 119347 poultry [33].

Study animals

Animals used in this study are equines (horses, donkeys, and mules) kept by individual farmers for cart pulling, packing and transport, for rent, ploughing and means of reserve capital. In the rural part of the study area, equines are kept with other species of animals specially oxen. When equines are used for transport or for other use they are supplied with supplementary feeding. In urban areas equines especially horses and mules are usually busy for pulling cart and for transporting water and stone donkeys are used. Therefore, equines are supplied with straw, crop residual from millets, hays and concentrates. In urban areas equines have better health care when they get sick and anthelimentics treatment as prophylaxis however, it is not un common to release equines free near rivers, road sides and passage of sewages to graze. Of the above populations of animals the study was conducted on equine populations which exist in and around Kombolicha and the existing equine species are almost extensively local. The study includes both sexes of male and female and also includes age range from two months of age to fourteen years.

Study design

Across sectional study was conducted from October, 2013 to April 2014 to estimate the prevalence of equine GIT helminthes infection and to identify the common GIT helminthes parasites of equines and their associated risk factors for the occurrence of GIT helminthes parasites. Information about species, age, sex, body condition scores and management systems of the study animals were gathered from the owners and those were considered as a risk factor for the occurrence of GIT helminthes infection in the area. During the study time the animals were categorized into three as young, adult and old and age of studied animals were estimated based on dentition pattern (Annexure II) and their body condition scoring was made (Annexure III).

Sampling method and sample size determination

The study was conducted by simple random sampling method to examine the prevalence of equines, GIT helminthes infections in and around Kombolcha. During the study time 384 fecal samples were collected from the rectum of equines or sometimes from freshly defected faeces if the animals were seen defecating. The age

of the selected animals was determined by dentition [34] and the body conditions scores were estimated based on guides published by Svendesen [13]. Equines less than two years of age were classed as young, those in range of two to ten years were classed as adults and those beyond ten years were classed as old. This way of age classing was based on age of first work, productive age and the life span of Ethiopia equines [13,35]. As a scientific work the study should have to be carried out by determining the sample size according to Thrusfield, [36] for an infinite population with 95% confidence level, 5% desired absolute precision by considering expected prevalence of the GIT helminthes infection in equines in the area. Therefore, according to Thrusfield, [36], the sample size was as follows:

$$n = \frac{(1.96)^2 p_{exp}(1 - p_{exp})}{d^2}$$

Where, n=required sample size; P_{exp}=expected prevalence; d=desired absolute precision

There was no previous study on the occurrence of GIT helminthes infection in equines in and around Kombolcha town. The sample size for this work therefore was determined using 50% expected prevalence, 50% expected prevalence and 5% absolute precision at 95% confidence level using the above formula, the minimum of 384 equines are intended to be sampled.

Study methodology

Fecal samples were collected from each selected animal directly from the rectum and from freshly dropped feces during defecation using disposal plastic globe and each sample was labeled and all description of the animal which is include species, age, sex, body condition scores and management were recorded on a paper corresponding to the label to exclude repetition of sample collection of the same animal. Then samples were transported to Kombolcha regional veterinary laboratory for analysis. Samples were kept in refrigerator at 4°C if immediate processing was not possible, but it had been processed within 48 hours. Direct fecal smear, sedimentation and floatation techniques were the utilized parasitological techniques to identify the eggs in feces and examined microscopically for presence of parasite ova following their procedures. Identification of the eggs was made on the basis of their morphology [27].

Sample processing and egg identification

In the laboratory, fecal samples were processed for examination of GIT helminthes eggs by flotation and sedimentation techniques. Every sample was examined simultaneously by both techniques. The presence of at least one parasite egg in either of the tests revealed that positive.

Methods of data management and statistical analysis

The data collected were entered and scored in Ms- excel worksheet. Before subjected to statistical analysis, the data were thoroughly screened for errors and properly coded. For analysis SPSS Microsoft software version 17.0 was used. Descriptive statistical analysis such as table was used to summarize and present the data collected. The prevalence of GIT helminthes infections were calculated as percentage by dividing total number of equine positive for GIT helminthes infection to the total number of equines examined. Pearson chi square (χ^2) test was employed to assess the existence of association between prevalence of the GIT helminthes infection and different potential risk factors considered. For (χ^2) test, p-value<0.05 were considered significant where as p-value >0.05 considered non significant.

Results

Coprological examination

Coprological examination of 384 equine fecal samples revealed that 281 (73.2%) of them are positive for GIT helminthes parasites and the prevalence in horses was 57%, in donkeys 82.5% and in mules 77.4%. The highest prevalence was recorded in donkeys followed by mules and then horses (Table 1). The parasites identified were *Strongyle* spp 54.7%, *Parascaris equorum* 7.6%, *Oxyuris equi* 2.3%, *Anoplocephala* spp 3.7% and mixed infections 4.9%. The prevalence of *Strongyle* spp was the highest among the detected helminthes parasites in the study.

The difference in the frequency GIT helminthosis between the species of animals was statistically significant (p<0.05) and it was highest in donkeys. The observed prevalence was higher in males than females but the difference was not statistically significant (P>0.05) (Table 2). The prevalence of helminthes infection was found to be significant among different age groups and the difference was statistically significant (P<0.05). The highest prevalence was observed in old equines (Table 3).

The result in Table 4 indicated that the prevalence was higher in poor body condition animals and the difference in the prevalence based on body condition was statistically highly significant (P<0.05). Related with management system the prevalence of GIT helminthes parasites was found to be higher in extensive system and the difference between different management system was statistically highly significant (P<0.05) as shown in Table 5.

Higher prevalence was recorded for *Strongyle* spp parasites of helminthes (Table 6). Mixed infestations were also found. Mixed infections were the occurrence of two or three parasites simultaneously and their prevalence is indicated in Tables 7 and 8.

Disscussion

In the present study the overall gastro intestinal helminth parasites in and around Kombolcha was 73.2% in equines. This was relatively lower than some of the earlier reports of 98.2% [35], 96.9% [37] and

Species	No. of animal examined	Positive	Prevalence %
Horse	128	73	57.0
Donkey	194	160	82.5
Mule	62	48	77.4
Total	384	281	73.2

P=0.001 and χ²=35.547

Table 1: The prevalence of GIT helminthes parasites based on species of animals.

Sex	No. of animal examined	Positive	Prevalence (%)
Male	267	198	74.2
Female	117	83	70.9

P=0.784 and χ²=3.965

Table 2: The prevalence of equine helminthes parasites based on the sex of animals.

Age	No. of animals examined	Positive	Prevalence (%)
Young (<2 years)	94	72	76.6
Adult (2-10 years)	213	146	68.5
Old (>10 years)	77	63	81.8

P=0.035 and χ²=24.928

Table 3: The prevalence of equine helminthes parasites based on the different age groups.

Body condition	No. of animals examined	Positive	Prevalence (%)
Good	55	32	58.2
Moderate	146	92	63.0
Poor	183	157	85.8

P=0.000 and χ²=40.823

Table 4: The prevalence of equine helminthes parasites based on the different body condition scores of animals.

Management System	No. of animal Examined	No. of positive animals	Prevalence (%)
Extensive	277	224	80.9
Semi intensive	65	39	60
Intensive	42	18	42.9

P=0.000 and χ² =45.374

Table 5: The prevalence of equine helminthes parasites based on different management systems.

Parasites detected	No. of positive animals	Prevalence (%)
Strongyle spp	210	54.7
Parascaris equorum	29	7.6
Oxyuris equi	9	2.3
Anoplocephala spp	14	3.7
Mixed infection	19	4.9
Total	281	73.2

Table 6: The prevalence of Gastro intestinal helminthes parasites based on coprological examination.

Mixed infection	No of positive animals	Prevalence %
Strongyle spp and *Parascaris equorum*	10	2.6
Strongyle spp and *Oxyuris equi*	4	1.0
and *Anoplocephala spp*	5	1.3

Table 7: The prevalence of mixed infections of Gastro intestinal tract parasitism.

92.71% [38] at Dugna Borena district, Hawassa town and around Gondar zone respectively. This difference could be attributed to the variation in sampling times as seasonality affects the occurrence of parasites. Additionally, accessibility of equines to grazing land, deworming of cart pulling horses and giving supplementary feed to these animals affect its occurrence. However the prevalence of important helminth parasites was recorded in the study area. Comparison was made regarding prevalence with respect of species, age, sex, body condition score and management systems.

The prevalence in donkeys was found to be higher followed by mules and horses and the difference was statistically significant (P<0.05) and this is due to difference in management especially horses and mules in the area. Most of the horses in the area were properly managed and dewormed regularly, whereas donkeys were the most neglected equine species in the area.

The current study revealed that the prevalence was higher in males than females but the difference was not statistically significant (P>0.05) and this agrees with the work of Alemayehu et al. [9] who reported no significant difference in GIT helminthes infection in relation to sex. The observed difference could be associated to more work load to males than females which could have caused stress and consequent immunosuppression in male facilitatating parasitism. Further in the study area, females usually have more care as they are used for breeding purposes.

The prevalence was higher in old equines than in young and adult equines. The observed difference was statistically significant (P<0.05).

Risk factors		Strongyle spp(%)	Parascaris equorum(%)	Oxyuris equi(%)	Anoplocepala spp(%)
Species	Horse	44.5	3.1	2.3	3.1
	Donkey	63.4	8.6	2.1	3.1
	Mule	48.4	12.9	3.2	6.5
Sex	Male	55.4	8.2	1.5	3.7
	Female	52.9	5.9	4.3	3.4
Age	Young	53.2	15.9	2.1	2.1
	Adult	53.5	4.2	2.3	3.3
	Old	59.7	6.5	2.6	6.5
Body condition	Good	43.6	5.5	1.8	1.8
	Medium	46.6	6.8	1.4	2.3
	Poor	64.5	8.7	3.3	4.9
Management	Extensive	61.4	7.9	3.2	2.9
	Semi-intensive	38.5	7.7	-	7.7
	Intensive	35.7	4.8	-	2.4

Table 8: The Prevalence of risk factors associated with Gastro intestinal tract helminthes parasites.

This findings disagrees with the work of Ibrahim et al. [37], Ayele and Dinka [39] in Hawassa and its surrounding and central Shoa, Ethiopia, respectively. But, it is in agreement with the work of Bewketu et al. [40]. The probable reason may be due to waning body conditions and immunity. Compared to the young equines, the immunity of the old equines is low as they are frequently exposed to different parasites, extensive work overload, and undernourished conditions.

The current study indicated that prevalence was significantly higher in those animals having poor body condition and it was 85.5% while equines with moderate and good body condition scores have prevalence of 63.0% and 58.2% respectively. The observed difference was statistically highly significant (P<0.05). This indicated that equine with poor body condition had higher chance of harboring the parasites. This could be due to the fact that animals with poor body condition might be immune-compromised probably due to malnourishment and higher workload and as a result of exposure to parasitism. On the other hand, poor body condition score could also be due to the parasitism and in such case, body condition score is considered as a dependent factor not as a risk factor. However, in the current study it is considered as a risk factor for the parasitism. This in agreement with Ayele et al. [35] and Alemayehu et al. [9] who reported more prevalence of helminth parasites in animals with poor body condition than well conditioned ones.

Regarding the management system there was highly statistically significant difference (P<0.05). In terms of helminthes infection prevalence was higher (80.9%) in extensive system while equines kept in semi intensive and intensive management system have prevalence of 60% and 42.5% respectively. This indicated that animals kept in extensive management system and used for packing and transport were found to harbour higher prevalence of parasitism than animals kept in semi intensive and intensive management system that were used for cart pulling and this might be confounded by the difference in the management care given to these groups of animals. There is a habit of giving especial care such as deworming and supplementary feed for the equines used for cart pulling. Moreover, the chance of grazing for these animals was less as they are on work, which actually reduces the chance of getting infection and it was similarly reported by Alemayehu et al. [9].

In this study three nematodes and one cestode parasite were identified following the methodology used. The overall prevalence of Strongyle spp spp was 54.7% and prevalence of Strongyle spp was 44.5%, 63.4% and 55.4% in horses, donkeys and mules respectively. The current finding, however, was lower than findings reported by other workers in Ethiopia. Yosef Shiferaw et al. [8], Fikru Regassa et al. [41],

Mulate [6], and Ayele Gizachew et al. [35] have reported the prevalence of helminthic parasites as 100%, 100%, 98.2% and 100% in equines of Wonchi, Highlands of Wollo provine, Western highlands of Oromia, and Dugda Bora district, respectively. The relative low occurrence of helminthic parasites in and around Kombolcha might be associated with the agro-ecological variations, better veterinary services provided by Kombolcha regional Veterinary clinic for equines and the diagnostic capacity of the parasitological techniques used [42].

The prevalence of Parascaris equorum was 7.6% which is in agreement with the study in Khartoum, Sudan by Seri et al. [43] but this study disagreed with Ayele et al. [35] and Belay [6] who recorded prevalence of 50% and 39.77% respectively.

Oxyuris equi was recorded with the prevalence of 2.3% and this agrees with Ayele et al. [35] and Getachew et al. [43] who reported a prevalence of 3% and 2% respectively. The present study indicated low prevalence of Oxyuris equi with 2.3% in horses followed by 2.1% in donkeys and 1.5% in mules. On the contrary, Alemayehu et al. [9] recorded 4.5%, 4% and 3.8% prevalence in donkeys, mules and horses respectively which indicated that the prevalence of Oxyuris equi was higher than the current work. This difference may due to the fact that the eggs of Oxyuris equi are laid in the perianal skin [14,20]. However, sample during the present study was taken from the rectum and the result might not have indicated the exact prevalence.

Anoplocephala spp parasites are the equine tape worms detected in the area and their prevalence was 3.7% which is in agreement with Belay [6] who reported 5.15% prevalence. Mixed helminthes infection of equines was observed with prevalence of 4.9% which is similar to that of Belay [6] who observed that polyparasitism was common finding.

Conclusions and Recommendations

The present study conducted on equine gastro intestinal tract helminth parasites in and around Kombolcha town of Amhara national regional state showed that gastro intestinal tract helminth parasites are an important health problem in the area affecting the well-being and productivity of equines. However, the attention given to the disease so far has not been sufficient. Horses are well managed in the area, while donkeys are neglected. Data showed that most of the horses in the area are used for cart purpose and are under proper care [44,45]. The study revealed the prevalence of helminthes like Strongyle spp, Parascaris equorum, Oxyuris equi, Anoplocephala spp and mixed infections. However the prevalence of equine trematodes was found to be nil in the present study. Generally GIT helminthes infection has great economic importance in equines and management was identified as a risk factor for the occurrence of helminthes infection of equines. Based on the above conclusion, the following recommendations were forwarded.

- To get clear epidemiological picture of parasitic helminthes, comprehensive study should be launched in the area

- Donkeys also require good management and awareness should be created regarding effective regular deworming.

- To control the burden of helminthes, regular and strategic deworming programmes with efficacious anthelminthics should be carried out regularly.

- Improved housing and feeding managemental system should be implemented to decrease the incidence of parasites in equines.

- The government should formulate and implement policies regarding management and health aspect of equines.

All newly introduced equines into the herd must be quarantined and properly screened and treated to prevent environmental contamination with helminth parasites.

References

1. FAO (1996) Production Year Book. Food and Agriculture Organization of the United Nation, Rome, Pp: 7-81.

2. FAOSTAT (2008) FAOSTAT statistical year book. The statistical division food and agricultural organization of the United Nations.

3. Upjohn MM, Shipton K, Lerotholi T, Attwood G, Verheyen KL (2010) Coprological prevalence and intensity of helminth infection in working horses in Lesotho. Trop Anim Health Prod 42: 1655-1661.

4. Tolossa YH, Ashenafi H (2013) Epidemiological study on Gastrointestinal Helminths of horses in Arsi-Bale highlands of Oromiya Region, Ethiopia. Ethiopian Vet J 17: 51-62.

5. Tegegne A, Crawford TW (2000) Draft animal power use in Ethiopia. Draught Animal News 33: 24-26.

6. Mulate B (2005) Preliminary study on helminthosis of equines in South and North Wollo Zones. J Vet Assoc 9: 25-37.

7. Kassa T (1999) Veterinary helminthology. Butterworth, New Delhi, Pp: 58-59.

8. Yoseph S, Feseha G, Abebe W (2001) Survey on helminthosis of equines in Wenchi. J Ethiopian Vet Assoc 5: 47-61.

9. Regassa A, Yimer E (2013) Gastrointestinal Parasites of Equine in South Wollo Zone, North Eastern Ethiopia. Glob Vet 11: 824-830.

10. Asefa Z, Kumsa B, Endebu B, Gizachew A, Merga T, et al. (2011) Endoparasites of donkeys in Sululta and Gefersa districts of Central Oromia, Ethiopia. J Anim Vet Adv 10: 1850-1854.

11. Stoltenow CL, Purdy CH (2003) Internal Parasites of Horses. NDSU Extension Service, North Dakota State University of Agriculture and Applied Science, and U.S. Department of Agriculture cooperating. 543: 1-6.

12. Mansman RA (1982) Equine medicine and surgery. 3rd edn. American Veterinary Publications: California, USA, Pp: 67.

13. Svendsen ED (1997) Parasites abroad. The professional handbook of the donkey. 3rd edn. Whittet Books Limited, London, Pp: 166-182.

14. Radostitis OM, Gay CC, Hincnchiff KW, Constable PD (2007) Veterinary Medicine: A text book of the disease of cattle, sheep pigs, goats and horses, 10th edn. WB Sounders Elsevier, London, Pp: 1556-1563.

15. Wosu MI, Udobi SO (2014) Prevalence of gastrointestinal helminths of horses (Equus caballus) in the southern guinea savannah zone of northern Nigeria. J Vet Adv 4: 499-502.

16. Pereira JR, Vianna SSS (2006) Gastrointestinal parasitic worms in equines in the Paraíba Valley, State of São Paulo, Brazil. Vet Parasitol 140: 289-295.

17. Lefevre CP, Blancou J, Chermette R, Uilenberg G (2010) Infectious disease of livestock. 1st edn. CABI Publishers, Paris, Pp: 1561-1588.

18. Hendrix CM (2006) Diagnostic Parasitology for Veterinary Technicians. 3rd edn. Mosby, USA, Pp: 47-50, 128-130.

19. Foreyt WJ (2001) Veterinary parasitology reference manual. 5th edn. Blackwell Science, London, Pp: 122-131.

20. Armour J, Duncan JL, Dunn AM, Jennings FW, Urquhart GM (1996) Veterinary parasitology. 2nd edn. University of Glasgow, Blackwell science Ltd., Scotland, pp: 3-137.

21. Krivoshein S (1989) Hand book of microbiology: laboratory diagnosis of infectious diseases. Mir publisher: Moscow, Russia, pp: 268-271.

22. Taylor MA, Coop RL, Wallers RL (2007) Veterinary parasitology. 3rd edn. Blackwell publishing, United Kingdom, Pp: 657-703.

23. Bowman DD (2003) Parasitology for veterinarians. 8th edn. Saunders Publishing, USA, pp: 115-116, 117-179, 202-206.

24. Saeed K, Qadir Z, Ashraf K, Ahmad N (2010) Role of intrinsic and extrinsic epidemiological factors on strongylosis in horses. J Anim Plant Sci 20: 277-280.

25. Kahn CM (2008) The Merk veterinary Manual. Merk and co. Inc., White House station, USA.

26. Kaufmann J (1996) Parasitic Infection of Domestic Animals. A Diagnostic Manual. Bir havsen Verleg, Germany, Pp: 5-21 and 224-227.

27. Soulsby EJL (1982) Helminthes, arthropods and protozoa of domesticated animals. 7th edn. Bailliere Tindall, London.

28. Kennedy J, Palmer J (2007) Parasitology of domestic animals. 5th edn. Saunders publishing: London.

29. Moximov VI (1982) A series of practical studies of the helminthes, arthropods and protozoa of domestic animals. By Gestetner in veterinary institute, Debrezeit, Ethiopia, pp: 48-51.

30. Sloss MW (1994) Veterinary Clinical Parasitology. 6th edn, Blackwell Publishers, USA, pp: 63-69.

31. Umur Ş, Acici M (2009) A survey on helminth infections of equines in the Central Black Sea region, Turkey. Turk J Vet Anim Sci 33: 373-378.

32. CSA (2008) Central statistical authority. Ethiopian agricultural sample enumeration, executive summary, Addis Ababa, Ethiopia.

33. SWZARD (2001) South Wollo Zone Agricultural and Rural Development Office Report.

34. Loch W, Bradely M (2000) Determining age of horses by their teeth. Department of Animal Science, University of Missouri, USA.

35. Ayele G, Feseha G, Bojia E, Joe A (2006) Prevalence of gastro-intestinal parasites of donkeys in Dugda Bora District, Ethiopia. Livestock Research for Rural Development 18: 1-5.

36. Thrusfield M (2005) Veterinary epidemiology. 3rd edn. Blackwell Science Ltd, UK, pp: 232-245.

37. Ibrahim N, Berhanu T, Deressa B, Tolosa T (2011) Survey of prevalence of helminth parasites of donkeys in and around Hawassa town, Southern Ethiopia. Glob Vet 6: 223-227.

38. Mezgebu T, Tafess K, Tamiru F (2013) Prevalence of gastrointestinal parasites of horses and donkeys in and around Gondar Town, Ethiopia. Open J Vet Med 3: 267-272.

39. Ayele G, Dinka A (2010) Study on strongyles and Parascaris parasites population in working donkeys of central Shoa, Ethiopia. Livestock Research for Rural Development 22: 1-5.

40. Takele B, Nibret E (2013) Prevalence of gastrointestinal helminthes of donkeys and mules in and around Bahir Dar, Ethiopia. Ethiopian Vet J 17: 13-30.

41. Fikru R, Reta D, Teshale S, Bizunesh M (2005) Prevalence of equine gastrointestinal parasites in western highlands of Oromia. Bull Anim Health Prod Afr 53: 161-166.

42. Seri HI, Hassan T, Salih MM, Abakar AD (2004) A Survey of Gastrointestinal Nematodes of Donkeys (Equus asinus) in Khartoum State, Sudan. J Anim Vet Adv 3: 736-739.

43. Getachew M, Trawford A, Feseha G, Reid SWJ (2010) Gastrointestinal parasites of working donkeys of Ethiopia. Trop Anim Health Prod 42: 27-33.

44. Pearson RA, Krecek RC (2006) Delivery of health and husbandry improvements to working animals in Africa. Tropical Anim Health Prod 38: 93-101.

45. Sheferaw D, Alemu M (2015) Epidemiological study of gastrointestinal helminths of equines in Damot-Gale district, Wolaita zone, Ethiopia. J Parasit Dis 39: 315-320.

10

Prevalence of Small Ruminant Trypanosomosis in Dangur District, Metekel Zone, Benishangul Gumuz Region, North Western Ethiopia

Kumela Lelisa[1]*, Adem Abdela[2] and Delesa Damena[3]

[1]National Institute for Control and Eradication of Tsetse Fly and Trypanosomosis, Addis Ababa, Ethiopia
[2]College of Veterinary Medicine, Haramaya University, Dire Dawa, Ethiopia
[3]National Animal Health Diagnostic and Investigation Center, Sebeta, Ethiopia

Abstract

A cross sectional study was conducted in Dangur district, North Western Ethiopia from February to June, 2013 to determine the prevalence of trypanosomosis in small ruminants using dark phase contrast buffy coat examination. Blood samples were collected from 312 randomly selected small ruminants including sheep (108) and goats (204) of different sexes and body conditions in five peasant associations. Of the total small ruminants examined during the study period, 8 animals (2.56%) were infected with trypanosomes. Out of the total examined, (3.70%) four sheep and four (1.96%) goats were found infected. Infections were due to *Trypanosoma vivax* (1.85%) and *Trypanosoma congolense* (0.98%) in both sheep and goats. There was no statistically significant difference (P>0.05) between season, body conditions, species and sexes on infection rate. The overall Mean Packed Cell Volume (PCV) value of examined animals was 27.66%. The difference in mean PCV of parasitaemic (23.13%) and aparasitaemic (27.78%) animals was not significant (P>0.05) although, lower mean PCV was recorded in parasitaemic animals. Although, the present study revealed low prevalence (2.56%) of trypanosomosis in small ruminants in the study area, the impact of this disease on production, and the role of these small ruminants as potential risk of transmission to other livestock should not be under estimated. Therefore, appropriate intervention measures need to be taken.

Keywords: Dangur; North west Ethiopia; Prevalence; Small ruminants; Trypanosomosis

Introduction

Ethiopia is endowed with huge and diverse livestock population that plays an important role in the economy and livelihoods of farmers and pastoralists. Livestock are a "Living bank" or "Living account" for rural and urban poor farmer, or livestock owners. They serve as a financial reserve for period of economic distress such as crop failure as well as primary cash income. Despite the large population of animal, productivity in Ethiopia is low and even below the average when compared to most countries in Sub-Saharan Africa. This is due to poor nutrition, reproduction insufficiency, management constraints and prevailing animal disease [1,2].

Although, livestock disease has beleaguered farmers worldwide, animal trypanosomosis was particularly detrimental [3,4]. It is a wasting disease in which there is a slow progressive loss of condition accompanied by increasing anemia and weakness to the point of extreme emaciation, collapse and death [5].

In tsetse fly infested areas, animal trypanosomosis is the most important livestock disease caused by variety of species and sub species of the genus *Trypanosoma* [6]. Six species of trypanosomes have been recorded in Ethiopia and most important trypanosomes in terms of economic loss in livestock are the tsetse transmitted species: *Trypanosoma congolense*, *Trypanosoma vivax* and *Trypanosom brucei* affecting cattle, sheep and goats [7]. Trypanosomosis is prevalent in two main regions of Ethiopia that is, the north-west and the south-west regions [8]. In these regions, tsetse fly transmitted animal trypanosomosis is a major constraint to utilization of the large land resources.

Tsetse flies (*Glossina* species) are the principal vectors of trypanosomosis in Sub-Saharan Africa. Other blood sucking flies such as *Stomoxys*, *Haematopota* and *Tabanus* species may also transmit the disease. Wild animal such as bush pigs, bush bucks, kudus, warthogs and buffaloes act as reservoir of infection in endemic areas. The influence of tsetse fly on Africa agriculture through the transmission of trypanosomosis continues to be a major constraint to the development of national economy, and their achievement of self-sufficiency in basic food production [9].

In Ethiopia, the tsetse flies are confined to the southern, south-western and north-western regions where there are five species of tsetse fly (*Glossina*): namely *G. morsitans submorsitans*, *G. pallidipes*, *G. f. fuscipes*, *G. tachnoids* and *G. longipennis*. Among these species the first four are widespread and most important while, *G. longipennis* is of minor economic importance [10,11]. Little is known about the prevalence of trypanosome infections in sheep and goats in the study area. Therefore, this study was carried out to determine the prevalence of trypanosomosis in small ruminants in Dangur district, Metekel zone, Benishangul Gumuz Region, North Western Ethiopia.

Materials and Methods

Study area

Dangur district is located in Metekel zone of Benishangul Gumuz regional state. It is situated at 563 km North-west Addis Ababa. The district has 837,700 ha of land. The agro- climate of the area alternates

*Corresponding author: Kumela Lelisa, National Institute for Control and Eradication of Tsetse Fly and Trypanosomosis, PO Box 19917, Addis Ababa, Ethiopia, E-mail: lelisakumela@gmail.com

with long summer rainfall (June to September) and winter dry season (December to March). The mean annual rainfall in the district ranges from 900 to 1400 mm. The annual temperature in Dangur district ranges from 30 to 38°C. The district is located in Blue Nile valley. The main rivers in Dangur district include: Beles and Ayma with many other tributaries that enter these rivers, including Hypapo, Manbuk, Anja, Anzibuka, kokel and Gublak. The distribution of tsetse fly is associated with the presence or absence of large game animals, which serve as sources of food for the tsetse fly. The area has got a number of wild animals which include African buffaloes, bush pigs, warthog, bush buck, lion, kudu, hippopotamus, crocodiles, hyena, velvet monkey and antelopes, many of which serve as reservoir of infection for trypanosomes.

Sample size and sampling method

The sample size was determined with 50% expected prevalence to increase the precision of the data using the formula described by Ref. [12].

$$N = \frac{1.96^2(P_{exp}(1 - P_{exp}))}{d^2}$$

Where, N: The sample size

d: The desired absolute precision

P: The expected prevalence

Accordingly, a total of 312 small ruminants were randomly sampled from five peasant associations to determine the prevalence of trypanosomosis in these small ruminants.

Study population

This study was carried on 108 local sheep and 204 goats selected using random sampling methods in the five peasant associations. Information obtained was on the sex, species, and body condition of the small ruminants, while packed cell volume was determined from collected blood samples. The body condition scoring of animals was based on Ref. [13].

Parasitological study

Blood samples were collected from the ear vein of sheep and goats after puncturing of the ear vein using lancet. The blood was channeled into a heparanized micro haematocrit tubes and then one end of the tube was sealed by crystal sealant and spun at 12,000 rpm for five minutes to separate the blood cells and to concentrate trypanosomes using centrifugal force as buffy coat. The PCV of each sample was recorded. Then the sample was examined under microscope using Buffy Coat technique. The trypanosome species were identified by observing under the microscope from Giemsa stained thin blood films [14].

Data analysis

Data obtained on individual animals and parasitological examination results were entered into Microsoft Excel program 2007, and later on analyzed with statistical package for the social sciences (SPSS) version 20 statistical software program. The prevalence of trypanosomes infection was calculated as the number of parasitological positive animals as examined by the Buffy coat method divided by the total number of animals investigated at that particular time and multiplied by 100. The association between the prevalence of trypanosome infection and risk factors were assessed using Chi-square test, whereas the student's t-test was used to assess the difference in mean PCV between trypanosome positive and negative animals. The

test result was considered significant when the calculated p-value was less than 0.05.

Results

Parasitological findings

The overall prevalence of trypanosomosis in small ruminant in the study area was 2.56%. Out of the total examined sheep (108), 4 were infected with trypanosomes while 4 goats were infected out of 204 goats examined. The prevalence of trypanosomosis in sheep and goats was 3.70 and 1.96%, respectively. The difference in the trypanosome prevalence between the two species was not statistically significant (P>0.05) (Table 1). Half (50%) of the parasitaemic animals were infected with *T. congolense,* and the rest were infected with *T. vivax.* Therefore, both *Trypanosoma* species were responsible for infection of sheep and goats in the study area. The prevalence on the basis of season was 3.01 and 2.05% in dry and rainy season, respectively. As to the infection rate between the two sex groups, an infection rate of 0.96 and 1.60% was recorded for male and female animals, respectively. There was no significance difference in the prevalence of trypanosomosis between the two sexes (P>0.05). The prevalence of trypanosomes among animals with poor, good and medium body condition was 7.69, 2.5 and 1.55%, respectively. The difference in prevalence among these three groups was not statistically significant (P>0.05).

Hematological findings

The overall mean PCV value of examined animals was 27.66%. The mean PCV values of parasitemic and aparasitemic animals were 23.13 and 27.78% respectively. The mean PCV value of sheep and goats were 28.59 and 27.17% respectively. The mean PCV in dry and rainy season were 27.99 and 27.29% respectively; while the mean PCV for male and female animals were 28.94 and 27.42%, respectively. Mean values of PCV, on the basis of body condition score were 25.44, 28.21, and 27.88% in poor, good and medium body conditioned animals, respectively.

Discussion

The overall prevalence of trypanosomosis in small ruminants recorded in the study area was 2.56%. Similar values (2.11%) were also reported by Tadese and Megersa [15] in small ruminants in Guto Gida district, Western Ethiopia. Samdi et al. [16] reported a prevalence of 2.10% at Kaduna abattoir, Nigeria. The present finding is lower to what was reported from other parts of Ethiopia by Mekonnen et al. [17] who reported 10.57% prevalence in goats in Abelti, Bede and Ghibe valley,

Variable	No. of examined (%)	No. of positive (%)	P-value	χ^2
Sex				
Male	50 (16.03)	3 (37.5)	0.12	2.81
Female	262 (83.97)	5 (62.5)		
Body condition				
Poor	39 (12.5)	3 (37.5)		
Medium	193 (61.86)	3 (37.5)	0.09	4.89
Good	80 (25.64)	2 (25)		
Species				
Caprine	204 (65.38)	4 (50)		
Ovine	108 (34.62)	4 (50)	0.28	0.86
Season				
Dry	166 (53.21)	5 (62.50)	0.43	0.29
Rainy	146 (46.79)	3 (37.50)		

Table 1: Prevalence of trypanosomosis and associated risk factors in small ruminants.

South-west Ethiopia. Dinka and Abebe [18] also reported a prevalence of 5.1% in Didessa and Ghibe Valley, south-west Ethiopia while Kebede et al. [19] reported 5.6% prevalence in Guangua district of north-western Ethiopia. The lower prevalence of trypanosomosis recorded in small ruminants in this study may be attributed to the practice of application of control measures such as spray of animals with acaricides and regular treatment of sick animals. The present value was relatively higher than the reports of Lemecha et al. [20] who reported 2.0 and 0.4% in sheep and goats respectively; while Kalu and Uzoigwe [21] observed a prevalence of 1.2% in sheep and 0.7% in goats. Ohaeri [22] had earlier reported 1.2% of trypanosomosis prevalence in goats and 1.1% in sheep in Abia, Nigeria. The higher prevalence of trypanosomosis could be due to differences in epidemiological factors.

Prevalence of infection among the infected animals indicated lower infection rate in goats (1.96%) than in sheep (3.70%). The higher prevalence in sheep than goats was also reported by Lemecha et al. [20] who reported 2.0 and 0.4% in sheep and goats, respectively; Kalu and Uzoigwe [21], observed a prevalence of 1.2 in sheep and 0.7% in goats; Bacha et al. [23] reported 3.6% in sheep and 3.17% in goats, and Ohaeri [22] reported 1.2% in goats and 1.1% in sheep in parts of Abia, Nigeria. However, the values for sheep and goats as reported in this study were lower than the findings of Dinka and Abebe [12] who reported 7.6% in sheep and 3.6% in goats. Several authors have shown that the prevalence was lower in goats than in sheep because of differences in susceptibility to infection between goat and sheep. This is usually related to tsetse feeding that means the anti-feeding behavior of goats and the docile nature and wool cover of the sheep [24,25].

Two species of trypanosomes, namely *T. vivax* and *T. congolense* were identified in the study area during the study period. Similar findings were also reported by Tadesse and Megersa [15] who concluded that *T. congolense* and *T. vivax* were the two trypanosomes which pose major threats to sheep and goats in Western Ethiopia.

Although, the difference in prevalence between dry and rainy seasons was not statistically significant (P>0.05), the current finding indicated higher prevalence in dry season than rainy season. This result is inconsistent with the report of Ameen et al. [26] in Ogbomoso Area of Oyo State, Nigeria. With regard to the infection rate among animals with different body condition scores, the highest prevalence of trypanosome infection was observed in animal of poor body condition which was followed by medium then good body condition. This indicates that trypanosomosis may be responsible for emaciation in animals thereby leading to poor body condition, although, there are also animals with poor body condition which are parasitologically negative.

The PCV value was calculated having considered (22-45%) as normal PCV for sheep and (22-38%) for goats. The difference in the mean PCV value of infected (23.13%) small ruminant was not statistically significant (P>0.05) from those of the non-infected (27.78%). This indicated that PCV value alone could not be used as diagnostic criterion for trypanosomosis because there are also other factors such as worm infestation and nutritional deficiency which may cause anemia [27]. Other diseases considered to be affecting the PCV values in animals include helmenthiasis and, tick borne diseases [28,29]. On the other hand, most of the parasitaemic animals in the low land areas were in good body condition despite having low PCV values. This could be attributed to the fact that animals in low altitude are always in good plane of nutrition due to availability of sufficient pasture [30].

Conclusion

The present study showed a relatively low prevalence of small ruminant trypanosomosis. However, this is an evidence not to be neglected that trypanosomosis has yet continued to pose a considerable threat to sheep and goats of the study area warranting attention to control this disease to in order to safeguard small ruminants' production.

References

1. Taddese A, Damene E, Kebede E, Birehanu T, Dabessa G, et al. (2012) Prevalence of Bovine Trypanosomosis and its Vector Density in Daramallo District, South Western Ethiopia. J Vet Adv 2: 266-272.

2. Bekele J, Asmare K, Abebe G, Ayelet G, Gelaye E (2010) Evaluation of Deltamethrin applications in the control of tsetse and trypanosomosis in the southern rift valley areas of Ethiopia. Vet Parasitol 168: 177-184.

3. Alsan M (2012) The effect of the Tsetse fly on African development. National Bureau of Economic Research. 105 Massachusetts, Avenue, Suite 418, Cambridge, MA 02138, USA.

4. Bal MS, Sharma A, Ashuma, Batth BK, Kaur P, et al. (2014) Detection and management of latent infection of Trypanosoma evansi in a cattle herd. Indian J Anim Res 48: 31-37.

5. Uilenberg G (1998) A field guide for diagnosis, treatment and prevention of African animal Trypanosomosis. Adapted from the original edition by Boyt WP. Food and Agriculture Organization of the United Nations (FAO), Rome.

6. Swallow BM (2000) Impacts of trypanosomosis in African agriculture. PAAT technical and scientific series No. 2, FAO, Rome.

7. Abebe G, Jobre Y (1996) Trypanosomosis: a threat to cattle production in Ethiopia. Rev Vet Med 147: 897-902.

8. Abebe G, Korme T, Habtewold D, Keno M (2004) Ethiopian Science and Technology Commission (ESTC), Southern Tsetse Eradication Project (STEP), Midterm Review Report.

9. Food and Agriculture Organization (1992) Training manual for tsetse control personnel: Use of attractive devices for tsetse survey and control. Food and Agricultural Organization of United Nations, Rome.

10. Abebe G (2005) Trypanosomosis in Ethiopia. Ethiop J Biol Sci 4: 75-121.

11. Keno M (2005) The current situation of tsetse and trypanomosis in Ethiopia, Ministry of Agriculture and Rural Development, Veterinary service department, in proceeding of 28th meeting of International Scientific Council for Trypanosomosis Research and Control (ISCTRC).

12. Thrusfield M (2007) Veterinary Epidemiology. 3rd edn. Black well science. Oxford, pp: 233.

13. Thompson J, Meyer H (1994) Body condition scoring of sheep, Oregon State University Extension Service offers educational programs.

14. Murray M, Murray PK, McIntyre WI (1977) An improved parasitological technique for the diagnosis of African trypanosomiasis. Trans R Soc Trop Med Hyg 71: 325-326.

15. Tadesse A, Megerssa G (2010) Prevalence of trypanosomosis in small ruminants of Guto Gidda district, East Wollega zone, Western Ethiopia. Ethiop Vet J 14: 67-77.

16. Samdi S, Abenga JN, Fajinmi A, Kalgo A, Idowu T, et al. (2008) Seasonal Variation in Trypanosomosis Rates in Small Ruminants at the Kaduna Abattoir, Nigeria. AJBR 11: 229-232.

17. Mekonnen B, Regasa F, Kahsay AG (2014) Epidemiology of trypanosomosis in goats at Abelti, Bede and Ghibe valley South-West Ethiopia. Int J Trop Med 9: 10-14.

18. Dinka H, Abebe G (2005) Small ruminants trypanosomosis in southwest of Ethiopia. Small Rumin Res 57: 239-243.

19. Kebede N, Fetene T, Animut A (2009) Prevalence of Trypanosomosis of small ruminants in Guangua district of Awi Zone, northwestern Ethiopia. J Infect Dev Ctries 3: 245-246.

20. Lemecha H, Hussein I, Lidetu D (2002) Prevalence and Distribution of major Vector born parasite Infections in Domestic Ruminants and Equine in Ethiopia. National animal health diagnostic center, Sebeta, Ethiopia.

21. Kalu AU, Uzoigwe NR (1996) Tsetse fly and trap on the Jos plateau. Observation on out breaks in B/Ladi L.G. Act Trop 14: 114-126.

22. Ohaeri CC (2010) Prevalence of trypanosomosis in ruminants in parts of Abia State, Nigeria. J Anim Vet Adv 9: 2422-2426.

23. Bacha B, Beyene Z, Woyessa M, Hunde A (2013) Prevalence of Small Ruminants Trypanosomosis in Assosa District of Benishalgul Gumuz Regional State, Western Part of Ethiopia. Acta Parasitol Glob 4: 99-104.

24. Bealby KA, Connor RJ, Rowlands GJ (1996) Trypanosomosis of goats in Zambia. ILRI, Nairobi, Kenya.

25. Snow WF, Wacher TJ, Rawlings P (1996) Observations on the prevalence of trypanosomosis in small ruminants, equines and cattle, in relation to tsetse challenge, in The Gambia. Vet Parasitol 66: 1-11.

26. Ameen SA, Joshua RA, Adedeji OS, Raheem AK, Akingbade AA, et al. (2008) Preliminary Studies on Prevalence of Ruminant Trypanosomosis in Ogbomoso Area of Oyo State, Nigeria. Middle-East J Sci Res 3: 214-218.

27. Radostitis DM, Gray CC, Blood DC, Arundel JH (2000) Veterinary Medicine: A textbook of the Diseases of cattle, sheep, pigs, goat and horses, 9th edn. Baillière Tindall, London, pp: 1329-1337.

28. Sharma A, Das Singla L, Tuli A, Kaur P, Bal MS (2015) Detection and assessment of risk factors associated with natural concurrent infection of Trypanosoma evansi and Anaplasma marginale in dairy animals by duplex PCR in eastern Punjab. Trop Anim Health Prod 47: 251-257.

29. Sharma A, Singla LD, Ashuma, Bath BK, Kaur P (2016) Clinicopatho-biochemical alterations associated with subclinical babesiosis in dairy animals. J Arthropod Borne Dis 10: 259-267.

30. Dagnachew S, Sangwan AK, Abebe G (2004) Epidemiology of bovine trypanosomosis in the Abay Basin Areas of Northwestern Ethiopia. Revue Élev Méd vét Pays trop 58: 151-157.

11

Gastrointestinal Nematodes in Ruminants: The Parasite Burden, Associated Risk Factors and Anthelmintic Utilization Practices in Selected Districts of East and Western Hararghe, Ethiopia

Dinaol Belina*, Abdurahman Giri, Shimelis Mengistu and Amare Eshetu

College of Veterinary Medicine, Haramaya University, PO Box 138, Dire Dawa, Ethiopia

Abstract

A cross-sectional study aimed to assess major GI nematode, parasite burden and associated risk factors as well as the current practices of anthelmintics utilization was conducted from September 2015 to August 2016 in selected districts of east and western Hararghe zones. In the study faecal samples were collected from randomly selected 768 ruminants' (cattle, sheep and goats) and coprological examinations and EPG techniques were employed. The study result indicated occurrence of GI nematode has statistically differences ($p < 0.05$) in all considered risk factors: age, sex, species, body condition and origin of animals and overall prevalence was 51.3% (394/7680). The infection rate was higher in ovine (63.33%) species than in bovine (36.84%) and caprine (52.67%). The current study also revealed the major GI nematodes at the study areas were *Strongyle* type (16.15%), Haemonchus (13.67%), Oesophagostomum (11.07%), *Strongyloides* (3.91%) and *Trichuris* (1.05%), whereas 5.47% (42/768) was recorded as mixed nematode infection. Questionnaire survey in this study indicated majority of the respondents had poor to no information on economic importance GI nematode (71.67%) and anthelmintic drugs utilization (83.61%). Albendazole, Tetramisole and Ivermectin are the commonly available anthelmintics for GI nematode infection treatment at our study area. On the other hand, about 35.83% of animal owners had free access to drugs from general shop (nonprofessional traders) and 24.17% (87/360) had used traditional medicinal plants of unknown doses. The study revealed that high prevalence of nematode infection in ruminates and majority of the people in the study area lack awareness on economic importance of GI nematode though they had free access to anthelmintics with no understanding of drug resistance. Therefore, there should be detail awareness creation and the need of further investigation to develop control and prevention strategies.

Keywords: Anthelmintics practices; Coprology; EPG; Nematode; Hararghe-Ethiopia

Introduction

The gastrointestinal (GI) nematodes are the important parasites of ruminants in all regions across the tropics and sub-tropic countries like Ethiopia. Helminthes infections in ruminants are currently triggering serious problems in the developing world, particularly where nutrition and sanitation are poor [1]. They cause low productivity due to stunted growth, poor weight gain, feed utilization, feeding and water intake, lower meat, wool and milk production, cost of treatment and mortality in young animals [2]. The nematode infections in other parts of the world also affect the health of millions of animals, causing huge economic loss in livestock farming [3].

Adult female nematodes produce eggs that are passed out of the host with the faeces. Under optimal condition in external environment first-stage larvae (L1) can develop and hatch egg within 24 hours. L1 grow and develop to the second stage larvae (L2) which in turn grow and develop in to third-stage larvae (L3), which is the infective stage. After ingestion L3 develop into fourth-stage larvae (L4), which then develop in to immature adults (L5). Sexually mature adult nematodes develop within 2 to 4 weeks after ingestion of the L3 unless arrested larvae development occurs [4].

There are many associated risk factors such as age, sex, weather condition and husbandry, anthelmintic application and etc. that influence the prevalence and burden of GI nematodes in ruminants [5]. The prevalence of GI helminthic parasites is quite different in different species and the severity of the infection also vary considerably depending on local environmental condition such as humidity, temperature, rainfall, vegetation and management practice [6].

The diagnosis of nematode infections in livestock has been based on the clinical signs and detection of nematode eggs or larvae in the faeces by direct microscopic examination. Quantifying number of egg per gram (EPG) of faeces is the best way of estimating parasite loads [7]. To take the control measures epidemiological surveillance of nematode parasite by different diagnostic methods like faecal examination, determination and identification of specific nematode species is important [8] and way of administering anthelmintic drugs is also advised in countries like Ethiopia. The eggs of the nematodes are most often diagnosed by floatation technique and the commonly used floatation solution for nematode and cestode eggs are sodium chloride or sometimes magnesium sulphate [9]. On the other hand, many parasitic helminths of veterinary importance have genetic features that favour development of anthelmintic resistance, this becoming a major worldwide constrain in livestock production. The development of anthelmintic resistance poses a large threat to future production and welfare of grazing animals [10]. The risk of under dosing and a continued use of one class of anthelmintics, irrespective of efficacy status are frequently encountered

***Corresponding author:** Dinaol Belina, College of Veterinary Medicine, Haramaya University, PO Box 138, Dire Dawa, Ethiopia
E-mail: belina.timketa@gmail.com (or) dinaol.belina@haramaya.edu.et*

factors enhancing development of anthelmintic resistances [11]. Reduced efficacy, that may reflect the development of resistance, can be detected by using the Faecal Egg Count Reduction Test (FECRT) though lack of sensitivity is its main limitation. Another disadvantage of FECRT is that it is not species-specific since eggs of different nematode species cannot be differentiated. Moreover, the interpretation of the test depends upon various factors including the detection limit of the method, the number of animals per group, the host species, and the level of egg excretion by the helminths [12].

In Ethiopia, the use of anthelmintics has been practiced for a long time, and constitutes a considerable share of the costs spent by the country in the control of helminthosis. Also, smuggling and misuse of veterinary drugs involving anthelmintics is a wide spread practice in the country [13]. Some of these drugs, particularly albendazole and tetramisole, have been continuously imported and distributed to every corner of the country under different trade names and by different manufacturers [14]. There was a complaint by the Regional Animal Health Officers and some animal owners with regard to the effectiveness of available anthelmintics, especially albendazole.

Considerable work has been done on prevalence of GI nematode of ruminants in many parts of Ethiopia. But, there was no previous study carried out on prevalence with parasite load of major GI nematodes and associated risk factors in ruminants at the present study area. On the other hand, knowing the current situation of the GI nematode in the area could be basis for the possible control and prevention of GI nematode. Therefore, the current study was designed to determine the load and associated risk factors of the GI nematode in ruminants and to assess the current anthelmintic utilization practices in selected districts of east and western Hararghe.

Materials and Methods

Study area description

The study was conducted in four selected districts of east (Haramaya

and Meta districts) and western (Tullo and Chiro woredas) Hararghe zones. East Hararghe zone is one of the 18 zones of Oromia National Regional State and boarderd by Somali Regional State from the east direction. Haramaya one of the east Hararghe district is located at 14 km north of Harari regional state capital city at 9°24′N 42°01′E and 9°24′N 42°01′E in the altitudinal range of 1400 to 2340 m a.s.l. with the mean annual temperature and relative humidity of 18°C and 65%, respectively. Its average temperature is 9.5-24°C with low temperature fluctuation. Climatically the district has two ecological zones of which 66.5% is midland and 33.3% is low land. According to Haramaya district agricultural statistics information, the district has about 63,723 cattle, 13,612 sheep, 20,350 goats, 15,978 donkeys, 530 camels and 42,035 chickens. Meta Woreda is also another districts of east Hararghe zone and situated in southwest of Harar along the road to Addis Ababa. Meta woreda covers three agro-ecological floors (dega 17 kebele, weina dega 15 kebele, kola 15 kebele) [15,16].

West Hararghe zone is bordered with Bale in the south, Arsi in the south west, East Hararghe in the east and Afar in the north West. Tullo one of the woredas in the west Hararghe zone is bordered by Mesela, Chiro, Doba and east Hararghe zone in south, west, north and in east, respectively. The district has 33 rural PAs, and Debeso and Hirna towns. The daily mean temperature of the district ranges from 18°C-26°C and mean annual rainfall 550 mm-800 mm. The agro-ecological zones of the district are highland (dega) 40%, medium high land (weynedega) 57%, kola 3% at elevation of 1500 m-2500 m a.s.l. The livestock populations of the district are 125,915 cattle, 37,973 goats, 13,177 sheep, 171,499 poultry, 5,905 donkeys, 338 horses and 274 mules. Chiro district/Zuria is of west harargeh is also another study site of the current investigation. it is bordered by tullo district in northeast It is part of former Chiro woreda what was divided for Chiro Zuria and Gemechis woredas and Chiro Town. The highest peak in Chiro is 3574 m. a.s.l. [17,18] (Figure 1).

Study design

A cross-sectional study was conducted from September 2015 to

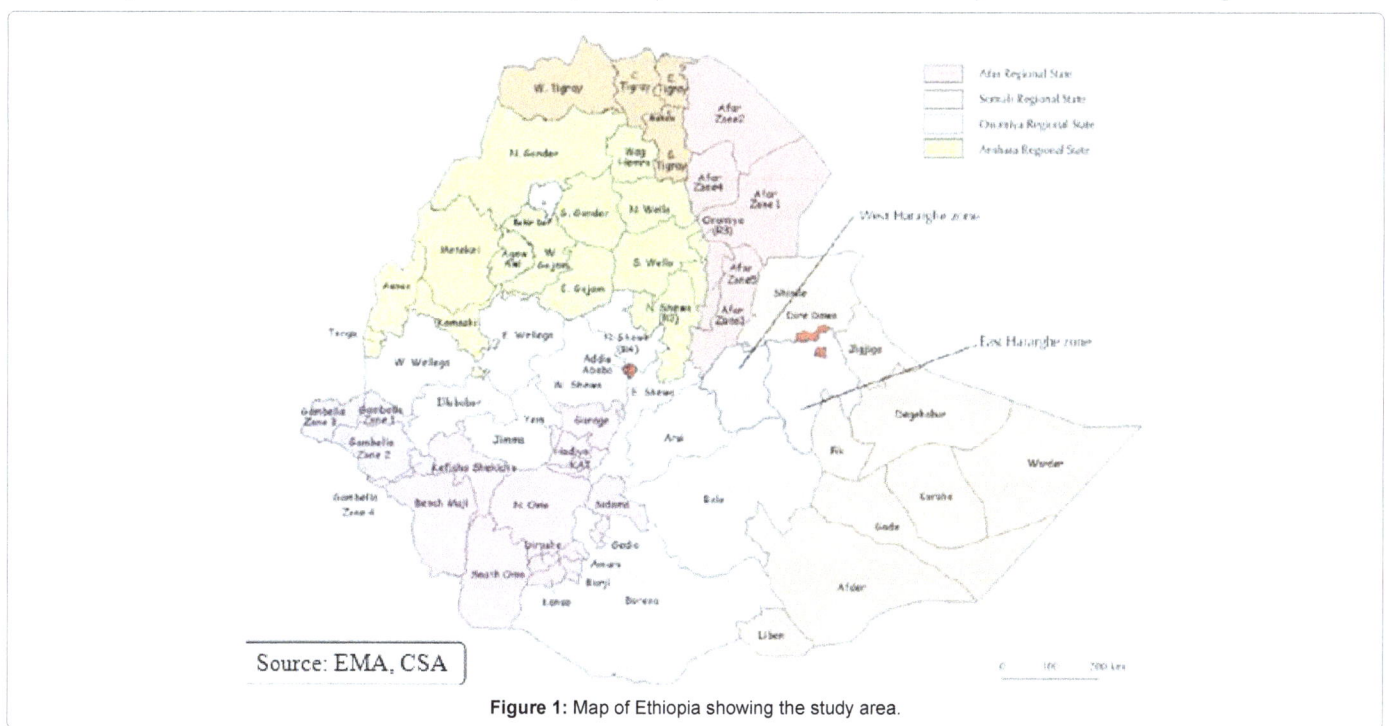

Figure 1: Map of Ethiopia showing the study area.

August 2016, on randomly selected cattle, sheep and goats from four purposely selected districts of both east and western Hararghe zones.

Study population

The study animals were local breeds of cattle, sheep and goats kept under mixed crop-livestock production system. The animals recruited to the study were also further categorized based on body condition score, locality, sex and age groups.

Concerning the current utilization practices of anthelmintics at our study areas questionnaires were distributed for representative respondents chosen from the four districts and retrospective data were also collected from animal health agency offices, veterinary clinics and drug shops in the areas.

Sample size determination and sampling method

The sample size was determined by the formula described by Thrusfield, at 95% confidence level and 5% precision, and considering 50% estimated prevalence as there was no previous such combined study at the current study area. However, to increase the precision of the study sample size was increase by two folds and a total of 768 animals (312 from east and 456 from western Hararghe zone) were included in to the study [19].

The 12 peasant associations (PAs) were purposively selected considering their distance from main road and equal proportions of samples were collected from each PAs. In line with this, 228 cattle, 240 sheep and 300 goats were included in to the study by simple random sampling technique within the species. Among animal species proportional sampling were applied based on estimated total number of each animal species in each PA, as taken from the respective agricultural offices the districts.

Study methodologies

Sample/data collection: Fresh faecal samples were collected directly from the rectum of 768 ruminant animals using gloved hand and placed in into universal bottles. In some cases when immediate faecal sample processing was impossible because distance from the laboratory, 10% formalin was added to the sample to preserve parasite eggs. Data on animal characteristics, management practices, Anthelmintic utilization practices and farmer status and knowledge on GI nematode infection impact in animal production were collected through survey questionnaires at the time of sampling. The faecal samples were transported to Hirna regional veterinary laboratory (HRVL) but samples from Haramaya areas were taken to Haramaya University CVM laboratory.

Parasitological examination: In the laboratory, faecal samples were examined for the detection of nematode eggs employing standard procedures of flotation as described by Charles M using sodium chloride (NaCl) as floatation fluid. This qualitative technique is followed by the quantitative technique McMaster egg counting. In which the positive samples further subjected to EPG counting to determine the number of eggs per gram of faeces and then the degree of infection was categorized as light, moderate and severe (massive) [20]. According to Soulsby egg counts from 50-799, 800-1200 and over 1200 per gram of faeces are considered as light, moderate and massive infection, respectively [21].

Questionnaire survey and or interviews and retrospective study: Evaluation of farmers and professionals awareness about GI nematodes impact and Anthelmintic drug utilization habits were done through designed questionnaires and interviews. In this a total of 360 participants i.e., 30 individuals from each PA (farmers of different ages and education levels, veterinarians, slaughter house personals, agricultural and rural development staffs) were contacted to collect data on: effect of GI nematode infection on animal production, clinical manifestation, control method and use of anthelmintic drugs (accessibility, source of drug, dose, professional administering the drug) and etc. Field observation and direct assessment was also conducted to support questionnaires and or Interviews data. During this period, common grazing sites, small scale farms, veterinary drug shops and clinics of the study areas were visited and the existing activities were investigated.

Data analysis: The data collected from field, laboratory tests and questionnaires and or interviews were analyzed using SPSS version 20.0. The study variables were analyzed by chi- square and descriptive statistics were also used to calculate the data prevalence or percentages by dividing positive samples for total examined. The confidence level was held at 95% and it was considered as significant when P-value is less than 0.05.

Results

In the present study out of 768 ruminant animals examined 394 (51.30%) were found to be positive for the gastrointestinal nematode eggs. In this age, sex, species, body condition and origin of animals were considered as risk factors and the result showed all risk factors were statistically significant (p<0.05). The infection rate was higher in ovine species (63.33%) than in bovine (36.84%) and caprine (52.67%) species. The result also indicated the GI nematode infection is more prevalent in adult, female animals with poor body condition than in young, male ruminants of good body condition. In relation to geographical origin of animals, significantly higher prevalence was found in ruminants from Genda Abdi of Chiro district (72.50%) than in other PAs (Table 1).

In the current study variation had been observed in the occurrence of different types of GI nematode parasites. The major GI nematodes observed in ruminants at the study area were Strongyle type, Haemonchus, Oesophagostomum, Strongyloides and Trichuris with the prevalence of 16.15%, 13.67%, 11.07%, 3.91% and 1.05%, respectively. In this mixed nematode eggs were also examined with prevalence of 5.47% (42/768) (Table 2).

To determine intensity of GI nematode infection among positive samples, the EPG count had employed using MC-master egg counting technique. The EPG counting result indicated majority of the study animals (18.86% bovine, 26.67% ovine and 33.67% caprine) were slightly infected. The study result also revealed ovine species had higher exposure to massive/severe infection (15%) than bovine and caprine species (Graph 1).

Based on questionnaire survey to assess community's current knowledge in the study area, majority of the respondents had poor to no information on economic importance of GI nematode (71.67%) and anthelmintic drugs utilization practices (83.61%). The result showed only 17.78% had deworming schedule and 68.33% of the respondents had no habit of even talking sick animals to veterinary clinics and also did not deworm their animals. Albendazole, Tetramisole and Ivermectin are the commonly accessible anthelmintics for GI nematode infection treatment at our study area. However, about 35.83% of animal owners got access (bought) the drugs from general shop (nonprofessional traders sold the drugs as any form goods) and 24.17% (87/360) had used traditional medicine (parts of plants and vegetables and seeds (Tables 3 and 4).

Risk factors			No. examined	No. positive (%)	X² (P-value)
Species		Bovine	228	84 (36.84)	33.21(0.00)
		Ovine	240	152 (63.33)	
		Caprine	300	158 (52.67)	
Sex		Male	350	162 (46.27)	6.47(0.01)
		Female	418	232 (55.50)	
Age		Young	264	120 (45.45)	5.51(0.02)
		Adult	504	274 (54.37)	
Body condition		Poor	292	218 (74.66)	109.39(0.00)
		Medium	260	110 (42.31)	
		Good	216	66 (30.56)	
Districts and PAs	Chiro	Chiro twon	43	12 (27.91)	17.21(0.00)
		Genda abdi	80	58 (72.50)	
	Tullo	Oda balina	84	48 (57.14)	
		Midhagdu	79	39 (49.37)	
		Kira-kufis	55	29 (52.73)	
		Rakata-fura	68	41 (60.29)	
		Hirna town	47	17 (36.17)	
	Meta	Chelenko main	95	64 (67.37)	
	Haramaya	Finkle	56	35 (62.50)	
		Gende tare	49	12 (24.49)	
		Damota	62	25 (40.32)	
		Adelle	50	14 (28.00)	
Total			**768**	**394 (51.30)**	

Table 1: Prevalence and associated risk factors of GI nematodes in ruminants.

Nematode egg type	No. examined	No. positive (%)
Styrongyloides	768	30(3.91)
Trichuris	768	8(1.04)
Oesophagostomum	768	85(11.07)
Haemonchus	768	105(13.67)
Other *Strongyle* type	768	124(16.15)
Mixed type/infection	768	42(5.47)
Total	**768**	**394(51.3)**

Table 2: Prevalence of GI nematode species in ruminants at the study areas.

Knowledge of respondents	No. interviewed	No. of respondents (%)
Knowledge on GI nematode		
Know about GI nematode	360	102 (28.33)
Don't Know	360	258 (71.67)
Level of individual's knowledge		
Well	360	27 (7.50)
Moderate	360	75 (20.83)
Poor/don't know	360	258 (71.67)
Level of knowledge on their clinical manifestation/signs		
Well	360	37 (10.28)
Moderate	360	62 (17.22)
Poor/don't know	360	261 (72.5)
Deworming schedule for the animals		
Yes	360	64 (17.78)
No	360	296 (82.22)

Table 3: Community Knowledge on GI nematode economic impact as animal disease at the study areas.

Discussion

The study showed of 768 ruminant animals examined 394 (51.30%) were found to be positive for the GI nematode eggs. This finding is higher than the findings of Muluneh et al. [22] who found 43.2% in small ruminants and Muktar et al. 41.5% in cattle from dire dawa [23]. In eastern Ethiopia, animals are managed under extensive pastoralism in which large numbers of the animals are kept together. This could increase the degree of pasture contamination leading to higher prevalence rate [24]. However, the current prevalence was lower than report of Mideksa et al. who found 88.8% GI nematode prevalence in small ruminants. The result also showed there was statistical difference in prevalence of GI nematode infections among animal species, age, sex, body condition score and geographical origins of the animals [25]. This deference could be due to varied knowledge in anthelmintic utilization practices by the farmers, difference in agro-climatic conditions that could support prolonged survival and development of infective larval stage of most nematodes [26]. Furthermore, sample size variation and management system of animals could also contribute in the differences of the prevalence. Supporting the current study [27] also reported highly varied GI nematode infections rate that had been reported by different authors from Ethiopia.

The species specific prevalence calculation in our study indicated highly significant infection in ovine 63.33%) than in bovine (36.84%) and in caprine (52.67%) which was in agreement with the report of

Dagnachew et al. [28] from Gondar area, and Waruiru et al. [29] from Kenya. This higher prevalence in ovine than caprine and bovine could be due to the grazing habit of the sheep where they might be grazing on contaminated pasture while goats are usually natural browsers. The higher prevalence in sheep than in cattle in this study might be due to small sample size (cattle) included to the current study; stress due to overcrowdings might also influence the immune status in sheep than in cattle. Contrary to this result reported that there is no significant difference in between sheep and goat in exposure to the GI nematode parasites [30].

Unlike the finding of Mideksa et al. statistical analysis of the current study showed there is difference in prevalence of GI nematode infections among animals with poor, medium and good body condition scores where the infection rate is significantly higher (p=0.00) in animals with poor body condition [25]. Muluneh J and

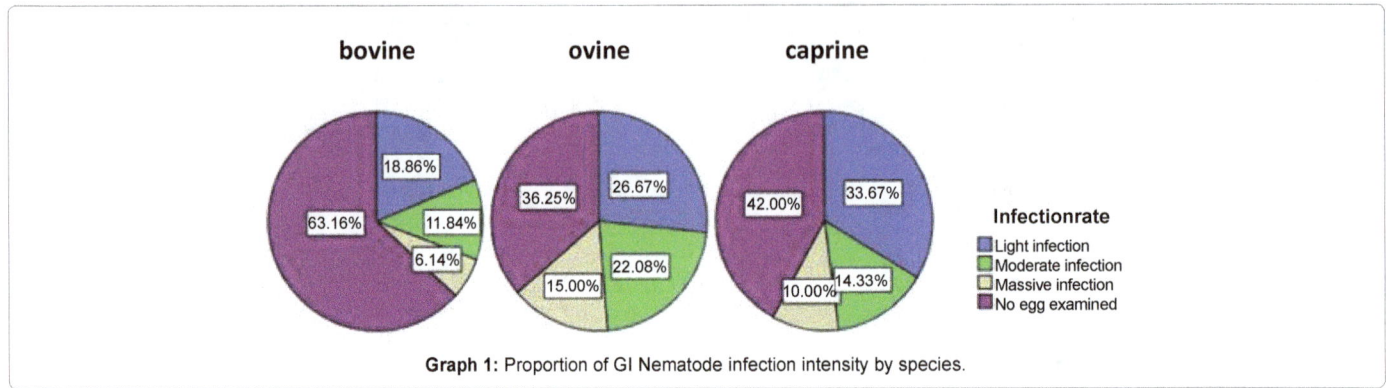

Graph 1: Proportion of GI Nematode infection intensity by species.

Knowledge and habit of respondents	No. interviewed	No. of respondent (%)
Knowledge on Anthelmintic drugs		
Know about anthelmintic	360	59 (16.39)
Don't know/poor	360	301 (83.61)
Level of individual's knowledge		
Well	360	23 (6.39)
Moderate	360	36 (10.00)
Poor/don't know	360	301 (83.61)
Source of anthelmintics drugs		
Licensed vet drug shop	360	72 (20.00)
Veterinary clinic	360	61 (16.94)
General shop/ nonprofessional trader	360	129 (35.83)
Awareness on talking animals to vet clinic and deworming		
Very good	360	36 (10.00)
Good	360	78 (21.67)
Poor/don't like	360	246 (68.33)
Mainly accessed anthelmintics		
Albendazole	360	90 (25.00)
Tetramisole	360	147 (40.83)
Ivermectin	360	123 (34.17)
Medicinal plants	360	87 (24.17)
Know about drug resistance		
Yes	360	76 (21.11)
No	360	284 (78.89)
Know about drug withdrawal period		
Yes	360	83 (23.06)
No	360	277 (76.94)

Table 4: Community Knowledge and status of anthelmintics utilization at the study areas.

Mohammed et al. also reported GI nematode infections is higher in animals with poor and medium body condition score than in animals with good body condition. This could be explained by the fact that loss of body condition in the study animals could be due to other factors, like parasitic infection and malnutrition or other concurrent disease which lead to lower immunological response against infective stage of the parasites [22,26].

Attributing to the Nana our study indicated higher prevalence of GI nematode infection in adult animals. This might also be because of the young animals are not exposed for grazing as adult and more time [31]. Chaparro also explained though most animals will stimulate a protective immunity against many species of nematodes after several months of exposure on pasture, there are certain parasites such as Ostertagia, for which an immune response is not so evident until at or after 2 years of age [32]. However, it contradicts with the report of Regassa and Mohammed et al. who found higher prevalence in young animals and justified their findings as that could be due to

the fact that younger animals are more susceptible than adult counter parts. Adult animals may acquire immunity to the parasites through frequent challenge and expel the ingested parasite before they establish infection. This variation may be due to all animals of age group in the present study were kept under outdoor grazing system [24,26].

Attributing our study Ibrahim also reported a significant difference of some GIT parasites infection among sex group of animals. The differences may be related with sample size variation and some female animals included in the current study being lactating, some others in pregnancy stages during the study period [33].

The coprological investigation in the present study revealed Strongyle type nematode infection was the predominant with 16.15% infection rate. Haemonchus, Oesophagostomum, Strongyloides and Trichuris were also examined as important nematodes accounting 13.67%, 11.07%, 3.91% and 1.05% prevalences, respectively. Attributing to our study Mohammed also reported Strongyle nematode as the most prevalent one in eastern Ethiopia [26]. This high prevalence of Strongyle type nematode may be related with the direct life cycle nature of this parasite as explained by Nana [31]. However, Mideksa found Haemonchus as the most and Trichuris as the second least significant nematodes with 55% and 10% prevalence rates in small ruminants [25]. The variation in the nematode prevalence might be due to differences among pasture contamination, because FECs usually used to predict pasture contamination.

In this study there was significant nematode variation among PAs (p>0.05) of the four districts of the two zones west Hararghe (Chiro and Tullo districts) east Hararghe (Meta and Haramaya districts). The highest prevalence was observed in Genda abdi PA (72.50%) followed by Rakata-fura (60.29%) in west Hararghe whereas the prevalence of 67.37% in Chelenko main and 62.50% from Finkle was recorded as the first and second most prevalences in eastern Hararghe zone. Supporting our study Bacha also reported GI nematode infection rate varies among localities, species and age of the animals, body condition and other risk factors [34]. Our study also revealed there were also important differences, not only in prevalence of infections among considered risk factors, but also in egg counts. The nematode infection severity/burden (massive and medium) was higher in sheep and followed by goats and cattle. Out 63.33% positive sheep 15% and 22.08% were severely and moderately infected. This study supports the assumption of earlier works in other part of Ethiopia [35] and Kenya [29] that higher parasite prevalence is more common in sheep than in goats due to the grazing habit of sheep. According to Regassa the higher prevalence rate observed in sheep and goats of eastern Ethiopia could be due to difference in management system of the animals and breeds of these animals [24]. In eastern Ethiopia, animals are managed under extensive pastoralism in which large numbers of the animals are kept together.

According to the result of the current questionnaire survey, 71.67% (258/360) of the interviewed respondents did not know the economic impact of GI Nematode on animal production as a disease; they even did not care about control and treatment of infected animals. On the other hand, about 7.5% of the participants had good information about the negative impact of GI Nematode on animal production and productivity. The study result indicated only 17.78% animal owners had deworming schedule for the animals. This implies that majority of respondents had poor understanding on GI Nematode infection which is inconsistent with the report of Aga, Kumsa and Melaku et al. [11,36,37]. These authors reported that frequency of treatments with anthelmintics varied among animal owners but most of the farmers treated their animals twice a year mainly at the beginning and end of the long rainy season. Even though they had bought anthelmintic drugs from licensed professionals and also from nonprofessional traders to treat GI Nematode infection, our study result revealed only 10.28% of participants were familiar with the clinical manifestation and signs the disease whereas 17.22% of the participants had moderate understanding on it. Educational backgrounds, lack of logistic, and inadequate veterinary infrastructure had its own impact to poor understanding on economic importance of animal diseases including GI Nematode in developing countries particularly rural areas.

The results of the current study disclosed that mainly available anthelmintic drugs at our study areas are albendazole, tetramisole and ivermectin. The data obtained from visited veterinary drug shops and clinics; and interviewed professionals also mentioned these three drugs accounts almost about 90% anthelmintics available and had been used to treat GI nematode infection at the investigated districts. Beside this

about 24.17% of animal owners had used mmedicinal plants (that had been believed to heal internal parasites) recommended by individuals whom locally experienced with ethno veterinary medicine to treat the nematode infection and other diseases. In line with this and free access in getting anthelmintics about 68.33% respondents had poor awareness of taking sick animals to clinics. Supporting this study, Wakayo explained even though Safe and effective use of anthelmintics requires professional regulation and supervision as also stipulated in Veterinary Drug and Feed Administration and Control (DACA) Proclamation No. 728/2011", widespread infringements such as: marketing of unknown formulation drugs, professionally unsupervised prescription and use of drugs, inappropriate calculation of drug doses and exhaustive use of few drugs is common in Ethiopia [38].

The current result indicated animal owners had free access in getting anthelmintic drugs from both licensed professionals and nonprofessional traders and sometimes treats their animals by themselves which enhance the development of anthelmintics resistance. Kumsa also found animal owners do not have information about anthelmintic rotation and the farmers treat their animals only by visual estimation of animals' body weight to determine the required doses [36]. Scientific information on GI parasites anthelmintics resistance problems prevailing under small holder farm settings is limited in Ethiopia [38]. The current study showed about 78.89% of interviewed respondents did not know the issue of anthelmintics resistance and its future impact. Waller Also reported anthelmintic resistance has become a global problem in the small ruminant industry during the last three decades [39]. According to Aga in western Oromia, the existing method to control endo-parasites has increased its dependence on the treatment with anthelmintics [11]. Meanwhile, the risk of under dosing and a continued use of one class of anthelmintics, irrespective of efficacy status are frequently encountered on many farms. Even though majority of the people at our study area depends on animal products (milk, meat etc.) as source food, 64.72% (233/360) participants had no understanding about residual effect of drugs (meat and milk drug withdrawal period). They prefer to slaughter sick animals when animals are unable to recover (poor response to treatment) from the disease they had been suffering with. This habit not only implies people poor understanding on drug residual effects but also lack of public health awareness including zoonosis.

In conclusion the study indicated Strongyle type nematode infection is more prevalent than Haemonchus, Oesophagostomum, Strongyloides and Trichuris at the study area though some animals suffer mixed nematode infection. On the other hand 51.3% overall prevalence of GI nematode parasites in ruminants at the study area indicated, the significance of these parasites in hampering animal production and productivity. However, the EPG counting result also indicated majority of the study animals (18.86% bovine, 26.67% ovine and 33.67% caprine) were slightly infected. The questionnaire survey analysis showed majority of the people had poor to no information on economic importance GI nematode (71.67%) and anthelmintic drugs utilization/practices (83.61%) to manage drug resistance. The result showed only 17.78% participants had deworming schedule and 68.33% of the respondents had no habit of even talking sick animals to veterinary clinics and also did not deworm their animals.

On the other hand, the role of ruminant animals in the realizing of the economy of the country and individual owners were very high. Hence there should be a need of more management practices in order to be benefit from these animals. At field level involving both veterinarians and animal owners, it is mandatory to increase awareness among them about rotational and minimum use of anthelmintics through enhancing the interaction among them by regular training programme. Further study should also be conducted to identify parasites species using the faecal culture and post mortem examination in study area.

Acknowledgements

The authors would like to thank the agricultural bureau officers of East and West Hararghe, Ethiopia, for their help in directing us to concerned individuals, Hirna Regional Veterinary Laboratory and College of Veterinary Medicine of Haramaya University for provision of research materials.

References

1. Odoi A, Gathuma MJ, Gachuiri KC, Omore A (2007) Risk factors of gastrointestinal nematode parasite infection in small ruminants kept in smallholder mixed farmers in Kenya. BMC Vet Res. 3: 1-11.

2. Paddock R (2010) Breed, Age and Sex Wise Distribution of *Haemonchuscontortus* in Sheep and Goats in and around Rawalpindi Region, Pakistan. Medical Veterinary Journals 12: 60-63.

3. Ahmed MAA (2010) Gastrointestinal (nematode) infections in small ruminants: Epidemiology, anthelmintic efficacy and the effect of wattle tannins. MSc Thesis submitted to School of Agricultural Sciences and agribusiness, University of KwaZulu-Natal Pietermaritzburg, pp: 1-6.

4. Smith BP (2009) Large Animal Internal Medicine. 4th edn. Mosby Elsevier: 1632-1633.

5. Muhammad NK, Mohammad SS, Mohammad KK, Zafar AH (2010) Gastrointestinal helminthiasis: Prevalence and associated determinants in domestic ruminants of district Toba Tek Singh, Punjab, Pakistan. Parasitol Res. 107: 787-794.

6. Lamy E, Harten SV, Baptista ES, Manuela M, Guerra M, et al. (2012) Factors Influencing Livestock Productivity. Environmental Stress and Amelioration in Livestock Production, Springer, pp: 19-34.

7. Roeber F, Jex RA, Gasser BR (2013) Impact of gastrointestinal parasitic nematodes of sheep and the role of advanced molecular tools for exploring epidemiology and drug resistance-an Australian perspective. Parasit Vectors. 6: 153.

8. Hiko A, Wondimu A (2011) Occurrence of nematdiasis in Holstein Friesian dairy breed. J Vet Med Anim Health. 3: 6-10.

9. Taylor MA, Coop RL, Wall RL (2015) Veterinary Parasitology. 4rd edn. Blackwell Publishing, pp: 700-701.

10. Skuce PJ, Morgan ER, van Dijk J, Mitchell M (2013) Animal health aspects of adaptation to climate change: beating the heat and parasites in a warming Europe. Animal. 7: 333-345.

11. Aga TS, Tolossa YH, Terefe G (2013) Parasite control practices and anthelmintic efficacy field study on gastrointestinal nematode infections of Horro sheep in Western Oromiya, Ethiopia. Afr J Pharm Pharmacol. 7: 2972-2980.

12. Graef JD, Claerebout E, Geldhof P (2013) Anthelmintic resistance of gastrointestinal cattle nematodes. Anthelminthicumresistentie of gastro-intestinal nematode bovine. Flemish Veterinary Magazine. 82: 113-123.

13. Biffa D, Jobre Y, Chakka H (2006) Ovine helminthosis, a major health constraint to productivity of sheep in Ethiopia. Anim Health Res Rev. 7: 107-118.

14. Kumsa B, Wossene A (2006) Abomasal nematodes of small ruminants of Ogaden region, Eastern Ethiopia prevalence, worm burden and species composition. Revue de Medicine Veterinary. 157: 27-32.

15. NMSA (2011) National meteorology service agency. Addis Ababa, Ethiopia.

16. EHARDO (2012) East Hararghe Agricultural and rural development office: climate change and livestock data recording book.

17. WHARDO (2013) East Hararghe Agricultural and Rural development office: Climate change and livestock data recording book.

18. CSA (2011) Ethiopian agricultural sample enumeration report on livestock and farm implement part IV. Addis Ababa, Ethiopia, pp: 29-136.

19. Thrusfield M (2007) Veterinary Epidemiology. 3rd edn. UK, Black well science, Wiley, pp: 178-197.

20. Charles M (2006) Diagnostic veterinary Parasitology. 3rd edn. St. Louis, MO. Elsevier Science.

21. Soulsby EJ (1982) Helminths, Arthropods and Protozoa of Domesticated Animals. 7th edn. London, Bailliere Tindall. 119-127.

22. Muluneh J, Bogale B, Chanie M (2014) Major Gastrointestinal Nematodes of Small Ruminants in Dembia District, Northwest Ethiopia. Europ J Appl Sci 6: 30-36.

23. Muktar Y, Belina D, Alemu M, Shiferaw S, Belay H (2015) Prevalence of Gastrointestinal Nematode of Cattle in Selected Kebeles of Dire Dawa Districts Eastern Ethiopia. Advan Biol Res 9: 418-423.

24. Regassa F, Sori T, Dhuguma R, Kiros Y (2006) Epidemiology of Gastro-intestinal Parasites of Ruminants in Western Oromia Ethiopia. Intern J Appl Res Vet Med 4: 51-57.

25. Mideksa S, Mekonnen N, Muktar Y (2016) Prevalence and Burden of Nematode Parasites of Small Ruminants in and Around Haramaya University. World Appl Sci J 34: 644-651.

26. Mohammed A, Disassa H, Kabeta T, Zenebe T, Kebede G (2015) Prevalence of Gastrointestinal Nematodes of Sheep In Gursum Woreda Of Eastern Hararghe Zone, Oromia Regional State, Ethiopia. Researcher, 7: 45-54.

27. Asmare K, Sheferaw D, Aragaw K, Abera M, Sibhat B, et al. (2016) Gastrointestinal nematode infection in small ruminants in Ethiopia: Asystematic review and meta-analysis. Acta Trop 160: 68-77.

28. Dagnachew S, Amamute A, Temesgen W (2011) Epidemiology of gastrointestinal helminthiasis of small ruminants in selected sites of North Gondar zone, Northwest Ethiopia. Ethiop Vet J 15: 57-68.

29. Waruiru RM, Mutune MN, Otieno RO (2005) Gastrointestinal parasite infections of sheep andgoats in a semi-arid area of Machakos District, Kenya. Bull Anim Health Prod Afr 53: 25-34.

30. Kantzoura V, Kouam MK, Theodoropoulou H, Feidas H, Theodoropoulos G (2012) Prevalence and Risk Factors of Gastrointestinal Parasitic Infections in Small Ruminants in the Greek Temperate Mediterranean Environment. Open J Vet Med 2: 25-33.

31. Nana T (2016) Prevalence of ovine gastrointestinal nematodes in Meskan district, Gurage zone, Southern Ethioipa. Int J Adv Multidiscip Res 3: 22-30.

32. Chaparro JJ, Ramírez NF, Villar D, Fernandez JA, Londoño J, et al. (2016) Survey of gastrointestinal parasites, liver flukes and lungworm in feces from dairy cattle in the high tropics of Antioquia, Colombia. ParasiteEpidemiology and Control. Elsevier 1: 124-130.

33. Ibrahim N, Tefera M, Bekele M, Alemu S (2014) Prevalence of Gastrointestinal Parasites of Small Ruminants in and Around Jimma Town, Western Ethiopia, Acta Parasitologica Globalis 5: 26-32.

34. Bacha A, Haftu B (2014) Study on Prevalence of Gastrointestinal Nematodes and Coccidian Parasites Affecting Cattle in West Arsi zone, Ormia Regional State, Ethiopia. J Veterinar Sci Technol 5: 207.

35. Teklye B (1991) Epidemiology of endoparasites of small ruminants in sub-saharan Africa. Proceedings of Fourth National Livestock Improvement Conference. Addis Ababa, Ethiopia, 13-15: 7-11.

36. Kumsa B, Debela E, Megersa B (2010) Comparative efficacy of Albendazole, Tetramisole and Ivermictin against gastrointestinal nematodes in naturally infected goat in Ziway Oromia Regional state (South Ethiopia). J Anim Vet Adv 9: 2905-2911.

37. Melaku A, Bogale B, Chanie M, Fentahun T, Berhanu A (2013) Study on utilization and efficacy of commonly used anthelmintics against gastrointestinal nematodes in naturally infected sheep in North Gondar, North-Western Ethiopia. Afr J Pharm Pharmacol 7: 679-684.

38. Wakayo BU, Dewo TF (2015) Anthelmintic Resistance of Gastrointestinal Parasites in Small Ruminants: A Review of the Case of Ethiopia. J Veterinar Sci Technol S10: 001.

39. Waller PJ (1994) The development of anthelmintic resistance in ruminant livestock. Acta Trop. 56: 233-243.

12

Pathological Investigation and Molecular Detection of Avian Pathogenic *E. coli* Serogroups in Broiler Birds

Azeem Riaz M*, Aslam A, Rehman M and Yaqub T

Department of Pathology, University of Veterinary and Animal Sciences, Lahore, Pakistan

Abstract

The objective of the present study the *rfb* gene clusters in avian pathogenic *E. coli* cardinal serotypes O1, O2 and O78 strains and to develop a multiplex polymerase chain reaction method for serotyping of the O-antigens. The multiplex polymerase chain reaction method was used for the identification of serotypes of APEC. The second part of the study was to study the pathological lesions caused by most prevalent sero group in experimentally infected broiler chicks. A total of 100 tissue samples (50 lungs and livers each) were collected from colibacillosis suspected broiler birds and subjected to isolation and identification of *E. coli* by conventional methods. Multiplex PCR was used for confirmation of three serogroups i.e., O1, O2 and O78. We found more O2 33% than O1 8% and O78 zero percent. These results suggested the prevalence of O2 sero group in our study. The prevalent sero group (O2) was experimentally inoculated in broiler birds at day 7 of their age. Lungs and liver samples from these experimentally infected birds were taken at days 14 and 21 of their age and subjected to histopathology. We found that there was hepatomegaly, coagulative necrosis, congestion and infiltration of inflammatory cells in infected livers. The lungs were congested and there were macrophages, lymphocytes and heterophils too. There was mostly hepatic form of colibacillosis with this infective strain.

Keywords: Colibacillosis; *E. coli* sero groups; Pathogenic *E. coli*; Multiplex PCR; Histopathology; Broiler birds

Introduction

Escherichia coli is a gram negative bacterium, uniform staining, non-acid fast, non-spore forming bacillus usually 2-3 × 10⁶ µm. Most of *E. coli* is non-pathogenic but some strains which can establish themselves outside of the intestine they lead to disease. *E. coli* serotypes which cause systemic diseases in birds are called avian pathogenic *E. coli* (APEC).

APEC is the causative agent of colibacillosis, distinguished by multiple organ lesions like pericarditis, airsacculitis, peritonitis, perihepatitis, salpingitis, osteomyelitis, synovitis, or yolk sac infection. One of the principal causes of morbidity and mortality in poultry worldwide is colibacillosis. Infection of the respiratory tract causes high economic losses followed by septicemia [1]. *Escherichia coli* are the normal intestinal inhabitant in poultry. It is opportunistic bacteria which attack when the immunity of the bird is compromised. It is not only pathogenic to avian species but recent studies have revealed that it has the zoonotic potential for human beings too as recent studies show the possibility of avian pathogenic.

Escherichia coli being incriminated in extra intestinal diseases in humans as well [2]. The present study was conducted to study the *rfb* gene clusters in avian pathogenic *E. coli* cardinal serotypes O1, O2 and O78 strains and to develop a multiplex polymerase chain reaction method for serotyping of the O-antigens. The multiplex polymerase chain reaction method was used for the identification of serotypes of APEC. The second part of the study was to study the pathological lesions caused by most prevalent serogroup in experimentally infected broiler chicks [3,4].

Materials and Methods

Isolation and identification

A total of 100 tissue samples (50 lungs and 50 livers) were collected from colibacillosis suspected broiler birds. Tissue samples were used for streaking on different growth media. MacConkey agar was used as primary culture media. Swabs from Colibacillosis suspected lungs and liver were taken and swabbing was performed on MacConkey agar. Colonial morphology and pink color colonies were observed. A single colony from positive MacConkey plates was taken and streaked on to EMB agar. This medium is selective for *E. coli*. Green metallic sheen was observed on EMB agar. Congo red media was used for differentiation between pathogenic and non-pathogenic bacteria. Pink colored colonies were considered as pathogenic [5].

DNA extraction

A Gene-Jet Genomic DNA Purification Kit (Thermo Fischer scientific catalog No. K0722-250) was used for the extraction of DNA from tissues samples. Purity and concentration of DNA was tested by using Nano Drop spectrophotometer (ND-2000 UV-Vis Nano Drop Technologies Wilmington, DE). For the present study, reported primers were used (Tables 1 and 2; Chart 1).

Amplification of bacterial nucleic acid

Amplification of *E. coli* DNA in the sample of broiler birds was conducted and then amplicons were confirmed with the help of agarose gel electrophoresis. It is a process in which various things of different charges and molecular weight are divided by an electric field. These substances undergo traveling various distances through agarose gels.

---

*Corresponding author: Muhammad Azeem Riaz, Department of Pathology, University of Veterinary and Animal Sciences, Lahore, Pakistan
E-mail: azeem.riaz786@outlook.com

Primers	Sequences (5' to 3')	Product size
ECO-F	5'CGATGTTGAGCGCAAGGTTG 3'	
ECO1-R	5'CATTAGGTGTCTCTGGCACG 3'	263 bp
ECO2-R	5'GATAAGGAATGCACATCGCC 3'	355 bp
ECO78-R	5'TAGGTATTCCTGTTGCGGAG 3'	623 bp

Table 1: Primer sequence and their details.

Stages	PCR Conditions	Cycles
Initial Denaturation	95°C for 5 min	1
Denaturation	95°C for 2 min	
Annealing	57°C for 30 seconds	30
Extension	72°C for 40 seconds	
Final Extension	72°C for 10 min	1

Table 2: Thermocycler Conditions for PCR.

Reagents	Volume (µL)			
DNA (50 ng/uL)	1.0			
PCR master mix (Fermentas, USA)	12.5			
Water	7.5			
Primers	ECO-F	ECO1-R	ECO2-R	ECO78-R
	1	1	1	1

Chart 1: PCR reaction mixture composition.

1.2% gel was prepared to check the PCR product by boiling 1.2 g of agarose powder in 100 mL of TAE Buffer (Tris, Glacial Acetic Acid and EDTA) in the microwave till the agarose was completely dissolved.

Then 5 µL of Ethidium bromide (Cons.10 mg/mL) was added into the gel solution. Ethidium bromide results in the staining of DNA by allowing the line to be look at under ultra-violet (UV) light. Gel was poured in a dual comb caster and stay for half-an-hour [6-8]. Then the gel was put in the electrophoresis tank and PCR products were suffused with it. Before loading the PCR products to the wells of the gel plate, tracking dye Bromophenol blue was added so that the distance traveled on the agarose plate could be seen more easily. For each row of wells, 4 µL PCR products with 3 µL loading dye were loaded. 100 volts charge was passed through the gel for 30 minutes. This resulted in the travelling of negatively charged DNA towards the positively charge electrode. The gel was then observed under UV light in Gel documentation system (Bio-Rad) and photographed.

Inoculum preparation

For Colony Forming Unit count (CFU), the organisms were grown in nutrient broth with yeast extract for overnight. Then 10 fold dilutions were made and 0.5 ml of each dilution will be transferred to the nutrient agar aseptically. The diluted samples were spread on the petri plate with sterile L-shaped glass spreader. The plates were then incubated at 37°C for 24-48 hours. Only those plates displaying 30-300 colonies were counted following incubation. The number of bacteria per ml of original sample was obtained by multiplying the diluting factor with the number of colonies. The results of CFU were expressed as number of organisms per ml of sample. Each bird was injected with 1 ml suspension of E. coli (4.5×10^7).

Experimental infection and pathological investigation

After confirmation of avian pathogenic E. coli by PCR, 2 groups

(20 chicks in each group) of broiler chicks were made. One group was infected with most prevalent serogroup of avian pathogenic E. coli via intra-tracheal route and second group was the control group which was not infected. Birds were inspected for any gross pathological lesions. After that postmortem study was performed on each group and difference of pathological lesions were noted. Histopathology of the organs affected was done by following schedule (Table 3) [3,9-12].

Histopathology

Tissue samples were collected for histopathological examinations. These were processed with standard techniques for fixation, dehydration, clearing, embedding, sectioning and staining.

Statistical design

Statistical analysis was conducted with the Statistical Package for Social Science, (SPSS for Windows version 20, SPSS Inc., Chicago, IL, USA). The data was analyzed by statistical analysis using chi square. $P<0.05$ was considered as level of significance [13,14].

Results

Results of isolation and identification

A total of 100 tissue samples (Lungs and Livers) were collected and streaked on different growth media. First of all, samples were streaked directly on MacConkey agar which was used as primary growth media. A total of 80 samples were found positive for E. coli on MacConkey agar out of 100 samples (80%). These were further streaked on EMB agar (Eosin Methylene Blue) out of which 60 petri plates (75%) were found positive which gave confirmatory metallic green sheen [15]. Congo red media was used for differentiation between pathogenic and non-pathogenic E. coli. Twenty four petri plates out of 60 EMB growth plates were found Pathogenic which were observed as pink colonies on Congo red media (40%) (Figure 1).

Results of PCR

DNA from 24 Congo red positive colonies was extracted and was confirmed by gel electrophoresis of 1.2% gel. Polaroid photo of the gel was taken by using Gel documentation system was used for recording the band of obtained. Twenty four samples were found pathogenic on the basis of pink colonies on Congo red media. These samples were further processed for confirmation of three serogroups of E. coli i.e., O1, O78 and O2 by PCR. Out of twenty four pathogenic isolates, 8 isolates were found to be of O2 serogroup on the basis of PCR. So out of total 100 tissue samples 8 samples were found pathogenic (8%). Two DNA samples were found to be of O1 serogroup on the basis of 263 bp bands on gel electrophoresis (2%) [16,17]. So, in our present study O2 serogroup was found in most of the extracted DNA samples i.e., 33% of 24 pathogenic isolates. O1 serogroup was only found to be 8% i.e., 2 samples out of 24 samples. No DNA sample of O78 serogroup was found in our study samples (Figure 2).

Results of histopathology

It was noted that there was mononuclear cells infiltration and thin

Days of Trial	Group 1	Group 2
Day 7	Infected by intra-tracheal route	Not infected
Day 14	Lungs and liver collection	Lungs and liver collection
Day 21	Lungs and liver collection	Lungs and liver collection

Table 3: Experimental Design.

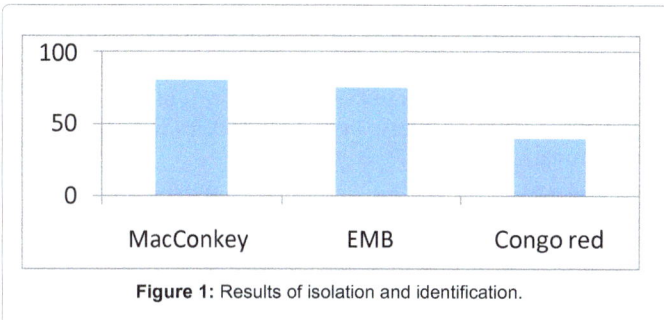

Figure 1: Results of isolation and identification.

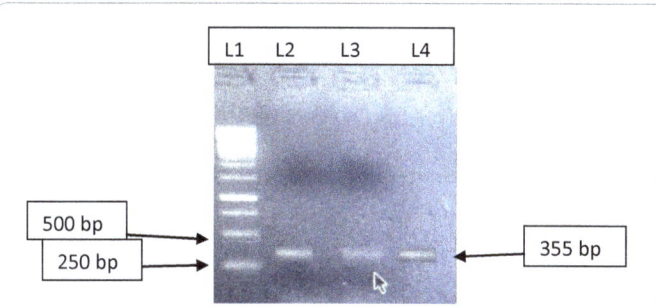

Figure 2: Gel electrophoresis of PCR product showing amplification of 355bp fragment of *E. coli serogroup O2*. Where in Lane; L1=Gene Ruler 250 bp DNA Ladder (Thermo scientific); L2=Sample with O$_2$ serogroup; L3=Sample with O$_2$; Serogroup L4=Sample with O$_2$ serogroup.

fibrinous layer over liver. Thickening of the liver capsule was noted due to invasion of mononuclear cells and there was marked congestion in hepatic portal areas and the central vein. There was atrophy of adjoining hepatic cords due to greatly distended and congested sinusoids. Besides these changes, hepatic cells in various phases of degeneration along with hemorrhages, areas of congestion and fatty changes in a few areas could be seen [18]. There was total demolition of hepatic cord settlement at some places. Necrotic areas were invaded predominantly by mononuclear cells and usual foci of necrosis were also observed. In chicks, the changes in liver were noticed at 14 and 21 days post infection. At first there was slight invasion of mononuclear cells in the portal areas, which was average to severe at subsequent intervals. Additionally, the deleterious changes and vacuolation in the hepatocyte were also observed in a few places [19-22]. There was infiltration of heterophils, severe congestion, lymphocytes and macrophages in the peribronchial alveoli as well as the wall of the bronchus. There was marked presence of granuloma in lungs. Some birds displayed thickening of the pleura and consolidated areas covered with yellowish fibrin in lungs (Figures 3a-3d).

Discussion

E. coli causes drastic types of ailments such as coli granuloma (Hjarre's disease), pericarditis, avian cellulites (inflammatory process), salpingitis, osteomyelitis, colisepticemia, swollen head, syndrome air sacculitis, panophthalmitis, peritonitis, enteritis, omphalitis / yolk sac infection and synovitis [1]. In this current study, all the described forms of colibacillosis were not observed [23]. However, the observed forms of colibacillosis could be classified as a fibrinous layer over the liver surface. *E. coli* alone does not fabricate typical gross lesions. The lesions are most eminent when concurrently affected with other organisms such as *Mycoplasma*. *E. coli* can cause disease by attaching with the mucosal

epithelia and another form by incursion to the mucosal epithelia. The observed lesions of liver were in the form of necrosis, degeneration, and severe inflammation associated with desquamation of mucosal epithelia [24]. Based on the observed lesions, the form of colibacillosis in the current study could be classified into hepatic form of colibacillosis. These types of histopathological lesions were reinforced by different

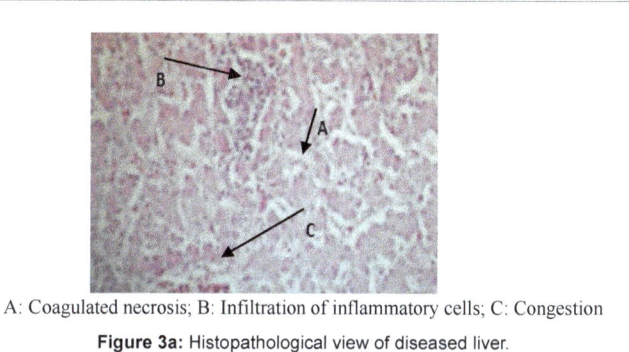

A: Coagulated necrosis; B: Infiltration of inflammatory cells; C: Congestion

Figure 3a: Histopathological view of diseased liver.

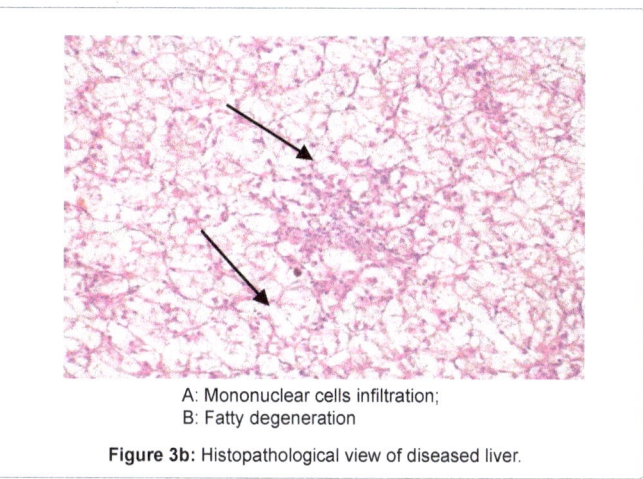

A: Mononuclear cells infiltration;
B: Fatty degeneration

Figure 3b: Histopathological view of diseased liver.

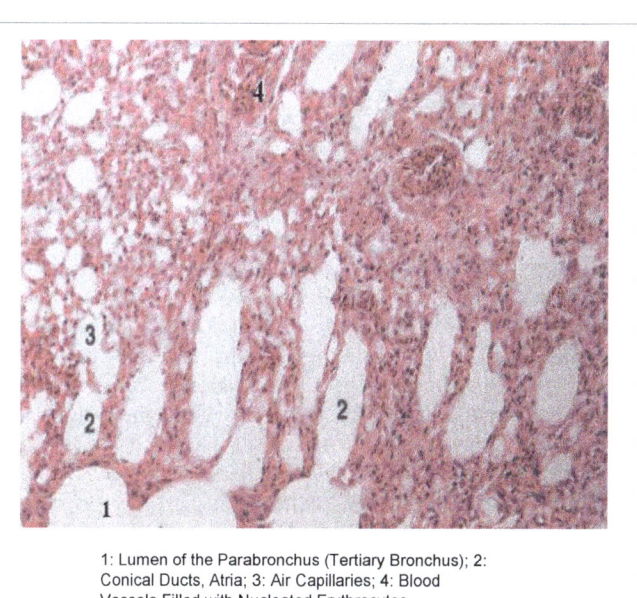

1: Lumen of the Parabronchus (Tertiary Bronchus); 2: Conical Ducts, Atria; 3: Air Capillaries; 4: Blood Vessels Filled with Nucleated Erythrocytes

Figure 3c: Histopathological view of normal lung.

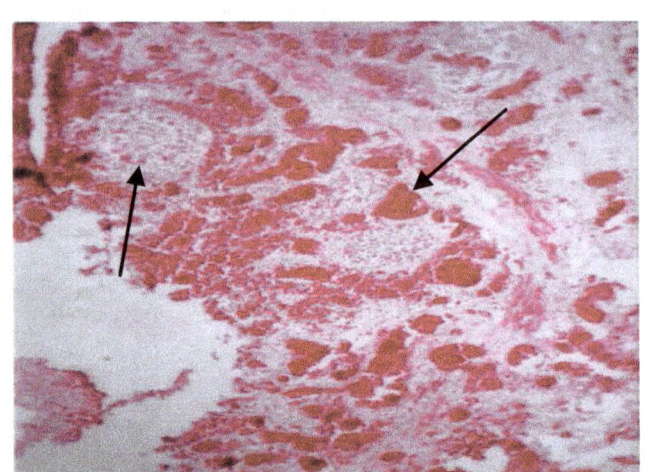

A: Severe Congestion; B: Infiltration of inflammatory cells

Figure 3d: Histopathological view of *E. coli* infected lungs.

authors. There was infiltration of heterophils, severe congestion, lymphocytes and macrophages in the peribronchial alveoli as well as in the wall of the bronchus. There was marked presence of granuloma in lungs. In liver, severe infiltration of leukocytes mononuclear cells were observed. Hepatomegaly and enlarged lungs were also noted. Microscopically, all deceased birds did not displayed analogous gravity of lesions in all organs in the current study correlated with the findings of others [4-6]. Colibacillosis is a contagious ailment of birds caused by *E. coli* [7] which is classified as one of the main reasons of morbidity and mortality, connected with huge financial losses to the poultry sector by its alliance with different disease conditions, either as primary pathogen or as a secondary pathogen [8,25,26]. Localized or systemic colibacillosis can have a variety of symptoms. In this study, there were same findings with the previous studies. Coli-granuloma is an infrequent form of colibacillosis, which is characterized by granulomas in caecum, duodenum, liver and mesentery. Coli-granuloma was found in liver and lung in our cases. The histopathological changes observed in the present study had similarities to observations in earlier [7]. It has been noted in the previous studies that there has been pitiful flock performance correlated with increased early mortality rates [9]. Hatchery practices have been reported as the cause of early mortalities of layer and broiler breeders. Twenty four locally isolated isolates of *E. coli* were tested by ECO-F, ECO1-R, ECO2-R and ECO78-R primers and showed 355-bp products from eight field samples after 1.2% agarose gel electrophoresis. Traditionally, isolation and identification of *E. coli* was used as the main tool for the diagnosis of colibacillosis. The isolation and identification rely upon the culture of the organism using various selective media and biochemical tests. PCR and its comparable methods have been reported to identify *E. coli,* instead of biochemical and ELISA tests. The PCR is used as a highly sensitive and peculiar test for the presence of pathogenic bacteria in clinical specimens [10]. PCR is also reliable and swifter than traditionally culture methods [11]. We also found the same results in the current study [27,28]. In this study, the isolated *E. coli* organisms from all collected birds were cultured in MacConkey agar, EMB agar and Congo red media, DNA was extracted and amplified by PCR using ECO-F, ECO1-R, ECO2-R and ECO78-R primers targeting *E. coli* DNA and found 355 bp amplicon after 1.2% agarose gel electrophoresis. The similar result also found by other authors [12]. This base pair is specific for *E. coli* O2 serogroup not for others [29-32].

The recent study assisted similar findings to those observed in layer flocks, with *E. coli* infections being due to multiple strains of *E. coli* [13]. This study supports the Koch's postulates for APEC according to which wild type pathogen originally isolated in an outbreak of APEC infection in the field could cause disease in healthy chickens infected with the cultured strain [33].

Conclusion

It was concluded with the results of present study that there are different serogroups of avian pathogenic *E. coli* in field and PCR is best technique to recognize the different strains of *E. coli*. The results of histopathology also confirmed that experimental infection of pathogenic serogroup O_2 produce pronounced lesions in lungs and livers of broiler birds and there is early mortality and decreased weight gain.

References

1. Barnes HJ, Gross WB (1997) Colibacillosis. In: Diseases of Poultry. Gross WB (ed.), Iowa State University Press, Ames Iowa, pp: 131-141.

2. Ewers C, Li G, Wilking H, Kiebling S, Alt K, et al. (2007) Avian pathogenic, uropathogenic, and newborn meningitis-causing *Escherichia coli*: how closely related are they? Intl J Med Microbiol 297: 163-176.

3. Kapakin KAT, Kapakin S, Kurt A, Iskender H, Altun S, et al. (2015) Histopathological Findings and Apoptosis Caused by *E. coli* in Layer Birds. Pak Vet J 35: 525-527.

4. Talha AFSM, Hossain MM, Chowdhury EH, Bari ASM, Islam MR, et al. (2001) Poultry diseases occurring in Mymensingh district of Bangladesh. The Bangladesh Veterinarian 18: 20-23.

5. Islam MR, Das BC, Hossain K, Lucky NS, Mostafa MG (2003) A study on the occurrence of poultry diseases in Sylhet region of Bangladesh. Int J Poult Sci 2: 354-356.

6. Ghosh RC, Hirpurkar SD, Suryawanshi PR (2006) Concurrent colibacillosis and infectious bursal disease in broiler chicks. Indian Vet J 83: 1019-1020.

7. Barnes HJ, LK Nolan, Vaillancourt JF (2008) Colibacillosis. 12th edn. In: Diseases of Poultry. Saif YM (Editor). Blackwell Publishing, USA, pp: 691-732.

8. Tonu NS, Sufian MA, Sarker S, Kamal MM, Rahman MH, et al. (2012) Pathological study on colibacillosis in chickens and detection of *Escherichia coli* by PCR. Bangla J Vet Med 9: 17-25.

9. Ugozzoli L, Wallace RB (1991) Allele-specific polymerase chain reaction. Methods 2: 42-48.

10. Cohen ND, Neibergs HL, McGruder ED, Whitford HW, Behle RW, et al. (1993) Genus-specific detection of salmonellae using the polymerase chain reaction (PCR). J Vet Diagnos Invest 5: 368-371.

11. Carli KT, Unal CB, Caner V, Eyigor A (2001) Detection of *Salmonellae* in chicken feces by a combination of tetrathionate broth enrichment, capillary PCR, and capillary gel electrophoresis. J Clin Microbiol 39: 1871-1876.

12. Kumar A, Jindal N, Shukla CL, Asrani RK, Ledoux DR, et al. (2004) Pathological changes in broiler chickens fed ochratoxin A and inoculated with *Escherichia coli*. Avian Pathol 33: 413-417.

13. Olsen RH, Stockholm NM, Permin A, Christensen JP, Christensen H, et al. (2011) Multi-locus sequence typing and plasmid profile characterization of avian pathogenic *Escherichia coli* associated with increased mortality in free-range layer flocks. Avian Pathol 40: 437-444.

14. Bauer AP, Dieckmann SM, Ludwig W, Schleifer KH (2007) Rapid identification of *Escherichia coli* safety and laboratory strain lineages based on Multiplex-PCR. FEMS Microbiol Lett 269: 36-40.

15. Blanco JE, Blanco M, Mora A, Jansen WH, García V, et al. (1998) Serotypes of *Escherichia coli* isolated from septicaemic chickens in Galicia (northwest Spain). Vet Microbiol 61: 229-235.

16. Blattner FR, Plunkett G, Bloch CA, Perna NT, Burland V, et al. (1997) The complete genome sequence of *Escherichia coli* K-12. Science 277: 1453-1462.

17. Chen J, Griffiths MW (1998) PCR differentiation of *Escherichia coli* from other Gram-negative bacteria using primers derived from the nucleotide sequences flanking the gene encoding the universal stress protein. Lett Appl Microbiol 27: 369-371.

18. Delannoy S, Beutin L, Burgos Y, Fach P (2012) Specific detection of enteroaggregative hemorrhagic *Escherichia coli* O104: H4 strains by use of the CRISPR locus as a target for a diagnostic real-time PCR. J Clin Microbiol 50: 3485-3492.

19. Ewers C, Janben T, Kiebling S, Philipp HC, Wieler LH (2004) Molecular epidemiology of avian pathogenic *Escherichia coli* (APEC) isolated from colisepticemia in poultry. Vet Microbiol 104: 91-101.

20. Fratamico PM, Briggs CE, Needle D, Chen CY, DebRoy C (2003) Sequence of the *Escherichia coli* O121 O-antigen gene cluster and detection of enterohemorrhagic *E. coli* O121 by PCR amplification of the wzx and wzy genes. J Clin Microbiol 41: 3379-3383.

21. Goren E (1978) Observations on experimental infection of chicks with *Escherichia coli*. Avian Pathol 7: 213-224.

22. Janben T, Schwarz C, Preikschat P, Voss M, Philipp HC, et al. (2001) Virulence-associated genes in avian pathogenic *Escherichia coli* (APEC) isolated from internal organs of poultry having died from colibacillosis. Int J Med Microbiol 291: 371-378.

23. Kemmett K, Williams NJ, Chaloner G, Humphrey S, Wigley P, et al. (2014) The contribution of systemic *Escherichia coli* infection to the early mortalities of commercial broiler chickens. Avian Pathol 43: 37-42.

24. Li G, Laturnus C, Ewers C, Wieler LH (2005) Identification of genes required for avian *Escherichia coli* septicemia by signature-tagged mutagenesis. Infect Immun 73: 2818-2827.

25. Mbanga J, Nyararai YO (2015) Virulence gene profiles of avian pathogenic *Escherichia coli* isolated from chickens with colibacillosis in Bulawayo, Zimbabwe. Onderstepoort J Vet Res 82: 1-8.

26. McPeake SJW, Smyth JA, Ball HJ (2005) Characterisation of avian pathogenic *Escherichia coli* (APEC) associated with colisepticaemia compared to faecal isolates from healthy birds. Vet Microbiol 110: 245-253.

27. Osek J (2001) Multiplex polymerase chain reaction assay for identification of enterotoxigenic *Escherichia coli* strains. J Vet Diagnos Invest 13: 308-311.

28. Parreira VR, Gyles CL (2003) A novel pathogenicity island integrated adjacent to the thrW tRNA gene of avian pathogenic *Escherichia coli* encodes a vacuolating autotransporter toxin. Infect Immun 71: 5087-5096.

29. Paton AW, Paton JC (1998) Detection and Characterization of Shiga Toxigenic *Escherichia coli* by Using Multiplex PCR Assays forstx 1, stx 2, eaeA, Enterohemorrhagic *E. coli* hlyA, rfb O111, and rfb O157. J Clin Microbiol 36: 598-602.

30. Rahman MA, Samad MA, Rahman MB, Kabir SML (2004) Bacterio-pathological studies on salmonellosis, colibacillosis and pasteurellosis in natural and experimental infections in chickens. Bangladesh J Vet Med 2: 1-8.

31. Rodriguez-Siek KE, Giddings CW, Doetkott C, Johnson TJ, Nolan LK (2005) Characterizing the APEC pathotype. Vet Res 36: 241-256.

32. Tenover FC, Arbeit RD, Goering RV, Mickelsen PA, Murray BE, et al. (1995) Interpreting chromosomal DNA restriction patterns produced by pulsed-field gel electrophoresis: criteria for bacterial strain typing. J Clin Microbiol 33: 2233.

33. Wang S, Meng Q, Dai J, Han X, Han Y, et al. (2014) Development of an allele-specific PCR assay for simultaneous sero-typing of avian pathogenic *Escherichia coli* predominant O1, O2, O18 and O78 strains. PloS one 9: e96904.

13

Seroprevalence of Peste Des Petits Ruminants Virus from Samples Collected in Different Regions of Tanzania in 2013 and 2015

Tebogo Kgotlele[1,2]*, Emeli Torsson[1,3], Christopher Jacob Kasanga[1], Jonas Johansson Wensman[1,4] and Gerald Misinzo[1]

[1]Department of Veterinary Microbiology and Parasitology, Sokoine University of Agriculture, Chuo Kikuu, Morogoro, Tanzania
[2]Molecular Biology Section, Botswana National Veterinary Laboratory, Gaborone, Botswana
[3]Department of Biomedical Sciences and Veterinary Public Health, Swedish University of Agricultural Sciences, SE-750 07 Uppsala, Sweden
[4]Department of Clinical Sciences, Swedish University of Agricultural Sciences, SE-750 07 Uppsala, Sweden

Abstract

Sero-surveillance was conducted to determine seroprevalence of peste des petits ruminant's virus (PPRV) in sheep and goats population of Tanzania using samples collected in 2013 and 2015. A total of 3,838 samples were collected from villages in 14 of the 25 mainland regions. Samples were tested by competitive ELISA for detection of antibodies against PPRV. Overall, 998 of the samples were found to be positive for antibodies against PPR, giving a seroprevalence of 27.1%. In this study, there was no statistical significant difference of getting PPR between sheep and goats (odds ratio of 1.06, 95% CI 0.89-1.25). The overall seroprevalence indicates that PPR is prevalent in small ruminants in the study areas. The study also confirms the presence of antibodies against PPR in sheep and goats in regions of Tanzania that previously had little to no data on the disease, an indication that PPR is spreading within Tanzania with the possibility of spreading to neighboring countries.

Keywords: Peste des petits ruminants; Seroprevalence; cELISA; Tanzania

Introduction

Peste des petits ruminants (PPR) is a highly contagious viral disease of goats and sheep characterized by oculo-nasal discharges, stomatitis, diarrhea and pneumonia [1]. It is a disease of economic significance because of its transboundary nature, high morbidity and mortality rates which result in loss of production, limitations on export and threat to human food chain [2]. The disease is caused by peste des petits ruminants virus (PPRV), belonging to the genus *Morbillivirus* of the family *Paramyxoviridae*. The virus is highly contagious and easily transmitted by direct contact through secretions and/or excretions of infected animals [3].

Peste des petits ruminants was first reported in West Africa in the early 1940s and later recognized as endemic in both West and Central Africa [4,5]. Currently, PPR is present in Central, Eastern and Western Africa, Asia, and the Near and Middle East [6]. In East Africa, PPR was detected serologically in Kenya and Uganda in 2007 [7].

Efforts to determine presence of PPR in sheep and goats in Tanzania can be traced back to Loliondo in 1995 through grey literature [8]. Three years later in 1998, the presence of antibodies against PPR was ruled out by a comprehensive study that did not find any antibodies against PPR in Tanzania sheep and goats [9]. A retrospective study done in Ngorongoro district using samples collected for Rift Valley fever virus and PPR surveys showed presence of antibodies against PPR in samples collected in 2004, suggesting the presence of PPRV at that period [8].

PPR was officially confirmed in Tanzania in 2008 and it was confined to the northern zone in districts bordering Kenya [10,11]. This follows the official confirmation of PPR in neighboring Kenya in 2007 [7]. The possible spread from Kenya to Tanzania may have been due to the difficulty in controlling transnational livestock movements across borders, especially where Maasai pastoralists are found on either side [12]. In 2011, an outbreak of PPR was reported in southern Tanzania [13]. In other areas of Tanzania, limited to no data is available about the disease. Therefore, the objective of this study was to determine seroprevalence of PPR in selected regions of Tanzania to have a current comprehensive view about the distribution of PPR in the country.

Materials and Methods

Samples

A total of 3,838 serum samples from 118 villages collected from sheep and goats in 14 regions of Tanzania (Figure 1) in 2013 and 2015 were used (Table 1). Samples were collected from apparently healthy animals, that is did not show any clinical signs associated with PPR. These serum samples were submitted to Sokoine University of Agriculture for official confirmation of PPR in Tanzania before a PPR vaccination campaign. Unfortunately, sex of sampled animals could not be retrieved from information stated in the submission forms.

Detection of PPR antibodies using competitive enzyme linked immunosorbent assay (cELISA)

Sera were tested for antibodies against PPRV using a competitive ELISA kit (cELISA) (CIRAD EMVT, Montpellier, France). The test was performed according to manufacturer's instructions. Samples presenting a competition percentage of less than or equal to 50% were considered positive for PPRV antibodies.

Statistical analysis

Apparent prevalence estimates were used to estimate true prevalence [14] and the kit's relative diagnostic sensitivity and specificity of 92.2% and 98.9% respectively [15]. The odds ratio was calculated to assess the association between being seropositive for PPR and animal species [16].

***Corresponding author:** Tebogo Kgotlele, Department of Veterinary Microbiology and Parasitology, Sokoine University of Agriculture, PO Box 3019, Chuo Kikuu, Morogoro, Tanzania, E-mail: tkgotlele@gmail.com

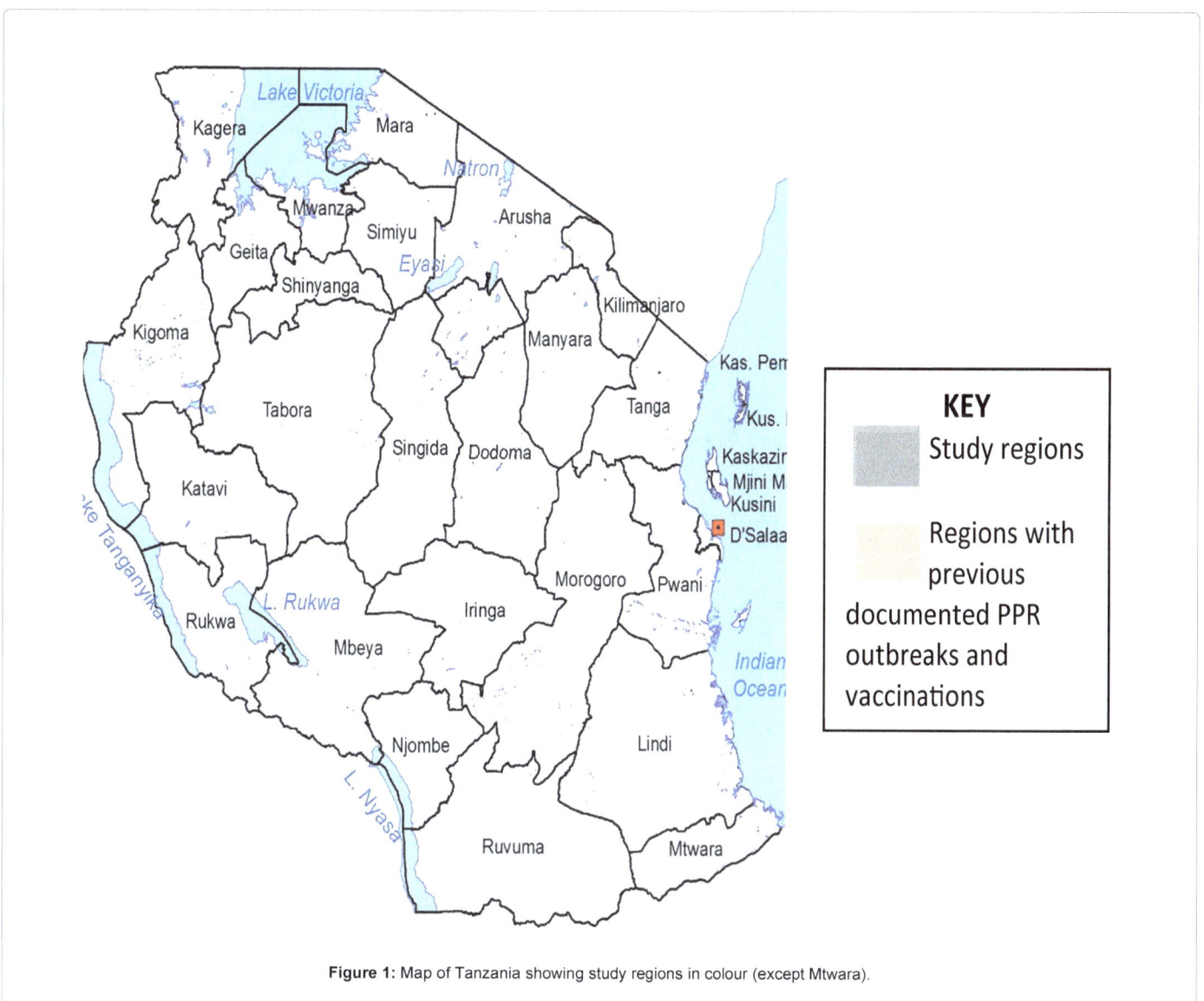

Figure 1: Map of Tanzania showing study regions in colour (except Mtwara).

Region	Districts (Villages)	Goats			Sheep			Total		
		Total	Positive (%)	TP (95% CI)	Total	Positive (%)	TP (95% CI)	Total	Positive (%)	TP (95% CI)
Morogoro	2 (10)	178	124 (69.7)	73.5 (66.4 - 81.7)	38	25 (65.8)	69.4 (53.4 - 85.5)	216	149 (70.0)	72.8 (66.3 - 79.4)
Shinyanga	3 (4)	217	16 (7.4)	7.2 (3.5 - 10.9)	33	0 (0)	<0	250	16 (6.4)	6.2 (2.9 - 9.4)
Coastal	3 (14)	310	90 (29.0)	30.3 (24.9 - 35.7)	41	13 (31.7)	33.1 (18 - 48.3)	351	103 (29.3)	30.6 (25.5 - 35.7)
Simiyu	3 (7)	202	15 (7.4)	7.3 (3.4 - 11.1)	59	6 (10.2)	10.2 (2 - 18.4)	261	21 (8.1)	7.9 (4.4 - 11.4)
Kagera	3 (16)	198	6 (3.0)	2.6 (0 - 5.1)	12	0 (0)	<0	210	6 (2.9)	2.4 (0 - 4.8)
Mwanza	7 (23)	414	15 (3.6)	3.2 (1.3 - 5.1)	92	0 (0)	<0	506	15 (3.0)	2.5 (0.9 - 4.1)
Kilimanjaro	1 (5)	80	29 (36.3)	38 (26.7 - 49.2)	66	12 (18.2)	18.7 (8.8 - 28.6)	146	41 (28.1)	29.3 (21.5 - 37)
Manyara	1 (5)	92	67 (72.8)	76.9 (67.2 - 86.6)	55	30 (54.5)	57.4 (43.4 - 71.5)	147	97 (66.0)	69.6 (61.5 - 77.8)
Arusha	1 (5)	97	66 (68.0)	71.8 (61.8 - 81.7)	56	37 (66.1)	69.7 (56.5 - 82.9)	153	103 (67.3)	71.1 (63.1 - 79)
Dodoma	3 (12)	420	240 (57.1)	60.2 (55.2 - 65.3)	180	104 (57.8)	60.9 (53.2 - 68.6)	600	344 (57.3)	60.4 (56.2 - 64.6)
Singida	2 (8)	167	39 (23.4)	24.2 (17.4 - 31.1)	79	0 (0)	<0	246	39 (15.9)	16.2 (11.4 - 21.1)
Tabora	3 (3)	245	31 (12.7)	12.8 (8.4 - 17.3)	115	11 (9.6)	9.5 (3.8 - 15.3)	360	41 (11.4)	11.5 (8 - 15)
Katavi	3 (3)	130	5 (3.8)	3.5 (-0.1 - 7)	62	0 (0)	<0	192	5 (2.6)	2.1 (-0.3 - 4.5)
Kigoma	3 (3)	136	16 (11.8)	11.9 (6.1 - 17.7)	64	2 (3.1)	2.7 (-1.9 - 7.2)	200	18 (9.0)	8.9 (4.7 - 13.2)
Total	**38 (118)**	**2 886**	**759 (26.3)**	**27.4 (25.7 - 29.1)**	**952**	**240 (25.2)**	**26.2 (23.3 - 29.1)**	**3 838**	**998 (26.0)**	**27.1 (25.6 - 28.5)**

Total: total number of animals sampled, Positive: number of animals tested positive with percentage given in parenthesis, TP: true prevalence with 95% confidence interval in parenthesis.

Table 1: Regions where serum samples from sheep and goats were collected in Tanzania.

Results

From 3,838 serum samples tested, 998 (26.0%) were positive; 759 (26.3%) of 2 886 from goats and 240 (25.2%) of 952 from sheep were positive (Table 2 and Figure 2). Overall true seroprevalence was 27.1% (95% CI, 25.6-28.5) and seroprevalence for goats and sheep was 27.4% (95% CI, 25.7-29.1) and 26.2% (95% CI, 23.3-29.1), respectively. Morogoro region had the highest overall seroprevalence (72.8%, 66.3-79.4) of antibodies against PPRV while Katavi region had the lowest (2.1%, -0.3-4.5). The odds of being seropositive to PPR was 1.06 (95% CI 0.89-1.25) times higher in goats compared to sheep, a figure that is not statistically significant (Table 3).

Discussion

This study shows that PPR was widely prevalent in small ruminants in the study areas. All regions had seropositive cases. The overall observed seroprevalence (27.1%, 25.6-28.5) (Table 2) is low compared to previous reports from northern and southern Tanzania performed in 2009 at 45.4% [11] and 2012 at 31.0% [13] respectively. There is a statistical significance (p<0.05) between the studies and years. This difference may be attributed to vaccination campaigns (Figure 1). Though the seroprevalence is low, the figure is highly significant in a

country with an estimated population of sheep around 8 million and goats around 16.7 million [17].

Though some regions registered seroprevalence of less than 20% (Figure 2), this indicates that PPR is widely prevalent in small ruminants in areas where the study was conducted. Data from studies in west, east and central Africa indicate that PPRV antibodies can be widespread among goats and sheep flocks raised in the tropics [9,3,18,19]. Studies also indicate cELISA as a preferred diagnostic test for screening antibodies against the PPRV. This is because the test is simple, rapid, specific and sensitive for intensive surveillance [20]. Screening for antibodies against PPRV in different geographical areas of a country with varying climatic conditions has been helpful in developing disease control strategies [21]. Hence these results can be helpful to government officials in developing control strategies for Tanzania.

The seropositivity difference between sheep and goats remains unclear in literature. In this study, prevalence between the two species was sheep 26.2% and goats 27.4%. The odds of being seropositive were 1.06 (95% CI 0.89-1.25) in goats than in sheep, which implies there is no difference between the species. This is in contradiction with some studies, including one carried out in Tanzania [11], which reported a

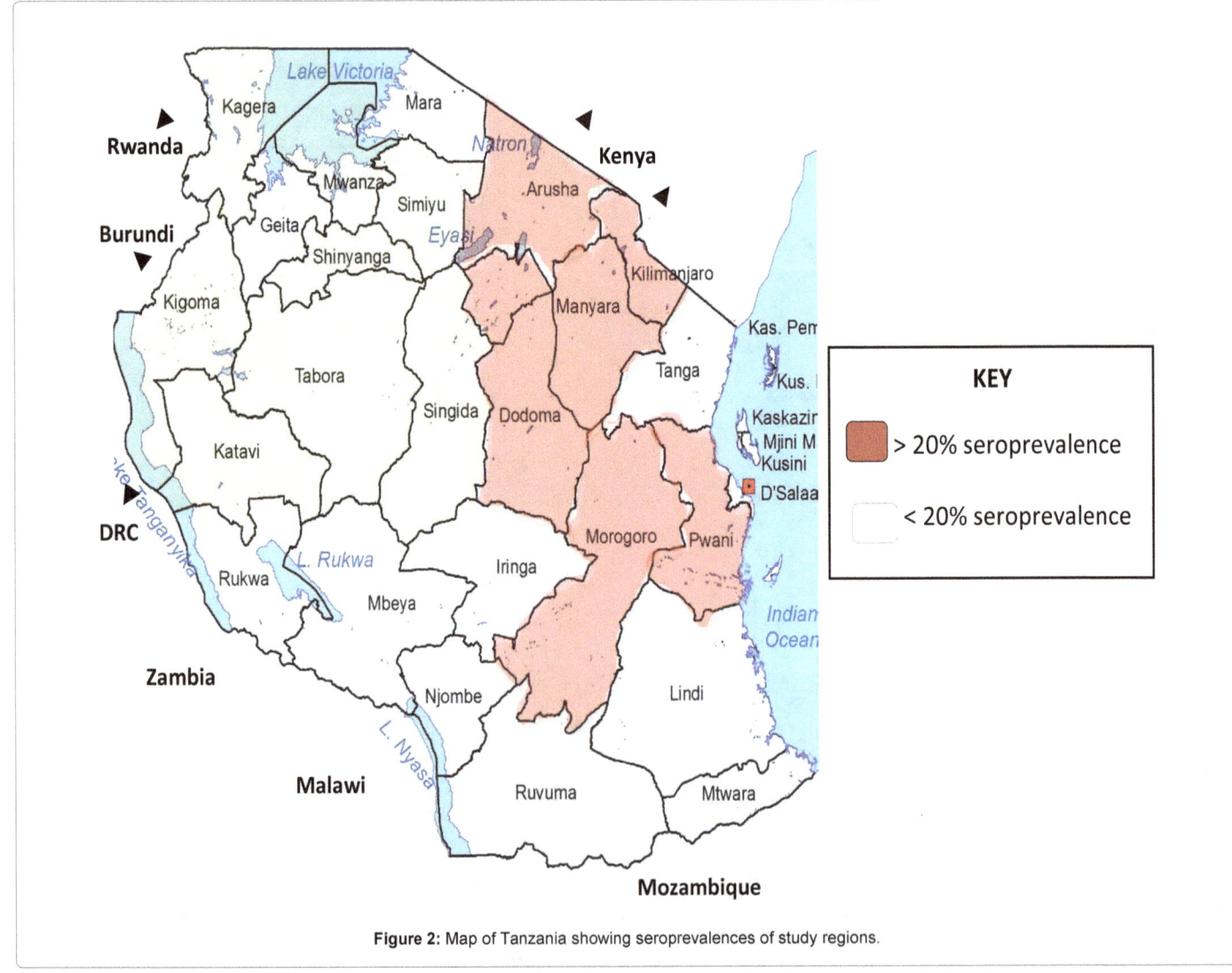

Figure 2: Map of Tanzania showing seroprevalences of study regions.

Region	Year collected	Sheep	Goats	Total
Morogoro	2013	38	178	216
Shinyanga	2013	33	217	250
Coastal	2013	41	310	351
Simiyu	2013	59	202	261
Kagera	2013	12	198	210
Mwanza	2013	92	414	506
Kilimanjaro	2015	66	80	146
Manyara	2015	55	92	147
Arusha	2015	56	97	153
Dodoma	2013	180	420	600
Singida	2013	79	167	246
Tabora	2013	115	245	360
Katavi	2013	62	130	192
Kigoma	2013	64	136	200
Total		952	2886	3838

Table 2: Regional seroprevalence of antibodies against PPRV in goats and sheep in Tanzania.

Variable	Odds ratio	95% CI	P value
Species (goats vs sheep)	1.06	0.89-1.25	0.507

Table 3: Association of species and being seropositive for PPR.

higher seroprevalence in goats than in sheep and linked it to higher fecundity in goats compared to sheep [2,18,22]. Other studies have reported higher seroprevalence in sheep than goats, attributing it to lower number of sheep sampled or due to the fact that goats are often affected more severely by the disease hence die prior to sampling [19,23]. Therefore, more investigations are needed to further determine the variation between the species.

In 2008 and 2010, PPR vaccination was carried out around the 2008 outbreak foci (Arusha region) with another vaccination ring in Morogoro and Mtwara regions, shown in Figure 1 [24]. Arusha and Mtwara regions were chosen because they had already been seen as hotspot areas while Morogoro region acted as a buffer zone for spread of the disease from south (Mtwara region) to north. The use of antibiotics in managing clinical cases is also believed to increase survival rate of sick animals [8] thus the surviving animals will carry antibodies against PPRV. These two factors may have contributed to the high seroprevalence because cELISA cannot discriminate from previously PPRV infected animals and vaccinated animals. Small ruminants vaccinated on a large scale with PPR vaccines will still test positive for antibodies against PPRV [25]. Despite this, presence of antibodies against PPR in regions that previously were thought to be free and no vaccinations have been performed, such as Mwanza, Shinyanga, Kigoma and Tabora, indicates that the disease is spreading (Figure 2). The data means future vaccinations should cover all regions of the country and not concentrate in known high risk areas. Small ruminants are easily moved especially for sale in markets. Live animal markets are an important vehicle for transmission of infectious diseases [25]. This was demonstrated in a study [13] that found out that lack of appropriate veterinary services and inadequate infrastructure especially in the local animal markets in Tanzania may be facilitating transmission of PPR. Trade also brings about livestock theft that has been found to play a major role in maintaining transmission of infectious diseases in many areas of East Africa [19].

In conclusion, this study has confirmed the presence of PPR in regions of Tanzania that previously had little to no data on the disease. This is a step forward to getting information about the disease situation that can help to properly put into place systems and proper control

measures to improve animal welfare and reduce episodes of disease outbreaks.

Acknowledgements

We would like to thank the Ministry of Livestock and Fisheries Development (MLFD) and District Veterinary Officers for sera collection. We also thank Miriam Richard Makange, Clara Yona and Margot Coudijzer for their help during sample analysis. The author is sponsored by a grant from the Wellcome Trust to the Southern African Centre for Infectious Disease Surveillance, SACIDS (grant WT087546MA), Swedish Research Council (grant nos. 348-2013-6402 and 348-2014-4293) and Sokoine University of Agriculture. The opinions expressed herein are those of the authors and do not necessarily reflect the view of Sokoine University of Agriculture.

Conflict of Interest Statement

The authors declare that there is no conflict of interests regarding the publication of this article.

References

1. Abubakar M, Rasool MH, Manzoor S, Saqalein M, Rizwan M, et al. (2016) Evaluation of Risk Factors for Peste des Petits Ruminants Virus in Sheep and Goats at the Wildlife-Livestock Interface in Punjab Province, Pakistan. BioMed Res Int 2016: 7826245.

2. Zahur AB, Ullah A, Hussain M, Irshad H, Hameed A, et al. (2011) Sero-epidemiology of peste des petits ruminants (PPR) in Pakistan. Prevent Vet Med 102: 87-92.

3. Banyard AC, Parida S, Batten C, Oura C, Kwiatek O, et al. (2010) Global distribution of peste des petits ruminants virus and prospects for improved diagnosis and control. J Gen Virol 91: 2885-2897.

4. Gargadennec L, Lalanne A (1942) La peste des petits ruminants. Bull Serv Zoo AOF 5: 15-21.

5. Abraham G, Sintayehu A, Libeau G, Albina E, Roger F, et al. (2005) Antibody seroprevalences against peste des petits ruminants (PPR) virus in camels, cattle, goats and sheep in Ethiopia. Prevent Vet Med 70: 51-57.

6. Libeau G, Diallo A, Parida S (2014) Evolutionary genetics underlying the spread of peste des petits ruminants virus. Anim Front 4: 14-20.

7. Karimuribo ED, Loomu PM, Mellau LSB, Swai ES (2011) Retrospective study on sero-epidemiology of peste des petits ruminants before its official confirmation in northern Tanzania in 2008. Res Opin Anim Vet Sci 1: 184-187.

8. Wambura PN (2000) Serological evidence of the absence of peste des petits ruminants in Tanzania. Vet Rec 146: 473-474.

9. Kivaria FM, Kwiatek O, Kapaga AM, Geneviève L, Mpelumbe-Ngeleja CAR, et al. (2009) Serological and virological investigations on an emerging Peste des Petits Ruminants Virus infection in sheep and goats in Tanzania. Proceedings of the 27th Tanzania Veterinary Association Scientific Conference.

10. Swai ES, Kapaga A, Kivaria F, Tinuga D, Joshua G, et al. (2009) Prevalence and distribution of Peste des petits ruminants virus antibodies in various districts of Tanzania. Vet Res Commun 33: 927-936.

11. Kivaria FM, Kwiatek O, Kapaga AM, Swai ES, Libeau G, et al. (2013) The incursion, persistence and spread of peste des petits ruminants in Tanzania: Epidemiological patterns and predictions. Onderstepoort J Vet Res 80: 01-10.

12. Muse EA, Karimuribo ED, Gitao GC, Misinzo G, Mellau LS, et al. (2012) Epidemiological investigation into the introduction and factors for spread of Peste des Petits Ruminants, southern Tanzania. Onderstepoort J Vet Res 79: 49-54.

13. Rogan WJ, Gladen B (1978) Estimating prevalence from the results of a screening test. Am J Epidemiol 107: 71-76.

14. Libeau G, Prehaud C, Lancelot R, Colas F, Guerre L, et al. (1995) Development of a competitive ELISA for detecting antibodies to the peste des petits ruminants virus using a recombinant nucleobrotein. Res Vet Sci 58: 50-55.

15. Altman DG (1991) Practical statistics for medical research, Chapman and Hall, London.

16. http://www.mifugouvuvi.go.tz/wp-content/uploads/2015/10/TLMI-electronic.pdf

17. Abdalla AS, Majok AA, El Malik KH, Ali AS (2012) Sero-prevalence of peste des petits ruminants virus (PPRV) in small ruminants in Blue Nile, Gadaref and North Kordofan States of Sudan. J Public Health Epidemiol 4: 59-64.

18. Megersa B, Biffa D, Belina T, Debela E, Regassa A, et al. (2011) Serological investigation of Peste des Petits Ruminants (PPR) in small ruminants managed under pastoral and agro-pastoral systems in Ethiopia. Small Rumin Res 97: 134-138.

19. Singh RP, Sreenivasa BP, Dhar P, Shah LC, Bandyopadhyay SK (2004) Development of a monoclonal antibody based competitive-ELISA for detection and titration of antibodies to peste des petits ruminants (PPR) virus. Vet Microbiol 98: 3-15.

20. Balamurugan V, Saravanan P, Sen A, Rajak KK, Bhanuprakash V, et al. (2011) Sero-epidemiological study of peste des petits ruminants in sheep and goats in India between 2003 and 2009. Rev Sci Tech 30: 889-896.

21. Rashid A, Asim M, Hussain A (2008) Seroprevalence of peste des petits ruminants (PPR) virus in goats, sheep and cattle at livestock production research institute Bahadurnagar Okara. J Anim Plant Sci 18: 114-116.

22. Khan HA, Siddique M, Arshad MJ, Khan QM, Rehman SU (2007) Sero-prevalence of peste des petits ruminants (PPR) virus in sheep and goats in Punjab province of Pakistan. Pakistan Vet J 27: 109-112.

23. Ministry of Livestock and Fisheries Development (2013) Peste des petits ruminants (PPR) progressive control and eradication strategy. The United Republic of Tanzania.

24. Libeau G (2015) Current Advances in Serological Diagnosis of Peste des Petits Ruminants Virus. In: Peste des Petits Ruminants Virus. Springer Berlin Heidelberg, Pp: 133-154.

25. Domenech J, Lubroth J, Eddi C, Martin V, Roger F (2006) Regional and international approaches on prevention and control of animal transboundary and emerging diseases. Ann NY Acad Sci 1081: 90-107.

14

Results from a U.S. Dog Owner Survey on the Treatment Satisfaction and Preference for Fluralaner against Flea and Tick Infestations

Robert P Lavan[1]*, Robert Armstrong[2], Dorothy Normile[3], Dongmu Zhang[4] and Kaan Tunceli[4]

[1]*Outcomes Research, Animal Health Center for Observational and Real-World Evidence, Merck & Co. Inc., Kenilworth, NJ 07033, USA*
[2]*Animal Health Global Marketing, Merck & Co. Inc., Madison, NJ 07940, USA*
[3]*Animal Health Technical Services, Merck & Co. Inc., Madison, NJ 07940, USA*
[4]*Center for Observational and Real-World Evidence, Merck & Co. Inc., Kenilworth, NJ 07033, USA*

Abstract

Background: Fluralaner is a potent acaricide and insecticide effective against flea and tick (F/T) infestations on dogs and cats. Fluralaner for dogs can be administered orally as a flavored chew with up to a 12-week re-dosing interval, about three-fold less frequently than monthly F/T medications. This study surveyed dog owners who currently administer fluralaner to their dogs to determine their level of satisfaction with the product and its perceived benefits compared to monthly medications, including the potential for on-time administration compliance.

Methods: In the period April to June 2016, dog-owner clients from 25 veterinary practices in 16 U.S. states completed a 10-item survey questionnaire (n=559) that asked respondents about their experience with fluralaner and monthly medications. In multivariate analyses, predictors of treatment satisfaction and predictors of preference with fluralaner have been estimated by an ordered logistic regression and a logistic regression, respectively.

Results: Seventy-three percent of survey respondents had used monthly F/T medications prior to fluralaner. Respondents identified convenience (74%), the 12-week dosing interval (69%), and less-frequent dosing (68%) as the three most important benefits of using fluralaner. Sixty six percent were very satisfied and 30% were satisfied with fluralaner and 89% preferred fluralaner versus monthly F/T medications. Pet owners who used monthly F/T products, 65% thought that they were more likely to give the next fluralaner dose on time compared to doses of monthly F/T products, and 88% said that giving repeat doses of fluralaner was more convenient than giving monthly F/T products. In multivariable models, "12 weeks dosing/convenience" and "female gender" were positively associated with treatment satisfaction and preference with fluralaner (*p*<0.05).

Conclusions: Overall satisfaction with fluralaner and preference for fluralaner compared to monthly F/T medications were high. The most significant factor predicting satisfaction and preference was perceived benefit with 12 weeks dosing or convenience.

Keywords: Bravecto; Canine; Compliance; Fleas; Ticks; Ectoparasite; Ectoparasiticide; Acaricide; Insecticide; Isoxazoline

Background

Canine flea-and-tick (F/T) medications in the United States are generally owner-administered and available for purchase from veterinarians or other retail locations. At this time, the isoxazoline class of F/T medications, including afoxolaner, fluralaner, and sarolaner, are only available by prescription through veterinarians. The high environmental and host prevalence and persistence of the target parasites, their role in flea allergy dermatitis (FAD) and vector-borne diseases, and the routine movement of infested dogs into previously non-endemic urban and suburban areas are factors that support the importance of ectoparasite control [1-3]. There is a wide assortment of approved oral and topical canine F/T medications with various modes of action and in various combinations, including some with insect growth regulator activity and some with canine heartworm (HW) indications. Fluralaner is a recently approved active ingredient in the isoxazoline class available in oral chewable formulation (Fluralaner, Merck Animal Health, Madison, NJ, USA) for dogs and a topical formulation for dogs and cats [4,5]. The fluralaner re-treatment interval is three times longer than the re-treatment interval for other flea/tick products that are dosed every 4 weeks. Fluralaner offers a new approach to canine F/T control, based on rapid and persistent acaricidal and insecticidal activity [6-8].

Clinical trials have demonstrated the ectoparasitic efficacy of fluralaner as a gamma-aminobutyric acid (GABA) and glutamate-gated chloride channel inhibitor with potent selectivity for arthropod

neuron receptors, resulting in excess neuronal stimulation and rapid insect death after feeding exposure [9,10]. After oral ingestion by the dog, fluralaner is rapidly absorbed and widely distributed, with a long half-life of 12-15 days. Fluralaner undergoes negligible host metabolism and is primarily excreted unchanged in the feces [11].

Fluralaner safety in dogs has been extensively evaluated, including dose tolerance studies with administration at up to five times the maximum label dose [4,12,13]. Fluralaner is unusual in the isoxazoline class of ectoparasiticides in that it has sustained activity that allows 12 week re-dosing [4] while the other isoxazolines are re-dosed at 4 week intervals.

Poor compliance is a leading cause of treatment failure in F/T and HW control as has been shown for other therapeutic regimens

*Corresponding author: Robert P Lavan, Outcomes Research, Animal Health Center for Observational and Real-World Evidence, Merck & Co. Inc., Kenilworth, NJ 07033, USA, E-mail: robert.lavan@merck.com

in veterinary and human medicine [14-17]. Compliance shortfalls are primarily influenced by the complexity and convenience of the therapeutic protocol. For example, Canadian investigators found that compliance declined significantly as the number of antimicrobial doses administered by dog owners increased [18]. Dog owners who were asked to give oral antimicrobial drugs once or twice daily to their dogs were nine times more likely to be fully compliant compared with owners who were asked to treat three-times daily. Similarly, in a European study, only 44% of dog owners (n=95) were fully compliant with a 10-day course of oral anti-infective therapy [19]. These results show that extended, multi-dose regimens are inherently more likely to be associated with missed doses and lack of on-time dosing. Simpler, less frequent dosing is directly related to better compliance across all therapeutic classes [20].

Monthly (or every 4 weeks) administration of oral or topical canine F/T and HW medications is common in companion animal veterinary practice and has become a standard dosing schedule. However, even a monthly dosing frequency does not lead to a high level of compliance in using these parasiticides, which are recommended for year round administration by animal health groups [21,22]. Recent data for canine patients (n=1,271) presented at a U.S. veterinary teaching hospital found that 74% were being treated with F/T preventive products and only 61% of those (45% of total population) received the products year around [16]. The authors considered this level of compliance for veterinary referral center patients to be much higher than that for the general dog population and suggested that improvement in owner compliance with treatment recommendations could provide better F/T control.

Using a cohort of dog owners who have recent experience giving fluralaner to their dogs, the objectives of this study were:

➢ To use a survey to assess treatment satisfaction and preference in dog owners that have given at least two doses of fluralaner and may have also given shorter acting (monthly) ectoparasiticides to their dogs.

➢ Describe predictors of satisfaction and preference.

➢ Assess dog owner difficulty adapting to 12 week dosing.

The survey included pet owners from geographically diverse regions of the U.S., including F/T endemic areas of the Eastern, Central, Southeastern and Western United States. Veterinarians in each of these clinics were also asked to provide the number of months that they routinely recommend flea/tick protection for their canine patients.

Methods

Survey population

Twenty-six veterinarians from 24 practices located in 16 states in various regions of the U.S. participated in the study (Table 1) during the period April to June, 2016. The veterinarians averaged 17.4 years in practice and included 11 male and 15 female practitioners. Each participating practice recruited dog owners whose pets were currently being treated with fluralaner and who had purchased ≥ 2 doses, and invited them to complete the survey questionnaire. Practices that dispensed various F/T products in addition to fluralaner were included in the study. Dog owners had various experiences with the prior use of flea and tick products although all were currently giving fluralaner to their dogs.

559 dog owners completed survey questionnaires after providing information on their age (10-year age block), gender, years as a

caretaker for their dog as well as their experience with fleas and ticks. Information for each dog included the dog's age, gender and neutering status, bodyweight, health assessment, summary of outdoor activities and time spent outdoors (Table 2).

Survey instrument

The dog owner questionnaire consisted of 10 questions related to utilization of F/T products, as shown in Table 3. The survey was developed and pretested in an iterative review process. Several survey questions invited the responder to make free-text written comments, thus providing an opportunity for more detailed, specific or alternate responses. The survey was designed to be completed in <5 minutes and was administered while they were in the veterinary clinic or by telephone if they had recently been in the clinic. The first survey question allowed the identification of a dog owner cohort subset who had used prior F/T products in addition to fluralaner. This cohort was particularly valuable in providing responses to questions 7-10 which compared 12 week dosing (fluralaner) to 4 week dosing (other monthly F/T products).

Data analysis

Responses to each survey question were examined for differences by pet owner gender, age, years as dog caretaker, geographic region, dog outdoor time and outdoor activities as well as the pet owners' F/T experience. Descriptive statistics (number/percentage or mean/SD) were used to describe responses for each survey question. All statistical analyses were performed using SAS version 9.3 (SAS Institute, Cary, NC). Significances of differences between variables were determined by analysis of variance (ANOVA) or Chi-Square test with values of $P<0.05$ considered statistically significant. Ordered logistic regression was

U.S. Region	Practices (#)	Surveys (#)	Participating veterinarians (#)	Mean years in practice
Northeast (NY, OH, PA)	4	92	5	6.0 ± 4.2
Central (AR, IL, IN, KS, KY, MO)	8	192	8	16.0 ± 8.6
South (AL, FL, GA, TX)	9	191	9	22.8 ± 10.6
West (AZ, CA, HI)	3	84	4	19.5 ± 1.4
Total	24	559	26	17.4 ± 10.7

Table 1: Location of veterinary practices participating in the dog-owner treatment satisfaction survey.

Population characteristics	Description
Owner Demographic Factors	
Gender	390 f, 140 m
Age 10-49 years	232 (41.5%)
50-69 years	223 (39.9%)
70+ years	41 (7.3%)
Years as Dog's Caretaker (Mean(SD))	5.5 (3.6)
Canine Demographic Factors	
Gender	288 m, 270 f
Neutered or spayed	89%
Age (Mean)	6.1 years
Owner reports good or excellent health	92%
Flea-and-tick exposure risk factors	
Ave. time spent outdoors	4.2 hours/day
Swims	1 in 4
Goes to dog park	1 in 3
Has access to woods	1 in 2.5
Walks off leash or has access to high or uncut grass	1 in 2
Owner reported seeing fleas on their dogs	41%
Owner reported seeing ticks on their dogs	31%
Owner reported seeing ticks on family members	11%

Table 2: Demographic profile and ectoparasite exposure risk factors for participating owners and their dogs.

Survey question and response options	Response rate	
Q1. Have you used flea-tick control products other than Fluralaner in the past?		
	% (n) dog owners (n=553 respondents)	
Yes	73 (406)	
No	20 (108)	
Don't know	7 (39)	
Q2. What is your level of satisfaction with Fluralaner?		
	% (n) dog owners (n=544 respondents)	
Very satisfied	66 (361)	
Satisfied	30 (161)	
Neutral	3 (19)	
Unsatisfied or very unsatisfied	1 (3)	
Q3. Which Fluralaner benefits are important to you (indicate any that apply)?		
	% (n) dog owners (n=559 respondents)	
Convenience	72 (405)	
12-week dosing interval	67 (373)	
Dosing less often than before	67 (372)	
Quickly kills F/Ts	45 (253)	
Easier dosing creates less stress	45 (251)	
Palatability	43 (240)	
Q4. If you had to select one benefit, which one is most important reason to use Fluralaner?		
	% (n) dog owners (n=559 respondents)	
12-week dosing interval	23 (131)	
Convenience	19 (106)	
Dosing less often	18 (102)	
Quickly kills F/Ts	17 (96)	
Easier dosing creates less stress	9 (49)	
Palatability	4% (25)	
Q5. Does using a product that lasts 12 weeks have an advantage over F/T products that require monthly dosing (indicate all that apply)?		
	% (n) of all dog owners (n=559 respondents)	% (n) of dog owners who have used Fluralaner and other F/T products (n=406 respondents)
Dogs is less likely to get fleas	54 (302)	54 (221)
Owner is less likely to forget a dose	52 (288)	53 (215)
Owner can give treatment less often	47 (263)	46 (188)
Dog is less likely to get ticks	44 (244)	44 (177)
Dog is less likely to bring fleas-ticks into house	41 (230)	42 (171)
Dog is more likely to be protected when it matters	35 (193)	34 (139)
Dog is less likely to itch	30 (169)	30 (123)
Q6. When you use Fluralaner during a given F/T season, is there a delay beyond the recommended 12-weeks in giving the next dose? I give the next dose:		
	% (n) dog owners (n=509 respondents)	
Mostly on time	75 (380)	
Delayed by a few days	17 (86)	
Delayed by weeks	6 (31)	
Delayed by months	2 (12)	
Q7. Are you more likely to give the next Fluralaner dose on time compared to monthly F/T products?		
	% (n) dog owners who have used Fluralaner and other F/T products (n=381 respondents)	
Yes	65 (246)	
No	4 (15)	
About the same	27 (102)	
Don't know	4 (18)	
Q8. With Fluralaner, my dog has (fewer/same/more) months of F/T protection in a year.		
	% (n) dog owners who have used Fluralaner and other F/T products (n=335 respondents)	
Fewer	8 (26)	
Same	56 (189)	
More	36 (120)	
Q9. Is it (more/equally/less) convenient to give repeat doses of Fluralaner than repeat doses of a monthly F/T product?		
	% (n) dog owners who have used Fluralaner and other F/T products (n=382 respondents)	
More	89 (339)	

Equally	10 (39)
Less	1 (4)
Q10. Do you prefer Fluralaner to other F/T product you have used?	
	% (n) dog owners who have used Fluralaner and other F/T products (n=383 respondents)
Yes	89 (341)
No	1 (5)
About the same	10 (37)

Table 3: Dog owner responses to a flea-and-tick (F/T) treatment survey.

used to understand the factors associated with pet owners' satisfaction of Bravecto. Satisfaction was measured as three levels: very satisfied, satisfied, and none-satisfied. Ordered logistic regression is an ordinal regression model-that is, a regression model for ordinal dependent variables. It is an extension of the logistic regression model that applies to dichotomous dependent variables, allowing for more than two ordered response categories. Binomial logistic regression was used to explore the factors associated with pet owners' preference of Bravecto. Preference was measured as two levels: Preferred *vs.* Non-preferred. The examined factors include pet owners' age, gender, number of years as a caregiver of the dog, seeing flee/tick on the dog, seeing tick on family members, identifying '12 weeks of dosing' or 'convenience' as one of Bravecto's benefits, dogs' age, weight, number of hours spending outside. Significant differences were noted with values of P<0.05.

Results

On average, veterinarians from 24 practices in 16 states reported that they recommended 12 months of flea and tick protection for their canine patients. Only two veterinarians had different opinions related to year-round coverage. One veterinarian in the Southern region recommended 9 months of tick control and one veterinarian in the Northeast region recommended 8 months of flea control.

Five hundred fifty nine pet owners submitted completed surveys although not all pet owners chose to answer every question. Survey respondents (Table 2) were most often female (70%, n=390) and in the 50-59 year age block and as seen from survey question 1, frequently were familiar with F/T medications other than Fluralaner (73%, 406/553).

The demographic profile of the canine patients is shown in Table 2. The canine population was evenly divided between male and female dogs, the great majority of which were neutered or spayed and in good or excellent health. The dogs had a relatively high risk of F/T exposure as indicated by access to various outdoor settings, an average of 4.2 hours/day spent outdoors, and a high percentage of on-animal ectoparasite sightings. Owners reported seeing fleas or ticks on their dogs in 41% and 31% of the cases, respectively, and 11% reported seeing ticks on family members.

A summary of responses are shown for the 10 survey questions (Table 3). While all participating pet owners were encouraged to answer all questions, the responses for a subset of pet owners who had used other flea/tick products were used to address questions 5 and 7 through 10, particularly because these questions compared current fluralaner use with prior use of F/T products that were dosed monthly.

The majority of dog-owners (96%) were either "satisfied" (30%) or "very satisfied" (66%) with their fluralaner experience. In the ordered logistic regression analysis of predictors of satisfaction (Table 4), female pet owners were significantly more likely to be "satisfied" compared to male pet owners (P=0.004), pet owners over 70 years of age were

less likely to be satisfied (P=0.036) compared to younger pet owners and pet owners who selected "12 week dosing" or "convenience" as preferred features of fluralaner were significantly more likely (P=0.001) to be satisfied compared to pet owners who has not selected "12 week dosing" or "convenience" after adjusting other variables in the model.

Questions 3 and 4 asked responders to identify any benefits they associated with using fluralaner. A majority of participating dog owners most often selected convenience (72%), 12-week dosing (67%), and dosing less often (67%) as important perceived benefits of fluralaner. Less frequently, respondents selected choices related to flea efficacy and their responsibility for giving the next dose on time. When asked about advantages associated with a longer lasting F/T product (question 5), dog owners most frequently chose responses related to "dog is less likely to get fleas" and "owner is less likely to forget a dose". Several questions (Questions 6-9) asked about the pet owner experience with 12 week dosing. Three quarters (75%) of dog owners stated that they thought that they gave fluralaner on time (question 6) and 17% reported that they administered the next dose with a few days delay suggesting that most pet owners thought that fluralaner was given in a more-or-less timely fashion (92% combined).

Questions 7-10 responses were drawn from dog owners who had used monthly F/T products in the past. Most respondents (65%) thought that they were more likely to give the next fluralaner dose on time compared to follow-on dose of monthly flea and tick medications (question 7). An smaller proportion (27%) said that they would be as just as likely to administer a dose of fluralaner on time as they would a dose of a monthly F/T medications. In terms of perceived months of F/T protection that their dogs received (question 8), approximately half of dog owners reported that their dogs got the same number of months of coverage, while approximately 1/3 of respondents thought that their dogs got more months of coverage with fluralaner. Most respondents (89%) found fluralaner to be more convenient (question 9) and preferred fluralaner compared to monthly F/T medications (question 10).

In the binary logistic regression analysis of predictors of preference (Table 5), female pet owners were significantly more likely to prefer fluralaner over monthly F/T products compared to male pet owners (P=0.047) and pet owners who selected "12 week dosing" or "convenience" as preferred features of fluralaner were significantly more likely (P=0.002) to prefer fluralaner compared to monthly F/T products after adjusting the other variables.

Discussion

Most veterinarians in this study recommended 12 months of flea and tick coverage for their canine patients. Ectoparasite exposure can be seasonal in the United States, depending on the region and harshness of the winter. In recent years, flea and tick control has been more important year-round because of the mildness and warming of

Variable	Value	Odds Ratio	95% CI	p-value
Owner gender	Male	Reference		
	Female	1.930	(1.241,3.002)	0.004
Owner age	10-49	Reference		
	50-69	0.843	(0.540,1.316)	0.453
	70+	0.454	(0.218,0.948)	0.036
Flea on the dog	No	Reference		
	Yes	0.779	(0.505,1.202)	0.259
Tick on the dog	No	Reference		
	Yes	0.934	(0.582,1.497)	0.775
Tick on family	No	Reference		
	Yes	1.232	(0.625,2.428)	0.547
Owner yrs of care		0.933	(0.821,1.059)	0.283
Dog age		1.030	(0.909,1.168)	0.643
Dog weight		0.997	(0.991,1.004)	0.459
Dog out door hours		1.013	(0.969,1.059)	0.575
12 Week dosing or convenience	No	Reference		
	Yes	2.754	(1.533,4.947)	0.001

*Treatment Satisfaction Categories: Very Satisfied, Satisfied, and Non-satisfied. Interpretation of odds ratios in the ordered logistic model: In the example with gender variable, 1.930 is the proportional odds ratio of comparing females to males on satisfaction adjusted with all other variables in the model. For females, the odds of very satisfied versus the combined satisfied and non-satisfied are 1.930 times higher than for males. Likewise, the odds of the combined categories of very satisfied and satisfied versus non-satisfied is also 1.930 times higher for females compared to males.

N=450 after excluding the pet owners with missing values for any of the variables

Table 4: Predictors of Pet Owners Satisfaction*.

Variable	Value	Odds Ratio	95% CI	p-value
Owner gender	Male	Reference		
	Female	1.977	(1.009,3.876)	0.047
Owner age	10-49	Reference		
	50-69	0.704	(0.348,1.425)	0.330
	70+	0.604	(0.195,1.867)	0.381
Flea on the dog	No	Reference		
	Yes	1.514	(0.745,3.076)	0.251
Tick on the dog	No	Reference		
	Yes	1.598	(0.711,3.591)	0.257
Tick on family	No	Reference		
	Yes	0.584	(0.226,1.510)	0.267
Owner yrs of care		0.846	(0.659,1.085)	0.188
Dog age		1.125	(0.874,1.447)	0.361
Dog weight		1.005	(0.994,1.016)	0.389
Dog out door hours		1.013	(0.936,1.096)	0.749
12 Week dosing or convenience	No	Reference		
	Yes	3.355	(1.564,7.198)	0.002

* Preferred: 1, Non-preferred: 0
N=450 after excluding the pet owners with missing values for any of the variables

Table 5: Predictors of Pet Owners' Preference.

the winters. In regions like the Southern and Western United States, ectoparasites are routinely found outdoors all year long. The year-round need for ectoparasite control is reflected in the recommendation by the U.S. veterinarians.

The dogs in this study faced assorted risks of flea and tick exposure, including an average of 4.2 hours a day spent outdoors and access to wooded or grassy areas in ≥ 40% of the cases. Seventy three percent of pet owners in this study indicated that they had used flea and tick control products other than fluralaner in the past and thus were well suited to render an informed opinion on the relative perceived merits of F/T medications.

The study participant pool was approximately 3/4 female / 1/4 male with the highest proportion of pet owners in the "middle aged" groups.

This may be more typical of the pet owner demographic that brings the dog to the clinic. The majority of pet owners were satisfied (30%) or very satisfied (60%) with their experience using fluralaner. It appears to be "12 week dosing" or "convenience" is an important perceived benefit for satisfaction with fluralaner. It is not clear why female pet owners were more likely to be satisfied compared to male pet owners. It is also not clear why older pet owners (70 years of age and older versus youngest age category "<49 years") were significantly less likely to be satisfied with fluralaner. Nevertheless, satisfaction was high across all age groups, regardless of the age of the pet owner or number of years that they had been the dog caretaker.

The three benefits of fluralaner that were most often selected were related to the longer dosing interval; convenience (72%), 12 week dosing interval (67%), and dosing less often (67%). The responses of "12 week dosing" was selected most often when dog owners were asked to select the single most important benefit of fluralaner. In a comparison to other F/T medications with monthly dosing, the majority of dog owners associated fluralaner with a reduced likelihood of getting fleas and a reduced likelihood of forgetting a dose. It is conceivable that pet owners might associate less forgotten doses with improved flea efficacy although there were no questions that specifically addressed this relationship. The next dose given "mostly on time" (75%) or "delayed by a few days" (17%) indicates that 12-weeks administration of fluralaner is easy to achieve by dog owners.

In comparisons with monthly F/T medications, most dog owners in our study appeared to favor fluralaner with regard to on time administration (65%), convenience for repeat doses (89%), and preference (89%) although the majority believes (56%) that dogs receive the same number of months of F/T protection in a year. The dog owners in this study did not seem to have any problem adjusting to the longer dosing interval.

As suggested in the analyses examining predictors of preference, dog owners who perceive "12 week dosing or convenience" as an important benefit of fluralaner were more likely to prefer fluralaner over monthly F/T medications. It is not clear why female pet owners were significantly more likely to state a preference for fluralaner over the monthly F/T products; a similar result found in the satisfaction analysis.

Medications with extended re-dosing intervals have been shown to improve patient compliance with veterinarian and physician recommendations when compared with medications that have shorter re-dosing intervals (15-17). Results from our study indicate that the 12 week re-treatment interval feature of fluralaner offering a longer approach to canine F/T control is associated with high satisfaction, convenience and preference scores in a group of dog owners that had currently been prescribed fluralaner for their dogs.

This study is based on the survey results of dog owners currently providing fluralaner to their own dogs. As such, it relies on pet owner opinion and is limited because it is a single-arm study design that did not directly compare fluralaner against specific monthly F/T products. Future studies that examine satisfaction, preference, and compliance comparing 12-week dosing to other F/T medications with monthly dosing are needed to fully evaluate the real-world experience of dog owners.

Conclusion

Overall satisfaction with fluralaner and preference for fluralaner compared to monthly F/T medications were high. The most significant factor predicting satisfaction and preference was the perceived benefit associated with 12 week dosing or convenience.

Acknowledgments

The authors thank Mark Dana of Scientific Communications Services, LLC for assistance in manuscript preparation.

References

1. Chomel B (2011) Tick-borne infections in dogs-an emerging infectious threat. Vet Parasitol 179: 294-301.

2. Shaw SE, Day MJ, Birtles RJ, Breitschwerdt EB (2001) Tick-borne infectious diseases of dogs. Trends Parasitol 17: 74-80.

3. Yancey CB, Hegarty BC, Qurollo BA, Levy MG, Birkenheuer AJ, et al. (2014) Regional seroreactivity and vector-borne disease co-exposures in dogs in the United States from 2004-2010: utility of canine surveillance. Vector Borne Zoonotic Dis 14: 724-732.

4. Fluralaner Chewable Tablets Dogs. Freedom of Information Summary. Original New Animal Drug Application (NADA 141-426). May 15, 2014.

5. Williams H, Young DR, Qureshi T, Zoller H, Heckeroth AR (2014) Fluralaner, a novel isoxazoline, prevents flea (Ctenocephalides felis) reproduction in vitro and in a simulated home environment. Parasit Vectors 7: 275.

6. Pfister K, Armstrong R (2016) Systemically and cutaneously distributed ectoparasiticides: a review of the efficacy against ticks and fleas on dogs. Parasit Vectors 9: 436.

7. Taenzler J, Wengenmayer C, Williams H, Fourie J, Zschiesche E, et al. (2014) Onset of activity of fluralaner (FLURALANER™) against Ctenocephalides felis on dogs. Parasit Vectors 7: 567.

8. Meadows C, Guerino F, Sun F (2014) A randomized, blinded, controlled USA field study to assess the use of fluralaner tablets in controlling canine flea infestations. Parasit Vectors 7: 375.

9. Crosaz O, Chapelle E, Cochet-Faivre N, Ka D, Hubinois C, et al. (2016) Open field study on the efficacy of oral fluralaner for long-term control of flea allergy dermatitis in client-owned dogs in Ile-de-France region. Parasit Vectors 9: 174.

10. Kilp S, Ramirez D, Allan MJ, Roepke RK, Nuernberger MC (2014) Pharmacokinetics of fluralaner in dogs following a single oral or intravenous administration. Parasit Vectors 7: 85.

11. Dryden MW, Smith V, Bennett T, Math L, Kallman J, et al. (2015) Efficacy of fluralaner flavored chews (Fluralaner) administered to dogs against the adult cat flea, Ctenocephalides felis felis and egg production. Parasit Vectors 8: 364.

12. Walther FM, Allan MJ, Roepke RK, Nuernberger MC (2014) Safety of fluralaner chewable tablets (Fluralaner), a novel systemic antiparasitic drug, in dogs after oral administration. Parasit Vectors 7: 87.

13. Walther FM, Paul AJ, Allan MJ, Roepke RK, Nuernberger MC (2014) Safety of fluralaner, a novel systemic antiparasitic drug, in MDR1(-/-) Collies after oral administration. Parasit Vectors 7: 86.

14. Rohdich N, Roepke RK, Zschiesche E (2014) A randomized, blinded, controlled and multi-centered field study comparing the efficacy and safety of Bravecto™ (fluralaner) against Frontline (fipronil) in flea- and tick-infested dogs. Parasit Vectors 7: 83.

15. Beck S, Schreiber C, Schein E, Krücken J, Baldermann C, et al. (2014) Tick infestation and prophylaxis of dogs in northeastern Germany: a prospective study. Ticks Tick Borne Dis 5: 336-342.

16. Gates MC, Nolan TJ (2010) Factors influencing heartworm, flea, and tick preventative use in patients presented to a veterinary teaching hospital. Prev Vet Med 93: 193-200.

17. Van VI, Nautrup BP, Gasper SM (2011) Estimation of the clinical and economic consequences of non-compliance with antimicrobial treatment of canine skin infections. Prev Vet Med 99: 201-210.

18. Adams VJ, Campbell JR, Waldner CL, Dowling PM, Schmon CL (2005) Evaluation of client compliance with short-term administration of antimicrobials to dogs. J Am Vet Med Assoc 226: 567-574.

19. Grave K, Tanem H (1999) Compliance with short-term oral antibacterial drug treatment in dogs. J Small Anim Pract 40: 158-162.

20. Claxton AJ, Cramer J, Pierce C (2001) A systematic review of the association between dose regimens and medication compliance. Clin Ther 23: 1296-1310.

21. Companion Animal Parasite Council: CAPC recommendations. Accessed Nov 22, 2016.

22. American Heartworm Society: Summary of the current canine guidelines for the prevention, diagnosis, and management of heartworm (Dirofilaria immitis) infection in dogs. Accessed Nov 22, 2016.

15

Epidemiological Studies on *Cysticercus bovis* at Gondar ELFORA Abattoir, North West of Ethiopia

Ezeddin Adem[1] and Tewodros Alemneh[2]*

[1]Metema Woreda Office of Agriculture and Rural Development, Metema, Gondar, Ethiopia
[2]Woreta City Office of Agriculture and Environmental Protection, S/Gondar, Woreta, Ethiopia

Abstract

A cross-sectional survey was undertaken in the abattoir to study the prevalence of *Cysticercus bovis* in cattle originated from different localities and to determine the cyst prevalence as well as distribution in different organs within infected animals in Gondar ELFORA abattoir from October, 2009 to March, 2010. Out of the total 450 cattle slaughtered and examined at Gondar ELFORA abattoir, 9 animals (2.0%) were identified positive for *Cysticercus bovis* infection. Predilection sites for *Cysticercus bovis* were observed and their relative infestation rates were recorded. As a result of this study, predominantly cysts were found on shoulder muscle (55.56%) followed by masseter muscle (33.33%) and tongue (11.11%). The prevalence and occurrence of *Cysticercus bovis* was also studied based on the geographical locations of slaughtered cattle. Accordingly, cattle from low lands and high lands had showed a prevalence of 6.45% and 0.307%, respectively. In conclusion, *C. bovis* is prevalent and is one of the major parasitic diseases that causes huge carcass condemnation of slaughtered animals and poses serious financial lose in the socio-economy of the study area. Therefore, public health awareness should be created on improving personal and environmental hygiene for breaking the life cycle of the disease.

Keywords: *Cysticercus bovis*; Gondar ELFORA; Prevalence; Epidemiological study

Introduction

Bovine cysticercosis is a muscular infection of cattle and is caused by larvae of the human intestinal cestode *Taenia saginata*. Its life cycle is entirely dependent on the link between man and cattle so that any break in this links can result in the total elimination of the parasite. Tapeworm infections have been recorded in history from 1500 BC and have been recognized as one of the earliest human parasite [1].

Cysts of *Cysticercus bovis* can be found anywhere in the carcass or meat and viscera [2]. The distribution of *Taenia saginata* is wider in developing countries where hygienic conditions are poor and where the inhabitants traditionally eat raw meat or insufficiently cooked meat [3,4]. Forty percent (40%) of the cases was reported in Africa [3,5]. Researchers reported that this disease being very common in developing countries like Ethiopia. It is associated with poor hygiene and local factors including cultural background, (eating raw meat "Kurt", Kitfo" semi cooked meat), economic condition and religious beliefs, close proximity of humans to cattle kept with little or no distinction between companion or utility functions [3].

Slaughtering is often carried out in open air in absence of abattoirs [3]. Transmission of the parasite occurs most commonly in the environment characterized by poor sanitation, primitive livestock husbandry practice and inadequate meat inspection, management, control police [6].

Bovine cysticerosis is responsible for considerable amount of economic losses which can approach 30% when allowance is made for the loss in the carcass weight and the cost of freezing for the infected meat [7]. The health caused by the adult worms in human gives rise to high medical costs [7]. Generally, the loss is determined by disease prevalence, grade of the animals infected, potential markets, prices of cattle and treatment costs for detained carcass [8] and medical costs for infected human beings [5]. The average annual loss due to taenicidal drugs for treatment in Ethiopia

was estimated to be 4,937,583.21 ETB or 225,036.97 USD [9-11]. Bovine cysticercosis is widely distributed in Ethiopia and a number of individuals reported the prevalence of bovine cysticercosis in different parts of the country. According to these reports, a prevalence of 9.7% in Debre Zeit by Amsalu [12], 21% in Nekemte by Ahmed [9], 13.85% in Debre Zeit by Getachew [13], 19.5% in Bahir Dar by Mulugeta [14], and 3.2% in different agro climatic zones by Tembo [15] was recorded.

The nation's domestic meat consumption of about 45% comes from cattle, which generates export income mainly from the sale of live animals [16].

On the other hand, the contributions of *Cysticercus bovis* to organ condemnation in slaughtered cattle at different abattoir have been reported [17,18]. It is a great problem in developing country like Ethiopia due to the cultural habit of eating raw meat in form of "kurt" and "kitffo" as routine dish and during holidays has promoted the spread of human taeniasis in Ethiopia [19]. The above mentioned problems allow the parasite to continue its life cycle till to date and in the coming future [20,21].

Therefore, the objective of this research is to determine the prevalence and occurrence of bovine cysticercosis in Gondar ELFORA abattoir and to see the association of the prevalence of the parasite with the risk factors.

*Corresponding author: Tewodros Alemneh Engdaw, Faculty of Veterinary Medicine, University of Gondar, PO Box: 196, Gondar, Ethiopia
E-mail: tedyshow@gmail.com (or) joteddy85@yahoo.com

Materials and Methods

Study area

The study was conducted in North Gondar, North western part of Ethiopia. It is divided into three major agro-climatic zones: highland, mid-highland and lowland. The altitude ranges from 4620 meters in the Semen Mountain in the North to 550 meters in the west. The rainfall varies from 880 mm to 1772 mm with a mono-modal distribution, while the minimum and maximum temperatures are in the order of -10°C in the highland and 44.5°C in the West. The area is also characterized by two seasons, the wet season from June to September, and the dry season from October to May (Figure 1).

The farming system of the study area is characterized by a mixed crop-livestock production system. Transhumance, from the highlands to western lowlands, is practiced as an important strategy to secure grazing resources for the highland livestock during the dry season of the year. In the case of the lowlands, crop farming is not as intensive as high and mid-highland areas and livestock has larger contributions to the farmer's livelihood.

Study population

According to the 2015 report of the Central Statistics Authority, there are 2,408,544 million cattle, 979,800 million sheep, 1,383,656 million goats, 31,456 million Horses, 272,655 Donkeys, and 2.9 million human populations. The herd size varies greatly, and it ranges from 2.11 to 7.15 animals (high and mid altitudes) to around 65 in the lowlands.

Sample size determination

The study animals were cattle coming to Gondar ELFORA abattoir for slaughter. Simple random sampling method was used for sampling and using the 95% confidence interval the sample size were determined by the formula [22]:

$$n = \frac{1.96^2 P_{exp}\left(1 - P_{exp}\right)}{d^2}$$

Where; n: required sample size; P_{exp}: expected prevalence; d: desired absolute precision

Study methodology

During the period of this study (October 2009 to April 2010), ante mortem and postmortem examinations were performed on 450 cattle in Gondar ELFORA abattoir. For the ante mortem examination, general condition of the animal was observed by visual inspection and age, breed as well as the origin of the animal were recorded. Out of the total 450 cattle, 124 were from low land localities and the rest 326 cattle were from high lands. All cattle that were subjected to the abattoir during the study period were old aged and males.

In this abattoir survey, random sampling technique was followed to select the animal to determine prevalence of bovine cysticerosis in the study area.

During the study period, bovine carcasses were randomly examined for the presence of C. bovis following the customary meat inspection procedure stipulated in the minister of agriculture meat inspection regulation [23]. There were visual inspections and palpations followed by multiple incisions of each organ (heart, tongue, shoulder, liver, masseter and diaphragm muscles) to examine the cysts of C. bovis. In positive cases the site and infestation of cyst were recorded. One deep incision in to triceps muscle of both sides was made. Similarly, tongue surface was examined by palpation then the inside part was examined by making deep incision in the ventral part of the tongue.

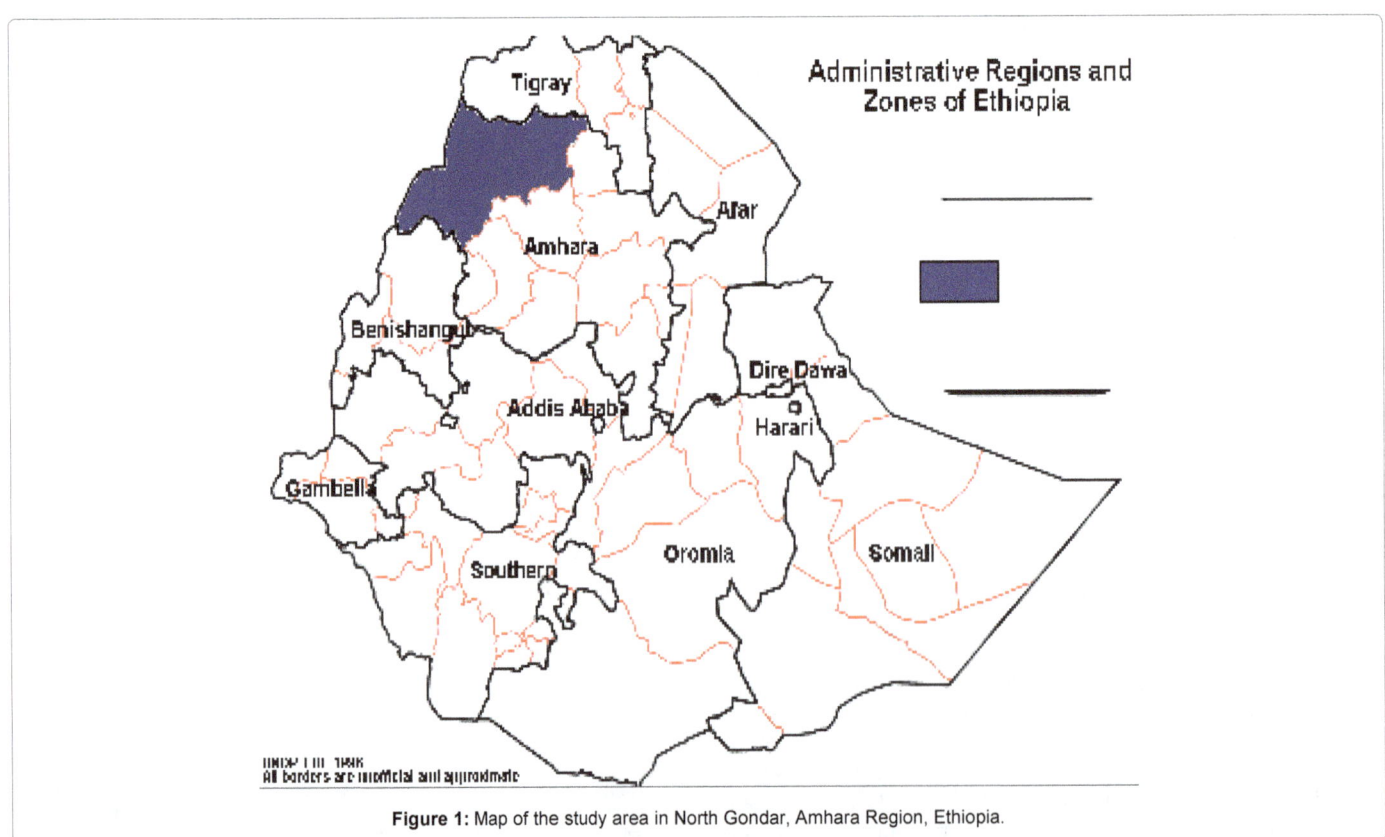

Figure 1: Map of the study area in North Gondar, Amhara Region, Ethiopia.

The pericardium of the heart was opened and incision was made in to the cardiac muscle from the base to the apex. When we come to masseter muscle, several deep incisions in to the internal and external muscle were made parallel to the plane of jaw. Moreover, the kidneys, spleen, liver and the lungs were inspected in the usual methods of inspection.

Results

Overall occurrence

Out of the total 450 cattle examined at the abattoir, 9 (2.0%) were found to be positive for *Cysticercus bovis*.

Occurrence of *Cysticercus bovis* in different agro-ecological zones

Among the 124 cattle examined, which came from low lands, 8 (6.45%) of them were found to be positive for *Cysticercus bovis* and from the 326 cattle, which came from high lands, only one (0.307%) was found to be positive (Table 1).

Occurrence of *Cysticercus bovis* in different organs of cattle

Shoulder muscle, tongue, masseter muscle, heart, liver and diaphragm were inspected. Among the nine (9) cattle that were confirmed positive, 5 (55.56%) were from shoulder muscle, 1 (11.11%) from tongue and 3 (33.33%) were from masseter muscle (Table 2).

Similarly, this study significantly showed that from the observed old aged cattle, the most affected organ was shoulder muscle, followed by masseter muscle and the tongue.

Discussion

Among the 450 carcasses of cattle inspected in Gondar ELFORA abattoir from October 2009 to March 2010, 5 carcasses were found to harbor cysts of *C. bovis* with an overall prevalence of 2.0% in various organs.

Though the prevalence of *Cysticercus bovis* is low in developed countries [24], the infestation rate is often around 30% in developing countries like Africa. However; in the present study, the rate of occurrence of *Cysticercus bovis* in Gondar was found to be 2.0% which was lower than the study made by Dawit [10]. This might be because of the differences in the experiences of meat inspectors as well as variations in veterinary services deliveries and peoples' awareness on the prevention of the disease in different localities. Moreover, in the routine inspection of beef carcasses, there was practical limitation to the degree of incision permissible for gross mutilation that decreased the marketability of the carcass as a result of which many infestations remained undetected.

In Ethiopia, various studies and reports revealed that the rate of infestation of cattle by *Cysticercus bovis* was different and higher than the current study in various agro-ecological zones; Natnael [25] in Debre zeit Elfora export abattoir reported 22.75%, Fufa [11] in Hawassa municipal abattoir reported 26.25%, Hailu [26] in East Shoa reported 17.5%, Ahmed [9] in Nekemte municipal abattoir reported 21%, Getachew [13] in Debre Zeit abattoir reported 13.8%. Likewise; in different African countries the occurrence is high. For instance, 20% in Senegal, 27% in Tanzania, and 38% in Kenya was recorded [27].

In this study, the assessment of occurrence of *Cysticercus bovis* based on the origin of cattle (high land and low land) had been done and among those animals submitted to the abattoir and inspected, 326 cattle (72.44%) were from highlands and the remaining 124 (27.56%) were from low lands. The rate of *C. bovis* occurrence in the highland animals were 0.307% and in the lowland cattle were 6.45%. The variation in the rate of occurrences in different altitudes might be related to the less resistance of the egg of the parasite (tape worm ova) to survive in the cold grazing environmental conditions of highlands for longer periods.

Cysticercus bovis is commonly found in muscle of mastication, particularly masseter muscle, shoulder muscle, heart, tongue, diaphragm and occasionally in fat, liver, lungs and lymph nodes. However, in the present study, cysts were found on shoulder (55.56%), masseter (33.33%) and tongue muscles (11.11%). From several reports, variation and deviation in localization of cysts were quite possible. For instance, in Addis Ababa abattoir, the infection rate of *Cysticercus bovis* was high as 16.3% in foreleg [28]. Some reports from Shoa Oromia Regional State showed 4.7% in liver and 0.7% in lungs [26]. On the other hand, Hailemariam [29], and Amsalu [12] indicated that examination of the tongue was the most effective means of detection for bovine cysticercosis.

Conclusion

The wide distribution of *C. bovis* is associated with several factors including: raw and under cooked beef consumption, bush defecation and poor waste disposal and sewage treatment system, low level of public awareness and presence of backyard slaughtering practices.

Geographical Location	No. of Carcass Inspected	Breed		Positive for *C. bovis*	Relative percentage among the total positive value (%)
		Local	Cross		
High land	326	322	4	1 (0.307%)	11.11
Low land	124	124	0	8(6.45%)	89.89
Total	450	446	4	9 (2%)	100

Table 1: Occurrence of *Cysticercus bovis* in relation to Animals' Origin.

Cyst Location	No. of Breeds Positive			Age			Origin	
	Exotic	Local	Cross	young	Adult	Old	High land	Low land
Shoulder muscle	0	5 (55.56%)	0	0	0	5 (55.56%)	1 (100%)	4 (50%)
Tongue	0	1 (11.11%)	0	0	0	1 (11.11%)	0	1 (12.5%)
Masseter muscle	0	3 (33.33%)	0	0	0	3 (33.33%)	0	3 (37.5%)
Heart	0	0	0	0	0	0	0	0
Liver	0	0	0	0	0	0	0	0
Diaphragm	0	0	0	0	0	0	0	0
Total	0	9 (100%)	0	0	0	9 (100%)	1 (100%)	8 (100%)

Table 2: Occurrence of *Cysticercus bovis* in different predilection sites of carcass.

This study confirmed the occurrence of bovine cysticercosis in different origin of cattle slaughtered at Gondar ELFORA abattoir. However, the prevalence was lower as compared to previous studies performed in other parts of Ethiopia. Although we couldn't compare the prevalence of *C. bovis* in relation to sex, age and body condition of animals, cattle from low lands were found more prevalently infected than those originated from high lands.

In general, veterinarians and medical professionals ought to work in collaboration for the control of this disease. Similarly, public health awareness should be created through public media on improving personal and environmental hygiene for breaking the life cycle of the disease. Further detailed study by considering various age groups, sex and breads shall be conducted to know the prevalence of the disease in the area in relation to different parameters.

Acknowledgements

The authors special thanks goes to Dr. Seleshe Nigatu (DVM, MVSc), Gondar ELFORA Abattoir and University of Gondar Faculty of Veterinary Medicine Instructors for their continual guidance to bring this research to completion.

References

1. Urquhart GMJ, Armour JL, Duncan AM, Dunn FW, Jennings (2013) Veterinary Parasitology. 8th edn. Black Well Science, London, pp: 120-137.

2. Collins DS, Huey RJ (2014) Gracey's Meat hygiene. 11th edn. Bailliere Tindall, 24-28. Oval roads, London NW 17X. pp: 412-420.

3. Fralova A (2014) Taeniosis. In: Zoonotic control. Lysenko A (ed), UNEP Publication, Moscow, pp: 192-239.

4. WHO (1996) Investigating in health research and development. Report of the Ad Hoc Committee on Health Research Relating to Future Intervention Options. WHO, Geneva, Switzerland, p: 268.

5. Fan PC (1997) Annual Economic loss caused by *Taenia saginata taenicysts* in East Asia. Parasitology Today 13: 194-196.

6. Mann I (1983) Environmental, hygiene and sanitation based on the concept of primary health care as a tool for surveillance, prevention and control of taeniasis/cysticercosis. Current Publication in Health Research in Tropics 36: 127-140.

7. Pawlowski Z, Schultz MG (1972) Taeniasis and cysticercosis (*Taenia saginata*). Advances in parasitology 10: 269-343.

8. Grindle RJ (2012) Economic loss resulting from bovine cysticercosis with special reference to Botswana and Kenya. Trop Anim Health Prod 10: 127-140.

9. Ahmed I (1990) Bovine cysticercosis in animals slaughtered at Nekemt abattoir. DVM Thesis, Addis Ababa University, Faculty of Veterinary Medicine, Debre Zeit, Ethiopia.

10. Dawit S (2004) Epidemiology of *Taenia saginata taeniasis* and cysticercosis in north Gondar zone, North West Ethiopia. DVM Thesis, Faculty of Veterinary Medicine, Addis Ababa University, Debrezeit, Ethiopia.

11. Fufa A (2012) Study on the prevalence of Bovine cysticercosis in Hawassa Municipal Abattoir and *T. saginata* in Hawassa town and its surrounding South Ethiopia. MSc Thesis, FVM, AAU, Debre Zeit, Ethiopia.

12. Amsalu D (2013) Prevalence and significance of *C. bovis* among slaughtered cattle at Debre Zeit abattoir. DVM Thesis, Debre Zeit, Ethiopia.

13. Getachew B (1990) Prevalence and significance of *C. bovis* among cattle slaughtered at Debre Zeit abattoir. DVM Thesis, Faculty of Veterinary Medicine, Addis Ababa University, Debre Zeit (Unpublished).

14. Alemu M (1997) Bovine Cysticercosis Prevalence Economic and Public Health Importance at Bahir Dar Municipality Abattoir. DVM Thesis. Faculty of Veterinary Medicine, Addis Ababa University, Ethiopia.

15. Tembo A (2001) Epidemiology of *T. saginatataeniasiscysticercosis* in three selected agro-climatic zone in central high land of Ethiopia. Doctoral Dissertation, Addis Ababa University, Deberzeit, Ethiopia.

16. EARO (Ethiopian Agricultural Research Organization) (2015) Beef Research Strategy. Animal Science Directorate. Addis Ababa, Ethiopia, pp: 241-243.

17. Fekadu D (2015) A study on cestodes and metacestode of sheep in Sheno agricultural Research (SHARC), North Shoa. DVM Thesis, Faculty of Veterinary Medicine, Addis Ababa University, Debre Zeit, Ethiopia.

18. Yimam M (2003) Major causes of organ condemnation in ruminants slaughtered at Gondar abattoir, Northwest Ethiopia. DVM thesis, Addis Ababa University, Faculty of Veterinary Medicine, Debre Zeit, Ethiopia.

19. Gebra-Emanuael T (1997) Food Hygiene - Principles and methods of food borne disease control with special Reference to Ethiopia. Faculty of Medicine, Department of Community Health, Addis Ababa University.

20. Eckert J (1996) Workshop summary: Food safety: meat-and fish-borne zoonoses. Vet Parasitol 64: 143-147.

21. Ethiopian Central Statistical Agency (CSA) (2015) Annual Ethiopian Animal Population Estimates.

22. Thrusfield M (2013) Veterinary Epidemiology. 3rd edn. Edinburgh, Blackwell, pp: 178-197.

23. MOA (2015) Meat inspection regulation. Negarit Gazeta, Addis Ababa, Ethiopia, p: 428.

24. Onyango-Abuje JA, Hughes G, Opicha M, Nginyi KM, Rugutt MK, et al. (1996) Diagnosis of *Taenia saginata* cysticercosis in Kenyan cattle by antibody and antigen ELISA. Vet Parasitol 61: 221-230.

25. Natnael T (2014) Prevalence and Economic Importance of *Cysticercus bovis* in Debre Zeit Elfora Export abattoir. DVM Thesis. JUCAVM.

26. Degefu H (2005) Prevalence and risk factors of *Taenia saginataTaeniasis/Cysticercosis* in three selection area of eastern shoe. Doctoral Dissertation, MSc Thesis, Addis Ababa University, Debrezeit, Ethiopia.

27. Over HJ, Jansen J, Van Olm PW (2012) Distribution and Impact of Helminth Diseases of Livestock in Developing Countries. FAO Animal Production and Health Paper 180, Rome.

28. Feseha G (1995) Zoonotic disease in Ethiopia. Ethiopian Society of Animal Production, Addis Ababa.

29. Hailemariam S (2013) Animal Health Review 1822-1969. Ethiopia, pp: 102-290.

16

Expert Views on Effectiveness, Feasibility, and Implementation of Biosecurity Measures for Mitigating Tier 1 Disease Risks in the U.S. Swine, Beef Cattle, and Dairy Industries

Qianrong Wu[1], Lee L Schulz[1]*, Glynn T Tonsor[2] and Julia M Smith[3]

[1]*Department of Economics, Iowa State University, Ames, Iowa, USA*
[2]*Department of Agricultural Economics, Kansas State University, Manhattan, Kansas, USA*
[3]*Department of Animal and Veterinary Sciences, The University of Vermont, Burlington, Vermont, USA*

Abstract

Understanding disease transmission routes and implications for biosecurity is critical to mitigating livestock disease outbreaks and maintaining efficient and profitable production. The goal of biosecurity is to eliminate pathogen exposure and minimize endemic pathogen impact, particularly important for foreign animal diseases that threaten U.S. animal health and the economy. We elicit swine, beef cattle, and dairy expert views on the effectiveness, feasibility, and implementation of both biosecurity measures targeting disease transmission routes and specific biosecurity measures. Biosecurity targeting direct animal-to-animal contact, semen, people, and vehicles and other fomites was identified as the most effective and feasible for the swine, beef cattle, and dairy industries. Efforts targeting airborne and arthropod transmission were ranked low for effectiveness and feasibility across all three industries. The swine industry had higher estimated implementation of biosecurity against most disease transmission routes. All-in and all-out production had the highest estimated implementation in the swine industry. In the beef cattle industry, performing daily observations by producer/employees had the highest estimated implementation. Reduced environmental viral load through pathogen reduction had the lowest estimated implementation in the swine and beef cattle industries. In the dairy industry, monitoring production records for health status changes had the highest estimated implementation, and line of separation in place for all employees entering premises had the lowest. Swine experts considered separation line for all animals entering/leaving premises and reduced environmental viral load through pathogen reduction the most and least effective and feasible, respectively. Stabilization and monitoring for affected premises and daily observations by producer/employees were identified as most effective and feasible by beef cattle and dairy experts, respectively. All-in and all-out production was rated least effective and feasible by both beef cattle and dairy experts.

Keywords: Beef cattle; Biosecurity; Dairy; Expert survey; Foreign animal disease; Swine

Introduction

State and federal animal health officials must be prepared to help deal with new, emerging, and foreign animal diseases characterized by uncertainty and complexity. Understanding disease transmission risks in light of current implementation of mitigating strategies can help identify opportunities for disease prevention and outbreak containment. In the event of a large, rapidly spreading foreign animal disease outbreak, biosecurity is the only tool realistically available as a means of control [1].

In this study we define biosecurity as "the implementation of measures that reduce the risk of disease agents being introduced and spread where biosecurity measures should be used to avoid the entry of pathogens into a herd or farm (external biosecurity) and to prevent the spread of disease to uninfected animals within a herd or to other farms, when the pathogen is already present (internal biosecurity)." [2].

Although biosecurity recommendations are often based on the risk of introduction of endemic diseases [3], there is always the risk of a new, emerging disease entering the United States that may circumvent current biosecurity recommendations [4,5]. An analysis of data from the National Animal Health Monitoring System (NAHMS) indicates 32.1% of beef cow-calf operations disagreed or strongly disagreed with the statement, "The United States is well prepared to handle outbreaks of livestock disease currently not found in this country, such as foot-and-mouth disease and rinderpest." [6].

Understanding the drivers of behavior is crucial to developing effective strategies that result in behavior changes [7] and greater protection against new, emerging, or foreign diseases or pests. Social science approaches are being employed to better understand the mindset of producers and influential professionals about biosecurity [8-11]. The literature includes a few assessments of expert views on factors influencing biosecurity decisions. Nissen and Krieter [12] compared risk factors in terms of importance for the introduction and spread of classical swine fever and foot-and-mouth disease in Germany. Kuster et al. [13] assessed the effectiveness and importance of individual on-farm biosecurity measures for preventing a host of infectious agents from entering and spreading on cattle and swine farms in Switzerland.

Given the size, structure, and extensive movement inherent in the U.S. livestock industry, which presents unprecedented challenges in the

*Corresponding author:** Lee L Schulz, Assistant Professor, Department of Economics, Iowa State University, 478D Heady Hall, 518 Farm House Lane, Ames, IA, 50011-1054, USA, E-mail: lschulz@iastate.edu

event of foreign animal disease outbreak [14], additional research is needed with respect to implementation of biosecurity measures. For example, no country with a livestock industry comparable to that of the United States has had to deal with an outbreak of foot-and-mouth disease [1].

As important as understanding the risk factors for the introduction and spread of disease is understanding the drivers of behavior to mitigate these risks [15]. Implementation of measures to protect animal health comes with a cost that must be weighed against potential effectiveness (and necessity). Feasibility and effectiveness are mentioned in most discussions of biosecurity at the producer level [16], thus we chose to focus on perceived effectiveness and feasibility in our study.

Stakeholders in the livestock industry are regarded as key players in the communication, selection, and implementation of biosecurity measures. Hernández-Jover et al. [17] found that successful livestock disease risk reduction depends on trust and co-management among stakeholders. We targeted livestock industry experts such as veterinarians, epidemiologists, animal scientists, and economists for an initial survey exploring the effectiveness, feasibility, and implementation of biosecurity measures in the swine, beef cattle, and dairy industries.

Our focus was to evaluate biosecurity practices currently recommended against endemic diseases for their role in protecting against new, emerging, and foreign diseases. The specific objectives were two-fold: firstly, to identify expert views on the effectiveness (extent of risk reduction), feasibility (practicality of affordable implementation), and current implementation (adoption) of biosecurity measures applicable to specific disease transmission risks (termed routes in this paper); and secondly, to identify expert views on the effectiveness, feasibility, and implementation of a set of specific biosecurity measures.

Materials and Methods

Questionnaire design and survey procedure

The survey procedures were approved by the Kansas State University Committee for Research Involving Human Subjects (#8132.1).

Three similar surveys were designed and circulated to swine, beef cattle, and dairy industry experts. Survey software, Qualtrics (Qualtrics, Provo, UT), was used to develop the surveys. Disease transmission routes and biosecurity measures were identified from the literature [2,18]. Nine disease transmission routes were examined: (1) direct animal-to-animal contact; (2) semen; (3) airborne transmission; (4) people; (5) vehicles and other fomites; (6) feed and drinking-water; (7) manure and bedding; (8) birds, bats, rodents, feral and wild livestock, and stray/domestic animals (hereafter referred to as wild carrying agents); and (9) arthropods. Nineteen biosecurity measures were examined (Tables 4, 5 and 6). All questionnaires included questions on all nine disease transmission routes. However, to minimize the risk of survey fatigue, questions on only five randomly selected biosecurity measures were presented to each respondent. To minimize the effect of order bias, items within each question were presented in random order. Demographic questions were also included to better identify the characteristics of the survey respondents.

To encourage the respondents to think in the context of disease risks that pose the most significant threat to U.S. agriculture as they have the highest risks and consequences, we defined and deliberately asked them to keep Tier 1 disease risks in mind when answering questions. Tier 1 diseases include African swine fever, classical swine

fever, foot-and-mouth disease, avian influenza, and virulent Newcastle disease [19].

The surveys were distributed by the National Institute for Animal Agriculture (NIAA) and the American Association of Swine Veterinarians (AASV). This sampling method relied on these two organizations to distribute the surveys to their members or subscribers using their preferred means of communication. Modes of recruitment were email list serves for NIAA members and online newsletters for AASV members. These communications included a link to the survey website and text describing the study. A reminder message was sent three weeks after the initial recruitment notice. One of the authors attended the 2016 National Institute for Animal Agriculture Annual Meeting during the study period to describe the study and encourage participation.

In March and April of 2016, communication of the survey was circulated to 778 NIAA members (226 registered for the 2016 NIAA Annual Conference and 552 past members) and 1,965 AASV members (1,350 U.S. members, 285 international members, and 330 student members). These NIAA and AASV members were asked to complete the survey best aligned with the industry they were most familiar and engaged with—swine, beef cattle, or dairy. Respondents were also welcome to complete a survey for more than one industry.

Statistical analysis

Data from the survey software were exported and analyzed in Excel (Microsoft, Redmond, WA) and STATA [20]. As commonly used for the analysis of this type of data [21-23], cross-tabulations were used to compare responses by effectiveness, feasibility, and implementation. For example, of interest is whether biosecurity measures targeting a specific disease transmission route are both highly effective and highly feasible or highly ineffective and highly infeasible or some combination of the extreme ratings. Similar assessments were performed for specific biosecurity measures.

Results

Response rate and respondent profile

Of the possible 2,743 experts contacted to complete the survey(s), 190 completed questionnaires—55 experts from the swine industry, 70 experts from the beef cattle industry, and 65 experts from the dairy industry (6.93% effective response rate). However, several surveys were only partially completed. For the analysis, 33, 38, and 37 surveys completed by swine experts, beef cattle experts, and dairy experts, respectively, were used. Descriptive statistics of the demographics (i.e., discipline, employment, and biosecurity expertise) of respondents are shown in Table 1.

Type of operation familiar to experts varied by species. Eighty-four percent of dairy experts most commonly interact with commercial operations and the rest of them with non-commercial operations. The beef cattle experts most commonly interact with cow-calf (79%), stocker (3%), feedlot (11%), and other operations (8%). Swine experts most commonly interact with farrow-finish (36%), farrow-wean (27%), feeder-finish (3%), wean-finish (9%), and other operations (24%).

Respondents interacted with operations in states with the largest number of operations and largest livestock populations. Approximately one-third of the swine experts most commonly interacted with operations in Iowa, and around one-sixth of experts most commonly interacted with operations in Illinois, with the remaining states including Ohio, Minnesota, Texas, Nebraska, Indiana, Oklahoma,

Respondent Characteristics	Swine	Beef cattle	Dairy
	%	%	%
Level of knowledge regarding animal disease development, spread, mitigation, or risk			
No expertise	0	0	0
Below average expertise	0	0	5
Average expertise	33	21	27
Above average expertise	33	42	38
Substantial expertise	33	37	30
Discipline or area of expertise and focus			
Animal Science	6	5	3
Economics	0	0	5
Epidemiology	6	11	5
Veterinary medicine	85	79	73
Other	3	5	14
Current employer			
University/academia	12	32	14
Government/public sector	18	37	38
Industry	64	21	22
Other	6	11	27
Contributions			
Presentations (at a producer meeting)	94	87	89
Non peer-reviewed publications	85	74	73
Peer-reviewed publications	55	50	43
Do you personally own or manage an operation	12	47	11
Number of observations	33	38	37

Table 1: Select survey respondent demographics.

Kansas, North Carolina, and Georgia. These states represent 48% of U.S. swine operations and 84% of the U.S. hog inventory. The states that beef cattle experts most commonly interacted with were Kansas, Nebraska, Mississippi, Missouri, Texas, Iowa, Kentucky, Alabama, Illinois, Arkansas, Colorado, Michigan, Ohio, Georgia, Washington, California, Oregon, North Dakota, Tennessee, Wyoming, and Pennsylvania. These states represent 67% of U.S. beef cow operations, 64% of the U.S. beef cow inventory, 61% of U.S. cattle on feed operations, and 83% of the U.S. cattle on feed inventory. Most of the dairy experts most commonly interacted with operations in Wisconsin, with a second tier including Texas, Washington, California, Ohio, New York, Minnesota, Pennsylvania, and a third tier including Vermont, Florida, Michigan, Virginia, New Mexico, Maryland, Missouri, Indiana, Arizona, Idaho, and New Jersey. These states represent 77% of U.S. dairy cow operations and 84% of the U.S. dairy cow inventory [24].

Assessment of routes of disease transmission

Rating of effectiveness, feasibility, and implementation of biosecurity measures targeting specific disease transmission routes are summarized in Table 2 for the swine, beef cattle, and dairy industries, respectively.

Biosecurity targeting four disease transmission routes—direct animal-to-animal contact, semen, people, and vehicles and other fomites—was identified as the most effective and feasible for the swine, beef cattle, and dairy industries. Biosecurity targeting manure and bedding was not far behind for all three industries. However, the swine industry, but not the beef cattle or dairy industries, indicated effectiveness and feasibility of controlling wild carrying agents as

Routes of disease transmission	Highly effective highly feasible %	Highly effective highly infeasible %	Highly ineffective highly feasible %	Highly ineffective highly infeasible %	Implementation[1]	
					Mean	Std. dev.
Swine Industry (N=33)						
Direct animal-to-animal contact	64	3	0	0	3.09	0.84
Semen	58	0	3	0	3.36	0.90
Airborne transmission	9	3	0	12	1.67	0.69
People	55	0	0	0	3.00	0.75
Vehicles and other fomites	58	3	0	0	2.67	0.69
Feed and drinking-water	27	3	0	0	2.24	0.94
Manure and bedding	33	0	6	0	2.52	0.83
Wild carrying agents	33	0	3	3	2.52	0.87
Arthropods	9	0	3	15	1.91	0.81
Beef Cattle Industry (N=38)						
Direct animal-to-animal contact	36	8	0	0	1.97	0.89
Semen	46	3	8	0	2.79	1.02
Airborne transmission	5	13	0	0	1.42	0.72
People	41	0	0	0	1.90	0.76
Vehicles and other fomites	46	3	0	0	1.74	0.83
Feed and drinking-water	15	0	5	3	1.87	0.88
Manure and bedding	33	3	3	3	1.82	0.77
Wild carrying agents	0	18	0	18	1.26	0.45
Arthropods	5	8	0	18	1.76	0.85
Dairy Industry (N=37)						
Direct animal-to-animal contact	37	5	0	3	1.92	0.98
Semen	42	0	11	11	2.73	1.15
Airborne transmission	5	8	0	37	1.30	0.62
People	45	0	3	3	1.68	0.75
Vehicles and other fomites	39	3	0	0	1.73	0.84
Feed and drinking-water	29	0	0	5	1.81	0.85
Manure and bedding	34	0	0	11	1.89	0.84
Wild carrying agents	0	11	3	16	1.68	0.75
Arthropods	11	8	0	18	1.73	0.87

[1]The survey instrument collected information on current implementation using categorical variables 1=25% or less, 2=26-50%, 3=51-75%, 4=76% or more.

Table 2: Summary of effectiveness, feasibility, and implementation of biosecurity measures targeting disease transmission route in the swine, beef cattle, and dairy Industry.

high as managing manure and bedding. Efforts targeting airborne and arthropod transmission were ranked low for effectiveness and feasibility across all three industries.

In terms of estimated current implementation, biosecurity measures targeting semen were highest followed by those targeting direct animal-to-animal contact as a route of disease transmission across the swine, beef cattle, and dairy industries. The lowest level of estimated implementation was against wild carrying agents in the beef cattle industry and against airborne transmission in the swine and dairy industries. Estimated current implementation and differences between industries are displayed in Table 3.

Assessment of biosecurity measures

The estimated implementation of specific biosecurity measures are shown for the swine, beef cattle, and dairy industries (Tables 4, 5 and 6 respectively) along with the percentage of experts ranking any measure at the extremes for effectiveness and feasibility. In the swine industry, the biosecurity measure of all-in and all-out production had the highest estimated current implementation; whereas protocols for pathogen reduction to reduce environmental viral load had the lowest estimated implementation. In the beef cattle industry, performing daily observations by producer/employees had the highest estimated

Route of disease transmission	Swine (N = 33)		Beef (N = 38)		Dairy (N = 37)		Swine-Beef		Swine-Dairy		Beef-Dairy	
	Mean	Std. dev.	Mean	Std. dev.	Mean	Std. dev.	t-stat	p-value	t-stat	p-value	t-stat	p-value
Direct animal-to-animal contact	3.09	0.84	1.97	0.88	1.92	0.98	5.42	0.00	5.32	0.00	0.25	0.80
Semen	3.36	0.90	2.79	1.02	2.73	1.15	2.51	0.01	2.56	0.01	0.24	0.81
Airborne transmission	1.67	0.69	1.42	0.72	1.30	0.62	1.46	0.15	2.36	0.02	0.80	0.43
People	3.00	0.75	1.89	0.76	1.68	0.75	6.13	0.00	7.39	0.00	1.26	0.21
Vehicles and other fomites	2.67	0.69	1.74	0.83	1.73	0.84	5.09	0.00	5.06	0.00	0.04	0.97
Feed and drinking-water	2.24	0.94	1.87	0.88	1.81	0.84	1.74	0.09	2.03	0.05	0.29	0.77
Manure and bedding	2.52	0.83	1.82	0.77	1.89	0.84	3.68	0.00	3.10	0.00	-0.41	0.68
Wild carrying agents	2.52	0.87	1.26	0.45	1.68	0.75	7.77	0.00	4.34	0.00	-2.91	0.00
Arthropods	1.91	0.80	1.76	0.85	1.73	0.87	0.74	0.46	0.89	0.38	0.17	0.87

[1]The survey instrument collected information on current national implementation using categorical variables 1=25% or less, 2=26-50%, 3=51-75%, 4=76% or more.

Table 3: Differences of swine, beef cattle, and dairy industry experts' assessment of implementation of biosecurity measures targeting disease transmission routes[1].

Biosecurity measure		Highly effective highly feasible	Highly effective highly infeasible	Highly ineffective highly feasible	Highly ineffective highly infeasible	Implementation[1]	
	Obs	%	%	%	%	Mean	Std. dev.
A communication/education plan is in place to inform visitors and service providers of disease status and biosecurity requirements	8	63	0	13	0	3.13	0.83
Line of separation is in place for all visitors and service providers entering premises	7	57	0	0	0	2.86	0.38
Protocols have been developed and implemented to contain and/or exclude the targeted virus within the affected premises	7	43	0	0	0	2.43	0.79
A communication/education plan is in place to inform employees of disease status and biosecurity requirements	10	30	0	0	0	2.60	0.70
Line of separation is in place for all employees entering premises	8	50	0	0	0	2.88	0.64
Protocols for monitoring employee biosecurity compliance have been developed	13	38	0	0	0	2.46	0.88
Timely visits by veterinarian(s)	7	29	0	0	0	3.14	0.38
Daily observations by producer/employees	9	22	0	0	0	3.00	0.87
Monitoring of production records for health status changes	14	38	0	8	0	3.00	0.71
Protocols: have been developed and implemented pertaining to transport biosecurity to contain or exclude the targeted virus within the affected premises	8	38	0	0	0	2.25	0.89
Protocols have been developed for cleaning and/or disinfecting vehicles for certain animal movements (required for verification of biosecurity payments)	8	25	0	0	0	2.38	0.74
Line of separation is in place for all animals entering and leaving premises	5	80	0	0	0	3.00	1.00
Protocols for loading/unloading animals that attempt to minimize virus introduction have been developed and implemented	9	33	0	11	0	2.89	0.78
Protocols for pathogen reduction have been developed and implemented to reduce environmental viral load	6	33	0	0	17	2.00	0.89
Use of an effective disinfectant (required for verification of biosecurity payments)	12	58	0	0	0	2.67	0.65
Follow appropriate downtimes after cleaning and disinfection	11	55	0	0	0	2.64	0.81
Where possible, use all-in and all-out production practices	14	43	0	0	0	3.29	0.73
Protocols have been developed and implemented to establish stabilization and monitoring for the affected premises (monitoring may include submission of samples to a diagnostic laboratory for testing)	6	50	0	0	0	2.33	0.52
Movements of animals on and off the premises are routinely recorded	4	75	0	0	0	3.25	0.50

[1]The survey instrument collected information on current implementation using categorical variables 1=25% or less, 2=26-50%, 3=51-75%, 4=76% or more.

Table 4: Summary of effectiveness, feasibility, and implementation of biosecurity measures in the swine industry.

Biosecurity measure	Highly effective highly feasible		Highly effective highly infeasible	Highly ineffective highly feasible	Highly ineffective highly infeasible	Implementation[1]	
	Obs	%	%	%	%	Mean	Std. dev.
A communication/education plan is in place to inform visitors and service providers of disease status and biosecurity requirements	9	33	0	0	0	1.78	0.67
Line of separation is in place for all visitors and service providers entering premises	10	80	0	0	0	1.50	0.85
Protocols have been developed and implemented to contain and/or exclude the targeted virus within the affected premises	10	55	0	0	10	1.70	0.67
A communication/education plan is in place to inform employees of disease status and biosecurity requirements	11	55	0	0	0	1.45	0.69
Line of separation is in place for all employees entering premises	8	63	13	0	0	1.38	0.52
Protocols for monitoring employee biosecurity compliance have been developed	8	0	0	0	0	1.75	0.46
Timely visits by veterinarian(s)	16	25	0	0	0	1.94	1.00
Daily observations by producer/employees	10	40	0	0	0	2.40	0.97
Monitoring of production records for health status changes	15	40	0	13	7	1.67	0.82
Protocols: have been developed and implemented pertaining to transport biosecurity to contain or exclude the targeted virus within the affected premises	8	38	0	0	0	1.63	1.06
Protocols have been developed for cleaning and/or disinfecting vehicles for certain animal movements (required for verification of biosecurity payments)	8	50	13	0	0	1.50	0.76
Line of separation is in place for all animals entering and leaving premises	10	50	10	0	0	1.30	0.67
Protocols for loading/unloading animals that attempt to minimize virus introduction have been developed and implemented	12	42	0	0	0	1.67	0.78
Protocols for pathogen reduction have been developed and implemented to reduce environmental viral load	8	50	0	0	0	1.13	0.35
Use of an effective disinfectant (required for verification of biosecurity payments)	6	67	17	0	0	1.67	0.82
Follow appropriate downtimes after cleaning and disinfection	13	46	0	0	0	1.69	0.63
Where possible, use all-in and all-out production practices	7	29	43	0	14	1.43	0.79
Protocols have been developed and implemented to establish stabilization and monitoring for the affected premises (monitoring may include submission of samples to a diagnostic laboratory for testing)	8	88	0	0	0	2.00	1.07
Movements of animals on and off the premises are routinely recorded	13	15	0	8	0	2.15	0.90

[1]The survey instrument collected information on current implementation using categorical variables 1=25% or less, 2=26-50%, 3=51-75%, 4=76% or more.

Table 5: Summary of effectiveness, feasibility, and implementation of biosecurity measures in the beef cattle industry.

current implementation. Similar to the swine industry, protocols for pathogen reduction to reduce environmental viral load had the lowest estimated implementation in the beef cattle industry. In the dairy industry, monitoring production records for health status changes and timely visits by veterinarian(s) had the highest estimated current implementation; whereas line of separation in place for all employees entering premises had the lowest estimated current implementation.

Swine experts considered the biosecurity measure of separation line for all animals entering and leaving premises as most effective and feasible (80% of experts identified as both highly effective and highly feasible) and protocols for pathogen reduction to reduce environmental viral load as the least effective and feasible (17% of experts identified as both highly ineffective and highly infeasible). Beef cattle experts identified protocols to establish stabilization and monitoring for the affected premises as most effective and feasible (88%); whereas the dairy cattle experts identified daily observations by producer/employees as most effective and feasible (71%). All-in and all-out production was rated the least effective and feasible by both beef cattle (14%) and dairy (8%) experts.

Discussion

Respondents

The low response rate necessitates caution when interpreting results. It is unknown whether asking these experts to respond based on number of operations versus number of animals would have affected the results. Also, industry experts were asked for global assessments even if their assessment would have differed by specific production segment (i.e., farrowing versus finishing or cow-calf versus feedlot). However, the number of responses from experts with beef cattle, dairy, or swine experience were fairly even and geographically representative of the areas of highest concentrations of production. Future producer surveys, informed by these results, will provide a more complete picture of the implementation of biosecurity practices on these types of livestock farms.

Biosecurity and disease transmission route

Across industries, the swine industry had higher estimated implementation of biosecurity against almost all disease transmission routes. This reflects the fact that the vast majority of commercially produced pigs do not have outside access, and therefore, are raised in more controlled environments than most cattle. Biosecurity against disease transmission by semen and direct animal-to-animal contact were consistently ranked highest in terms of implementation by experts from all three industries. Biosecurity against these routes of transmission was also considered effective and feasible. The implementation of biosecurity against two routes of disease transmission, airborne and arthropod-borne, was estimated to be less than 25% nationally by the swine industry and was not different from the implementation estimate for the beef industry (and beef was not different from dairy). In general, estimated current implementation of biosecurity measures targeting disease transmission routes was found to be more strongly correlated with feasibility than with effectiveness in the disease transmission routes across the three industries (data not

Biosecurity measure		Highly effective highly feasible	Highly effective highly infeasible	Highly ineffective highly feasible	Highly ineffective highly infeasible	Implementation[1]	
	Obs	%	%	%	%	Mean	Std. dev.
A communication/education plan is in place to inform visitors and service providers of disease status and biosecurity requirements	9	11	0	22	0	1.89	0.93
Line of separation is in place for all visitors and service providers entering premises	11	27	9	9	0	1.18	0.40
Protocols have been developed and implemented to contain and/or exclude the targeted virus within the affected premises	8	13	0	0	0	1.25	0.46
A communication/education plan is in place to inform employees of disease status and biosecurity requirements	7	57	0	14	0	1.71	0.95
Line of separation is in place for all employees entering premises	9	11	0	0	0	1.11	0.33
Protocols for monitoring employee biosecurity compliance have been developed	6	50	0	0	0	1.33	0.52
Timely visits by veterinarian(s)	9	33	0	0	0	2.22	0.44
Daily observations by producer/employees	7	71	0	0	0	2.14	0.90
Monitoring of production records for health status changes	7	57	0	0	0	2.29	1.11
Protocols: have been developed and implemented pertaining to transport biosecurity to contain or exclude the targeted virus within the affected premises	7	43	0	0	0	1.57	0.79
Protocols have been developed for cleaning and/or disinfecting vehicles for certain animal movements (required for verification of biosecurity payments)	9	44	0	0	0	1.89	1.05
Line of separation is in place for all animals entering and leaving premises	8	50	0	13	0	1.38	0.74
Protocols for loading/unloading animals that attempt to minimize virus introduction have been developed and implemented	10	20	0	0	0	1.60	0.70
Protocols for pathogen reduction have been developed and implemented to reduce environmental viral load	21	38	5	0	0	1.62	0.80
Use of an effective disinfectant (required for verification of biosecurity payments)	11	18	0	0	0	1.36	0.50
Follow appropriate downtimes after cleaning and disinfection	14	43	0	0	0	2.07	1.00
Where possible, use all-in and all-out production practices	12	8	42	0	8	1.25	0.62
Protocols have been developed and implemented to establish stabilization and monitoring for the affected premises (monitoring may include submission of samples to a diagnostic laboratory for testing)	10	60	0	0	0	1.60	0.84
Movements of animals on and off the premises are routinely recorded	10	50	0	0	0	2.10	0.99

[1]The survey instrument collected information on current implementation using categorical variables 1=25% or less, 2=26-50%, 3=51-75%, 4=76% or more.

Table 6: Summary of effectiveness, feasibility, and implementation of biosecurity measures in the dairy industry.

shown). This is not surprising as producer implementation decisions are likely to reflect privately absorbed costs and perhaps only partially internalize the broader, social values of more effective biosecurity measures.

Biosecurity measures

Swine industry experts estimated that over 50% of the industry was implementing all-in all-out production (where possible), recording movements of animals, accessing veterinary services in a timely manner, communicating biosecurity requirements with visitors and service personnel, monitoring production records for changes in health status, observing animals daily, and maintaining a line of separation for animals entering and leaving the premises. Of these practices, maintaining a line of separation for animals entering and leaving, was ranked as being both highly effective and highly feasible by the greatest number of experts (80%). However, maintaining a line of separation for all visitors and service providers and for all employees was ranked as highly effective and highly feasible by fewer experts (57% and 50%, respectively) and is estimated to be implemented by fewer than 50% of the industry. Establishing a premises line of separation for people and animals is a key component of Secure Food Supply guidance to support continuity of operations in the event of a foreign animal disease outbreak (http://www.securepork.org/plan-components.php). As such it is an important biosecurity measure to mitigate a Tier 1 disease risk.

Another key component of Secure Food Supply guidance is observation and reporting of animal health status. Accessing veterinary services in a timely manner, monitoring production records, and observing animals daily are all implemented widely by the industry, despite being ranked highly effective and highly feasible by fewer than 50% of expert respondents. Managed movements of animals would be part of a foreign animal disease response. Recording of movements is important for tracing disease (forward or back) and has been implemented by more than 50% of the industry.

All-in all-out production is used by over 70% of nursery pig [25] and over 80% of feeder-to-finish farms [26] and has been shown since the early 1990s to improve health and performance [27], primarily by facilitating the control of respiratory diseases and reducing variability within lots of hogs marketed. Premises with all-in all-out production were able to implement protocols to eliminate porcine epidemic diarrhea virus from herds (personal communication). The integration of movement between premises specializing in different production phases requires pre-planning to address movement management in the event of a foreign animal disease outbreak.

Interestingly, the list of biosecurity measures, informed by the literature, from which experts were asked to evaluate a subset does not include any practices designed to minimize disease transmission risk by means of airborne or arthropod-borne spread. Efforts to minimize feed and water contamination do not appear on this list either. Manure management as a measure to prevent feed and water contamination and vector control in general do commonly appear in biosecurity recommendations in the United States [28].

Conclusion

Experts report differences in effectiveness, feasibility, and current implementation of biosecurity measures targeting disease transmission routes and recommended biosecurity measures among swine, beef, and dairy industries. With this information, a targeted set of disease transmission routes and biosecurity measures can be examined that would allow for a more in-depth and refined study, enhancing the power of future studies, and improving the ability to formulate recommendations. All biosecurity measures come with a cost and ineffective and infeasible methods should be avoided. Likewise, transmission routes that impose the greatest risk should be the focus, rather than low-risk transmission routes.

The information and infrastructure needed to achieve adequate biosecurity can vary significantly by industries. Variations in the management and marketing structure of each livestock industry, including size and reliance on extensive movement of animals, can complicate progress towards achieving sufficient biosecurity. Prioritization of the most effective and feasible biosecurity measures will ensure resources are applied where biosecurity advances are of the highest importance and that will offer the greatest return on investment.

Acknowledgements

This material is based upon work that is supported by the National Institute of Food and Agriculture, U.S. Department of Agriculture, under award number 2015-69004-23273.

References

1. Roth JA, Spickler AR (2014) FMD vaccine surge capacity for emergency use in the United States. Vet Microbiol and Prev Med Rep, Paper 8. Accessed on: 8 August 16.

2. Food and Agriculture Organization of the United Nations/World Organisation for Animal Health/World Bank (2010) Good practices for biosecurity in the pig sector – Issues and options in developing and transition countries. FAO Animal Production and Health Paper No. 169. Rome, FAO.

3. Lewerin SS, Österberg J, Alenius S, Elvander M, Fellström C, et al. (2015) Risk assessment as a tool for improving external biosecurity at farm level. BMC Vet Res. 11: 171-181.

4. Sutherst RW (2001) The vulnerability of animal and human health to parasites under global change. Int J Parasitol. 31: 933-948.

5. Dee S, Clement T, Schelkopf A, Nerem J, Knudsen D, et al. (2014) An evaluation of contaminated complete feed as a vehicle for porcine epidemic diarrhea virus infection of naïve pigs following consumption via natural feeding behavior: proof of concept. BMC Vet Res. 10: 176.

6. US Department of Agriculture Animal and Plant Health Inspection Service Veterinary Services (2010) Beef 2007-08, Part IV reference of beef cow-calf management practices in the United States. February 2010. Accessed on: 29 October 2016.

7. Smith WA, Strand J (2008) Social marketing behavior: A practical resource for social change professionals. Academy for Educational Development, Washington DC, USA.

8. Gunn GJ, Heffernan C, Hall M, McLeod A, Hovi M (2008) Measuring and comparing constraints to improved biosecurity amongst gb farmers, veterinarians and the auxiliary industries. Prev Vet Med. 84: 310-323.

9. Heffernan C, Nielsen L, Thomson K, Gunn G (2008) An exploration of the drivers to bio-security collective action among a sample of UK cattle and sheep farmers. Prev Vet Med. 87: 358-372.

10. Delgado AH, Norby B, Scott HM, Dean W, McIntosh WA, et al. (2014) Distribution of cow–calf producers' beliefs about reporting cattle with clinical signs of foot-and-mouth disease to a veterinarian before or during a hypothetical outbreak. Prev Vet Med. 117: 505-517.

11. Delgado AH, Norby B, Scott HM, Dean W, McIntosh WA, et al. (2014) Distribution of cow–calf producers' beliefs regarding gathering and holding their cattle and observing animal movement restrictions during an outbreak of foot-and-mouth disease. Prev Vet Med. 117: 518-532.

12. Nissen B, Krieter J (2003) Relative importance of risk factors concerning the introduction and spread of classical swine fever and foot-and-mouth disease in Germany. Arch Tierz. 46: 535-546.

13. Kuster K, Cousin ME, Jemmi T, Schüpbach-Regula G, Magouras I (2015) Expert opinion on the perceived effectiveness and importance of on-farm biosecurity measures for cattle and swine farms in Switzerland. Plos One. 10: e0144533.

14. Jochimsen AA (2015) The vulnerability of U.S. agriculture to foot and mouth disease. Master's thesis. Monterey, CA: Naval Postgraduate School.

15. Mankad A (2016) Psychological influences on biosecurity control and farmer decision-making. A review. Agron Sustain Dev. 36: 40.

16. Dewey C, Bottoms K, Carter N, Richardson K (2014) A qualitative study to identify potential biosecurity risks associated with feed delivery. J Swine Health Prod. 22: 232-243.

17. Hernández-Jover M, Gilmour J, Schembri N, Sysak T, Holyoake PK, et al. (2012) Use of stakeholder analysis to inform risk communication and extension strategies for improved biosecurity amongst small-scale pig producers. Prev Vet Med. 104: 258-270.

18. US Department of Agriculture Animal and Plant Health Inspection Service Veterinary Services (2014) Veterinary services herd/premises management plan requirements for Swine Enteric Coronavirus Disease (SECD) reported herds. Accessed on: 23 November 2015.

19. US Department of Agriculture Animal and Plant Health Inspection Service (2013) High-consequence foreign animal diseases and pests. Accessed on: 12 November 2015.

20. Stata Corp LP (2016) Stata Statistical Software Release 14. StataCorp, LP, College Station, TX, USA.

21. Cross P, Rigby D, Edwards-Jones G (2012) Eliciting expert opinion on the effectiveness and practicality of interventions in the farm and rural environment to reduce human exposure to escherichia coli O157. Epidemiol Infect. 140: 643-654.

22. Erdem S, Rigby D (2013) Investigating heterogeneity in the characterization of risks using best worst scaling. Risk Anal. 33: 1728-1748.

23. Tonsor GT, Schroeder TC, Mintert J (2014) Using expert knowledge to guide commodity promotion and research program investments: A US beef industry example. J Agribus. 32: 1.

24. US Department of Agriculture National Agricultural Statistics Service (2014) 2012 census of agriculture, United States summary and state data. May 2014. Accessed on: 5 September 2016.

25. US Department of Agriculture Animal and Plant Health Inspection Service Veterinary Services Centers for Epidemiology and Animal Health (2009) Nursery and grower/finisher management in swine 2000 and swine 2006. Accessed on: 16 December 2016.

26. McBride WD, Key N (2013) US Hog production from 1992 to 2009: Technology, restructuring, and productivity growth, ERR-158. US Department of Agriculture, Economic Research Service. Accessed on: 16 December 2016.

27. Scheidt AB, Cline TR, Clark LK, Mayrose VB, Van Alstine WG, et al. (1995) The effect of all-in-all-out growing-finishing on the health of pigs. J Swine Health Prod. 3: 202-205.

28. Moore DA, Merryman ML, Hartman ML, Klingborg DJ (2008) Comparison of published recommendations regarding biosecurity practices for various production animal species and classes. J Amer Vet Med Assoc 233: 249-256.

17

Bovine Trypanosomosis and Tsetse Fly Vectors in Abobo and Gambela Districts, Southwestern Ethiopia

Mohamed Kedir[1], Kumela Lelisa[2]* and Delesa Damena[3]

[1]National Tsetse and Trypanosomosis Investigation and Control Center, Bedele, Ethiopia
[2]National Institute for Control and Eradication of Tsetse Fly and Trypanosomosis, Ethiopia
[3]National Animal Health Diagnostic and Investigation Center, Sebeta, Ethiopia

Abstract

The study was conducted from October 2015 to November 2015 in Gambela and Abobo districts of Gambela Peoples Regional State, southwestern Ethiopia. It was designed to avail information on prevalence of bovine trypanosomosis and apparent densities of vectors of the trypanosomosis. A parasitological study using buffy coat technique was employed for the determination of prevalence of trypanosomosis while baited mono pyramidal traps were used for the vector survey. A total of 862 cattle randomly selected from the study population were examined for the parasitological study. The result of parasitological study revealed that the overall prevalence of trypanosomosis was found to be 16.59%, 95% CI=14.10-19.08 indicating trypanosomosis is a serious problem in the area. Three Trypanosoma species were identified during the study period: *Trypanosoma brucei*, *T. vivax* and *T. congolense*. Highest trypanosome prevalence (18.67%) was seen in animals with poor condition than that of those with medium (16.76%) and good (14.20%) body condition for the concerned blood parasite but no significant difference was observed (P>0.05). Higher infection rate was occurred in male (18.35%) than female (14.79%) cattle without significant difference (P>0.05). Prevalence was significantly higher in adult animals (17.95%) than younger ones (7.27%) (P>0.05). The study suggested that mean PCV values of parasitaemic (21.13%) cattle was significantly lower than aparasitaemic (22.26%) animals (P<0.05). During entomological survey, four species of tsetse fly: G. tachnoides, G. morsitsns submorsitans, G. pallidipes and G. fuscipes fuscipes and three genera of other biting flies: Tabanus, Haematopota and Stomoxys spp. were caught. The overall apparent density of tsetse flies was 0.75 fly/trap/day. Trypanosomosis and tsetse fly pose great threat to cattle residing in study areas. Thus, appropriate intervention measures need to be taken.

Keywords: Abobo; Density; Gambela; Prevalence; Trypanosomosis; Tsetse fly

Introduction

Trypanosomosis is an endemic disease to east Africa including Ethiopia [1]. Bovine trypanosomosis is one of the diseases that are caused by flagellated protozoan parasites belong to the genus Trypanosoma [2]. Trypanosomosis limits the extension of natural herds in Africa where the presence of tsetse fly density access to woody land and savannah areas with good grazing potential. It is a serious constraint to agricultural production in extensive areas of the tsetse infested regions [3] which accounts over 10 million square kilometers of the tropical Africa. The reduced capacity for work animals is also a very important factor where 80% of the traction power in African agriculture is provided by animals. In general, there is a great threat of trypanosomosis which impedes the economic development of Africa.

Out of six species of trypanosomes are recorded in Ethiopia, three are the most important trypanosomes in terms of economic loss in domestic livestock and are tsetse transmitted species. These include *Trypanosoma congolense*, *T. vivax* and *T. brucei*. Tsetse flies are principal vector of African animal trypanosomosis and Sleeping Sickness. Tsetse flies in Ethiopia are confined to southwestern and northwestern regions between longitude 33° and 38° E and latitude 5° and 12° N covers an area of 220,000 km². Tsetse infested areas lie in the river basins of Blue Nile, Baro-Akobo, Didessa, Ghibe, and Omo. Five species of Glossina (*G. m. submorsitans*, *G. pallidipes*, *G. tachinoides*, *G. f. fuscipes* and *G. longipennis*) have been investigated in Ethiopia [4] out of which the first four are distributed widely in western and south western part of the country. Tsetse transmitted animal trypanosomosis still remains as one of the major causes of livestock mortality and production losses in western, southwestern and northwestern lowlands

of Ethiopia [5], although trypanosomosis can also be transmitted by other blood sucking insects.

Currently, trypanosomosis is found to be one of the factors hampering livestock production and productivity in most parts of western and south western Ethiopia. An understanding of the prevalence of the disease and magnitude of the vector population is crucial for designing appropriate control strategies. Therefore, the aim of this research was to estimate the infection rate of trypanosomosis in cattle and relative abundance of Glossina species and other biting flies responsible for transmitting the disease in Gambela and Abobo districts, Southwestern Ethiopia.

Materials and Methods

Study area

The study was conducted from October to November 2015 in five peasant associations of Gambela district and five peasant associations of Abobo district located in Gambela regional sate. The districts are situated at 766 and 811 Kilometers South West of Addis Ababa respectively. The

*Corresponding author: Kumela Lelisa Dera, National Institute for Control and Eradication of Tsetse Fly and Trypanosomosis, PO Box 19917, Addis Ababa, Ethiopia, E-mail: lelisakumela@gmail.com

mean annual rain fall in both Gambela and Abobo districts ranges from 1000-2000 mm. The annual temperature ranges from 27-40°C. Both districts have altitudes ranging from 400-520 meters above sea level. The areas are well known by their diversified wildlife such as buffaloes, elephants, lions, leopards, cheetahs, giraffes, hartebeest, baboons, Bush pigs, warthog, bush buck, kudu, hippopotamus, crocodiles, and antelopes etc. which might be claimed to serve as sources of food for tsetse fly and as reservoir for trypanosomes (Figure 1).

Study population, sampling design and sample size determination

The cattle in the study areas are local breeds that are kept under traditional extensive husbandry systems with communal herding. The animal population of the Gambela district is estimated to be 1752 cattle, 325 sheep, 1194 goats, and 13 equines and Abobo has an estimated 4049 cattle, 44 sheep, 2141 goats, 116 equines population.

A cross-sectional study was conducted in ten purposively selected villages of Gambela and Abobo districts, Gambela Peoples Regional State, southwest Ethiopia. Then simple random sampling technique was followed to select individual study animals. The number of animals required for the study was determined using the formula given by Thrusfield [6] for simple random sampling. The size of sample was determined using 95% level of confidence, 50% expected prevalence and 0.05 desired absolute precision. Therefore, a total of 384 cattle were needed for the study even though, samples collected from 862 cattle was examined. The sex, body condition and origin of cattle including districts and peasant associations were explanatory variables used to associate with the prevalence. Body condition for each cattle was

estimated based on Nicholson and Butterworth [7]. Whilst, age of study animals was determined by dentition according to De Lahunte and Habel [8] and categorized into two age groups as adult (>3 years) and young (≤ 3 years).

Study methodology

Survey of trypanosomes: Blood samples were collected in to heparinized micro hematocrit tubes (Deltalab S.L, Bercelona, Spain) after piercing the ear vein using lancet. Then one end of the capillary tube was sealed with sealant (Hawksley Ltd, Lancing, UK) and centrifuged at 12,000 revolutions per minute (rpm) for five minutes to separate the blood cells and to concentrate trypanosomes using centrifugal force as buffy coat. Then Packed Cell Volume (PCV) was determined using hematocrit reader and recorded. The capillary tubes were then broken just below buffy coat and expressed on microscopic slide, mixed and covered with a 22 × 22 mm cover slip. Then it was examined under x40 objective of microscope using dark ground Buffy coat technique to detect the presence of motile trypanosomes and for positive samples Geimsa stain of thin blood smears were made, fixed with methanol for 5 minutes, and examined under oil immersion using x100 objective to identify the species of trypanosomes [9].

Entomological study: A total of 145 baited mono-pyramidal traps were deployed along suitable tsetse habitats to assess the apparent densities, distributions and species of tsetse flies and other haematophagus flies involving in transmission of trypanosomes. All traps were baited with acetone, Octenol (1-3-Octane) and cow urine filled in separated bottles and labeled and deployed at an interval of 200-250 meters. After 48 hours of trap deployment time the cages

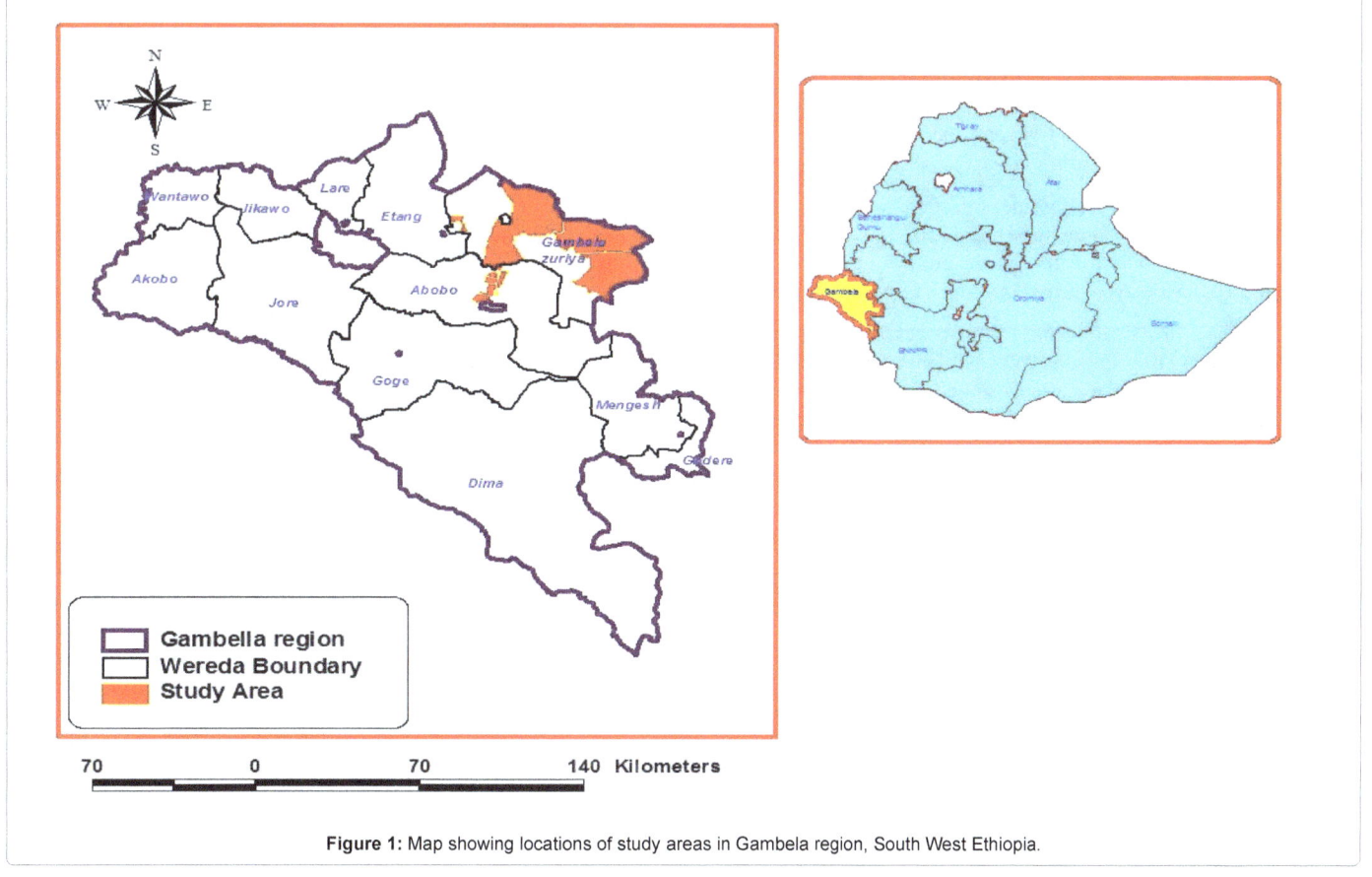

Figure 1: Map showing locations of study areas in Gambela region, South West Ethiopia.

were collected and captured flies were identified and sexed according to morphological characteristics and counted. The tsetse flies were identified to species level and the other biting flies to the genus level [10].

Data management and analysis

The data collected were entered in to Microsoft Excel Data base system. The entered data were analyzed using STATA version 10 statistical software program. The prevalence of trypanosomosis was calculated by dividing the proportion of cattle infected with one and/or more trypanosome species by the total number of cattle examined multiplied by 100. The association between the prevalence of trypanosome infection and associated risk factors were assessed by logistic regression, whereas the student's t-test was used to assess the difference in mean PCV between trypanosome positive and negative animals. A statistically significant association between variables was said to exist if the calculated P<0.05 at 95% confidence level. Finally, the density of fly population is calculated by dividing the number of flies caught by the number traps deployed and number of days of deployment, and expressed as fly/trap/day (FTD).

Results

Parasitological findings

From the total examined cattle (n=862), 143 (16.59%, 95%CI=14.10-19.08) were found to be infected with trypanosomes. Out of the total 580 cattle examined, 105(18.10%) cattle were positive for trypanosomosis in Abobo district, while 38 (13.48%) were infected with trypanosomes out of the 282 examined cattle in Gambela district (χ^2=2.94; P=0.09). The prevalence was varying from 12.50% to 29.82% in Abobo district. In Gambela district the infection rate of bovine trypanosomes was ranging from 9.64% to 58.82% (Tables 1 and 2).

Infection rate was 18.35% and 14.79% in male and female respectively. Higher prevalence of trypanosomosis was recorded in adult animals (17.95%) than younger ones (7.27%). Similarly, anemic cattle (PCV ≤ 24%) had higher trypanosomes prevalence than those with PCV values within the normal range (25_48%) (Table 3).

The proportion of trypanosome infection with species level indicated 94 (65.73%) were found to be infected by *T. vivax*, 36 (25.17%) were found to be infected by *T. congolense*; 3(2.10%) were infected by *T. brucei* and 10 (6.99%) were mixed infections (χ^2=862; P=0.00).

The prevalence in male and female animals was 18.35% and 14.79%, respectively. Of the 110 young and 752 adult animals examined, 7.27% and 17.95% tested positive for trypanosome infection, for young and adults, respectively. Significantly higher prevalence was recorded in adult animals as compared to the young ones. Higher prevalence of

trypanosomosis was recorded in animals with a poor body condition (18.67%) than in those in medium (16.76%) and good body condition (14.20%).

Hematological findings

The overall mean PCV values of examined cattle was 22.07 ± 4.83 (/t/=00, DF=8, SE=0.16, p=0.00, 95%CI=21.75-22.39). Cattle with good body condition had highest (23.78%, SE=0.38, 95%CI=23.04-24.51) mean PCV value followed by medium (20.02 SE=0.20, 95%CI=21.63-22.41) and poor (22.43, SE=0.39, 95%CI=19.56-21.10). The mean PCV of parasitaemic and aparasitaemic animals was 21.13%, 95% CI=20.39-21.86 and 22.26%, 95% CI=21.90-22.62 respectively.

Entomological findings

The tsetse flies found during the study period were *Glossina m. submorsitans*, *G. pallidipes*, *G. fuscipes fuscipes* and *G. tachnoides* and other biting flies particularly genus Stomoxys, Haematopota and Tabanus. A total 3154 blood sucking flies were caught during the study period of which 218 (6.91%) were tsetse fly, 14(0.44%) were Stomoxys, 11 (0.35%) were Haematopota and 2911 (92.30%) were Tabanids. The overall fly species caught was 10.88 fly/trap/day. The apparent densities of Glossina, Tabanus, Haematopota and Stomoxys were 0.75, 10.04, 0.04 and 0.05 flies/trap/day respectively. The apparent densities of Glossina species was 0.24 and 1.09 fly/trap/day in Gambela and Abobo districts, respectively. The sex category indicated male and female tsetse fly account for 36.70% and 63.30% of total caught Glossina species, respectively.

Discussion

Bovine trypanosomosis affects cattle which have a major role in the economy of Ethiopia. Prevalence of trypanosomosis in Gambela and Abobo areas, located in Baro Akobo water basin during the study period was found to be 16.59%. This result is fairly similar with earlier report from different parts of Ethiopia and from abroad: 14.68% in north western Ethiopia [11], 16.44% in northern Cameroon [12] and 17.33% in southern Ethiopia [13]. Infection rate is significantly higher in Bonga village (58.82%) (P<0.05). This might be related with high density of blood sucking insects in the village. The prevalence of trypanosomosis in Gambela and Abobo districts was 13.48% and 18.10%, respectively. However, there was no statistically significant difference (p>0.05) between these two districts. This may be related with similarity of the two districts in vegetation and other epidemiological factors such as cattle breed and management system.

The present result revealed that the trypanosome species encountered in the area were *T. vivax, T. congolense* and *T. brucei*.

BC result	Peasant Associations					Total
	Village 17	Village 14	Village 13	Village 11	Village 7	
Negative	92 (86.79%)	40 (70.18%)	60 (74.07%)	124 (78.98%)	84 (87.50%)	475 (81.90%)
Positive	14 (13.21%)	17 (29.82%)	21 (25.93%)	33 (21.02%)	12 (12.50%)	105 (18.10%)
Total (N)	106	57	81	157	96	580

Table 1: Prevalence of bovine trypanosomosis in different peasant associations of Abobo district.

BC result	Peasant Associations					Total
	Village 8	Bonga	Elchiwe	Abol	Opanga	
Negative	75 (90.36%)	7 (41.18%)	17 (70.83%)	136 (97.14%)	84 (83.17%)	244 (86.52%)
Positive	8 (9.64%)	10 (58.82%)	7 (29.17%)	4 (2.86%)	17 (16.83%)	38 (13.48%)
Total (N)	83	17	24	140	101	282

Table 2: Prevalence of bovine trypanosomosis in different peasant associations of Gambela district.

Variables	No. of negative	No. of positive	Total	X^2	P-value
Districts					
Gambela	244(86.52%)	38(13.48%)	282 (32.71%)		
Abobo	475(81.90%)	105(18.10%)	580 (67.29%)	2.94	0.09
	719(83.41%)	143(16.59%)	862 (100%)		
Sex					
Male	356(81.65%)	80(18.35%)	436 (50.58%)		
Female	363(85.21%)	63(14.79%)	426 (49.42%)	1.97	0.16
	719 (83.41%)	143 (16.59%)	862 (100%)		
Body Condition					
Good	145(85.80%)	24(14.20%)	169 (19.61%)		
Medium	452(83.24%)	91(16.76%)	543 (62.99%)	1.18	0.56
Poor	122(81.33%)	28(18.67%)	150 (17.40%)		
	719 (83.41%)	143 (16.59%)	862 (100%)		
Age					
Young	102 (97.73%)	8(7.27%)	110 (12.76%)		
Adult	617(87.05%)	135(17.95%)	752(87.24%)	7.91	0.01**
	719(83.41%)	143(16.59%)	862 (100%)		
PCV					
≤24%	502 (81.76%)	112 (18.24%)	614 (71.23%)		
>24 %	217 (87.50%)	31 (12.50%)	248 (28.77%)	4.21	0.04**
	719 (83.41%)	143 (16.59%)	862 (100%)		

Table 3: Prevalence of bovine trypanosomosis and associated risk factors in Gambela and Abobo districts.

These three species of trypanosomes were also reported from western and south western part of Ethiopia by Lemecha et al. [14] in Ghibe valley, Tilahun et al. [15] in Dale Sadi district; Habte et al. [16] in Darimu district and Lelisa et al. [17] in southwestern Ethiopia. The study showed that *T. vivax* was the predominant (65.73%) species in the area. Similar reports were made previously by Mhiret and Mamo [18] in East Gojjam, North West Ethiopia and Tadesse et al. [19] in Northwestern Ethiopia. This may be associated to the presence high density of biting flies that are mechanical vector of trypanosomes (*T. vivax*) which can be transmitted by tsetse flies and/or other blood sucking insects like *Tabanus, Haematopota* and *Stomoxys* spp. [20].

The prevalence of trypanosomosis in male and female animals was 18.35% and 14.79%, respectively. The difference in prevalence between the sex groups was not statistically significant (p>0.05). Of the 110 young and 752 adult animals examined, 7.27% and 17.95% tested positive for trypanosome infection, respectively. Significantly higher prevalence was recorded in adult animals as compared to the young ones (P<0.05). This might be due to increased exposure of adult cattle to vectors of trypanosomes. Dagnachew [21], Tekle and Mekonen [22] and Mulatu et al. [23] also reported significantly higher infection rate in older cattle. Although the difference is not significant (p>0.05), higher prevalence of trypanosomosis was higher in animals in a poor body condition (18.67%) than in those in medium (16.76%) and good body condition (14.20%) indicating weight loss is one of the symptoms of trypanosomosis [24].

The study also indicated that the mean PCV values of investigated cattle of the study area was negatively correlated (r=-0.09) with trypanosomosis prevalence, that is, mean PCV was decreased with increasing prevalence of infection. The mean PCV value of parasitaemic animals was 21.13%, SE=0.38, 95%CI=20.39-21.86 and aparasitaemic animals was 22.26%, SE=0.18, 95% CI=21.90-22.62. Measuring the mean PCV value is one of the indicator of a herd infected with trypanosomosis and hence the anemic status of sampled animals showed reduced PCV values. Such result was also reported by Lelisa et al. [25]; Tasew and Duguma [26]; Zecharias and Zeryehun [27]; Kassaye and Tsegaye [28]. Thus, the development of anemia is the most

reliable indication of the progress of the trypanosome infection. There are also parasitoloically negative animals within the PCV values of less than the threshold value (≤ 24%). This may be due to in adequacy of detection method (Buffy coat technique) or delayed recovery of anemic situation after current treatment with trypanocidal drugs. Other blood parasites infection like babesiosis and theileriosis [29] and malnutrition can also lead to the development of anemia. Whilst, the occurrences of parasitologically positive cattle with PCV greater than 25% might be thought of recent infections of animals with trypanosomes.

In this study, the entomological findings revealed that four species of Glossina (*Glossina m. submorsitans, G. pallidipes, G. fuscipes fuscipes* and *G. tachnoides*) out of five reported in Ethiopia and other biting flies of genera Stomoxys, Haemtopota and Tabanids occur Gambela and Abobo districts, Gambela Peoples Regional State, South west Ethiopia. These four tsetse specie also reported by Duguma et al. [30] in western and Southwestern Ethiopia. The apparent densities of Glossina species was 0.24 and 1.09 fly/trap/day in Gambela and Abobo districts respectively. This result is in agreement with different reports in western, south, south western and north western part of the country: 1.45 and 0.58 fly/trap/day in two districts of East Wollega zone, western Ethiopia [31], and 1.14 fly/trap/day in Southern Rift Valley of Ethiopia [32]. The sex category indicated male and female tsetse fly account for 36.70% and 63.30% of total caught Glossina species, respectively. The higher number of female than males might be related with the longer lifespan of female than male tsetse flies.

In conclusion, the present study indicated that tsetse transmitted trypanosomosis is a potential threat for cattle residing in the area. Thus, trypanosomosis and tsetse control methods should be expanded to reach all infested areas in sustainable manner besides participatory extension packages to create public awareness. Further epidemiological investigation is also a necessity to synchronize control efforts at national level and detail survey of human African trypanosomosis also should be undertaken.

References

1. Shaw APM, Cecchic G, Wintd GRW, Mattiolie RC, Robinson TP (2014) Mapping the economic benefits to livestock keepers from intervening against bovine trypanosomosis in Eastern Africa. Prev Vet Med 113: 197-210.

2. Uilenberg G (1998) A field guide for the diagnosis, treatment and prevention of African animal trypanosomosis, Food and Agriculture Organization of the United Nations, Rome.

3. Slingenbergh J (1992) Tsetse control and agricultural development in Ethiopia. World Anim Rev 70-71: 30-36.

4. Abebe G (2005) Trypanosomosis in Ethiopia. Ethiop J Biol Sci 4: 75-121.

5. NTTICC (2004) Annual Report on Tsetse and Trypanosomosis Survey, National Tsetse and Trypanosomosis Investigation and Control Center, Bedele, Ethiopia.

6. Thrusfield M (2005) Veterinary epidemiology. 3rd edn, Black well science, Oxford, p: 233.

7. Nicholson MJ, Butterworth MH (1986) A guide to body condition scoring of zebu cattle. International Livestock Research Center for Africa, Addis Ababa, Ethiopia.

8. DeLahunta A, Habel RE (1986) Teeth. In: Applied Veterinary Anatomy. DeLahunta A and Habel RE (eds.). W.B. Saunders Company, Philadelphia, USA.

9. Murray M, Trail JCM, Turner DA, Wissocq Y (1983) Livestock productivity and trypanotolerance: Network training manual. International Livestock Centre for Africa (ILCA), Addis Ababa.

10. Wall R, Shearer D (1997) Veterinary Entomology. Arthropod Ectoparasites of Veterinary Importance. London, UK, Champman and hall, pp: 141-193.

11. Dagnachew S, Sangwan AK, Abebe G (2005) Epidemiology of bovine trypanosomosis in the Abay (Blue Nile) Basin Areas of Northwest Ethiopia. Rev D"Elev Et De Med Vet Des Pays Trop 58: 151-157.

12. Achukwi MD, Musongong GA (2009) Trypanosomosis in the Doayo/Namchi (*Bos taurus*) and zebu White Fulani (*Bos indicus*) cattle in Faro Division, North Cameroon. J App Biosci 15: 807-814.

13. Zeleke G (2011) Preliminary survey on tsetse flies and trypanosomosis at grazing fields and villages in and around the Nech Sar National Park, Southern Ethiopia. Ethiop Vet J 15: 59-67.

14. Lemecha H, Mulatu W, Hussein I, Rege E, Tekle T, et al. (2006) Response of four indigenous bovine breeds to natural tsetse and trypanosomosis challenge in the Ghibe valley of Ethiopia. Vet Parasitol 141: 165-176.

15. Tilahun Z, Jiregna D, Solomon K, Haimanot D, Girma K, et al. (2014) Prevalence of Bovine Trypanosomosis, its Vector Density and Distribution in Dale Sadi District, Kellem Wollega Zone, Ethiopia. Acta Parasitol Glob 5: 107-114.

16. Habte F, Kebede A, Desta T (2015) Study on Spatial Distribution of Tsetse Fly and Prevalence of Bovine Trypanosomosis and other Risk Factors: Case Study in Darimu District, Ilu Aba Bora Zone, Western Ethiopia. J Pharmacy and Alt Med, p: 7.

17. Lelisa K, Damena D, Tasew T, Kedir M, Megersa M (2016) Prevalence of Bovine Trypanosomosis and Vector Distributions in Chewaka Settlement Area of Ilubabor Zone, Southwestern Ethiopia. Adv Biol Res 10: 71-76.

18. Mhiret A, Mamo G (2007) Bovine trypanosomosis in three districts of East Gojjam zone bordering Blue Nile River in Ethiopia. J Infect Dev Ctries 1: 321-325.

19. Tadesse E, Gashaw G, Assaye M (2015) Prevalence of Bovine Trypanosomosis in Bure and Womberma Districts of West Gojjam Zone, North West Ethiopia. Acta Parasitol Glob 6: 164-173.

20. Gooding RH, Krafsur ES (2005) Tsetse Genetics: Contributions to Biology, Systematics, and Control of Tsetse Flies. Annu Rev Entomol 50: 101-123.

21. Dagnachew S (2004) Epidemiology of bovine trypanosomosis in the Abay Basin Areas of Northwestern Ethiopia. Addis Ababa University, Faculty of Veterinary Medicine, MSc Thesis, Debre Zeit, Ethiopia

22. Tekle Y (2013) Prevalence of Bovine Trypanosomosis in Tsetse Controlled and Uncontrolled Areas of Eastern Wollega, Ethiopia. J Sci and Innov Res 2: 61-75.

23. Mulatu E, Lelisa K, Damena D (2016) Prevalence of Bovine Trypanosomosis and Apparent Density of Tsetse Flies in Eastern Part of Dangur District, North Western Ethiopia. J Vet Sci Technol 7: 347.

24. Radostitis OM, Gay C, Blood DC (2007) Veterinary Medicine: A text book of diseases of cattle, horse, sheep, pigs and goats. Balliere Tindal London, pp: 1531-1540.

25. Lelisa K, Shimelis, Bekele J, Shiferaw D (2014) Bovine trypanosomosis and its fly vectors in three selected settlement areas of Hawa-Gelan district, western Ethiopia. Onderstepoort J Vet Res 81: 715.

26. Tasew S, Duguma R (2012) Cattle anaemia and trypanosomiasis in western Oromia State, Ethiopia. Revue Méd. Vét 163: 581-588.

27. Zecharias A, Zeryehun T (2012) Prevalence of Bovine Trypanosomosis in Selected District of Arba Minch, SNNPR, Southern Ethiopia. Glob Vet 8: 168-173.

28. Kassaye BK, Tsegaye D (2016) Prevalence of Bovine Trypanosomosis, Tsetse Density and Farmers Perceptions on the Impact of Control Program in Kellem Wollega Zone, Western Oromia, Ethiopia. J Veterinar Sci Technol 7:295.

29. Sahinduran S (2012) Protozoan Diseases in Farm Ruminants. In: A Bird's-Eye View of Veterinary Medicine. Carlos C Perez-Marin (Ed.). INTECH Open Access Publisher.

30. Duguma R, Tasew S, Olani A, Damena D, Alemu D, et al. (2015) Spatial distribution of Glossina species and Trypanosoma species in south-western Ethiopia. Parasites & Vectors 8: 430.

31. Tafese W, Melaku, A, Fentahun T (2012) Prevalence of bovine trypanosomosis and its vectors in two districts of East Wollega Zone, Ethiopia. Onderstepoort J Vet Res 79: 1-4.

32. Muturi KS, Msangi S, Munstermann S, Clausen P, Getachew A, et al. (2000) Trypanosomosis Risk Assessment in Selected Sites of the Southern Rift Valley of Ethiopia. I. Distribution, Density and Infection Rates of Tsetse Flies. II. Epidemiology of Bovine Trypanosomosis. In: International Scientific Council for Trypanosomiasis Research and Control (ISCTRC). Proceedings of the 25th meeting held in Mombassa, Kenya. OAU/STRC No. 120.

Prevalence of *Melophagus ovinus* and *Bovicola ovis* infestation in sheep in Wogera District, North Gondar Zone, Ethiopia

Amare Eshetu*, Tilahun Ayele, Shimelis Mengistu, and Dinaol Belina

College of Veterinary Medicine, Haramaya University, PO Box-138, Dire Dawa, Ethiopia

Abstract

The study was conducted from October, 2015 to May, 2016 in Wogera district, North Gondar zone, Ethiopia with the objectives of identifying and estimating the prevalence of sheep ked and lice infestation and to appraise potential risk factors of their attachment to sheep. Out of 423 sheep examined 71.6% were infested either by *Melophagus ovinus* (*M. ovinus*) or *Bovicola ovis* (*B. ovis*) or both. The prevalence of *M. ovinus* and *B. ovis* was 33.57% and 12.07% respectively. Mixed infestation of *M. ovinus* and *B. ovis* (25.53%) was also recorded. The overall prevalence of *M. ovinus* and *B. ovis* infestation was significantly varied among the age (x^2=56.52; P=0.00), sex (x^2=14.71; P=0.00) and body condition (x^2=22.52; P=0.00) categories of sheep. The prevalence of *M. ovinus* in sheep of poor (70.1%) and medium (64.5%) body condition was significantly (x^2=23.29; P=0.00) higher as compared to those of good body (40.5%) condition. Furthermore, the prevalence of *M. ovinus* was significantly varied with age (x^2=99.26; P=0.00). Similarly, *B. ovis* prevalence was significantly (x^2=16.56; P=0.00) highest in poor (52.9%) and medium (38.2%) than in good (25%) body condition score group. Moreover, the prevalence of *B. ovis* was significantly (x^2=7.44; P=0.008) higher in rams (46.5%) than in ewes (33%) but, did not significantly varied with age (p>0.05). Significant differences were noted in harboring mixed *B. ovis and M. ovinus* infestations among the age (x^2=23.42; P=0.00), sex (x^2=18.41; P=0.00) and body condition (x^2=21.74; P=0.00) groups. In conclusion, further studies on prevalence and economic impacts of infestation of sheep with *M. ovinus* and *B. ovis* are recommended.

Keywords: *Bovicola ovis;* Ethiopia; Ectoparasites; *Melophagus ovinus;* Sheep

Introduction

In Ethiopia nearly 25.5 million sheep are reared in varied agro-ecologies and production systems for multiple purposes such as meat production, income generation, and as a source of skin [1,2]; contributing significantly to small scale farmers' livelihoods [3]. Contribution from sheep production to Ethiopian economy is adversely affected by several constraints. The subclinical parasitism due to endoparasites and ectoparasitism form the main factors [4]. Ectoparasites are however being more important in the changing scenario as they have a range of direct and indirect consequences on their hosts [5]. Ked and lice of small ruminant feeds on the blood of their hosts thus cause blood loss leading to anaemia [6]. They cause irritation to the skin and stimulate scratching, rubbing, and licking leading to restlessness, damage to the fleece and skin and reduction in carcass weight [6,7]. Furthermore, Ked and lice of sheep cause downgrading and rejection of sheep skins [8] thus, adversely affect productivity and reproductive efficiency. Ectoparasites are also vector for various diseases [9]. Furthermore, ectoparasites have major impact on welfare of their hosts [10]. In general, external parasitism adversely affect economic production of sheep resulting in poor sheep products particularly skins thus causes huge losses in terms of income to producers, the skin processing and export industries and the country at large [7,11,12].

Ethiopia used to get the second largest foreign currency earnings from the export of skins and hides which has been deteriorating due to the decrease in skin quality owing to the increase in external parasite infestations [11]. Annually, sheep skin contributes about 30% of skins and hides production based on off take rate [7]. However, studies in the country indicated that ectoparasites are becoming growing threat for small ruminant production and export of skin in Ethiopia and it has been reported that about 35% of sheep skin rejections in the country are due to external parasitism [12,13]. Both lice and ked are considered as a cause of 'ekek' in Ethiopian sheep skins thus, play a major role in

the continuous declining in quality of skin of small ruminants including sheep [14].

In Ethiopia national control program against ectoparasites and skin diseases have been designed by the Ministry of Agriculture and Rural Development of Ethiopia in 2005 and launched in Tigray, Amhara and Afar regions [15]. Regardless of which, reports from different parts of country indicated that ectoparasitism of sheep is still alarming condition [4,7,12,16,17]. Additionally, to the best of our understanding, all the earlier reports on ked and lice of sheep in Ethiopia originated from studies of other ectoparasites, especially ticks and mites or based on examination of fresh sheep skins after slaughter. Therefore, the objectives of this study were to identify and estimate the prevalence of sheep ked and lice infestations in their hosts' natural environment and to appraise potential risk factors of their attachment to sheep in Wogera District, North Gondar Zone, Ethiopia.

Materials and Methods

Study area

The present study was conducted from October, 2015 to May, 2016 in Wogera district, located between 37.36° East and 12.46° North longitude and at an altitude of 2900 m. a. s. l in the North Gondar zone highlands, 781 km from Addis Ababa and 41 km from Gondar town in

*Corresponding author: Amare Eshetu, College of Veterinary Medicine, Haramaya University PO Box-138, Dire Dawa, Ethiopia
E-mail: amare.eshetu@yahoo.com

Amhara National Regional State, Ethiopia. It has annual average rainfall of 700 mm of bimodal pattern, which long rainy season that extends from June to September and a short rainy season from March to May and its average annual temperature is 12.7°C.

Study animals and design

The study employed a cross sectional design using simple and systemic random sampling. The total sample size was calculated as per the formula given by Thrusfield [18] using 95% confidence interval, 5% desired absolute precision and with the assumption of 50% expected prevalence of ectoparasites accordingly a total of 423 sheep were included in this study. Five peasant associations (PAs) of the study district including Ambagiorgis, Ketema, Koseye, Kurajic, Sankatikim, and Sakbesak were randomly selected. The study animals were randomly selected using a systemic sampling technique from sheep population traditionally managed under extensive production system. Sheep of different age, sex, and body condition were included in this study. The animals were grouped into three age categories as young (<1 year), adult (1-3 years) and old (>3 years) based on dentition. Animal body condition score on scale of 0-5 was classified as starving, very thin, thin, moderate, fat and very fat on bases of criteria set by Ethiopian Sheep and Goats Productivity Improvement Program [3]. However, in this study sheep with animal body condition score less than 2 considered as poor; animal body condition score 2 and 3 were considered as medium and animals with body condition scores above 3 considered as good.

Ectoparasites collection and identification

Following proper restraining of the animals clinical examination was performed as described by Kumsa et al. [12]. The skin was palpated across all parts of the animal for the presence of parasites, and gross lesions suggestive of a clinical form of sheep ked and lice infestations and animals found infested were considered positive [12]. Visual inspection of the skin and wool were conducted to detect parasites. The parasite was removed carefully and gently by hand and forceps to avoid any damage on the body. The collected ked and lice from their attachment site inserted into universal bottles containing 70% ethyl alcohol labeled with animals particularities and transported to University of Gondar (UOG) Faculty of Veterinary Medicine (FVM) Parasitology laboratory were further identification of the parasites were conducted under stereomicroscope according to the identification keys of Urquhart et al. and Wall and Shearer [19,20].

Statistical analysis

Collected data were entered into Microsoft Excel 2003 spreadsheets (Microsoft Corp., Redmond, WA, USA) and analyzed using SPSS for Windows version 15.0 (SPSS Inc., Chicago, IL, USA). The animals were divided into different groups: according to their sex as female and male; age groups that is, as young (<1 year), adult (1 to 3 years) and old (>3 years) and body condition score was rated as poor, medium and good. Prevalence was determined based on the formula described by Thrusfield [18] as the rate of number of infested animals and total number of study animals. Associations between the explanatory variables (sex, age and body condition) and prevalence was evaluated by fisher's exact test analysis. Parameters recognized as significant in fisher's exact test analysis were then subjected to logistic regression analysis to investigate the associations between prevalence and explanatory variables. Differences were considered significant at value of P<0.05.

Results

Out of 423 sheep examined 303 (71.6%) were infested by M. ovinus,

B. ovis or both Table 1. The overall prevalence of M. ovinus and B. ovis was 33.57% and 12.07% respectively. In this study mixed infestation of (25.53%) of M. ovinus and B. ovis was also recorded.

The common sites of M. ovinus infestation were the skin of neck, flank, shoulder, back, ramp and belly with the proportion of 57.21%, 32.62%, 11.11%, 8.27%, and 5.91% respectively. For B. ovis infested sheep, the commonly parasitized sites were neck (31.91%), flank (29.55%), back (16.8%), shoulder (14.42%), ramp (11.35%) and belly (4.49%) as shown in Figure 1.

The overall prevalence of M. ovinus and B. ovis based on sex, age, and body condition of the study animals is summarized in Table 2. The overall prevalence of M. ovinus and B. ovis infestation in young (<1 years), adult (1-3 years) and old (>3 years of age) sheep was 86.8%, 67.5% and 46.1% respectively. It was observed that an overall prevalence of sheep ked and lice infestation was significantly (χ^2=56.52; P<0.001) varied among the age categories of sheep. Logistic regression revealed that younger sheep was more likely to be infested with ked and lice than older sheep (OR=4.86; 95% CI: 2.59-9.13).

The overall prevalence of sheep ked and lice in sheep with poor, medium and good body condition was 85.1%, 74.5% and 56% respectively. The study showed that the overall prevalence of the infestation was significantly (χ^2=22.52; P=0.00) higher in poor (85.1%) conditioned sheep than in good (56%) body condition score group. Logistic regression revealed that sheep of poor body condition were more likely to be infested by ectoparasites compared to sheep of good body condition (OR=4.36; 95% CI: 2.06-9.21). Furthermore, sheep of medium body condition were also more likely to be infested by ectoparasites compared to sheep of good body condition (OR=1.71; 95% CI: 1.01-2.88). Also, sex of sheep had a significant effects on overall prevalence of sheep ked and lice infestation (P<0.001).

Prevalence and summery of binary logistic regression analysis for M. ovinus on sheep based on explanatory variables were computed Table 3. The prevalence of M. ovinus was significantly (χ^2=99.26; P=0.00) higher in young (80.9%) and adult (52.1%) sheep compared to old (23.5%) sheep. The odds of the infestation of M. ovinus in young sheep were more times likely than in sheep of older age with 95% CI=4.28-15.13. Likewise, a significantly higher prevalence of M. ovinus in sheep with poor 70.1% (OR=3.46, p<0.001) and medium 64.5% (OR=1.94, p<0.05) body condition was recorded as compared to 40.5% in sheep with good body condition. Sheep with poor body condition were 3.46 times more at risk of infestation of M. ovinus than sheep with good body condition with 95% CI=1.73-6.89. Higher prevalence of M. ovinus in rams than in ewes was recorded (OR=1.16, p=0.05) however, it was not marginally significant among the sex groups of animals. Moreover, sheep with medium body condition were 1.94 times more at risk of infestation of M. ovinus than sheep with good body condition with 95% CI=1.14-3.31.

Prevalence and results of binary logistic regression analysis for B. ovis on sheep against explanatory variables were also computed Table 4. Body condition had a significant effect on prevalence of B. ovis infestation of sheep (χ^2=16.56; P=0.00) with B. ovis infestation being significantly higher in sheep with poor (52.9%) body condition

Ecto-parasites	No. positive	Prevalence (%)
M. ovinus	142	33.57
B. ovis	51	12.07
Mixed infestation	108	25.53
Overall	303	71.63

Table 1: Overall prevalence of M. ovinus and B. ovis in sheep in the study area.

Risk factors		Examined	Positive (%)	χ2	p	OR	p	95%CI for OR
Age	Young	204	177 (86.8)	56.52	0	4.86	0	2.59-9.13
	Adult	117	79 (67.5)			1.83	0	1.02-3.29
	Old*	102	47 (46.1)			1		
Sex	Female*	279	183 (65.6)	14.71	0	1	-	-
	Male	144	120 (83.3)			2.63	0	0.95-2.95
Body condition	Poor	87	74 (85.1)	22.52	0	4.36	0	2.06-9.21
	Medium	220	164 (74.5)			1.71	0.046	1.01-2.88
	Good*	116	65 (56)			1	-	-

OR: Odds Ratio; CI: Confidence Interval; *: reference category

Table 2: Overall prevalence of *M. ovinus* and *B. ovis* according to sex, age and body condition of sheep.

Risk factors		Examined	Prevalence (%)	χ2	p	OR	p	95%CI for OR
Age	Young	204	80.9	99.26	0	8.05	0	4.28-15.13
	Adult	117	52.1			2.53	0.003	1.36-4.50
	Old*	102	23.5			1	-	-
Sex	Female*	279	50.9	22.83	0	1	-	-
	Male	144	75			1.68	0.051	0.09-2.84
Body condition	Poor	87	70.1	23.29	0	3.46	0	1.73-6.89
	Medium	220	64.5			1.94	0.015	1.14-3.31
	Good*	116	40.5			1	-	-

OR: Odds Ratio; CI: Confidence Interval; *: reference category

Table 3: Prevalence and results of binary logistic regression for *M. ovinus* on sheep based on age, sex and body condition.

Risk factors		Examined	Prevalence (%)	χ2	p	OR	p	95%CI for OR
Age	Young	204	41.2	3.37	0.18	1.21	0.53	0.67-2.17
	Adult	117	37.6			1.16	0.63	0.64-2.11
	Old*	102	30.4			1	-	-
Sex	Female*	279	33	7.44	0.008	1	-	-
	Male	144	46.5			1.83	0.009	1.17-2.87
Body condition	Poor	87	52.9	16.56	0	3.49	0	1.89-6.44
	Medium	220	38.2			1.8	0.025	1.08-3.03
	Good*	116	25			1	-	-

OR: odds ratio; CI: confidence interval; *: reference category

Table 4: Prevalence and results of binary logistic regression for *B. ovis* on sheep based on age, sex and body condition.

than in those with good (25%) body condition and logistic regression analysis revealed that sheep with poor body condition were 3.49 times more likely to be infested by *B. ovis* compared to sheep with good body condition (OR=3.49, 95% CI: 1.89-6.44). With regard to the effect of sex on the *B. ovis* infestation of it was observed that sex had a significant (χ^2=7.44; P=0.008) influence on the prevalence of *B. ovis* where the prevalence of *B. ovis* was highest in rams (46.5%) than in ewes (33%). Additionally, logistic regression analysis pointed out that rams were more likely to be infested by *B. ovis* as compared to ewes (OR=1.83; 95% CI: 1.17-2.87). Prevalence of *B. ovis* infestation was highest in young (41.2%) sheep `compared to adult (37.6%) and older (30.4%) sheep but did not significantly vary among age categories (P>0.05).

Discussion

The result of the present study showed that the overall prevalence of *B. ovis* and *M. ovinus* infestation was high (71.63%) in the sheep reared in extensive production system. This is in accordance with the reports of Kumsa et al., Desta et al., Seyoum et al. and Bekele et al. who reported high prevalence of ectoparasites in sheep and goats in different parts of Ethiopia, where prevalence as high as 81.5% [12,14,21,22]. This might be due to ideal climatic condition, poor husbandry practices, less awareness of the animal owners, minimal attention given to the ectoparasites and their effects on animals' health, and inadequate flock health program in the area [12,14,16]. *B. ovis* and *M. ovinus* might also

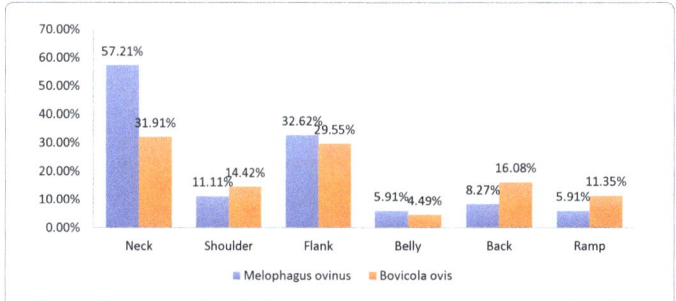

Figure 1: Common sites of *Melophagus ovinus* and *Bovicola ovis* infestations in sheep.

be unnoticed because of their small size but, can multiply before being discovered [11].

M. ovinus infestation and distribution is restricted to cooler highlands in hot and humid tropics, with temperature playing role in its dynamics [23]. In this context, *M. ovinus* infestation in sheep is reported to be prevalent in highland areas of Ethiopia [24]. The prevalence of *M. ovinus* in this study was 33.57% this is in accordance with the reports of Desta, Chanie et al. and Kumsa et al. who reported 36.5%, 32.99% and 31.7% in highland areas of Oromia and Ahmara regions of Ethiopia [12,14,16]. In contrast, the current finding also differs with the findings of some other studies, where lower overall prevalence of *M. ovinus* 9.2% [21] and 8.07% [22] were reported from different parts of the country. The prevalence of *M. ovinus* infestation up to 52.4% was also reported in highland area of Tigray region [25]. These differences might be due to variations in climatic condition, season of the studies and access to veterinary service in the study areas [12]. Moreover, these differences between current and earlier studies might also be due to the large differences in susceptibility to ked infestation between sheep breeds [26].

The prevalence of *B. ovis* (12.07%) noted in this study is in agreement with 15.3% reported by Mulugeta et al. in Tigray region but it is lower than that of Kumsa et al. who reported a prevalence of 27.2% in Oromia region, 83.23% reported by Bekele et al. in central Ethiopia, 37.4% reported by Sertse and Wossene in eastern Amhara region, 47.86% and 34.43% reported by Chanie et al. in Yemenz Gera Midir and Kalu districts of Amhara region respectively and the prevalence of *B. ovis* (12.07%) in this study is higher than 8.9% reported by Seyoum et al. in Sekela and 6.17% reported by Chanie et al in Bati district of Amhara region [12,16,17,21,22,25]. These differences in prevalence of *B. ovis* infestation of sheep might be due to dissimilarities in climatic conditions, animal husbandry and health care of sheep in the study areas [17].

Significantly (χ^2=56.52; P=0.00) varied differences in the overall prevalence of the ked and lice infestation on sheep between adult and young animals was observed and sex (χ^2=14.71; P=0.00) and body condition score (χ^2=22.52; P=0.00) of sheep had a significant effect on an overall prevalence of *B. ovis* and *M. ovinus* infestation in sheep. These findings agree with the reports of Mulugeta et al., Amare et al. and Kumsa et al [12,15,25]. It has also been reported that age differences in ectoparasite infestation is evident in sheep, where young animals are more susceptible to ectoparasite infestations, partly due to a higher proportion of accessible surface to body volume and poor grooming behavior of young animals [26,27]. The higher prevalence of ectoparasites in the poor body condition scores than good body condition scores could be due to lowered immune response as a predisposing factor and/or the poor body condition could be the result of chronic ectoparasite infestation [19].

The present study indicated that *M. ovinus* was prevalent in sheep accounting for 33.52% prevalence. Significantly higher prevalence of *M. ovinus* infestation (χ^2=23.29; P=0.00) was observed in poor (70.1%) and medium (64.5) compared to sheep of good body condition group (40.5%). Logistic regression analysis indicated that poor body condition sheep were 3.46 times more at risk for *M. ovinus* infestation than those with good body condition (OR=3.46, p=0.00). This is in accordance with the report of Kumsa et al. who reported that significantly higher prevalence of *M. ovinus* in sheep with poor (23.4%) than good body condition (13.7%) [12]. It has been reported that sheep in poor conditions suffer most from ked infestation and sheep ked have been reported to cause a reduction in carcass weight [23].

Furthermore, significantly (χ^2=99.26; P=0.00) varied differences in the prevalence of the *M. ovinus* between age groups of sheep was also observed. The result of this study indicated that young sheep were more vulnerable to *M. ovinus* infestation than old animals. The odds of *M. ovinus* infestations in young sheep were 8.05 times compared to older sheep. The observation of significantly higher prevalence of *M. ovinus* in young than in old sheep is described by the movement of ked from ewe to lamb as an important source of infestation [12]. It has also been documented that, young animals are generally more susceptible

to ectoparasites because of their immature immunity, a higher ratio of accessible surface to the body volume and poor grooming behavior [27]. Furthermore, logistic regression analysis revealed that sex of animals did not significantly affect the prevalence of *M. ovinus* infestation in sheep (P>0.05) which agrees with the findings of Kumsa et al. and Bekele et al. yet, the prevalence of *M. ovinus* infestation was higher in rams (75%) than in ewes (50.9%) [12,22].

B. ovis has tendency to move on body surface thus, can spread over the whole body causing considerable irritation, restlessness, interrupted feeding and loss of condition and is responsible for development of nodular hypersensitivity reaction lesions (cockle or 'ekek') in pickled pelts [20,28]. With regard to *B. ovis* infestation, significantly higher prevalence of *B. ovis* infestation (χ^2=16.56; P=0.00) was observed in poor (52.9%) and medium (38.2%) compared to sheep of good body condition group (25%). Poor body condition sheep were 3.49 times more at risk for *B. ovis* infestations than good body conditioned sheep. This is in agreement with the reports of Kumsa et al. and Amare et al. [12,15]. The higher prevalence of ectoparasites in the poor body condition scores than good body condition scores might be due to lowered immune response as a predisposing factor and/or the poor body condition could be the result of chronic ectoparasite infestation.

Furthermore, animals with poor condition and that are improperly feed and exposed to cold and debilitating diseases carry the heaviest infestations of lice, since debilitated animals do not groom themselves and leave the lice undisturbed [19]. Sex was significantly (χ^2=7.4; P=0.01) associated with the prevalence of *B. ovis* in sheep where the prevalence was higher in rams (46.5%) than in ewes (33%). Logistic regression indicated that rams were 1.83 times more likely to harbor *B. ovis* than ewes. This might be due to the close contact the rams made with multiple ewes for longer time for mating during the breeding seasons which might increase the risk of acquiring lice from infected ewes as it has been reported that clinically affected and carrier animals are the sources of infection [29].

In the current study high 25.53% prevalence of concurrent infestation of *M. ovinus* and *B. ovis* in sheep was recorded. It was documented that the effects of ectoparasite infestations are more pronounced in heavy and mixed infestations [30-32]. Thus, this high dual infestation of *M. ovinus* and *B. ovis* in sheep in this study suggests that the effects of infestations were so pronounced on the animals.

Conclusion

This study concludes that the prevalence of *M. ovinus* and *B. ovis* in the study area is high with this high prevalence of *M. ovinus* and *B. ovis* infestation in the study area and considering effects of *M. ovinus* and *B. ovis* on health, welfare and productivity of sheep further studies on prevalence and economic impacts of infestation of sheep with *M. ovinus* and *B. ovis* are recommended. Furthermore, sanitation and hygiene of good standard of animal pens and houses are also recommended. To reduce and control *M. ovine* and *B. ovis* infestation appropriate flock health reprograms and control measures should also be implemented to improve the health and productivity of sheep.

Acknowledgments

The authors would like to thank University of Gondar (UOG), Faculty of Veterinary Medicine (FVM) Parasitology laboratory staffs for their kind support. We are also very gratefully to the animals' owners in the study area for their cooperation during the study.

References

1. CSA (2013) Livestock and livestock characteristics survey 2012-13 (private peasant holdings) Statistical bulletin no. 570, Addis Ababa, Ethiopia.

2. Mengesha M, Tsega W (2012) Indigenous sheep production in Ethiopia: A review Iranian. J Appl Anim Sci 2: 311-318.

3. ESGPIP (Ethiopian Sheep and Goats Productivity Improvement Program) (2009) Sheep breeds of Ethiopia: guide for identification and utilization. Technical Bulletin no.28.

4. Berhanu W, Negussie H, Alemu S, Mazengia H (2011) Assessment on major factors that cause skin rejection at Modjo export tannery, Ethiopia. Trop Anim Health Prod 43: 989-993.

5. James-Rugu NN, Jidayi S (2004) A survey of the ectoparasities of some livestock from some areas of Borno and Yobe States. Nigerian Vet J 25: 48-55.

6. Radostatits OM, Gray K, Hinchcliff H, Constable P (2007) A Textbook of the Disease of Cattle, Horses, Sheep, Pigs and Goats. 10th ed. WB Saunders, Edinburgh, UK.

7. Kebebew G (2015) Experimental study on sheep infested with *B. ovis* and *M. ovinus* of pathological changes, processed skin defect and effect of treatment in improving skin quality. MSc Thesis submitted to College of Veterinary Medicine and Agriculture, Addis Ababa University.

8. Phillips CJC (2005) The Effects of External Parasites and their Control on the Welfare of Livestock. Center for Animal Welfare and Ethics School of Veterinary Science, University of Queensland, p 63.

9. Petney TN, Kolonin GV, Robbins RG (2007) Southeast Asian ticks (Acari: Ixodida): a historical perspective. Parasitol Res 101: 201-205.

10. Colebrook E, Wall R (2004) Ectoparasites of livestock in Europe and the Mediterranean region. Vet Parasitol 120: 251-274.

11. (ESGPIP) Ethiopian Sheep and Goats Productivity Improvement Program (2010) Control of external parasites of sheep and goats. Technical Bulletin no. 41.

12. Kumsa B, Beyecha K, Geloye M (2012) Ectoparasites of sheep in three agro-ecological zones in central Oromia, Ethiopia. Onderstepoort J Vet Res 79: 1-7.

13. Kassa B (2006) Cockle, manage and pox: major threats to the leather industry in Ethiopia in Ethiopian Leather Industry: Prevalence towards Value Addition. Proceedings of the National Workshop, December 14-15, 2006, Addis Abeba, Ethiopia, pp 71-92.

14. Desta TS (2004) Investigation on ectoparasites of small ruminants in selected sites of Amhara regional state and their impact on the tanning industry. MSc Thesis submitted to Faculty of Veterinary Medicine, Addis Ababa University.

15. Amare S, Asfaw Y, Tolossa YH (2013) Ectoparasites of sheep and goats in North-West Amhara Regional State, Ethiopia. Ethiopian Vet J 17: 55-67.

16. Chanie M, Negash T, Sirak A (2010) Ectoparasites are the major causes of various types of skin lesions in small ruminants in Ethiopia. Trop Anim Health Prod 42: 1103-1109.

17. Sertse T, Wossene A (2007) A study on ectoparasites of sheep and goats in eastern part of Amhara region, northeast Ethiopia. Small Ruminant Res 69: 62-67.

18. Thrusfield M (2007) Veterinary Epidemiology. 3rd ed. UK, Black well science, Wiley, New Jersey, USA, pp 178-197.

19. Urquhart GM, Armour J, Duncan AM, Jennings FW (1996) Veterinary Parasitology. 4th ed. Blackwell Science, Glasgow, Scotland.

20. Wall R, Shearer D (2001) Veterinary External Parasites: Biology, Pathology and Control. 2nd ed. Blackwell Science LTD, New Jersey, USA.

21. Seyoum Z, Tadesse T, Addisu A (2015) Ectoparasites Prevalence in Small Ruminants in and around Sekela, Amhara Regional State, Northwest Ethiopia. J Vet Med 4: 2015.

22. Bekele J, Tariku M, Abebe R (2011) External parasite infestation in small ruminants in Wolmera district of Oromiya region, central Ethiopia. J Anim Vet Adv 4: 518-523.

23. Radostits OM, Blood DC, Gay CC (1994) Veterinary Medicine, Textbook of Cattle, Sheep, Pigs, Goats and Horses. 8th edn. Bailliere Tindall, UK, pp 1280-1308.

24. Kebede MC (2013) Effect of small ruminant ectoparasites in the tanning industry in Ethiopia: a review. J Anim Sci Adv 3: 424-430.

25. Mulugeta Y, Yacob HT, Ashenafi H (2010) Ectoparasites of small ruminants in three selected agro-ecological sites of Tigray Region, Ethiopia. Trop Anim Health Prod 42: 1219-1224.

26. James PJ (1999) Do sheep regulate the size of their mallophagan louse populations? Int J Parasitol 29: 869-875.

27. Lehman T (1993) Ectoparasites: Direct Impact on Host Fitness. Parasitol Today 9: 8-13.

28. Heath AC, Cooper SM, Cole DJ, Bishop DM (1995) Evidence for the role of the sheep-biting louse *B. ovis* in producing cockle, a sheep pelt defect. Vet Parasitol 59: 53-58.

29. Mekonnen S, Pegram RG, Gebre S, Mekonnen A, Jobre Y, et al. (2007) A synthesis of ixodid (Acari: Ixodidae) and argasid (Acari: Argasidae) ticks in Ethiopian and their possible roles in disease transmission. Ethiopian Vet J 11: 1-17.

30. Mohammad AN, Agbede IRS (1980) Control of ectoparasites of ruminants in Nigeria. In proceedings of the national seminar on the current problems facing the leader industry in Nigeria, NSCPFLIN'80, Nigeria.

31. Singla LD (1995) A note on sub-clinical gastro-intestinal parasitism in sheep and goats in Ludhiana and Faridkot districts of Punjab. Indian Vet Med J 19: 61-62.

32. Singh E, Kaur P, Singla LD, Bal MS (2017) Prevalence of gastrointestinal parasitism in small ruminants in western zone of Punjab, India. Vet world 10: 61-66.

19

Identification of Tick and Tick Borne Hemo-Parasites in Tiyo District, Arsi Zone, Oromia Region

Tolosa Shane[1], Teshome Gunse[1] and Fanos Tadesse Woldemariyam[2]*

[1]Arsi Zone Livestock and Fisheries Development Office, Ethiopia
[2]College Veterinary Medicine and Agriculture, Addis Ababa University, Ethiopia

Abstract

This study was conducted between November 2014 to march 2015 in Tiyo district and the surrounding peasant associations to determine the prevalence of tick and tick- born haemo-parasites in local and exotic cattle. A total of 384 local, exotic and cross breed cattles of all age group and sex group were included in this study. Four genera of ticks namely Amblyoma, Boophilus, Rhepicephalus and Hyaloma were identified with prevalence rate of (72%, 15%, 3%, 6.5%) respectively. From these ticks Boophilus constituted a high percentage of prevalence (72%) followed by Amblyoma(15%), Rhepicephalus(6.5%) and Hyaloma (3%) respectively. Out of 371 animals which were infested with ticks thin blood smears were examined for tick-borne protozoan parasites. From this 8 out of 371 were positive and 6 animals were found to be positive for Babesiosis while 2 of them for Anaplasmosis with prevalence rate of 1.6% and 0.5% respectively. Although it is difficult to deduct conclusive ideas about the general incidence and prevalence of hemo-parasites due to the short interval of the survey period, especially which did not include the wet season, it is clear that tick and tick borne haemoparasites constitutes a very important place in the area.

Keywords: Cattle; Haemo-parasite; Tick-born; Tiyo district; Tick species

Introduction

Ethiopia a country located in the horn of Africa has an extremely diverse topography which is suitable for different agricultural production (crop, livestock). The livestock population of Ethiopia is estimated to be about 50 million cattle, 23 million sheep, 18 million goats, 1.65 million equines and 42 million poultry representing 45% of agricultural output/GDP in Ethiopia. Export commodities (meat, live animals, hides and skins as well as drought power, milk production and as source of manure are the main outputs of livestocks [1,2].

Ticks effects on animals include loss of blood (anemia), Tick toxicosis, tick worry bite wound, wounds and myiasis, tick-borne diseases [3,4]. Studies conducted on the ticks and tick-borne diseases of cattle in Ethiopia showed several species of ticks belonging to genus Amblyomma, Boophilus, Rhipicephalus, Hyalomma and Haemaphysalis [5].

It has been estimated that about 80% of the world population of cattles are infested with ticks [6]. Tick and tick borne diseases causes a tremendous economic importance in livestock production in tropical and subtropical countries [7]. From animal health and economic point of view tick borne disease of ruminants are certainly the most important [8] but no realistic prospects for the eradication of tick and tick-borne diseases has been developed elsewhere in the world [9].

These economically most important haemo-parasitic tick borne diseases of ruminant on a global scale are Babesiosis, Anaplasmosis, Theileriosis and Cowdriosis of cattle and small ruminants [10]. According to FAO (1984) global estimation on tick and tick-borne diseases and with the assumption of 80% infestation of world 1226 million cattle were infested by ticks with estimated to annual loss from each animal to be of US$ 7.36. Accordingly, Ethiopia with 50 million cattle population may suffer an annual loss of US $ 368 million only from large ruminants [11].

In Ethiopia, various surveys showed the abundance of tick species on livestock in different regions of the country. More than 60 species of ticks have been recorded infesting both domestic and wild animals among which about 33 species are widespread and are important parasite of livestock [12-16]. However, the statuses of ticks and tick-borne hemo-parasites are not thoroughly studied in Tiyo District of Arsi Zone and information are so far scanty. Some reports from the veterinary clinics reveal the existence of ticks and haemo-parasites using routine parasitological examination technique.

There for, the objectives of this study were to:

- Determine the prevalence of tick-borne haemo-parasites in cattle coming to Tiyo District Veterinary clinic and fattening farms in and around Assela.

- Identify the major tick species infesting cattle coming to Tiyo District Veterinary clinic and fattening farms.

Materials and Methods

Study area

Arsi Zone is in Oromia region. It is located in south east of Ethiopia within 6° 59' and 8° 49' N latitude and 38° 41' and 40° 44' E longitude. Tiyo dstrict, is located 175 km south east of Addis Ababa and It comprises of Assela town and Villages around it. The altitude of the district ranges from 1650-3000 meters above sea level (Masl). About 37% of the total area is highland (>2400 m); 52% mid-land (1800-2400 m) 11% is low-land (<1800 m) (Central planning Authority, 1994). The area has daily maximum temperature that reaches up to 28°C and

***Corresponding author:** Woldemariyam FT, College Veterinary Medicine and Agriculture, Addis Ababa University, Ethiopia
E-mail: fanos.tadesse@aau.edu.et

minimum temperature of 10°C with an annual rainfall that ranges from 700-1658 mm and annual average relative humidity, ranging from 43-60%. The area has a bimodal rainfall occurring form March to April (a short rainy season) and from July to October (long rainy season). The common and widely used livestock production system in the area is an extensive type of production system where animals are kept only on grazing with no extra supplementary feed except crop residues during dry season. But there are few indoor, intensive animal production systems particularly in Assela town.

Study design

A cross-sectional study was designed to address the objective of this investigation. Both district veterinary clinics and Animal health posts as well as small scale farms were selected for the study. Simple random sampling was used for both infected and non infected animals irrespective of their age, breed, sex, and agro-ecology to collect ticks and blood sample.

Study animal

For this study the sample size from Assela and the surrounding area is determined for definite precision and level of confidence. A 95% CI and 5% with 50% expected prevalence was used in determining the sample size.

i.e., $N = \dfrac{1.96^2\,Pexp\,(1-)exp)}{d^2}$

$$\dfrac{1.96^2 0.5\,(1-05)exp)}{0.05^2}$$

For this study a total of 384 animals were sampled to collect tick and blood.

Sampling and sample processing

Ticks were collected gently from half body regions of the selected cattle and their species were identified and thin blood smears were taken from the ear vein of cattle coming to Tiyo district veterinary clinic, Veterinary health posts found in the district and farms. History of all cattles were recorded. This samples were brought to Assela regional laboratory and were processed as follows.

Collection and examination of blood sample: Thin blood smears were taken from one of the small blood vessels of the ear making sure to take the first drop so as to not miss the parasites. The blood smears stained with 10% Geimsa solution and the haemo-parasites were looked for in the red blood cells of the smear under the oil immersion objective of the microscope.

Collection and identification of ticks: Ticks which were collected from the animals and preserved in 10% formalin solution and identified under stereomicroscope using key morphological characteristics as describd by Urquhart et al. and Soulsby [17,18].

Data Analysis

Descriptive data analysis was employed in summarizing the data regarding haemo-parasitic disease and major tick isolated in cattle of different sex, breed, altitude and group of animal. Chi-square test of independence was employed in comparing the prevalence of haemo-parasitic diseases with respect to altitude; sex and age as well as breed to determine the association of risk factors and occurrence of haemo-pasitic disease in cattle.

Results

Out of 384 cattle examined (Cross n=41, Exotic n=6, Local n=337) 371 (96.5%) were found to be infected with different genera of ticks. Four general of ticks namely; *Boophilus* (72%), *Amblyomma* (15%), *Rhipicephalus* (6.5%) and *Hyalomma* (3%) were identified (Table 1). Similarly from 384 blood samples collected thin blood smears were stained and examined for the presence of haemo-parasites out of which, 8(2.1%)were found to be infected with different haemo-parasites (Table 4).

Boophilus takes the largest share in infesting all the three Agro-ecology of cattles with more than 70% prevalence which is followed by Aambylyoma species except the midland having 66% (Table 3). With respect to breed, sex and age tick infestation it was *Boophilus* tick species which took the largest share except the youner cattles were found to be infested with *Amblyomma* species (Table 2).

From the total of 384 cattles examined 371 animals were found to be infested with ticks from this cattles blood sample (smear) were collected and examined for the presence of haemo-parasites. Of which 8(2.1%) prevalence was found to be positive for hemo-parasite. From this it was found that 6 out of 371(1.61%) were positive for *Babesia* and 2 (0.53%) were found to be positive for Anaplasmosis (Table 4).

Discussion

In this study period (November 2014 to March 2015) a total of 384 cattle were examined and found four genera of ticks in 371(96%) cattles. These 371 heads of cattles were again subjected to thin smear preparation and examined for the presence of hemo-parasites. In this regard 8(2.1%) of blood smears were found to be haemo-parasite. Two haemo-paraites namely, *Babesia* (1.6%) and Anaplasma(0.5%) were identified during the study.

Boophilus was the dominate tick identified followed by Amblyomma, Rhipicephalus and Hyalomma respectively. This findings disagree in figure but agrees with the genera identified with Mekonen and partially agreed with Belew and Mekonin who reported that the major tick genera recorded in tick distribution survey, made in Ethiopia were Amblyomma (40%), Rhipicephalus (37%), Boophilus(21%) and Hyalomma (1.5%). This could be due to difference in the season during which the study was conducted [19,20]. Even though the percentage between Amblyomma and Boophilus differs it is common to find the four genera of ticks which were prevalent in Ethiopia. Pawlos Wasihun and Derese Doda, were also stated that three out of four of our tick genera were prevalent in Ethiopia [21]. But our finding was in agreement with the explanation that Boophilus tick is present in areas with long rainy season which is true for Tiyo district [22]. This was also in agreement with the findings of Sinshaw at Metekel ranch which found tick in wet season [23].

Ticks species	Agro-ecology		
	Highland (n=178)	Mid land (n=50)	Low land (n=156)
Rhipicephalus	8(4.6%)	3(6%)	14(9%)
Amblyomma	25 (14%)	9(18%)	24(16%)
Boophilus	133 (74.7%)	33(66%)	110(70.5%)
Hayalomma	7(4%)	2(4.2%)	3(2%)

Table 1: Over all prevalence of ticks species identified in Tiyo district, Arsi Zone.

Ticks species	Breed			Sex		Age	
	Cross n=41	Exotic n=6	Local n=337	Female n=75	Male n=300	Adult n=363	Young n=21
Rhipicephalus	3(7.3%)	0	22(6.5%)	3(4%)	22(7.3%)	22(6.1%)	3(14.3%)
Amblyomma	6 (14%)	1 (17%)	51 (15%)	**25** (33%)	33 (11%)	**40** (11 %)	**18** (85.7%)
Boophilus	30 (73.2%)	5 (83%)	241 (71.5%)	53 (70.7%)	223 (74.3%)	260 (71.6%)	16 (76.2%)
Hayalomma	2 (4.9%)	0	10 (3%)	3 (4%)	9 (3%)	11 (3.03%)	1 (4.8%)

Table 2: The prevalence of ticks among, breed, sex and age group of cattle.

Ticks species	Agro-ecology			
	Highland (n=178)	Mid land (n=50)	Low land (n=156)	
Rhipicephalus	8(4.6%)	3(6%)	14(9%)	
Amblyomma	25 (14%)	9(18%)	24(16%)	
Boophilus	133 (74.7%)	33(66%)	110(70.5%)	
Hayalomma	7(4%)	2(4.2%)	3(2%)	

Table 3: The prevalence of ticks among agro-ecology of Tiyo District.

Haemo-parasite	Agro-ecology			Breed			Sex		Age	
	High land tn=178	Mid land n=50	Low land n=156	Cross n=41	Exotic n=6	Local n=337	Female n=75	Male n=300	Adult n=363	Young n=21
Babesia	4 (2.2%)	0	2 (1.3%)	1 (2.4%)	0	5 (1.5%)	3 (4%)	3 (1%)	5 (1.4%)	1 (4.8%)
Anaplasma	0	0	2 (1.5)	0	0	2 (0.6)	0	2 (0.6%)	2 (0.6%)	0

Table 4: The prevalence of haemo-parasites among agro-ecology, breed, sex and age.

Rhipicephalus is the 3rd and Hyalomma is the 4th encountered tick genera in the area. Rhipicephalus is the most common tick genera in the study area during the period covered. It was more identified in the low land and followed by high land and midland. It was highly dominate in the low land areas in Dera around 50 km distance form Assela town. In general; Boophilus, Amblyomma and Rhipicephalus ticks constitutes highest percentage of the total collection. The Hyalomma and other tick species were found in limited number or not found in our study site this is in agreement with the finding of Mekonin et al. [19]. In the present study only 8 positive cases were observed for hemo-parasite, of which six animals were positive for *Babesia* parasite and the other two were positive for Anaplasma parasite.

Infection by *A. marginale* is wide spread in the country as its major tick vector is *B. decoloratus* [24]. Babesiosis is mainly a disease of cattle in Ethiopia and is caused by *Babesia bigemina* whose vector is *B. decoloratus* and *Babesia bovis* whose vector is *B. annualtus*.

Our finding was in agreement with a report of Mekonnen, which states that Clinical cases of Babesiosis are encountered rarely [19]. Additionally rare prevalence of tick born diseases this could be due to the fact that thin blood smear examination and other simple laboratory procedures were not very efficient procedures were not very efficient means of identifying tick-borne haemoparasites [7]. Anaplasmosis, Babesiosis, Cowdriosis and theileriosis together with a range of vector tick species are found in Ethiopia [24].

A 1992 serological survey of tick-borne diseases in private and state dairy farms with their cross –breed cattle reported high percentage of antibodies against *A. marginal* (>90%). *Babesia begemina* (60%) and *T. mutans* (30%) indicating a fair level of enzootix stability in respect to those tick-borne diseases each tick-borne haemo-parasites may have a restricted number of tick species which acts as effective vector [19].

Conclusion and Recommendations

Ticks and the disease they cause and transmit are among the important livestock problem. They are the main causes of decreased productivity and they expose animals to a number of diseases out breaks in the area. Although it is difficult to deduct conclusive ideas about the general incidence and prevalence due to the short interval of the survey period, especially which did not include the wet season, it is clear that tick borne haemo-parasites constitutes a very important place in the area. Taking into account the demand for livestock in the region and that the ticks are the main problems in upgrading animals productivity of ticks and tick borne diseases are among remarkable problems in the study area.

Based on the above conclusive remarks, the following recommendations are given:

➢ Detailed epidemiological studies should be conducted on ticks and tick born disease in different season's indifferent species of domestic animals.

➢ Country wide effective tick and tick-born disease control strategies should be designed

➢ Efforts to be made to introduce community based tick controlling strategies

➢ Veterinary professionals mainly technicians should be trained on the effective and modern field diagnostic techniques of tick borne diseases.

References

1. Kidane C (2001) Hides and skins defects, nature and effects on the industry technical work shop on good practices for the Ethiopian hides and skins industry. Addis Ababa, Ethiopia, December 4-7, 2001. p: 8.

2. Solomon G (2005) Agriculture in Ethiopia: ICIPE tick modeling work shop held at Duduviell   Report on 9-19 October 1997. Nairobi, Kenya.

3. Daniel ES, Robert SL, William LN (2012) Medical and Veterinary Entomology. Elsevier Science, USA, pp: 517-558.

4. Bowman DD (2009) Class Arachnida: Georgis' Parasitology for Veterinarians. 9th edn. Saunders Elsevier, USA, pp: 40-60.

5. Nibret MB, Basaznew B, Tewodros F (2012) Hard Ticks (Ixodidae): Species Composition, Seasonal Dynamics and Body Site Distribution on Cattle in Chilga District, Northwest Ethiopia. Asian J Agric Sci. 4: 341-345.

6. Minjauw B, McLeod A (2003) Tick borne diseases and poverty. The impact of ticks and tick borne diseases on livestock owners in India and Eastern health program center for tropical veterinary medicine. University of Edinburgh, UK, pp: 24-57.

7. FAO (1984) Ticks and tick born diseases control. A practical field manual. Vol 1. I FAO, Rome, pp: 1-30.

8. Kocan KM (1995) Targeting tick for control of selected haemopatasite disease cattle. Veterinary Parasitology 57: 121-151.

9. Eshetu Y (1986) Prevalence of tick born hemo-parasitie in Bahirdar Awraja. DVM Thesis. FVM, AAU, Debre zeit, Ethiopia.

10. Uilenberg G (1995) International collaborative research significance of tick borne. Vet Parasitol 57: 19-41.

11. FAO (1991) Tick and tick born diseases control. A particular field manual Vol. II. Tick Born disease control. FAO, Rome, pp: 301-362.

12. Morel PC (1980) Study of Ethiopia ticks. Acarina, ixodidael. Ministry of Foreign Affairs, IEMCT, France.

13. Pegram RE (1981) Tick (Ixodoidea) of Ethiopia with special reference to cattle and a critical review of the taxonomic status of species within the and Rhipicephalus sanguineus gros. M Phil Thesis, Burnel University, Uxbridge, England, UK.

14. Feseha F (1983) Notes on tick species and tick born diseases of domestic animals. In: Ethiopia, FVM, AAU, Debre zeit, Ethiopia.

15. Kasier MN (1987) Report on tick taxonomy and biology AG: DP/ETH/83/023 Consultants Report FAO. p: 92.

16. De castro JJ (1994) Sustainable tick and tick-born disease control in livestock improvement in developing countries. Vet Parasitol 71: 77-97.

17. Urquhart GM, Armour A, Duncan JL, Dunn AM, Jennings FW (1996) Veterinary Parasitlogy. 2nd edn. Black Well Sciences Ltd., p: 231.

18. Soulsby EJ (1982) Helminthes, Arthropods and Protozoa of domestic animals. 7th edn. Lea and Febiger, Philadelphia, USA, pp: 40-52.

19. Mekonnen S (1995) Ticks, Tick-borne diseases and control strategies in Ethiopia. In: Tick borne pathogens at the host vector interface.

20. Mekonen S (1991) Tick and tick-borne disease control in Ethiopia. In: Proceeding of Joint OAU, FAO and ILRDA work shop held in Liongwe, Alwi, pp: 19-20.

21. Pawlos W, Derese D (2013) Study on prevalence and identification of ticks in Humbo District, Southern Nations, Nationalities and People's Region (SNNPR), Ethiopia. J Vet Med Anim Health 5: 73-80.

22. Aiello SE (1998) Ticks. In: The Merck Veterinary Manual. 8th edn. Merck and Co. Inc., Whitehouse Station. USA, pp: 670-686.

23. Sinshaw A (2000) Distribution of ticks and tick-borne disease at Metekel ranch Ethiopia. Ethiop Vet J 4: 40 -59.

24. Behailu B (2004) A survey of ticks and tick-borne blood protista in cattle at Asselas, Arsi zone. DVM Thesis FVM, AAU.

20

Prevalence and Associated Risk Factors to Lice Infestation in Sheep of Arsi High Land, Oromiya Regional State, Ethiopia

Eyob Eticha[1]*, Diriba Lemma[1], Birhanu Abera[1] and Hani Selemon[2]

[1]*Asella Regional Veterinary Laboratory, PO Box 212, Asella, Ethiopia*
[2]*Arsi University School of Agricultural and Environmental Science, Asella, Ethiopia*

Abstract

This study was done from November 2011 to March 2012. A total of 384 sheep from Tiyo District of Arsi Zone, around High land area of Asella were selected for the study. A cross sectional study was conducted to determine the prevalence of lice in sheep and to identify major species of lice in the study area. The densities of lice were determined through counting after parting of the fleece/wool at five (5) points on a length of 10 cm in different regions of the body (neck, shoulder, back, rump and flank) on both sides. The overall prevalence of lice infestation was found 53.9% (n=384). From this *Damalina ovis* takes the highest prevalence in each variable (sex, age, body condition and month) whereas *Linognathus ovillus* had lower prevalence in each variable. The prevalence of lice for female and male was 53.26% and 56.4%, respectively. Adult and young infestation rate of lice was 51.52% and 57.5%, respectively. Prevalence of lice infestation in good, medium and poor body condition was 36.8% (64), 62.7% (94) and 81.7% (49), respectively. The prevalence of lice in November was 74.44% (94), in January 32.8% (42) and in February 55.5% (71). There is statistically significant difference in the occurrence of lice infestation between body condition scores and months (p<0.05) but there is no statistically significant difference between age and sex (p>0.05). These result shows that lice infestation has a great effect on the skin quality and on the production of meat and milk. From this result it can be concluded that occurrence of lice depends on body condition and climatic factor. Therefore, owners should practice good management system by keeping the hygiene of animal and by avoid mixing of healthy animals from diseased once with the use effective acarcide control.

Keywords: Asella; Lice; Prevalence; Sheep

Introduction

In Ethiopia, small ruminants comprise large proportion of livestock resources, constitute about 30% of the total livestock population of the country and are among important contributors to food production in Ethiopia, providing 35% of meat consumption and 14% of milk consumption [1]. And the country is an ideal case for studying livestock diversity in the context of developing regions. It is route of sheep migration from Asia into Africa, has large population [2] and diverse traditional sheep breeds spread across diverse ecology, communities, and production system. At the national level, sheep/goat account for about 90% of the live animal/meat and 92% of skin and hide export trade value [3]. At the farm level sheep contribute as much as 22-63% to the net cash income derived from livestock production in the crop-livestock production system [4].

Lice are among the major disease of sheep and cause serious economic loss to farmers through mortality, decreased production and reproduction, down grading and rejection of skins which also affect the tanning industries. According to tanneries report, skin diseases due to external parasites cause 35% sheep skin rejection [5], among highly prevalent and pathogenic ectoparasites of sheep. Both biting and sucking lice affect small ruminants. The important species of lice found in sheep and goats are the genus Damalina and Linognathus and the important species in sheep being *L. ovillus* (sucking face louse), *L. aficanus*, *L. spedalis* (sucking foot louse) and *Bovicola ovis* (biting louse). In goats *L. stenopsis* (sucking blue louse), *L. africanus*, *B. caprae* (biting louse), *B. alimbata* and *B. crassiceps* are reported [6].

All species cause irritation of the skin, stimulate scratching, rubbing, and licking leading to restlessness, these have great effect on sheep production and skin quality [5]. Accordingly, the enormous economic losses induced by Lice in sheep necessitate detailed investigation on their incidence in order to organize efforts to at least minimize these losses. This study is therefore aimed for assessing the prevalence of lice and determining the magnitude of lice infestation in relation to associated risk factors.

Materials and Methods

Study area

The present study was conducted from November 2011 to March 2012 in Tiyo district of Arsi Zone, around highland area of Asella, capital town of Arsi zone, which is located at 175 km southeast of Addis Ababa, and the altitude and annual rainfall of the area ranges from 502-4130 meters above sea level and 200-400 mm with mean annual temperature of 22.5°C, respectively. It is one of the highly-populated areas in Ethiopia with estimated human population of 2,521,349 and livestock population of cattle-82,190; sheep-51,292; goat-8, 11,479; poultry- 5, 62,915; equine- 22,055 [7].

Study design and sampling strategies

A cross sectional study was conducted to determine the prevalence of lice in indigenous sheep in the study areas. With the assumption of possible prevalence rate of the disease 50%, absolute desired precision

*Corresponding author: Fanos Tadesse Woldemariyam, College of Veterinary Medicine and Agriculture, Addis Ababa University, Addis Ababa, Ethiopia, E-mail: fanos.tadesse@aau.edu.et

of 5% and confidence level of 95% was considered for estimation prevalence in the simple random sampling according to Thrusfield, [8] the total sample size was 384 sheep.

Study population

The present study involved sheep kept under extensive (mixed-crop livestock production) production system in selected peasant associations of Tiyo district. A total 384 sheep was randomly selected from 19,453 sheep population in the district. The sampling was made by 3 rounds in different months of the study period.

Clinical examinations

The animals were randomly selected and clinically examined for presence of the ectoparasites. Prior to clinical examination, the sex, ages, body condition scores of the selected animals were recorded. The different age groups such as young and adult have been selected for the present study and the age group was done as per standard method of Hamito [9]. Body condition score of the animals will be considered as poor, medium, and good by modifying the system described by Johns [10] for sheep. The clinical examination was performed by multiple fleeces parting in the direction opposite that in which hair or wool normally rests and visual inspection and palpation of the skin for parasites on neck, shoulder, wither, flank and ramps are sites of concern. In each of the mentioned body parts both on the either sides /left and right/ a place 10 cm long is parted for the presence of lice and if found in all or one of the 10 cm long place. Those sheep found infested by parasites was considered positive. The type of parasites was identified on the basis of their morphological structure as described in Wall and Shearer [11].

Specimen collection and examination

Those detected lice that are unidentified during clinical examination was collected by forceps/hand picking, with hairs from their attachment site, put into a clean separate container(universal bottles), labeled and kept preserved with 70% ethyl alcohol before transportation to Asella regional veterinary laboratory for detailed laboratory examination as described by Urquhart et al. [12]. Then the collected ectoparasites was examined by stereomicroscope and identification was performed according to the identification key given by wall and shearer [11].

Data management and analysis

The data was subjected for statistical analysis by entry in to Microsoft Excel spread sheet and descriptive statistics like prevalence and analytical statistics such as chi- square (χ^2) was conducted by using SPSS 17.0 for determining the significance of association between age groups, sex, body condition scores, and month with lice infestation. For the purpose of this study, 95% confidence level and $P<0.05$ was used for significance.

Results

Overall prevalence of lice

Out of the total sheep population examined for lice infestation, 53.9% (207) sheep were infested with lice. The major species of lice were *D. ovis* and *L. ovillus* species, from this the most prevalent species was *D. ovis* with an overall prevalence of 86.9% (180) while *L. ovillus* species was only 1.9% (4) and mixed lice infestation was 11.6% (23). The commonest site of lice attachment was the skin of neck, shoulder, flank and rump.

Prevalence of lice in sheep by different age groups

Out of the total population of sheep examined for lice infestation 60.2% (231) sheep was adult and 39.8% (153) was young. The overall prevalence of lice infestation in adult was 51.52% (119) where as in young it was 57.5% (88) of this the most prevalent lice species were *D. ovis* with the prevalence of 89.1%(106), where as *L. ovillus* species have 0 prevalence and mixed lice infestation was 10.9% (13) in adult and in case of young (lamb) *D. ovis* 84.09% (74), *L. ovillus* species 4.54%(4) and mixed lice infestation 11.36%(10) (Table 1). In both age groups there is no statistically significant difference ($p=0.248$)

Prevalence of lice in sheep by different sex group

Out of the total population of sheep examined for lice infestation 79.7% (306) sheep were female and 20.3% (78) are male. The overall prevalence of lice in female is 53.26% (163) and in male are 56.4% (44). The most prevalent species is *D. ovis* with the prevalence of 87.12% (142), whereas *L. ovillus* 1.23% (2) and mixed 11.66% (19) in female sheep. In male sheep the prevalence of *D. ovis* was 100% (44), *L. ovillus* 9.1% (4) and mixed infection is 9.1% (4) (Table 2). In both sex groups there is no statistically significant difference ($p= 0.619$).

Prevalence of lice infestation in sheep by different body condition

From the total population of sheep examined for lice infestation 45.3% (174) sheep have good body condition, 39.1% (150) sheep have medium body condition and 15.6% (60) sheep have poor body condition. The overall prevalence lice infestation of good, medium and poor body conditions was 36.8% (64), 62.7% (94) and 81.7% (49), respectively. The most prevalent species was *D. ovis* with the prevalence of 90.6% (58), *L. ovillus* 3.13% (2) and mixed lice infestation 6.25% (4) in good body conditioned animal. In medium body condition animal the prevalence of *D. ovis* was 84.04% (79), *L. ovillus* 1.064% (1) and mixed lice infestation 14.89% (14). In poor body condition prevalence of *D. ovis* was 87.76% (43), *L. ovillus* 2.04% (1) and mixed lice infestation 10.2% (5) (Table 3). There is statistically significant difference in the occurrence of lice infestation between body condition sores ($p=0.000$).

Prevalence of lice infestation in sheep by month wise

Out of the total population of sheep examined for lice infestation equal numbers of sheep were taken in each month (i.e., 33.3% (128), in November, 33.3% (128) in January and 33.3% (128) in February). Out of this the overall prevalence of lice in November was 73.44% (94), in January 32.8% (42) and in February 55.5% (71). Out of this prevalence of *D. ovis* was found 85(90.42%), *L. ovillus* 0 prevalence and mixed lice infestation 9.6% (9) in November. In January the prevalence of *D. ovis* was 83.33% (35), *L. ovillus* 0 prevalence and mixed lice infestation 16.66% (7). In February prevalence of *D. ovis* was 84.5% (60), *L. ovillus* 4.22% (3) and 15.5% (11) and mixed lice infestation 9.86% (7) (Table 4). There is statistically significant difference in between the three months ($p=0.000$).

Lice	Adult	Young
D. ovis	89.1%(106)	84.09%(74)
L. ovillus	0% (0)	4.54%(4)
Mixed lice	10.9% (13)	11.36%(10)
Overall lice	51.52%(119)	57.5%(88)

For Total infestation Chi square (df=1)=1.334, *P*=0.248

Table 1: Prevalence of lice in sheep by age wise.

Prevalence of lice in sheep by severity

Out of the total population of sheep infected with lice 41.06% (85) sheep were severely infected, 101(48.79%) sheep with moderate infection and 10.14% (21) were with slight infestation. The most prevalent species was *D. ovis* with the prevalence of 97.65% (83), 79.2% (80) and 85.71% (18) in severe, moderate and slight infestation respectively. While for *L. ovillus* 1% (1) was slight infestation and 14.29% (3) was moderate infestation. In mixed lice infestation 2.35% (2) was for severe infestation and 20.79% (21) for moderate infestation (Table 5).

Discussion

The high prevalence of lice was 53.9%, recorded in the study, which is suggestive of the importance of the parasite in sheep population of the study area. Poor management and poor level of awareness of sheep owners on the effect of ectoparasites particularly lice infestation are believed to have contributed to wide spread occurrence of the parasites. *D. ovis*is the most prevalent lice species recorded with a prevalence of 86.9%, from the 207 sheep infected with lice infestation where as *L. ovillus* species and mixed lice infestation were 1.9% and 11.6% respectively.

The overall prevalence obtained in this study is higher than observations made in North western Amhara Region [13] which is 30.9% for *D. ovis,* by Tadesse et al. [14] 22.28% for *B. ovis* in around Kombolcha and by Sertse [15] 25.7% in Amhara region. But the present findings indicates lower prevalence than prevalence of 63.5% as reported in Amhara National Regional State [16] and by Yacob et

Lice	Female	Male
D. ovis	87.12% (142)	100% (44)
L. ovillus	1.23% (2)	9.1% (4)
Mixed lice	19(11.66%)	9.1% (4)
Over all lice	53.26% (163)	56.4% (44)

For Total infestation Chi square (df=1)=0.247, *P*=0.619

Table 2: Prevalence of lice in sheep by sex wise

Lice	Poor	Medium	Good
L. ovillus	2.04% (1)	1.064% (1)	90.6% (58)
D. ovis	43(87.76%)	84.04% (79)	36.8% (64)
Mixed lice	10.2% (5)	14.89% (14).	3.13% (2)
Overall lice	81.67% (49)	62.7% (94)	6.25% (4)

For Total infestation Chi square (df=6)=43.778, *P*=0.000

Table 3: Prevalence of lice in body condition.

Lice	November	January	February
D. ovis	90.42% (85)	83.33% (35)	84.5% (60)
L. ovillus	0%	0%	4.22% (3)
Mixed lice	9.6% (9)	16.66% (7)	15.5% (11)
Overall lice	73.44% (94)	32.8% (42)	55.5% (71)

For Total infestation Chi square (df=2) 42.698, *P*=0.000

Table 4: Prevalence of lice by month wise.

Lice	Severe	Moderate	Slight
D. ovis	97.65% (83)	79.2% (80)	85.71% (18)
L. ovillus	0%	3(14.29%)	1% (1)
Mixed lice	2.35% (2)	20.79% (21)	0%
Overall lice	41.06% (85)	48.79% (101)	10.14% (21)

Table 5: Prevalence of Lice by Severity.

al. [17] in Southern Ethiopia, Sodo, and in the Zone of this study area, Arsi, which was 75.5%. Such difference in prevalence with the above observations may arise from differences in agro climate, management, health care of animal and the sensitivity of the diagnostic method used to reveal ectoparasites. Similarly, lice infestation was greater in winter and spring similar to the findings of Colwel et al. [18].

In addition to skin damage, lice infestation also has a significant effect on production and productivity of animals because the presence of lice interferes with nutrition of animal. Due to itching and scratching the animal spend more time by grooming on fixed objects rather than taking feed which result in decreased body Condition. Body condition has also contribution for the occurrence of lice infestation because there is also evidence that immune response may be involved in regulating louse numbers and may underlie differences amongst sheep in susceptibility to lice [19,20]. Impaired immune response may explain the greater susceptibility to lice of animals in poor condition or under stress.

In the present study sex and age are not statistically significant in the occurrence of lice infestation but in male animal the prevalence of lice is slightly higher than female animal and in young the prevalence of lice infestation is higher than in adults this is because the lambs doesn't mixed with ewes therefore transmission from ewe to lamb doesn't occur.

The other factor for the occurrence of lice is climatic condition. In this study the occurrence of lice is higher in November than February and January, which shows infestation of lice is high in cooler time. According to Wilkinson et al. [21]; Niven and Pritchard [22] lice infestation is very high in spring time in European countries where the temperature is low during that time.

Considering the importance of skin and hides as a main source of foreign currency to the country, the prevailing ecto parasites mainly in different sheep reared in Arsi zone requires attention in order to minimize the spread of infestation and increase income earnings of farmers and small scale holders whose livelihood is dependent on their animals.

Conclusion

Lice infestation is among the major causes of sheep production constraints and quality deteriorations of exported skin in Ethiopia. Lice are easily overlooked because of their small size but they have the capacity to multiply very fast before being discovered. In this study the overall prevalence of lice infestation was very high (86.9%), this can be resulting in high economic losses through decreased production of meat and milk due to interference with nutrition and skin damages. Lice have a significant effect on body condition. Whereas sex and age of the host animals were not determinant factors for the prevalence variation. Therefore, based on the above points the following recommendations are forwarded: The effect of lice on production, productivity and skin quality is not appreciated by farmers. Therefore farmers should have enough awareness and effective extension programs that raise public awareness on effect of lice, reducing the prevalence of Lice mainly relies on treatment of affected animals with appropriate acaricides and improving the management system and detailed study on economic losses associated with lice infestation and investigation of other causes of skin downgrading and rejection should be conducted.

Acknowledgements

Authors are grateful for the technical and material support of the staffs of Asella regional veterinary laboratory.

References

1. Asfaw B (1998) The Tanning Industry. Proceedings of control of sheep and goat skin disease to improve quality of hides and skin, Addis Ababa, Ethiopia.

2. CSA (2006) Ethiopian Agricultural Sample Enumeration. Statistical report on Livestock and Farm Implements, Addis Ababa, Ethiopia.

3. Gizaw G (2008) Sheep resources of Ethiopia: Genetic Diversity and Breeding Strategy. PhD Thesis, Wageningen University, The Netherlands, pp: 2-145.

4. Zelalem A, Feltcher IC (1993) Small Ruminant Productivity in the central Ethiopian Mixed Farming System. In: Processing of the Fourth National livestock Improvement Conference, Addis Ababa, Ethiopia.

5. Bayou K (1998) Overview of sheep and goat skin diseases, treatment trial for improved quality of hides and skins (phase II). Addis Ababa, Ethiopia, pp: 13-20.

6. Radostits OM, Blood DC, Gay CC (1994) Veterinary Medicine. Text Book of Cattle, Sheep, Pigs, Goats and Horses. 8th edn, Bailliere Tindall, UK, pp: 1280-1308.

7. Deselegn TB, Gangwar SK (2011) Seroprevalence study of bovine brucellosis in Assela government dairy farm of Oromia Regional State, Ethiopia. Int J Sci Nat 2: 692-697.

8. Thrusfield M (2005) Veterinary Epidemiology. 3rd edn, Blackwell Science Ltd., UK, pp: 229-245.

9. Hamito D (2009) Estimation of Weight and Age of Sheep and Goats. ESGPIP, Technical Bulletin 23: 8-10.

10. Suiter J (1994) Body condition scoring of sheep and goats. Farmnote, p: 69.

11. Wall R, Shearer D (1997) Veterinary Entomology. 1st edn, Chapman and Hall, UK, pp: 1-438.

12. Urquhart GM, Armour J, Duncan JL, Dunn AM, Jennings FW (1996) Veterinary Parasitology. 2nd edn., Blackwell Science Ltd., UK, pp: 141-205.

13. Mariam SW (2011) Impact of ectoparasite control campaign on quality of processed skins in tanneries of the Amhara Regional Government: a rapid assessment. Ethiopian Veterinary Journal 15: 103-115.

14. Tadesse A, Fentaw E, Mekbib B, Rahmeto A, Mekuria S, et al. (2011) Study on the prevalence of ectoparasite infestation of ruminanats in and around Kombolcha and damage to fresh goat pelts and wet blue (pickled) skin at Kombolch Tannary, Northestern Ethiopia. Ethiop Vet J 15: 87-101.

15. Sertse DF (2004) Investigation on Ectoparasites of Small ruminants in Selected Sites of Amhara Regional State and their Impact on the Tanning industry. MSc Thesis, Faculty of Veterinary Medicine, Addis Ababa University, DebreZeit, Ethiopia, pp: 40-47.

16. Kebede N, Fetene T (2012) Population dynamics of cattle ectoparasites in Western Amhara National Regional State, Ethiopia. Journal of Veterinary Medicine and Animal Health 4: 22-26.

17. Yacob TH, Yalew AT, Dinka AA (2008) Ectoparasite Prevalence's in Sheep and in Goats in and around Wolaita soddo. South Ethiopia Revue Med Vet 159: 450-454.

18. Colwel DD, Bill Clymer B, Booker WC, Guichon TP, Jim KG, et al. (2001) Prevalence of sucking and chewing lice on cattle entering feedlots in southern Alberta. Can Vet J 42: 281-285.

19. James PJ, Garrett JA, Moon RD (2002) Sensitivity of two stage sampling to detect sheep biting lice (*Bovicola ovis*) in infested flocks. Veterinary Parasitology 103: 157-166.

20. James PJ (1999) Do sheep regulate the size of their mallophagan louse populations. International Journal for Parasitology 29: 869-875.

21. Wilkinson FC, de Chaneet GC, Beetson BR (1982) Growth of populations of lice, *Damalinia ovis*, on Sheep and their effects on Production and Processing Performance of wool. Veterinary Parasitology 9: 243-252.

22. Niven DR, Pritchard DA (1985) Effects of control of the sheep body louse (*Damalinia ovis*) on wool production and quality. Australian Journal of Experimental Agriculture 25: 27-31.

21

Epidemiology and Economic Importance of Sheep and Goat Pox: A Review on Past and Current Aspects

Nesradin Yune* and Nejash Abdela

School of Veterinary Medicine, College of Agriculture and Veterinary Medicine, Jimma University, PO Box 307, Jimma, Ethiopia

Abstract

Sheep and goat pox is highly devastating viral systemic disease of sheep and got. This disease is manifested by skin and internal lesions, fever, conjunctivitis, with oculonasal discharge and excess salivation. The objective of this paper was to review epidemiology and economic importance sheep and goat pox with special emphasis on both the past and currents aspects. The causative agent of Sheep and goat pox is sheep and goat pox virus of family poxoviaride, genus capripoxvirus. The poxviruses of Sheep pox and goat pox viruses are distinct, but hard to differentiate and Recombination can occur. Sheep and goat virus can survive in the environment for prolonged time. Today, Sheep and Goat Pox is found in most parts of Africa (mainly north of the equator), portion of India, central Asia (including south Russia and western China) and the Middle East. In Ethiopia, the disease is distributed in all regions and in endemic areas the disease are economically important due to production losses because of decreased weight gain, milk yield, damage to wool and hides, cause abortion, and increased susceptibility to other disease, while also being a direct cause of death. The diseases are more severe in young animal then adults. Infected animals can acts as the main cause of spreading SGP viruses. Since these diseases have no effective drug the treatment should be directed at preventing secondary bacterial infection. Furthermore, the animal should be vaccinated with commercially available attenuated vaccine as the main control measure in endemic regions.

Keywords: Sheep and goat pox; Epidemiology; Economic importance; Vaccination

Introduction

Ethiopia is believed to have the largest livestock population in Africa with sheep and goat populations exceeding 49 million, which is one of the largest populations of small ruminants in Africa [1]. Small ruminants (sheep and goats) have a unique role in smallholder agriculture as they require small investments; faster growth rates, have shorter production cycles, and greater environmental adaptability as compared to large ruminants. They are important protein sources in the diets of the poor and help to provide extra income and support survival for many farmers in the tropics and sub-tropics [2,3]. In Ethiopia, sheep are the second most important livestock species next to cattle [4]. Sheep and goat play an important economic role and make a significant contribution to both domestic and export markets through provision of food (meat and milk) and non-food (manure, skin and wool) products [5,6]. Although sheep and goat plays a significant role in national economy of the country to date the benefit obtained from these livestock are hampered by different constrains. Livestock diseases are among the important technical constraints that have hindered the development of the sector by decreasing production and hampering trade in animal and animal products [7,8]. Of which infectious disease like Sheep and goat pox are major and widely distributed in all region of the country [9].

Sheep pox and goat pox (SGP) are a group of viral disease that causes highly infectious disease in sheep and goats. Generally the disease is less commonly seen in indigenous breeds in area where it's endemic as compared with exotic breeds. Indigenous animals are more likely infected from the disease in areas where it has been not found or dormant for a period of time, when intensive husbandry methods are introduced, or in association with other disease agents such as or Foot and Mouth disease or Peste des Petits Ruminants [10]. The virus that causes sheep and got pox is Sheep and goat pox virus of family poxoviaride, genus capripoxvirus, one of the largest (170-260 nm by 300-450 nm), enveloped double stranded DNA viruses [11]. Mostly the disease is transmitted by direct contact, but indirect contact with infected object and mechanical insect can also transmit. Aerosol and nasal secretions can also spread sheep and got pox virus [12]. Sheep and goat pox (SGP) highly devastating viral systemic of sheep and goats characterized by widespread skin eruption, fever, generalized papules or nodules, vesicles (rarely) on non wool skin, internal lesions in the lungs, respiratory and gastrointestinal mucosa and cause death [13,14].

In Middle East, Africa, the Indian subcontinent, and much of central Asia Egypt, Turkey, Iraq, Iran, Afghanistan, Africa north of the equator, and in South-Eastern Europe, sporadic outbreaks occur [13]. Recently outbreaks have been recorded in Kazakhstan, Mongolia, and Azerbaijan and in Turkey, Greece and Bulgaria. Although the gene sequence of Mongolian goat pox (GP) virus in 2008 P32 was distinct as compared to sequences of several other GP viruses originated from China, it has not been identified the source of Mongolian outbreak [15].

Regarding the Ethiopian situation sheep and goat pox is found all region of the country [10]. Sheep and Goat Pox (SGP) is a disease that results in a substantial loss in the production and productivity of sheep and goats in Ethiopia. This disease is comparably more serious in lowland arid areas than in midland and highland agro ecologies [16]. According to Woldemeskel and marsha [17], of 1432 sheep and 1128 goats examined the prevalence of pox (22% in sheep and 18% in goats).

*Corresponding author: Nesradin Yune School of Veterinary Medicine, College of Agriculture and Veterinary Medicine, Jimma University, Jimma, Ethiopia, E-mail: Nesradin.90@gmail.com

In recent study around Gonder a total of 1296 ruminants studied for skin disease, the prevalence of sheep and goat pox is 77(48.12%) or 64(40%) or 13(8.12%) respectively [18].

Generally, Sheep and Goat pox result in economic losses due to high morbidity and mortality rate, decrease production, damage to the quality of skins and other production losses [10]. Despite the huge economic loss of sheep and goat pox in endemic area there is paucity of information. Therefore, the objective of this paper is to review the epidemiology, economic impact and control technique of sheep and goat pox.

Literature Review

Sheep and goat pox (SGPX) are serious, fatal viral systemic diseases. Characterized predominantly by skin lesions extending all over the skin, but are most obvious on face, eyelids and ears, perineum and tail and internal lesions [19]. Sheep and goat pox in endemic areas are associated with significant production losses because of reduced milk yield, decreased production, abortion, damage to wool and hides, and increased susceptibility to other disease, while also being a direct cause of mortality [20].

Etiology

The disease is result from infection caused by sheep pox virus (SPV) or goat pox virus (GPV), of family poxoviaride, Subfamily *Chrodopoxvirinae*, genus capripoxvirus. Is DNA virus. The poxviruses of sheep and goats (capripoxviruses) are closely related, both antigenically and physicochemically. We have unable to distinguish poxvirus from each with serological techniques (including serum neutralization), and were once thought to be strains of a single virus. SGP viruses are usually species specific; however, strains do exist that can infect both sheep and goats. Genetic sequencing has now confirmed that these viruses are distinct, but recombination can occur between them, however some capripoxivirus are not host specific. Kenya sheep and goat pox virus and Yeman and Oman infect both sheep and goat [12].

capripoxvirus are highly stable in normal environment condition and can survive for prolonged time, with or without susceptible animal. They are inactivated by sun light and heat, but can survive in cool dark environment for up to 6 month [21]. The sheep pox and goat pox viruses are generally considered host specific, but some strains affect both species [22].

Family poxoviride contain, Entomopoxvirinae, the poxviruses of insects, and Chordopoxvirinae, the poxviruses of vertebrates. The subfamily Chordopoxvirinae is comprised of eight genera, namely orthopoxivirus, parapoxvirus capripoxvirus, avipoxvirus, Leporipoxvirus, Suipoxvirus, Molluscipoxvirus and Yatapoxvirus. Genetic recombination within genera results in extensive serological cross-reactions and cross-protection [23] (Figure 1).

Epidemiology

Distribution and transmission

Sheep and Goat Pox are prevalent in parts of, central Asia, Africa except in South Africa, and the Middle Eastern countries. Goat pox is first reported in 879 in Norway and was later observed in Macedonia during the First World War. Capripoxvirus is found in the middle east, in Africa north of equator India, Pakistan, Turkey and Iran. Recent outbreak was occurred in 2008 and 2009 in Mogolia. Other outbreak have occurred in 2008 and 2009 is in Greece and Kazakhstan and Azerbaijan respectively. In Vietnam goat pox has been introduced in

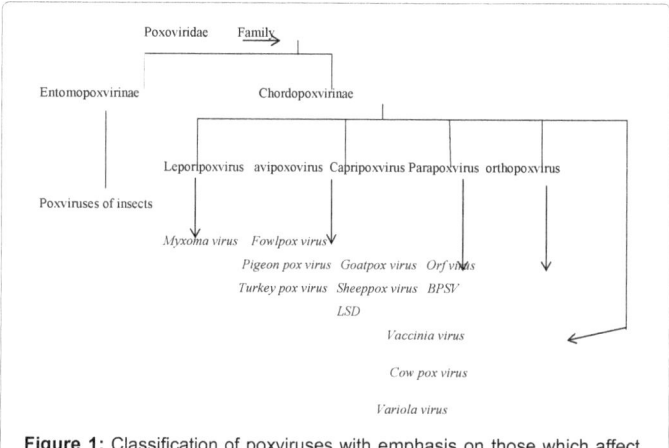

Figure 1: Classification of poxviruses with emphasis on those which affect domestic animals [23].

2005. The outbreak of goat pox was occured in Chinese Taipei in 2008 and in 2010 the disease reoccurred and was declared endemic [24]. In Ethiopia, the disease is distributed in all regions [25].

The virus of sheep and got pox is highly contagious. Virus enters via respiratory tract and transmission is mostly by aerosol through contact with infected animal or fomite. Vectores like, stomoxys calcitrans and tsetse flay can transmite virus mechanically [25]. Most experimental transmission and pathogenesis studies have used intradermal inoculation of the virus. Disseminated infection of the skin following either experimental intradermal inoculation or after respiratory infection is the result of viraemia and subsequent systemic viral spread to the skin [26,27].

The virus can survive for several weak in oral and nasal secretion after infection and also can live in scabs that have fallen off the animal for several months. Spread can also occur from contact with contaminated materials and through skin abrasions produced iatrogenically or by insects [28-30].

Risk Factor

Pathogen risk factor: The poxviruses are thought to have prolonged survival in environment and inactivated by drying, freezing, thawing, and remain viable for months in the lyophilized state. But its sensitive to 1% of formalin and extreme PH. can remain infectious for up to six months in sheep pens, and may also be found on the wool or hair for as long as three months after infection [31]. Capripoxvirus are highly stable in normal environment condition and can survive for prolonged time, with or without susceptible animal. They are inactivated by sun light and heat, but can survive in cool dark environment for up to 6 month [21].

Host risk factor: Group of Sheep and goat of all age, breed and sex are susceptible to sheep and goat pox. In areas where sheep pox is enzootic, imported breeds such as Merinos or some European breeds may show greater susceptibility than the native stock. Sheep and goat pox infect only sheep and goat and have no zoonosis. Wild ungulate is not reservoir for this disease [10]. Capripoxvirus can affect sheep, goat and cattle. Virus of goat pox is highly host-specific, infecting only goats, but from isolate to isolate host specificity varies. It is possible that the host preference shown by different strains is due to their adaptation to the presence of either sheep or goat alone in a limited geographical area. Isolates of Capripoxvirus are not host-specific; cattle, goats, and sheep who have recovered from infection with Capripoxvirus isolates from a heterologous host hav immune to any challenge with a virulent homologous virus [32].

There are two types of sheep pox virus [33], in which, one affects both sheep and goats (Kenyan sheep and goat (KSG) strain while the other is host specific. Recent records indicate that strains of sheep pox do pass between sheep and goats, although most cause more severe disease in sheep. Recombination also occurs between strains of SPV producing a spectrum, showing intermediate host preferences and a range of virulence [34].

Environment risk factor: Environmental determinants play a great role in the occurrence of sheep and goat pox. It had impact on the agent, host and vectors as well as interaction between them. These predisposing factors have a great role in maintenance of Stomoxys calcitrans and the tsetse fly to susceptible animals which are the vectors for transmission of disease [25].

Pathogenesis

Incubation period of sheep pox is 4-8 of that of goat pox is 4-15 days. After it inters, goat pox virus replicates locally in the tissues. Since the virus is epitheliotropic, it will infest the epithelium tissues of the organism. On the 7th day post-inoculation, the virus titer reached to its peak. The virus spread to the regional lymph nodes, after 3-4 days of primary viremia. The viremia spread in the body, and affected spleen, lungs and liver. The virus inhaled may also cause lungs lesions. In skin nodules from 7 to 14 days after inoculation, the virus titers persisted and decreased with the development of serum antibodies. Within 24 hours of the appearance of generalized papules, affected animals develop conjunctivitis, rhinitis and enlargement of all the superficial lymph nodes, in particular the prescapular lymph nodes. Excessive salivation can also occur after infection [24].

There are five stages in the development of pox infection. Roseola stage is stage in which Skin lesions typically begin with small red spots with in three days of infection which is followed by papules. The affected animals are febrile at this stage. The second stage of pox lesion is Papules wich develops after 3 days of roseola stage. Nodular skin lesions that are devcloped from roseola stage (red spots) those are hard during palpation. Papules with in 5-6 days are changed to vesicles and known as vesicular stage. Pustular stage develops after 3 days of vesicular stage. The last stage of pox lesion is scab. Quantitative analysis using real-time PCR and isolation of the pathogenesis of Sheep pox virus and Goat pox virus in their respective hosts revealed high viral loads in skin [35].

Clinical Sign and Finding

Both sheep and goat pox have similar clinical sign [22]. The incubation of SGP is between 4-15 Days in field condition [36]. The clinical sign of sheep pox can be either malignant or benign. The malignant form of sheep pox is mostly common in lamb. Affected lambs may die without observable pox lesion. Fevers which peak at 40-42°C, dyspnea, and occulonasal discharge and pox lesion on unwooled skin are manifested in malignant form of sheep pox. The diseases are more severe in young animals than adults. In benign form of sheep pox only skin lesions occur particularly under the tail. This form of sheep pox is common adult. There is no systemic reaction and the animal recovers in 3-4 weeks. Abortion and secondary pneumonia are complications. In young the mortality rate may reach 100% while the overall mortality may be 50% of the flock. Lesions may be seen on the vulva, prenium, nostril and mucous membranes of the mouth. If lesion is present in the lung acute respiratory distress occurs [37] (Figures 2 and 3).

Post mortem Lesions of sheep and goat pox can develop in lung, spleen, lymph node and other internal organs. Lesion may also present in the mouth, nares, eye or eyelid. Affected mucous membranes may become ulcerate or slough and necrotic. Nodules occur in digestive, respiratory and urogenital system. Animals with lung lesions may have respiratory signs including coughing, nasal discharge and dyspnea. Nodules in the digestive system can cause diarrhea. Depression and emaciation may be seen in some animals. Abortions can occur but are not common. In acute disease some breeds of sheep can die before the characteristic skin lesions develop [12]. At necropsy, skin lesions have congestion, hemorrhage, edema, vasculitis, and necrosis and will be seen to involve all layers of the epidermis, dermis, and, in severe cases, extend int the adjacent musculature. Histologically, pox lesions have extensive inflammatory, necrotic and proliferative changes. The presence of Borrel cells, and intracytoplasmic inclusion bodies similar to the inclusions found with all poxviruses, are characteristic of Sheep and goat pox. Poxvirus of sheep and got pox can be seen under electron microscope and can be readily differentiated from the virus particles of contagious pustular dermatitis, but indistinguishable from the orthopoxviruses [37].

Diagnosis

Sheep and goat Pox can be diagnosed based on observable clinical sign like, fever, dyspnea and pox lesion in different parts of the unwoolen skin. Clinical pathology and species of affected host are also important in the diagnosis of this disease. Epidemiology of the disease is also important in diagnoses of sheep and goat pox. As the virus of sheep and goat pox are very closely related it's indistinguishable by serologically. It appears that the host preference shown by these viruses with respect to either sheep or goats, accompanied by the case history, may be regarded as partially affirmative for either sheep pox or goat pox, but confirmatory diagnosis requires laboratory studies. It is also known that heterologous diagnostic reagents tend to be less efficient than homologous reagents for confirmatory diagnosis [38].

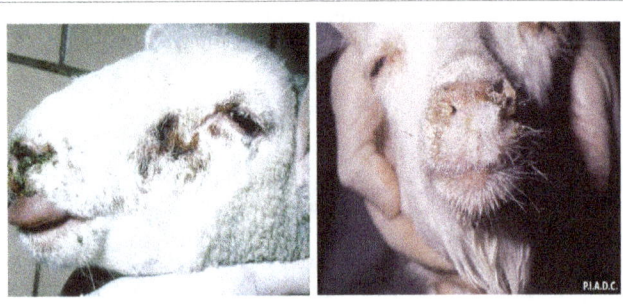

Figure 2: Malignant form of sheep pox.

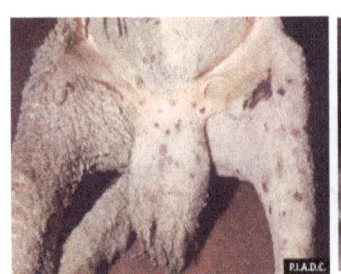 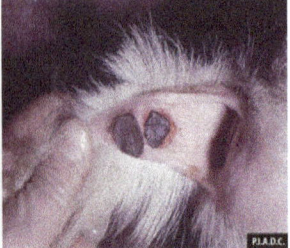

Figure 3: Benign form of sheep and goat pox.

Before collecting or sending any samples, the proper authority's samples should only be sent under secure conditions and to authorized laboratories to prevent the spread of the disease. Samples for virus isolation must be sent to the laboratory as soon as possible. They should be kept cold and shipped on gel packs. If these samples must be shipped long distances without refrigeration, glycerol (10%) can be added; tissue samples must be large enough that glycerol does not penetrate into the centre of the tissue and destroy the virus. Sheep and goat antigen can be detected using routine laboratory procedure. Direct fluorescent antibody test using edema fluid, Agar gel immuno Diffusion (AGID) using biopsies of lymph nodes using specific immune sera and ELISA are used to detect sheep and goat pox antigens. Other laboratory diagnoses of sheep and goat pox include observation of the virus using electron microscope, virus isolation, and indirect fluorescent antibody and detection of antibody by virus neutralization test [27], or both; and characteristic histopathologic lesions [21].

Sheep and goat pox may have similar clinical sign with contagious ecthyma (orf), bluetongue, Parasitic pneumonia, caseous lymphadenitis, Insect bites, Sheep scab, Mange and Photsensitization, Peste des petits ruminants [10].

Economic Importance

Sheep and goat pox is highly devastating viral systemic disease of sheep and got. Sheep and goat pox are among the commonest disease of sheep and goat entailing a huge economic loss of the country. These two diseases are limiting international trade of animals and animal product [13,14]. This disease is fatal in newly introduced animal, but may be mild in indigenous breeds from endemic region. The outbreak of sheep and goat pox may cause serious stock and economic loss in sheep and goat industries [39].

In endemic areas the disease are economically important due to production losses because of decreased weight gain, milk yield, damage to wool and hides, cause abortion, and increased susceptibility to other disease, while also being a direct cause of death. In naïve animal's mortality and Morbidity rates can be very high, approaching 100% [40]. In India mortality rate had been 49.5 and took 6 years to recover from an outbreak [41].

Sheep and goat pox (SGP) disease can affect trade, import, export and intensive production of animals. Flock size, number of adult animals and number of days of illness play significantly in influencing the economic losses due to Sheep Pox [42,43].

Management Strategies

Sheep and goat pox has no effective treatment so treatment of sheep and goat pox should be directed to control secondary bacteria infection. So parenteral administration of abroad spectrum antibiotic is important to control secondary bacterial infection. Clean, well ventilated enclosure and balanced diet should be provided. If Animals are unable to feed 100/o glucose saline should be given parentally. To limit secondary bacterial complication all diseased animal should be treated with antibiotics. Wash and clean the nostril with weak solution of potassium permanganate (1:10000) to relieve respiratory related sign. Topically applying antibiotic ointment is important for skin lesion [42]. Heating at 56°C (133°F) for 2 hours, or to 65°C (149°F) for 30 minutes are reported to destroy Capripoxviruses. Although some strains are resistant to ether, capirpoxvirus are generally inactivated by chloroform, formalin and ether 20%. Capripoxviruses are generally sensitive to ether (20%), formalin and chloroform [12].

Vaccination with commercially available live attenuated vaccines has been applied as the main control measure for SPP/GTP in endemic regions. Annual vaccinations using live attenuated SPP vaccines provide good protection and are able to control the outbreaks when the minimal coverage of 75 % is reached and maintained. Experience obtained from the FAO Regional Animal Disease Surveillance and Control Network for SPP eradication programme in 2000 within Maghreb countries demonstrated that a considerable reduction in SPP cases was achieved when the goal for vaccination coverage was set between 75 and 90 % [44]. To control loss from sheep and goat pox vaccination is an effective means of controlling in area where disease is endemic. As they do not provide long lasting immunity, killed vaccine have not yet proven to be practical under field condition. For protection of sheep and goat pox modified live vaccine can also used. Roman strain vaccine has been used effectively for many years for the control of sheep and goat pox [45,46].

As per the guidelines OIE, eradication of sheep and goat pox can be adopted the same strategy as followed incase of rinder pest. This can be applied after serological surveillance for a period of 2 years and cessation of vaccination program followed by an initial mass vaccination. In general, to declare a country free from SGP about ten years is required [47-49].

Conclusion

Sheep and goat pox are the most serious viral disease of sheep and goat. It is economically important disease as it causes high morbidity and mortality rate in sheep and goat industries. These diseases are widely distributed in Middle East, Africa, central Asia and Indian content. Direct or indirect contact with infected animal or fomite, and vectors are some important means of this disease. Since these diseases have no effective drug the treatment should be directed at preventing secondary bacterial infection. Movement of animals and animal products should be restricted during disease outbreak. Carcass and any skins, wool or fiber which may have been contaminated should be either burned or buried. Furthermore, insects that are potential vectors to transmit virus should also be controlled and animal should be vaccinated with commercially available attenuated vaccine as the main control measure in endemic regions.

References

1. CSA (Central Statistic Authority) (2013) Agricultural sample survey Volume II, Central Statistic Authority, Addis Ababa, Ethiopia.

2. Tibbo M, Philipsson J, Ayalew W (2006) Sustainable sheep breeding programmes in the Tropics: Framework for Ethiopia.

3. Nottor DR (2012) Genetic Improvement of reproductive efficiency of sheep and goat. Animal reproduction Science. 130: 147-151.

4. Gizaw S, van Arendonk JAM, Komen H, Windig JJ, Hanott O (2007) Population structure, genetic variation and morphological diversity in indigenous sheep of Ethiopia. Animal Genetics 38: 621-628.

5. Alvarez I, Traore A, Tamboura HH, Kabore A, Royo LJ, et al. (2009) Microsatellite analysis characterizes Burkinafaso as a genetic contact zone between Sahelian and Djallonke sheep. Anim Biotechnol 20: 47-57.

6. Duguma G, Mirkena T, Haile A, Iñiguez L, Okeyo AM, et al. (2011) Identification of smallholder farmers and pastoralists' p references for sheep breeding traits: choice model approach. Animal 5: 1984-1992.

7. Jilo K, Abdela N, Adem A (2016) Insufficient Veterinary Service as a Major Constrants in Pastoral Area of Ethiopia: A Review. Journal of Biology, Agriculture and Healthcare 6: 94-101.

8. Abdela N (2016) Important Cattle Ticks and Tick Born Haemoparasitic Disease in Ethiopia: A Review. Acta Parasitologica Globalis. 7: 12-20.

9. Tsegaye D, Belay B, Haile A (2013) Prevalence of Major Goat Diseases and Mortality of Goat in Daro-Labu District of West Hararghe, Eastern Ethiopia. Journal of Scientific and Innovative Research 2: 665-672.

10. Sheep, Ethiopian (2009) Goats Productivity Improvement Program (ESGPIP), "Common defects of sheep and goats skin in Ethiopia and their causes". Technical Bulletin 19.

11. Matthews RE (1982) Classification and nomenclature of viruses. Intervirology. 17: 1-99.

12. CFSPH (2008) The Center for Food Security Public Health, Iowa State University, College of Veterinary Medicine and Institution of International cooperation in Animal Biologics, an OIE collaborating center.

13. OIE (2008) Peste Des Petits Ruminants. Terrestrial Manual. Pp: 1036-1046.

14. OIE (2008). Sheep Pox and Goat Pox. Terrestrial Manual. Pp: 1058-1068.

15. Beard PM, Sugar S, Bazarragchaa E (2010). A description of two outbreaks of capripoxvirus disease in Mongolia. Vet Microbiol. 142: 427-431.

16. Sileshi Z (2009) Sheep and goat pox: causes, prevention and treatment. In: Technical bulletin no.29 sheep and goat pox: causes, prevention and treatment.

17. Woldemeskel M, MarshaG (2010) Study on caprine and ovine dermatophilosis in Wollo, Northeast Ethiopia. Trop Anim Health Prod. 42: 41-44.

18. Daniel T (2016) Prevalence of Major Skin Diseases in Ruminants and its Associated Risk factors at University of Gondar Veterinary Clinic, North West Ethiopia. Austin J Vet Sci Anim Husb. 3: 1019.

19. Bhanuprakash V, Moorthy ARS, Krishnappa G, Srinivasagowda RN, Indrani BK (2005) An epidemiological study of sheep pox in Karnataka state, Révue Scientific et, Technique (Office International des Epizooties). 24: 909-920.

20. Yeruham I, Yadin H, Van Ham M, Bumbarov V, Soham A, et al. (2007) Economic and epidemiological aspects of an outbreak of sheeppox in a dairy sheep flock. Vet Rec. 160: 236-237.

21. Davies FG (1981) Sheep and Goat pox. In: Virus diseases of food Animals. London: Academic Press. pp: 733-748.

22. Kitching RP, Taylor WP (1985) Clinical and antigenic relationship between isolates of Sheep and goat pox viruses. Tropical Animal Health and Production. 17: 64-74.

23. Quinn PJ, Markey BK, Carter ME, Donnelly WJ, Leonard FC (2002) Veterinary Microbiology and Microbial Disease. Black well publishing company: Blackwell Science, London, UK, pp: 137-143.

24. OIE Terrestrial Manual (2012). Chapter 2.7.14 Sheep pox and goat pox.

25. Webbs G (1980) Sheep and goat pox, transmission of capripox viruses by various flies indicated the need for a reassessment of the methods of controlling this disease. Annual Report, Institute for Animal Health, Pirbright, UK.

26. Afshar A, Bundza A, Myers DJ, Dulac GC, Thomas FC (1986) Sheep pox: Experimental studies with a west african isolate. Canadian Veterinary Journal 27: 301-306.

27. Davies FG, Otema C (1978) The antibody response in sheep infected with a Kenyan sheep and goat pox virus. J Comp Path. 88: 205-210.

28. Swanepoel R, Coetzer JAW (2004) Rift valley fever. Infectious diseases of livestock 2: 1037-1070.

29. Radostits OM, Gay CC, Hinchcliff KW (2006) Veterinary Medicine. 10th edn. Saunders, pp: 1430-1431.

30. Animal Health Australia (AHA) (2011) Disease Strategy Sheep pox and goat pox, Available at: www.animalhealthaustralia.com.au/programs/emergency-animal Disease preparedness/ausvetplan

31. Sharma B, Negi BS, Pandey AB, Bandyopadhyay SK, ShankarH, et al. (1988) Detection of goat pox antigen and antibody by the CIE test. Tropical Animal Healtb and Production 20: 109-113.

32. Kitching RP, Bhat PP, Black DN (1989) The characterization of African strains of capripoxviruses. Epidemiology and Infection. 102: 335-343.

33. Singari NA, Moorthy AS, Rama Rao P (1990) Sheep pox. Livest Adviser 15: 40-42.

34. Manual OIE (2000) Manual of standards for diagnostic tests and vaccines. 4th edn.

35. Bowden TR, Babiuk SL, Parkyn GR, Copps JS, Boyle B (2008) Capripoxvirus tissue tropism and shedding: A quantitative study in experimentally infected sheep and goats. Virol. 371: 380-393.

36. House JA (1992) Sheep and goat pox. In: Veterinary Diagnostic Virology: Practitioners Guide, Mosby Year Book, pp: 217-219.

37. AUSVETPLAN (1996) Australian Veterinary Emergency Plan. Disease Strategy, Lumpy skin disease.

38. Pandey R, Singh P (1972) Soluble antigens of sheep pox and goat pox viruses as Determined by immunodiffusion inagar gel. Acta Virologica16: 47-46.

39. Garner MG, Lack MB (1995) Modelling the potential impact of exotic diseases on regional Australia. Australian Vet J. 72: 81-87.

40. Bhanuprakash V, Indrani BK, Hosamani M, Singh RK (2006) The current status of sheep pox disease. Comp. Immunol Microbiol Infect Dis. 29: 27-60.

41. Garner MG, Sawarkar SD, Brett EK (2000) The Extent and Impact of Sheep Pox and Goat Pox in the State of Maharashtra India. Tropical Animal Health and Production 32: 205-223.

42. Senthilkumar V, Thirunavukkarasu M (2010) Economic losses due to sheep pox in sheep farms in Tamil Nadu. Tamil Nadu Journal of Veterinary and Animal Sciences 6: 88-94.

43. Nandi S, Rao TVS, Poonam M (1999) Sheep pox - a scourge to sheep industry in India. Indian Farming 49: 29-31.

44. FAO (Food and Agriculture Organization) (2001) RADISCON workshop on sheep pox eradication programme. EMPRES Transboundary Animal Diseases Bulletin 18/13.

45. Ramyar H (1965) Studies on the immunogenic properties of tissue culture sheep pox virus. Zentralbl. Veterinar Med. 123: 537-540.

46. Sabban MS (1957) The cultivation of sheep pox virus on the chorioallantoic membrane of the developing chicken embryo. AJVR 18: 618.

47. Kitching RP (1986) The control of sheep and goat pox. Revue Scientifique et Technique de l'OIE (France) 5: 503-511.

48. Rweyemamu MM, Roeder PL, Taylor WP (2006) Towards the global eradication. In: Barret T (ed). Cambridge: Institute of Animal Health, Biology of Animal.

49. Bhanuprakash V (2011) Prospects of control and eradication of capripox from the Indian subcontinent: A perspective. Antiviral Research 91: 225-232.

22

Antibiotic Resistance of Aerobic Bacteria Isolated from Uteri of Slaughtered Cows in and around Addis Ababa, Ethiopia

Solomon Abreham[1]*, Merry Hailu[1], Ali Worku[1] and Solomon Tsegaye[2]

[1]Veterinary Drugs and Feed Administration Control Authority, Addis Ababa, Ethiopia
[2]College of Agriculture, Woldia University, Woldia, Ethiopia

Abstract

Uterine samples were collected from Addis Ababa abattoir with the objective of isolating aerobic bacteria and determine the antibiotic sensitivity profiles of the isolates. A total of 38 uteri of cows were collected and samples were processed for bacteriology and isolates identified by morphological, staining and biochemical tests. At least one species of bacteria was isolated from each uterine sample. The highest isolate found in this study was *Escherichia coli* (42.1%) followed by *Bacillus* species (17.1%), *Staphylococcus spp.* (15.7%), *Arcanobacterium pyogens* (7.9%) and *Streptococcus spp.* and *Proteus spp.* (3.9% each). Other isolates include *Corynebacterium, Rhodococcus equi, Klebsiela* and *Citrobacter*. Among all bacteria screened, sensitivities for selected drug were: chloramphenicol (98.6%), amikacin (90.8%), nitrofurantoin (82.9%) and trimethoprim-sulfamethoxasole (81.5%), tetracycline (71%) and polymixin-B (67.1%). Contrary to this, penicillin-G, methicillin and erythromycin showed highest resistance to the isolates identified respectively.

Keywords: Abattoir; Addis Ababa; Antibiotic sensitivity; Biochemical tests; Uterine bacteria

Introduction

Cattle production is the main component of livestock production in most sub-Saharan Africa farming systems [1]. Tropical African countries have been reported to have 147 million heads of cattle. However the current milk and meat production of these countries, including Ethiopia, is still low and relies on the import of livestock products from other sources [2].

Bovine uterine diseases is mainly caused by the contamination of uterus after parturition which contribute to a great economic losses due to longer calving intervals, lower conception rates and increased rate of culling. *E. coli* is the most relevant pathogenic bacteria involved in the puerperal uterine infection and persistence of uterine disease, it is resistant to many antibiotics and mostly have synergetic action with other uterine bacteria such as A. pyogenes [3].

Different part of genital organs infections in ruminant animals are often caused by opportunistic bacteria, especially *E. coli* species, majorly isolated from uterus of ewes, goats and cows. Fecal origin coliforms and non-specific bacteria are also opportunistic invaders of the reproductive tract. Genital infection resulting reproductive failure in ruminants can be caused by opportunist bacteria under stressful conditions [4].

After parturition, mostly three weeks later a diverse group of bacteria including *Bacillus* spp. *Trueperella pyogenes, Streptococcus uberis* and *Escherichia coli* can be frequently isolated from the cattle uterus. Many bacteria including those pathogens are known to cause bovine endometritis, but also other bacterial species invade cattle uterus after delivery. The uterine clearance is a unique process, during which a progression of bacteria and their interactions will result the occurrence of endometritis [5].

Much effort to improve the productivity of cattle by cross breeding local breeds with improved breeds has been implemented for long time in Ethiopia. However, the result of cross breeding was not successful related to several reproductive abnormalities. Due to less performance cows are culled and sent to abattoir for slaughter [6].

Antimicrobial agents (antibiotics) are used either to control infection or prevent disease progression. Antibiotic compounds like tetracyclines, sulfonamides, aminoglycosides, β-lactams and cephalosporins have been used together or in single for the treatment of postpartum metritis. Extensive use of antimicrobial agents in dairy cattle could result bacterial resistance, milk-residue effect and human health risk [7]. The antimicrobial susceptibilities of these isolates in tropical zones may vary; that limit the efficacy of the common antibiotic treatment protocols in use in these areas [4].

Naturally, specific and non-specific bovine uterine infections occur. Unlike the specific infections, the non-specific infections require a predisposing factor. Hence, different species of bacteria cause uterine infection under favorable conditions [8]. Even though, a variety of antibiotic have been used against uterine infections; the disease is gradually becoming refractory and incurable in Addis Ababa and its surroundings. Antibiotic resistance can result from different factors such as bacterial adaptations and faulty administrations. However, sensitivity tests on uterine bacterial isolates for different antibiotic preparations have rarely been conducted.

The objectives of this study were therefore:

To isolate the common aerobic bacteria from normal and infected uterus of cattle slaughtered in Addis Ababa Abattoir's Enterprise.

To determine Antibiotic susceptibility patterns of those aerobic bacterial isolates.

*Corresponding author: Solomon Abreham, Veterinary Drugs and Feed Administration Control Authority, Addis Ababa, Ethiopia
E-mail: sollatta@gmail.com

Materials and Methods

Study area

The study was conducted from November 2004 to 2005. Uterine samples were obtained from Addis Ababa Abattoir's Enterprise, Addis Ababa. Bacteriological study was then conducted at Addis Ababa University, Faculty of Veterinary Medicine (FVM), Debrezeit, 47 km southeast of Addis Ababa. Addis Ababa was located at an altitude of 2408 meter above sea level. It has an average minimum and maximum temperature of 9.4°C and 32.2°C respectively. It receives an annual rainfall of 1200 mm.

Sampling methods

The study was conducted on 38 uterine samples with different physiological and pathological statuses as: apparently healthy, endometrities with pus, endometrities without pus and gravid uterus. The whole uterus was separated and opened aseptically with sterile scalpel blades and scissors and endometrial tissues of all apparently healthy and abnormal uteri were sampled from both right and left horns. Samples labeled and immediately transported, keeping the cold chain, to microbiology laboratory of FVM, Debrezeit.

Bacterial isolation and identification

Different laboratory procedures were adopted for bacterial isolation and identification according to different literatures [9-13].

The surface of samples was heated with hot scalpel blade and chopped with sterile blade on a sterile petridish. Chopped samples were first incubated in to brain-Heart-Infusion broth and incubated at 37°C overnight and then a loop full of the suspension was inoculated on 7% sheep-blood agar. After overnight incubation at 37°C, aerobically, representative colonies were isolated on another blood agar. Cellular morphology and Gram's reaction, from gram stained smears, and growth on MacConkey agar were then made from pure cultures and further biochemical tests were conducted.

The following biochemical tests were employed: Catalase test, using 3% H_2O_2, Oxidase test, using aqueous solution of tetramethyl-p-phenylenediamine dihydrochloride, Motility test by SIM (Sulfide Indole Motility) medium and modified Hugh Liefson's medium was used for Oxidation-Fermentation test.

Further secondary biochemical tests were applied to identify the bacteria to species level. These tests include: Citrete utilization test, Voges-Proskauer test, Methyl Red test, Indole test, Urease test, Gas production test and also by inoculating on different medias like TSI (Triple Sugar Iron) agar, Manitol salt agar, Eosin- Methylene blue agar and Edward's media.

Antibiotic susceptibility tests

Agar disk diffusion (Kirby-Bauer) method was used as described in Quinn et al. [13] and Ikram [14] to determine the antibiotic susceptibility patterns of each bacterial isolates.

A suspension was made from an 18 hour pure culture colonies from nutrient agar in sterile distilled water using a sterile plastic loop. The inoculums density in the suspension was adjusted to 0.5 McFarland using a device called colorimeter, which detects turbidity by UV (Ultra Violet) light. The standardized bacteria suspension was inoculated on Mueller Hinton II agar plates, which has 4-5 mm thickness. For Streptococci and Arcanobacterium pyogens, the agar was supplemented with 5% sheep blood. The bacterial suspensions were inoculated on the

agar plates with sterile cotton swabs. The plates were allowed to dry for at least 15 minutes. Then antibiotic discs were placed on the plates using sterile forceps.

The isolates were subjected to disc assay testes using, Penicillin-G (10 units), Tetracycline (30 µg), Erythromycin (5 µg), Amikacin (30 µg), Nitrofurantoin (300 µg), Methicilin (5 µg), Chloramphenicol (30 µg), polymixin-B (300 units), Trimethoprim-Sulfamethoxazole (1.25/23.75 µg). Regularly spaced antibiotics were placed on two different Mueller Hinton agar plates (4 discs on the first and 5 on the second plate) for each isolate using paper templates under these plates. The plates are then incubated at 37°C within 15 minutes after the discs were placed on the plates. Zone of inhibitions of the antibiotic discs were measured after 18-24 hours of incubation, using a transparent ruler to the nearest mm. The inhibition zone diameters were then interpreted as Resistance, Intermediate and Susceptible as described by Ikram [14].

Data analysis

Descriptive statistics were used to analyze the findings of this study. This includes: Bar-graphs, Tables and percentage descriptions.

Results

Gross uterine examination findings

A total of 38 uterine samples were collected. Gross examination on apparently healthy 21 (55.2%), endometritis 5 (13.1%), endometrities with pus 7 (18.4%) and gravid uterus 5 (13.1%) was done as indicated in Table 1.

Bacterial isolates

All uterine samples were positive for bacteria, 16 (42.1%) of which were mixed infections with two bacteria, 11 (28.9%) were mixed infection of three bacteria. E. coli was the most common isolated bacteria from 32 (84.2%), followed by Bacillus species from 13 (34.2%) uterus samples, Staphylococcus species from 12 (13.6%) and Arcanobacterium pyogenes from 6 (15.6%) uterus samples (Table 2).

Antimicrobial susceptibility profiles of bacterial isolates

As shown on Figure 1, isolates of all apparently healthy and abnormal uterine samples are commonly sensitive to chloramfenicol (98.6%), amikacine (90.8%), nitrofurantion (82.9%) and trimethoprim-sulfamethoxazole (81.5%); where as they were less sensitive to tetracycline (71%) and polymixin-B (67.1%). Relatively, many isolates show resistance for the rest of the antibiotics used on this study: penicillin-G (80.3%), methicillin (65.8%) and erythromycin (48.7%).

Resistance to one antibiotic was found in 5 (6.6%) isolates, for two antibiotics in 21 (27.6%) isolates and 47 isolates (61.8%) showed mixed resistance for at least three antibiotics. However, 3 isolates (3.9%) were found to be sensitive to all antibiotics in this study.

Antibiotic sensitivity of gram-negative isolates

As illustrated on Figure 2, all of the gram-negative isolates are sensitive to amikacin (100%) followed by chloramphenicol (97.4%),

Types of Abnormality	Total examined	%
Apparently healthy	21	55.2
Endometritis	5	13.1
Endometritis with pus	7	18.4
Gravid uterus	5	13.1

Table 1: Different uterine status of cattle examined.

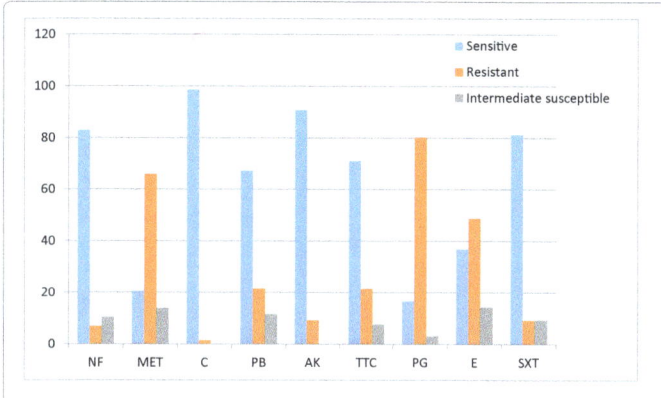

NF- Nitrifurantoin; MET- Methicillin; C- Chloramphenicol; PB- Polymixin-B; AK- Amikacin; TTC Tetracycline; PG- Penicillin; E- Erythromycin; SXT-Trimethoprim-Sulfamethoxazole.

Figure 1: Percentage sensitivity of bacterial isolates to different Antibiotics.

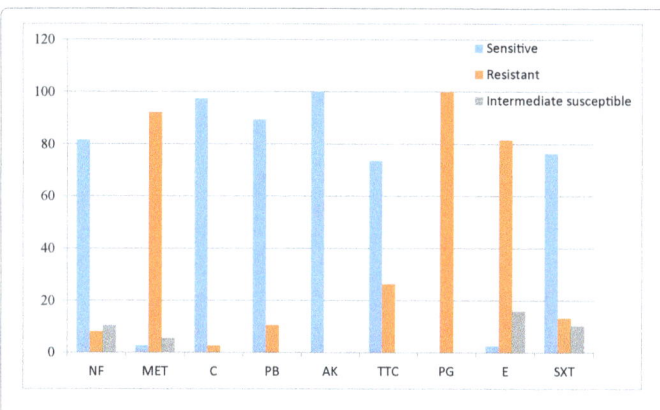

NF- Nitrifurantoin; MET- Methicillin; C- Chloramphenicol; PB- Polymixin-B; AK- Amikacin; TTC Tetracycline; PG- Penicillin; E- Erythromycin; SXT-Trimethoprim-Sulfamethoxazole

Figure 2: Sensitivity patterns of Gram -ve bacterial isolates.

polymixin-B (89.5%) and nitrofurantoin (81.65%) in that order. Meanwhile, they were resistant to penicillin-G (100%), methicillin (92.1%) and erythromycin (81.6%). Some resistance to other antibiotics was also seen on tetracycline (26.3%) and trimethoprim-sulfamethoxazole (13.2%).

Antibiotic sensitivity of gram-positive isolates

The sensitivity patterns of all gram-positive uterine isolates are illustrated in Figure 3. Among the antibiotics used in this study gram positive isolates were highly sensitive to Chloramphenicol (100%), Trimethoprim-sulfamethoxazole (86.8%), Nitrofurantoin (84.2%) and Amikacine (81.6%); and less sensitive to Erythromycin (73.7%), Tetracycline (68.4%) and Methicillin (55.3%). Complete resistance was seen on some isolates to, Penicillin-G (60.5%), Methicillin (39.5%) and Polymixin-B (34.2%). Resistance to Tetracycline, Amikacin and Erythromycin is observed to the extent of 23.7%, 18.4% and 15.8%, respectively.

Antibiotic resistance of uterine isolates

Antibiotic resistances of different bacterial isolates were tested in this study. *E. coli*, *Bacillus* species and *Corynebacterium* species 100% resisted Penicillin and different rates of resistance found as indicated in Table 3.

Discussion

Nonspecific infection of a bovine uterus relates to the endocrine state at time of infection. Even if massive invasion occurs, during estrus and parturition, infection is not established unless there is a serious problem. However, during diestrus and pregnancy, uterine infections are more likely to establish [15]. Common organisms in cattle, that can be isolated aerobically, are *Arcanobacterium* (Actinomyces) *pyogenes*, *E. coli*, *Staphylococci*, *Streptocci* and less frequently proteus species and others [15,16]. In the present study different types of bacterial isolates from endometrial tissue samples were identified. Moharana et al. [17] from India has also reported similar bacterial isolates from uterine mucus samples.

Among all the bacterial isolates *E. coli* was the most dominant bacterium followed by *Bacillus* Species and *Staphylococci*. This finding agrees with previous work done by Baishya et al. [18] in India, who reported *E. coli* was the most dominant uterine isolate (29.7%). The report also agrees with the findings in this study regarding the dominant species in the second order, which were *Bacillus* species, *Staphylococci* and *Streptococci* species.

Gram positive bacteria isolated in this particular study, there was multi-drug resistance to various levels. For *A. pyogenes* it was high, which was resistance to 8 of them. This organism shared higher resistance to Tetracycline, which was also seen on another similar study, on uterine isolates in Israel [19].

Likewise, significant levels of resistance were also found for one other important antibiotic (Tetracycline) in this study. Supporting the current study *E. coli* isolated from uterus was found to be resistant to Oxytetracycline and Sulfonamides [20]. Pejsak and Kolodziejcxyk [21] observed a similar resistance pattern against Teracycline on *E. coli* isolated from diseased lungs. According to Adegoke [22] resistance develops owing to the use of the drug as food additive and mass treatment in different outbreaks.

Penicillin-G is considered as an appropriate drug for systemic treatment of cows with endometritis. However, isolates of this study showed resistance to penicillin-G to a high level, which makes it ineffective for the treatment of uterine infections. Resistance to penicillin may be likely due to β-lactamase production. It is mentioned that, of veterinary isolates, 50-60% of Staphylococcus strains and 40-70% of *E. coli* strains are resistant to Penicillin–G due to similar effect [23]. Similarly, other studies on uterine isolates of cattle reported the resistance of these isolates against Penicillin-G [24,25].

Although Tetracycline has showed considerable resistance against isolates from this study, a study done by Cohen et al. [19], on *in-vitro* antibiotic sensitivity of uterine isolates from post parturient dairy cows, showed a high level of resistance of the isolates (*E. coli*, *A. pyogenes*, *Streptococci* and *Bacteroides* species) to tetracycline. It was suggested that, the use of the drug for treating post- parturient cows is inconsistent, in Israel. Resistances of uterine isolates against tetracycline were also mentioned by other authors [18,20]. Tetracycline resistance could result from mutation of plasmid mediated resistance [26]. But most commonly it is easily developed through indiscriminate drug usage.

Trimethoprim-sulfamethoxazole is the most recommended drug when compared to the other drugs tested in this study. It is better than Amikacin in that, its effect against anaerobic pathogens of uterus and resistant bacteria which could be isolated from uterus and development of resistance to this drug is not common to occur [23].

	No. of isolates (%)	Apparently healthy	Endometritis with pus	Endometritis without pus	Gravid uterus	Total Rate of isolation
E. coli	32 (42.1%)	21	2	4	3	84.2%
Bacillus species	13 (17.1%)	7	3	3	-	34.2%
Staphylococcus aures	7 (9.2%)	2	3	1	1	18.45
- other staph.	5 (6.6%)	3	2	-	-	13.2%
A. pyogenes	6 (7.9%)	-	5	1	-	15.8%
Streptococci	3 (4%)	1	2	-	-	7.9%
Corynebacterium sp.	2 (2.6%)	1	1	-	-	5.3%
Rhodococcus Equi	2 (2.6%)	1	-	-	1	5.3%
Proteus	3 (4%)	2	1	-	-	7.9%
Salmonella	1 (1.3%)	1	-	-	-	2.6%
Klebsiela	1 (1.3%)	1	-	-	-	2.6%
Citrobacter	1 (1.3%)	1	-	-	-	2.6%
Total	76 (100%)	41	19	9	6	

Table 2: Bacterial species isolated from different status of uteri from cows slaughtered.

Bacterial Isolate	Antibiotics applied								
	NF	MET	C	PB	AK	TTC	PG	E	SXT
E. coli	4 (2.4%)	31 (93.7%)	1 (3.1%)	2 (6.3%)	-	9 (28.2%)	32 (100%)	31 (93.7%)	9 (28.1%)
Bacillus Species	3 (23.1%)	10 (76.9%)	-	11 (84.6%)	-	3 (23.1%)	13 (100%)	5 (38.5%)	
Staphylococcus	-	1 (8.3%)	-	2 (16.7%)	-	5 (41.7)	6 (50%)	2 (16.7%)	2 (16.7%)
Arcanobacterium pyogenes	1 (16.7%)	3 (50%)	-	4 (66.7%)	4 (66.7)	2 (33.3%)	2 (33.3%)	(33.3%)	3 (50%)
Streptococcus	-	-	-	3 (100%)	3 (100%)	-	-	-	1 (33.3%)
Corynebacterium species	1 (50%)	2 (100%)	-	1 (50%)	-	-	2 (100%)	1 (50%)	-
Rhodococcus egui	1 (50%)	1 (50%)	-	-	-	-	1 (50%)	-	-
Other Enterobacteriacae	3 (50%)	6 (100%)	-	2 (33.3%)	-	1 (16.7%)	6 (100%)	6 (100%)	-

Tetracycline; PG- Penicillin; E- Erythromycin; SXT- Trimethoprim-Sulfamethoxazole.
Table 3: Antibiotic resistance (%) profiles of aerobic bacteria isolated.

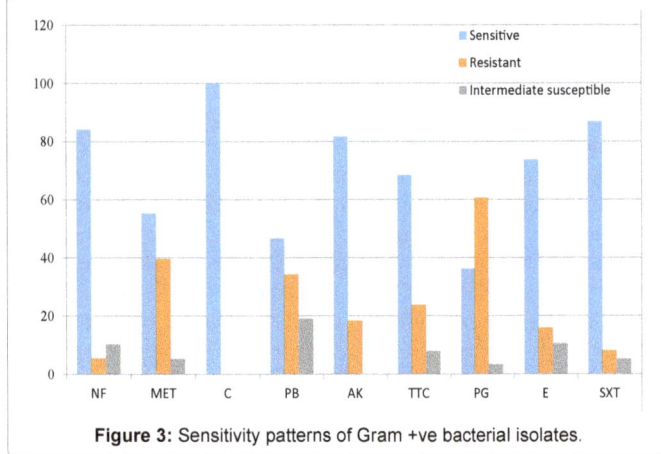

Figure 3: Sensitivity patterns of Gram +ve bacterial isolates.

The finding of this study, indicating the drugs as the most effective, agrees with studies by other authors. Prahland et al. [27] mentions Chloramphenicol and Nitrofurantoin being the most effective on uterine isolates. The study by Anjaneyulu et al. [24] shows Trimethoprim-sulfamethoxazole and Chloramphenicol are the most effective with levels of 69% and 62%, respectively. Uterine isolates in a study by Moharanan et al. [17] were highly sensitive to Chloramphenicol, whereas isolates of Rajangam et al. [25] shows highest sensitivity to Nitrofurantoin.

In conclusion, cattle uteri are free from bacteria due to several defensive factors. But all the sampled uteri harbor bacteria during isolation. *E. coli, Bacillus* species, *Staphilococcus, A. pyogenes* and *Streptococci*, which are environmental contaminants, were the dominant isolates from the uterus. Among these isolates *E. coli* and

A. pyogenes found to be highly resistant. Tetracycline and penicillin-G are commonly available drugs on market in Ethiopia. However, the use of these drugs for uterine infections are not recommended, due to the resistance showed by the isolates and side effects, particularly by tetracycline after extensive use for many infectious diseases.

Conflict of Interest

No conflict of interest declared.

Acknowledgements

The authors would like to thank Faculty of Veterinary Medicine and Agriculture, Addis Ababa University and Addis Ababa Abattoir's Enterprise for their material and laboratory support.

References

1. Tekelye B, Kassali O (1988) Reproductive problems in cattle. International foundation for science. Joint seminar on Animal Reproduction for African countries, ILCA, Addis Ababa, Ethiopia, pp: 1-8.

2. Jahnke H (1982) Livestock production systems and livestock development in tropical Africa. Kielerwissen Chafts-VerlaVauk, Kiel, pp: 253.

3. Yang L, Wang Y, Peng Y, Min J, Hang S, et al. (2015) Genomic characterization and antimicrobial susceptibility of bovine intrauterine Escherichia coli and its relationship with postpartum uterine infections. J Integr Agr 15: 1-20.

4. Mshelia G, Bilal V, Maina1 V, Okon K, Mamza S, et al. (2014) Microbiological studies on genital infections in slaughtered ewes from tropical arid zone of Nigeria. Sokoto Journal of Veterinary Sciences. 12: 18-22.

5. Wagener K, Grunert T, Prunner I, Ehling-Schulz M, Drillich M (2014) Dynamics of uterine infections with Escherichia coli, Streptococcus uberis and Trueperella pyogenes in post-partum dairy cows and their association with clinical endometritis. Vet J 202: 527-532.

6. Singleton G, Dobson H (1995) A survey of the reasons for culling pregnant cows. Veterinary Record 136: 162-164.

7. El-Khadrawy H, Wahid M, Zaabal M, Emtenan M (2015) Strategies for diagnosis and treatment of uterine infection in bovines. Global Veterinaria 15: 98-105.

8. Arthur G, Noakes O, Person H (1989) Veterinary Reproduction and Obstetrics, 6th edn. Bailliere Tinelall, London, pp: 341-416.

9. Carter G (1984) Diagnostic procedures in veterinary bacteriology mycology, 4th edn. pp: 12-47.

10. Koneman E, Allen S, Dowell V, Janda W, Sommers H, et al. (1988) 3rd edn. J.B Lippincott Company, Philadelphia, pp: 311-390.

11. Baron E, Peterson L, Finegold S (1994) Bailey and Scott's Diagnostic Microbiology. 9th edn. Clanrinda company, USA, pp: 79-96.

12. Barrow G, Feltham R (1995) Cowan and steel's manual for identification of medical bacteria. 3rd edn. Cambrige University Press.

13. Quinn P, Carter M, Markey B, Carter G (1999) Clinical veterinary microbiology. Mosby International Limited, London, pp: 13-236.

14. Ikram M (2002) Diagnostic microbiology. In: Laboratory procedures for veterinary technicians. 4th edn. Mosby Publishing Company, pp: 105-115.

15. Hafez E, Jainudeen M (1993) Reproductive failure in females. Reproduction in Farm Animals. 6th edn. Lea & Febiger, Philadelphia, pp: 261-286.

16. Linda LS (2006) The Merck Veterinary Manual Online. 8th edn, Reference Reviews, pp: 40-49.

17. Moharanan H, Pradhan R, Patro D, Sahoo P, Nanda K, et al. (2000) Antibiotic sensitivity studies on repeat breeder crossbred sersey cows in coostal districts of Orissa. Indian Veterinary Journal 77: 809-810.

18. Baishya S, Das K, Rahman H, Borgohain B (1998) Antibiogram of bacteria isolated from uterine discharge of repeated cattle. Indian Journal of Comparative Microbiology, Immunology and infectious Diseases 19: 130-131.

19. Cohen R, Ziv G, Winkler M, Saran A, Bernstein M, et al. (1997) Sensitivity to antibiotics of bacteria isolated from uterine secretion of dairy cows with retained fetal membranes and post parturient metrites and concentration of tetracycline in uterine secretions after intra uterine administration. Israel Journal of veterinary Medicine 52: 30.

20. Ziv G, Cohen R, Winkler M, Saran A (1996) Antimicrobial susceptibility of Escherichia coli and streptococcus species recovered from the uterus of dairy cows with post parturient metritis. Israel Journal of Veterinary Medicine 51: 63-66.

21. Pejsak Z, Kolodziejezyk P (2002) Incidence and drug sensitivity of bacteria isolated from diseased lungs in pigs. Medycyna Veterynaryjna 57: 480-485.

22. Adegoke G (1991) Antibiotic resistance in Staphylococci isolated from goats. Bulletin of Animal health. Production in Africa 29: 361-364.

23. Aiello S, Mays A (1998) Metritis in large animals, antibacterial agents. The Merck Veterinary Manual. 8th edn. Merck & Co Inc., White house station, USA, pp: 1016-1788.

24. Anjaneyulu Y, Wilson J, James R (1999) Antibiogram in bovine endometritis, a field studies. Indian Veterinary Journal 76: 351-352.

25. Rajangam R, Jeyaram N, Rajeswar J (2001) Treatment of repeated breeding crossbred cattle. Indian Journal of Animal Reproduction 22: 172 -173.

26. Haryh D, Zee Y (1999) Laboratory Diagnosis, Antimicrobial Drugs. Veterinary Microbiology, Blackwell Science Inc., pp: 15-50.

27. Prahland R, Nanda A, Arora A (1997) Bacteriology and therapeutics of placental retention in buffaloes (Bubalus bubalis). Indian veterinary Journal 74: 660-661.

23

Review on Newcastle Disease of Poultry and its Public Health Importance

Tagesu Abdisa* and Tolera Tagesu*

Jimma University College of Agriculture and Veterinary Medicine, Jimma, Ethiopia

Abstract

Newcastle disease is a contagious bird disease affecting many domestic and wild avian species and which can be transmissible to humans. It is caused by avian paramyxovirus serotype 1 virus which, with viruses of the other eight serotypes (avian paramyxovirus 1-9) has been placed in the genus *Avulavirus*, sub-family Paramyxovirinae, family Paramyxoviridae. Virulent Newcastle disease virus strains are endemic in poultry in most of Asia, Africa, and some countries of North and South America. Other countries, including the united states of America and Canada, are free of those strains in poultry. Highest prevalence of Newcastle disease is recorded in cross breeds of chickens than local breed and the low altitudes do have higher prevalence than the mid and high altitudes. The transmission of Newcastle disease occurs through respiratory aerosols, exposure to fecal and other excretions from infected birds, through newly introduced birds, selling and giving away sick birds and contacts with contaminated feed, water, equipment and clothing. The strain of Newcastle pathogenicity can be classified into five pathotype: Asymptomatic enteric strain; Lentogenic strain; Mesogenic stain; Viscerotropic velogenic strain and Neurotropic velogenic strain. Clinical signs are extremely variable depending on the strain of virus, species and age of bird, concurrent disease, and preexisting immunity caused by paramixovirus with worldwide distribution affecting chickens (all poultry and birds are susceptible) of All age group are susceptible. Symptoms from the respiratory tract are gasping, coughing, sneezing and rales. Signs from the nervous system include tremors, paralyzed wings and legs, twisted necks, circling, clonic spasms and sometimes complete paralysis. Other general symptoms that can be seen are greenish diarrhea, depression and inappetence, partial or complete drop in egg production and an increased production of deformed eggs. Clinical diagnosis based on history, signs and lesions may establish a strong index of suspicion but the laboratory confirmation must be done. The general approaches to the control of Newcastle disease are hygiene and vaccination. Humans are among the many species that can be infected by Newcastle disease in addition to avian species. Newcastle disease may cause conjunctivitis in humans, when a person has been exposed to large quantities of the virus. Mostly, Laboratory workers and vaccinators are affected. Recently, the disease which decreases the development of poultry production for industry is the infectious diseases, among infection disease Newcastle is the one which causes economical lose of poultry and its product. The objective of this review is to understand the Newcastle disease causative agent, pathogenicity, clinical sign and how to prevent and control the Newcastle disease, which concerned with the currently published or reported research.

Keywords: Newcastle disease; Pathogenicity; *Avulavirus*; Poultry; Vaccination

Abbreviations: PMV: Avian Paramyxovirus; C terminus: Cleavage terminus; ELISA: Enzyme Linked Immune Sorbent Assay; END: Exotic Newcastle Disease; HA: Hemagglutinin; HN: Hemagglutinin Neuraminidase; HPAI: Highly Pathogenic Avian Influenza; loNDV: Low virulence Newcastle disease virus; M: Matrix; mRNA: Messenger Ribonucleic Acid; NP: Nucleoprotein; NDV: Newcastle disease Virus; NVND: Neurotropic velogenic Newcastle disease; P: Phospho Protein; PCR: Polymerase Chain Reaction; RBC: Red Bood Cell; RT-PCR: Reverse- transcriptase polymerase chain reaction; vNDV: Virulent Newcastle Disease.

Introduction

Poultry, the largest livestock group, account for more than 30% of all animal protein. However, this production is mainly based on commercial poultry, which accounts for only 20% of the total poultry population [1]. Based on the number of animals, poultry represents the largest domestic animal stock in the world [2]. Poultry represents an important sector in animal production, with backyard flocks representing a huge majority, especially in the developing countries. In these countries, villagers raise poultry to meet household food demands and as additional sources of incomes. Backyard production methods imply low biosecurity measures and high risk of infectious diseases, such as Newcastle disease or zoonosis such as HPAI [3]. Newcastle disease is a contagious bird disease affecting many domestic and wild

avian species; it is transmissible to humans [4]. Newcastle disease is an important infectious disease of the poultry that is caused by virulent strains of Avian Paramyxovirus -1, which is a single strand non-segmented negative sense RNA virus (Figure 1) [5].

The epizootics of Newcastle Disease in poultry continue to occur in Asia, Africa, Central and South America while in Europe, sporadic epizootics occur [6]. In developing countries, human diet is deficient in the animal proteins; approximately 66% population has protein deficient diet [7]. Newcastle disease is an economically important disease and also a major threat to poultry industry [8]. According to variation in strains of NDV, the rate of mortality and morbidity in a flock is variable [9]. Pathotyping of Newcastle disease viruses by RT-PCR and restriction enzyme analysis along with decrease in egg production [10]. Isolation of

*Corresponding authors: Tagesu Abdisa, Jimma University College of Agriculture and Veterinary Medicine, Jimma, Ethiopia
E-mail: abdisatagesu@gmail.com

Tolera Tagesu, Jimma University College of Agriculture and Veterinary Medicine, Jimma, Ethiopia, E-mail: toleratagesu3@gmail.com

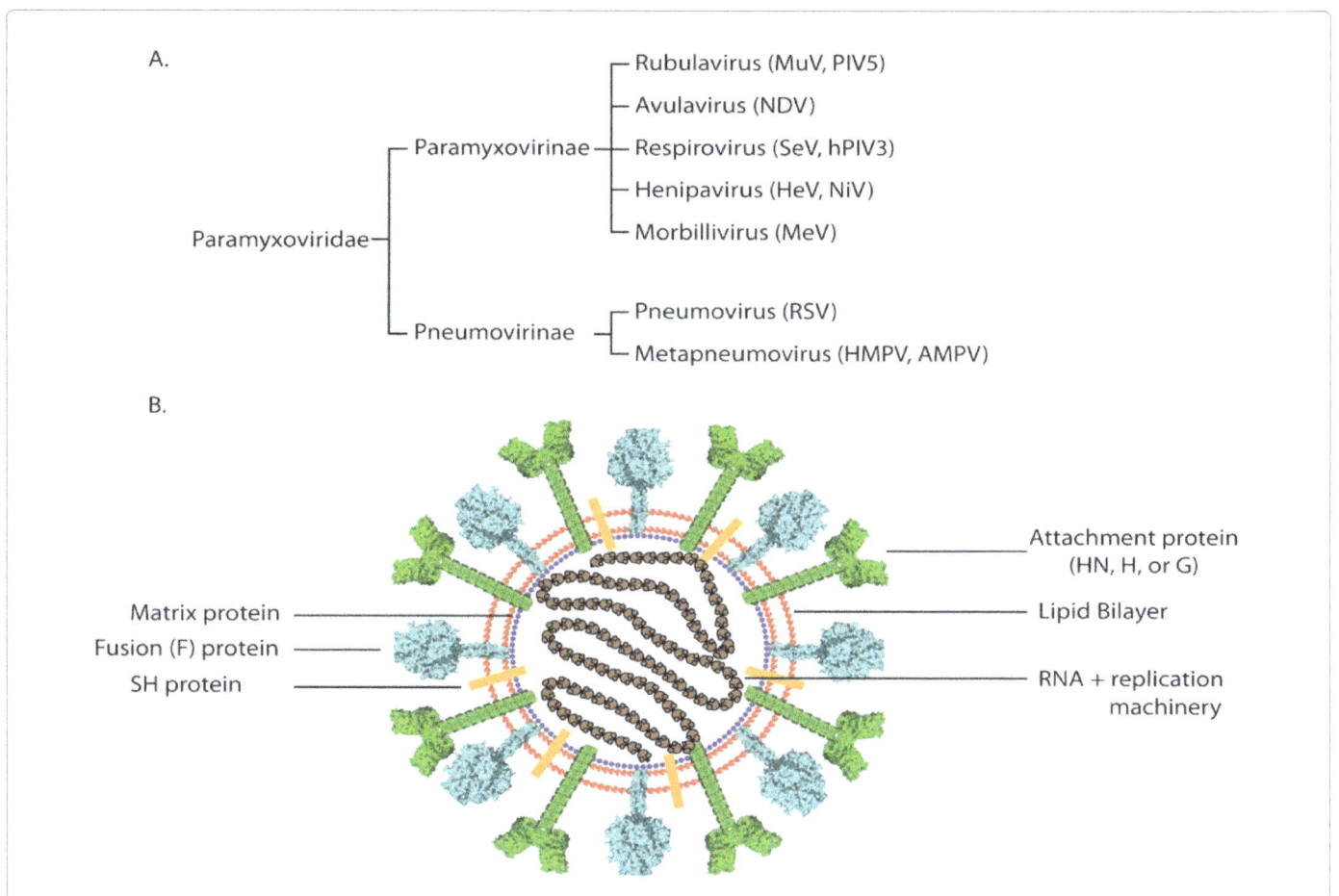

Figure 1: (**A**) Classification of representative members of the paramyxovirus family, the genus of ND Avulavirus. (**B**) Schematic of a paramyxovirus. Genomic RNA is wrapped by nucleocapsid core proteins (brown), which are connected to the viral envelope (red) by the matrix protein (blue). The attachment (green), small hydrophobic (present only in certain paramyxoviruses, orange), and fusion proteins (cyan) are depicted at the virus surface [34].

virus and serological diagnostics, such as HI Test, ELISA and molecular diagnostic tests like real time PCR confirmed the presence of velogenic Newcastle Disease Virus [11]. The economic importance of Newcastle disease may affect on the meat quality of poultry. In developing countries, the broiler meat is the cheapest source of animal protein. Availability of egg is increasing at rate of round about 4% annually [12] White meat's essential nutrients are same as red meat, but white meat has the advantage of containing less cholesterol and saturated fat. In most developing countries, meat is a very important protein sources in diet of people because it is affordability and has high quality protein [13]. In developing countries; the broiler meat is the cheapest source of animal protein. The objective of this review is to understand the Newcastle disease causative agent, pathogenicity, clinical sign and how to prevent and control the Newcastle disease, which concerned with the currently published or reported research. Recently, the disease which decreases the development of poultry production for industry is the infectious diseases, among infection disease Newcastle is the one which causes economical lose of poultry and its product.

Literature Review

General description of poultry Newcastle disease

Newcastle disease is a contagious viral disease of birds and considered one of the most important poultry diseases worldwide. The disease can vary from mild to severe. A highly contagious and severe form of the disease, called exotic Newcastle disease (END), is so deadly that many birds die suddenly without showing any signs of disease [14].

Etiology

Newcastle disease is caused by avian paramyxovirus serotype 1 [APMV-1] viruses, which, with viruses of the other eight APMV serotypes [APMV-2 to APMV-9], have been placed in the genus *Avulavirus*, sub-family Paramyxovirinae, family Paramyxoviridae, in the current taxonomy [15,16]. Newcastle disease belongs to order Mononegavirales, family Paramyxoviridae, sub family Paramyxovirinae and genus *Avulavirus* which are negative sense, single stranded and non-segmented RNA genomes [17]. All the avian paramyxoviruses APMVs are part of genus *Avulavirus*. Virions are roughly spherical;150 nm or more in diameter and filamentous [18]. The genome is about 15.2 kb in length [19,20] that codes for six structural and two non-structural proteins [10]. Rule of six should be followed by genome because it should be of poly hexametric length to replicate rapidly. It encodes for six proteins in 3' to 5' direction; these are Nucleoprotein (NP), Large RNA polymerase (L), Fusion (F), Hemag-glutinin Neuraminidase (HN), Matrix (M) and phosphor protein (P) [21,22]. The proteins W and V are additionally created within the P gene during transcription of mRNA at editing site by insertion of guanines [22,23]. In virus particles, NP is the most abundant protein which provides the NDV score helical nucleocapsid structure. NP is the main regulator in replication of viral genome [25]. The genomic RNA is associated with NP, P and L proteins to form RNP complex, which serve as template for RNA synthesis [24]. NP is found to be highly immunogenic, as it induces antibody responses in chickens [26].

Molecular basis for pathogenicity

During the replication of NDV, the functionally important fusion protein is produced as a precursor glycoprotein, F0, which has to be cleaved to F1 and F2 for the progeny virus particles to be infectious [27]. This post translation cleavage is mediated by host cell proteases [28]. If cleavage fails to take place, noninfectious virus particles are produced. Trypsin can cleave F0 for all NDV strains, and *in vitro* treatment of non-infectious virus will restore infectivity [29]. The importance of F0 cleavage was easily demonstrated, because viruses normally unable to replicate or produce plaques in cell culture systems were able to do both if trypsin was added to the agar overlay or culture fluid. Although all viruses could replicate and produce infectious progeny in the allantois cavity, the viruses pathogenic for chickens could replicate in a wide range of cell types *in vitro* with or without added trypsin, whereas strains of low virulence could replicate only when trypsin is added [30]. Thus, F0 molecules of virulent viruses can be cleaved by a host protease or proteases found in a wide range of cells and tissues, but F0 molecules in viruses of low virulence were restricted in their sensitivity to cleavage by specific host enzymes. Consequently, these viruses can grow only in certain host cell types. Early reports of the deduced amino acid sequences of the F0 precursor, obtained from nucleotide sequencing of the F gene fora number of NDV strains [31,32], enabled comparison of viruses of low virulence to those that were velogenic or mesogenic. For all viruses, the amino acid at residue 116, the C terminus of the F2 protein at the site of cleavage, was arginine. The viruses of low virulence all had leucine at residue 117, the N-terminus of the F1 protein, and another basic amino acid at residue 113. In contrast, all velogenic or mesogenic viruses had phenylalanine at residue 117 and, with one exception, basic amino acids at residues 115 and 112 in addition to those at 113 and 116. The exception was the pigeon variant PMV-1 virus, which was identical to the virulent viruses but lacked a basic amino acid at position 112.

The strain of Newcastle pathogenicity: The strain of Newcastle pathogenicity can be classified into five pathotype:- Asymptomatic enteric strain a form that has sub-clinical enteric infection without clear symptoms; Lentogenic strain which virus present with the mild respiratory infections; Mesogenic stain which virus presents with rare nervous and respiratory signs while mortality rate is related with the age of susceptible birds (young birds are more susceptible as compare to adults); Viscerotropic velogenic strain which virus cause haemorrhagic intestinal lesions and it is highly pathogenic; Neurotropic velogenic strain which virus cause high mortalities followed by respiratory and nervous signs [33].

Epidemiology of Newcastle disease: Virulent NDV strains are endemic in poultry in most of Asia, Africa, and some countries of North and South America [34]. Other countries, including the USA and Canada, are free of those strains in poultry and maintain that status with import restrictions and eradication by destroying infected poultry. Cormorants, pigeons, and imported psittacine species are more commonly infected with vNDV and have also been sources of vNDV infections of poultry. NDV strains of low virulence are prevalent in poultry and wild birds, especially waterfowl. Infection of domestic poultry with loNDV contributes to lower productivity [35]. ND virus is infective for almost all avian species, both domestic and wild. Chickens are higly susceptible to infection with Newcastle disease virus, including the pigeon variant of APMV-1. Considered to be the most susceptible of domestic poultry species. Newcastle disease virus is heat stable when compared with most of paramyxovirus. It remain infectious in bone marrow and muscle of slaughtered chicken at least six month at -20°C and for up to four month in refregrator temperature and also infectious virus may survive for months at room temperature in eggs laid by infected hens and for over year at 4°C [36]. Higher prevalence of ND is during dry season than wet season. However, rare higher prevalence of ND is also seen during wet season that may be related to Ethiopian Holidays (Filseta, Enkutatesh etc) celebrated during wet season. Human activity and increased turnover in the chicken markets during dry season could leads to outbreaks of NCD that have been attributed to high prevalence during dry season [37,38]. As studies reported on Newcastle disease that indicated high significant difference in NCD prevalence between local and cross breeds of chickens. Highest prevalence's are recorded in cross breeds of chickens than local breed [39]. The low altitudes do have higher prevalence than the mid and high [38-40]. Mortality may be very high, often reaching 50 to 100%. The prevalence of NCD varies among years in Ethiopia.

Transmission

The transmission of NDV occurs through respiratory aerosols, exposure to fecal and other excretions from infected birds, through newly introduced birds, selling and giving away sick birds and contacts with contaminated feed, water, equipment and clothing. The usual source of virus is an infected chicken, and spread is usually attributed to the movement of chickens through chicken markets and traders [41]. Newcastle disease is very contagious and is easily spread from one bird to another. The infection is usually transmitted by direct contact with sick birds or unaffected birds carrying the virus. Even vaccinated birds that are clinically healthy can excrete virulent virus after they have been exposed. Virus can also be transmitted indirectly by people, other animals, equipment, vehicles, contaminated poultry products, feed and water [42].

The infection takes place by inhalation or ingestion of the virus or by contact with mucous membranes, specially the conjunctiva. Infected birds shed virus in aerosol, respiratory discharge and faeces. Infected birds start to excrete virus during the incubations period and continue to excrete virus for a varying but limited time during convalescence [42].

During the course of infection of most birds with NDV, large amounts of virus are excreted in the feces. Ingestion of feces results in infection; this is likely to be the main method of bird-to bird spread for avirulent enteric NDV and the pigeon variant virus, neither of which normally produces respiratory signs in infected birds [43]. Vertical transmission (i.e., passing of virus from parent toprogeny via the embryo) remains controversial. The true significance of such transmission in epizootics of ND is not clear. Experimental assessment using virulent viruses is usually hampered by cessation of egg laying in infected birds. Infected embryos have been reported during naturally occurring infections of laying hens with virulent virus [44], but this generally results in the death of the infected embryo during incubation.

Cracked or broken infected eggs may serve as a source of virus for newly hatched chicks, as may virus-laden feces contaminating the outside of eggs. Virus may also penetrate the shell after laying [45], further complicating the assessment of true vertical or transovarian transmission. Infected chicks may be hatched from eggs infected with vaccinal or other lentogenic viruses that do not necessarily cause death of the embryo [46].

Pathogenicity

The virulence of NDV strains varies greatly with the host. Chickens are highly susceptible, but ducks may be infected and show few or no clinical signs, even with strains lethal for chickens [47]. In chickens, the pathogenicity of ND is determined chiefly by the strain of virus, although dose, route of administration, age of the chicken, and environmental conditions all have an effect. In general, the younger the chicken, the more acute the disease. With virulent viruses in the field, young chickens may experience sudden deaths without major clinical signs; however, in older birds the disease may be more protracted and with characteristic clinical signs. Breed or genetic stock does not appear to have a significant effect on the susceptibility of chickens to the disease [48].

Clinical Sign

The clinical signs in birds infected with ND virus vary greatly from very high morbidity and mortality to asymptomatic carriers. The severity of an infection is dependent on factors like the virulence and tropism of the virus, host species, age of host, immune status, other diseases and environmental conditions [49]. Symptoms from the respiratory tract are gasping, coughing, sneezing and rales. Signs from the nervous system include tremors, paralyzed wings and legs, twisted necks, circling, clonic spasms and sometimes complete paralysis. Other general symptoms that can be seen are greenish diarrhoea, depression and inappetence, partial or complete drop in egg production and an increased production of deformed eggs [49]. Clinical sign and course of disease can be grouped into four different pathotypes based on the strains of Newcastle disease virus [50]. These all four pathotypes are listed as follow:

Viscerotropic velogenic: That can be seen are obvious depression, inappetence, substantial drop in egg production, increased respiration, a profuse greenish-yellow diarrhoea that rapidly leads to dehydration and collapse, swollen heads and cyanotic combs. Mortality can be up to 90% and infected birds usually die within one or two days. Birds that survive the initial phase often develop nervous signs. Sometimes birds desperately without previous clinical signs.

Neuroptopic velogenic: Acute signs from the respiratory tract and nervous system dominate. Sudden depression, inappetence and drop in egg production are seen together with coughing and other signs from the respiratory tract, followed by nervous signs within a few days. Mortality is usually around 10-20% for adult birds but can be higher for young birds.

Mesogenic: Coughing and other signs from the respiratory tracts dominate. Other symptoms are depression, loss of weight and decreased egg production for up to three weeks. Signs from the nervous system can develop late in the disease. Mortality is around 10%.

Lentogenic: Are often subclinical but mild respiratory signs and a small drop in egg production can be seen. No nervous signs and mortality is usually negligible.

Pathology

Gross lesions: As with clinical signs, the gross lesions and the organs affected in birds infected with NDV are dependent on the strain and pathotype of the infecting virus, in addition to the host and all the other factors that may affect the severity of the disease. No pathognomonic lesions are associated with any form of the disease. Gross lesions may

also be absent. Nevertheless, the presence of hemorrhagic lesions in the intestine of infected chickens has been used to distinguish VVND viruses from NVND viruses [51]. These lesions are often particularly prominent in the mucosa of the proventriculus, ceca, and small and large intestine. They are markedly hemorrhagic and appear to result from necrosis of the intestinal wall or lymphoid tissues such as cecal tonsils and Peyer's patches. Generally, gross lesions are not observed in the central nervous system of birds infected with NDV, regardless of the pathotype [52]. Gross pathologic changes are not always present in the respiratory tract, but when observed they consist predominantly of mucosal hemorrhage and marked congestion of the trachea [53]. Air sacculitis may be present even after infection with relatively mild strains and thickening of the air sacs with catarrhal or caseous exudates is often observed in association with secondary bacterial infections [44].

Diagnosis

Clinical diagnosis based on history, signs and lesions may establish a strong index of suspicion but the laboratory confirmation must be done. Hemagglutination and hemagglutination inhibition test, virus neutralization test, Enzyme linked immune-sorbent assay, plaque neutralization test and reverse-transcriptase polymerase chain reaction (RT-PCR) can be used for confirmation of the ND virus [54]. Now RT-PCR is the most exclusively used method to detect AIVs and NDVs [9,55,56]. RT-PCR assay is more sensitive, specific and less labor intensives as compare to other conventional methods used for lab diagnoses such as virus isolation, Immuno-Fluorescence Staining, Neuraminidase Inhibition and ELISA [57,58]. Using modern technologies, new diagnostic techniques are being developed for identification and differentiation of NDV strains [59]. Other molecular diagnostic tests like real time PCR and nucleotide sequence analysis are also important in viral disease diagnosis [58,60].

Isolation and identification of causative agent

Direct detection of viral antigens: Immuno histologic techniques offer a rapid method for the specific demonstration of the presence of virus or viral antigens in organs or tissues. Immunofluorescence techniques for thin sections of trachea [61], or impression smears [62] and an immunoperoxidase technique for thin sections [63,64] have been reported and used in NDV infections.

Virus isolation of NDV: Although molecular techniques, especially those developed to employ RT-PCR directly on samples from affected birds [65], mean that a positive diagnosis at least can be obtained rapidly without virus isolation, it is still important that, for primary outbreaks especially, the virus is isolated for proper characterization and future work.

Culture system: Virulent ND viruses can be propagated in many cell culture systems, and viruses of low virulence can be induced to replicate in some of them. It is possible to use primary cell cultures or even cell lines for routine isolation of NDV. The embryonated chicken egg, however, represents an extremely sensitive and convenient vehicle for the propagation of NDV and is used almost universally in diagnosis. Embryonated chicken eggs should be obtained from a specific pathogen free (SPF) flock and incubated for 9-10 days at 37°C before use. If SPF eggs cannot be obtained, eggs from a flock free of NDV antibodies should be used. NDV strains in eggs containing yolk antibodies can be propagated, but the virus titer is usually greatly reduced, and such eggs should be avoided for diagnostic use.

Serologic tests for Newcastle disease virus antibodies: Antibodies to NDV may be detected in poultry sera by a variety of tests including single radial immune diffusion [66], single radial hemolysis [67], agar gel precipitin [68], VN in chick embryos [69], and plaque neutralization [44]. Sera from other species (including turkeys) may cause low-titer, nonspecific agglutination of chicken RBCs, complicating the test. Such agglutination may be removed by adsorption with chicken RBCs before testing. Although the HA and HI tests are not greatly affected by minor changes in the methodology [70].

Differential diagnosis of Newcastle disease: Differential diagnosis is the process of differentiating Newcastle disease with other disease which share similar signs or symptoms. The disease which have similar clinical sign with Newcastle disease are as the follow: Fowl cholera, Highly pathogenic avian influenza, Laryngotracheitis, Fowl pox (diphtheritic form), Psittacosis (psittacine birds), Mycoplasmosis, Infectious bronchitis, Aspergillosis, Also management errors such as deprivation of water, lack of or nutritionally deficient feed and poor ventilation. In pet birds:- Pacheco's parrot disease (psittacine birds), salmonellosis, adenovirus, and other Paramyxoviruses, In cormorants and other wild waterfowl: botulism, fowl cholera and conformational abnormalities [71].

Prevention and Control

The general approaches to the control of Newcastle disease are hygiene and vaccination, this is always important, especially in the control of NCD in semi-intensive systems where birds are confined within a fenced yard or house. Hygiene includes measures such as cleaning, disinfection, limiting access to wild birds, and personal hygiene of the farm staff. Vaccination in combination with appropriate hygiene measures, this remains the most effective way of controlling NCD [72]. Vaccination against vND would result in immunity against infection and replication of the virus. Realistically, ND vaccination usually protects the bird from the more serious consequences of disease, but virus replication and shedding may still occur [73,74].

NCD vaccines are available in either "live" or "dead" forms: Live vaccines are fragile and have very precise rules for use, requiring a cold chain up to the point of application to the bird. Their effectiveness is reduced if there are residual antibodies in the chickens. The immune response increases as the pathogenicity of the live vaccine increases [75]. Therefore, to obtain the desired level of protection without serious reaction, vaccination programs are needed that involve sequential use of progressively more virulent viruses or live virus followed by inactivated vaccine. Killed vaccines give good immunity but require priming with a live vaccine for best results, unless a natural infection has already served this purpose. In Ethiopia, vaccination has been reported as the only safeguard against endemic NCD. However, vaccines currently in use are mainly of benefit to commercial poultry producers whose chickens are kept in large, single age, confined flocks. Manufacturers produce heat labile NCD vaccines in multidose vials, often containing 1,000 or 2,500 doses, which must be kept cold (within 19a 'cold chain') from manufacture until administration to the chickens. In contrast, village chickens are raised in small, multi-age, free-range flocks and large multi-dose vials of vaccine are inappropriate. The cold chain is difficult to maintain under village conditions and purchase of commercial vaccines is a drain on foreign exchange [76].

Vaccines are being used to control and prevent ND. Currently, many inactivated and live ND vaccines are available around the world [77,78]. Chickens and turkeys are immunized against New-castle disease. Live virus vaccines are administered by variety of routes and schedules from hatching till grow-out [79]. Killed virus oil emulsion vaccines are administered parentally prior to the onset of egg production.

Although proper vaccination protects the birds from clinical disease but it does not prevent virus replication and shedding, which results in a source of infection [80]. In developing countries, there is wide use of vaccines on commercial flocks [81]. Anti NDV antibody titers of flocks are continuously monitored and flocks are revaccinated to maintain the protective antibody titers. The breeders and layers are vaccinated against NDV and oil based vaccines are being used prior to onset of egg production for long term immunity [82,83]. Anti NDV antibody titers of breeder flock is also important to maintain the anti NDV maternal antibody titers of pro-geny. These maternal antibodies protect chicks from the disease during the first week of life. In spite of extensive vaccination, outbreaks are continuously occurring [60]. To overcome this problem poultry producers are using different combinations of live and killed vaccines in a flock. Good biosecurity measures are essential to prevent Newcastle disease in poultry flocks. Commercial flocks should not have any contact with domesticated poultry or wild birds or any pet birds. Workers should avoid contact with birds outside the farm. Biosecurity measures include bird-proof houses, feed and water supplies, minimizing travel on and off the facility, disinfecting vehicles and equipments that enter the farm. Pests such as insects and mice should also be controlled. If possible, employees should shower and change into dedicated clothing prior entry into the poultry farm.

Public Health Important

Humans are among the many species that can be infected by NDV in addition to avian species. NDV may cause conjunctivitis in humans, when a person has been exposed to large quantities of the virus [84]. Mostly, Laboratory workers and vaccinators are affected. The use of personnel protective equipment and biological safety cabinet has reduced the exposure of laboratory workers. Infection is rarely seen in the workers of a farm; moreover, persons handling or consuming poultry products do not appear to be at risk [85]. The conjunctivitis usually resolves rapidly, but the virus will be shed in the ocular discharges from 4 to 7 days. In some cases, mild, self-limiting influenza like disease with fever and headache has also been reported in humans [83,84]. There is no evidence found to support human to human transmission but the potential for human to bird transmission exists [84].

References

1. Pemin A, Pedersen G, Riise JC (2001) Poultry as a tool for poverty alleviation: Opportunities and problems related to poultry production at village level. In ACIAR proceedings, pp: 143-147.

2. FAO (2012) Faostat. Production. Live animals.

3. Conan A, Goutard FL, Sorn S, Vong S (2012) Biosecurity measures for backyard poultry in developing countries: a systematic review. BMC Vet Res 8: 240.

4. Nelson CB, Pomeroy BS, Schrall K, Park WE, Lindeman RJ (1952) An outbreak of conjunctivitis due to Newcastle disease virus (NDV) occurring in poultry workers. Am J Public Health Nations Health 42: 672-678.

5. Ashraf A, Shah MS (2014) Newcastle Disease: Present status and future challenges for developing countries. African J Microbiol Res 8: 411-416.

6. Naveen KA, Singh SD, Kataria JM, Barathidasan R, Dhama K (2013) Detection and differentiation of pigeon paramyxovirus serotype-1(PPMV-1) isolates by RT-PCR and restriction enzyme analysis. Trop Anim Health Prod 45: 1231-1236.

7. Maqbool A (2002) Marketing of commercial poultry, poultry meat and eggs in Faisalabad City. MSc Thesis, University of Agriculture Faisalabad, Pakistan.

8. Narayanan MS, Parthiban M, Sathiya P, Kumanan K (2010) Molecular detection of Newcastle disease virus using Flinders Molecular detection of Newcastle disease virus using Flinders Tehnology Associates-PCR Technology Associates-PCR. J Veterinarski Arhiv 80: 51-60.

9. Haque MH, Hossain MT, Islam MT, Zinnah MA, Khan MSR, et al. (2010) Isolation and Detection of Newcastle disease virus from field outbreaks in Broiler and Layer chickens by Reverse transcription Polymerase chain reaction. Bangl J Vet Med 8: 87-92.

10. Choi KS, Lee EK, Jeon WJ, Kwon JH (2010) Antigenic and immunogenic investigation of the virulence motif of the Newcastle disease virus fusion protein. J Vet Sci 11: 205-211.

11. Munir S, Hussain M, Farooq U, Zabid Ullah Jamal Q, Afreen M, et al. (2012) Quantification of antibodies against poultry haemagglutinating viruses by haemagglutination inhibition test in Lahore. Afr J Microbiol Res 6: 4614-4619.

12. Numan M, Zahoor MA, Khan HA, Siddique M (2005) Seroligical statusof Newcastle disease in broilers and layers in Faisalabad and surrounding districts. Pakistan Vet J 25: 55-58.

13. Thomazelli LM, Araujo JD, Ferreira CS, Hurtado R, Oliveira DB, et al. (2012) Molecular Surveillance of the Newcastle Disease Virus in Domestic and Wild Birds on the North-Eastern Coast and Amazon Biome of Brazil. Brazilian J Poult Sci 14: 01-07.

14. USDA- APHIS-VS (2008) Website.

15. Lamb RA, Collins D, Kolakofsky JA, Melero Y, Nagai MBA, et al. (2000) Family Paramyxoviridae. In: van Regenmortel MHV (ed.), Virus Taxonomy, Seventh Report of the International Committee on Taxonomy of Viruses. Academic Press: New York, USA, pp: 549-561.

16. Mayo MA (2002) A summary of the changes recently approved by ICTV. Arch Virol 147: 1655-1656.

17. Cattoli G, Susta L, Terregino C, Brown C (2011) Newcastle disease: are view of field recognition and current methods of laboratory detection. J Vet Diagn Invest 23: 637-656.

18. Catroxo MHB, Martins AMCRPF, Petrella S, Curi NA, Melo NA (2011) Research of viral agent in free-living pigeon feces (Columba livia) in the City of Sao Paulo, SP, Brazil, for transmission electron microscopy. Int J Morphol 29: 628-635.

19. Cao Y, Gu M, Zhang X, Liu W, Liu X (2013) Complete Genome Sequences of Two Newcastle Disease Virus Strains of Genotype VIII. Genome Announc 1: 01.

20. Zhang Y, Zhang S, Wang X, Zhang G (2012) Complete genome sequence of a sub genotype viid Newcastle disease virus circulating predominantly in chickens in China. J Virol 86: 13849-13850

21. Al-Habeeb MA, Mohamed MHA, Sharawi S (2013) Detection and characterization of Newcastle disease virus in clinical samples using real time RT-PCR and melting curve analysis based on matrix and fusion genes amplification. Vet World 6: 239-243.

22. Linde AM, Munir M, Zohari S, Stahl K, Baule C, et al. (2011) Complete genome characterization of a Newcastle disease virus isolated during an outbreak in Sweden in 1997. Virus Genes 41: 165-173.

23. Qiu X, Sun Q, Wu S, Dong L, Hu S, et al. (2011) Entire genome sequence analysis of genotype IX Newcastle disease viruses reveals their early-genotype phylogenetic position and recent-genotype genome size. Virol J 8: 01-11.

24. Kho CL, Tan WS, Tey BT, Yusoff K (2003) Newcastle disease virus nucleocapsid protein: self-assembly and length-determination domains. J Gen Virol 84: 2163-2168.

25. Kho CL, Tan WS, Tey BT, Yusoff K (2004) Regions on nucleocapsid protein of Newcastle disease virus that interact with its phosphoprotein. Arch Virol 149: 997-1005.

26. Ahmad-Raus R, Ali AM, Tan WS, Salleh HM, Eshaghib M, et al. (2009) Localization of the antigenic sites of Newcastle disease virus nucleocapsid using a panel of monoclonal antibodies. J ResVet Sci 86: 174-182.

27. Radhavan VS, Kumanan K, Thirumurugan G, Nachimuthu K (1998) Comparison of various diagnostic methods in characterizing Newcastle disease virus isolates from Desi chickens. Trop Anim Health Prod 30: 287-293.

28. Nagai Y, Klenk HD, Rott R (1976) Proteolytic cleavage of the viral glycoproteins and its significance for the virulence of Newcastle disease virus. Virology 72: 494-508.

29. Nagai Y, Ogura H, Klenk HD (1976) Studies on the assemblyof the envelope of Newcastle disease virus. Virol 69: 523-538.

30. Rott R 1979. Molecular basis of infectivity and pathogenicity of myxoviruses. Arch Virol 59: 285-298.

31. Collins MS, Bashiruddin JB, Alexander DJ (1993) Deduced amino acid sequences at the fusion protein cleavage site of Newcastle disease viruses showing variation in antigenicity and pathogenicity. Arch Virol 128: 363-370.

32. Toyoda T, Sakaguchi T, Imai K, Mendoza IN, Gotoh B, et al. (1987) Structural comparison of the cleavage-activation site of the fusion glycoprotein between virulent and avirulent strains of Newcastle disease virus. Virol 158: 242-247.

33. OIE (2012) Newcastle disease. Manual of Diagnostic Tests and Vaccines for Terrestrial Animals. Chapter 2.3.14.

34. Chang A, Dutch RE (2012) Paramyxovirus fusion and entry: multiple paths to a common end. Viruses 4: 613-636.

35. Merck (1995) Newcastle disease. Merck & Co. Inc., Kenilworth, NJ, USA. Available from: http://www.merckvetmanual.com/poultry/newcastle-disease-and-other-paramyxovirus-infections/newcastle-disease-in-poultry

36. Fenner FF, Bachmann PA, Gibbs EPJ, Murphy FA, Studdert MJ, et al. (1987) Paramyxoviridae. In: Veterinary Virology, Academic Press, Orlando, Florida, 493.

37. Nega M, Moges F, Mazengia H, Zeleke G, Tamir S (2012) Evaluation of I2 thermostable Newcastle disease vaccine on local chickens in selected districts of Western Amhara. J Anim Feed Res 2: 244-248.

38. Zeleke A, Sori T, Gelaye E, Ayelet G (2005) Newcastle Disease in Village Chickens in the Southern and Rift Valley Districts in Ethiopia. Int J Poultry Sci 4: 507-510.

39. Belayheh G, Moses NK, Melese B, Fufa D (2014) Seroprevalence of Newcastle Disease Virus Antibodies in Village Chickens in Kersana-kondalaity District, Ethiopia. Global Veterinaria 12: 426-430.

40. Serkalem T, Hagos A, Zeleke A (2005) Seroprevalence Study of Newcastle Disease in Local Chickens in Central Ethiopia. Int J Appl Res Vet Med 3: 1.

41. Desalegn JM (2015) Epidemiology of Village Chicken Diseases: A Longitudinal Study on The Magnitude and Determinants of Morbidity and Mortality- The Case of Newcastle And Infectious Bursal Disease. Addis Ababa University College of Veterinary Medicine and Agriculture, Department of Clinical Study.

42. Caupa I, Alexander DJ (2009) Avian Influenza and Newcastle Disease a Field and Laboratory Manual. Milan: Springer-Verlag.

43. Alexander DJ, Parsons G, Marshall R (1984) Infection off owls with Newcastle disease virus by food contaminated with pigeon feces. Vet Rec 115: 601-602.

44. Beard CW, Hanson RP (1984) Newcastle disease. In: Hofstad MS, Barnes HJ, Calnek BW, Reid WM, Yoder HW (eds.), Diseases of Poultry, 8th edn. Iowa State University Press: Ames, IA, USA, pp: 452-470.

45. Williams JE, Dillard LH (1968) Penetration patterns of Mycoplasma gallisepticum and Newcastle disease virus through the outer structures of chicken eggs. Avian Dis 12: 650-657.

46. Coman I (1963) Possibility of the elimination of strain F virus of Asplin (1949) in the eggs of inoculated hens. Lucr Inst Past Igiena Anim Buc 12: 337-344.

47. Higgins DA (1971) Nine disease outbreaks associated with myxoviruses among ducks in Hong Kong. Trop Anim Health Prod 3: 232-240.

48. Cole RK, Hutt FB (1961) Genetic differences in resistance to Newcastle disease. Avian Dis 5: 205-214.

49. Kahn CM (2005) The Merck Veterinary Manual. 9th edn. Philadelphia: National Publishing Inc.

50. Alexander DJ, Bell JG, Alders RG (2004) A Technology Review: Newcastle Disease. With Special Emphasis on its Effect on Village Chickens. FAO Animal Production and health Paper (FAO).

51. Hanson RP (1980) Newcastle disease. In: Hitchner SB, Domermuth CH, Purchase HG, Williams JE (eds.), Isolation and Identification of Avian Pathogens. American Association of Avian Pathologists: Kennett Square, PA, USA, pp: 63a-66a.

52. McFerran JB, McCracken RM (1988) Newcastle disease. In: Alexander DJ (ed.), Newcastle Disease. Kluwer Academic Publishers, Boston, MA, USA, pp: 161-183.

53. Alexander DJ, Allan WH (1974) Newcastle disease virus pathotypes. Avian Pathol 3: 269-278.

54. Chaka H, Goutard F, Gil P, Abolnik C, Almeida R, et al. (2013) Serological and molecular investigation of Newcastle disease in household chicken flocks and associated markets in Eastern Shewa zone, Ethiopia. Trop Anim Health Prod

45: 705-714.

55. Liu H, Zhao Y, Zheng D, Lv Y, Zhang W, et al. (2011) Multiplex RT-PCR for rapid detection and differentiation of class I and class II Newcastle disease viruses. J Virol Methods 171: 149-155.

56. Wakamatsu N, King DJ, Seal BS, Brown CC (2007) Detection of Newcastle disease virus RNA by reverse transcription polymerase chain reaction using formalin fixed, paraffin-embedded tissue and comparison with immune histochemistry and in situ hybridization. J Vet Diagn Investigation 19: 396-400.

57. Tang Q, Wanga J, Bao J, Sun H, Sun Y, et al. (2012) A multiplex RT-PCR assay for detection and differentiation of avian H3, H5, and H9 subtype influenza viruses and Newcastle disease viruses. J Virol Methods 181: 164-169.

58. Shahzad M, Rizvi F, Khan A, Siddique M, Khan MZ, et al. (2011) Diagnosis of avain paramyxovirus type-1 infection in chicken by immunoflourescence technique. Int J Agric Biol 13: 266-270.

59. Rezaeianzadeh G, Dadras H, Safar A, Ali M, Nazemshirazi MH (2011) Serological and molecular study of Newcastle disease virus circulating in village chickens of Fars province, Iran. J Vet Med Anim Health 3: 105-111.

60. Shabbir MZ, Goraya MU, Abbas M, Yaqub T, Shabbir MA, et al. (2012) Complete Genome Sequencing of a Velogenic Viscerotropic Avian Paramyxovirus 1 Isolated from Pheasants (Pucrasia macrolopha) in Lahore, Pakistan. J Virol 86: 13828-13829.

61. Hilbink F, Vertommen M, Van't Veer JTW (1982) The fluorescent antibody technique in the diagnosis of a number of poultry diseases: Manufacture of conjugates and use. Tijdschr Diergeneeskd 107: 167-173.

62. McNulty MS, Allan GM (1986) Application of immunofluorescence in veterinary viral diagnosis. In: McNulty MS, McFerran JB (eds.), Recent Advances in Virus Diagnosis. Martinus Nijhoff: Dordrecht, The Netherlands, pp: 15-26.

63. Hamid H, Campbell RSF, Lamihhane CM, Graydon R (1988) Indirect immunoperoxidase staining for Newcastle disease virus (NDV). Proc 2nd Asian/Pacific Poult Health Conf. Australitan Veterinary Poultry Association: Sydney, Australia, pp: 425-427.

64. Lockaby SB, Hoerr FJ, Ellis AC, Yu MS (1993) Immunohistochemical detection of Newcastle disease virus in chickens. Avian Dis 37: 433-437.

65. Gohm DS, Thur B, Hofmann MA (2000) Detection of Newcastle disease virus in organs and feces of experimentally infected chickens using RT-PCR. Avian Pathol 29: 143-152.

66. Chu HP, Snell G, Alexander DX, Schild GC (1982) A single radial immunodiffusion test for antibodies to Newcastle disease virus. Avian Pathol 11: 227-234.

67. Hari Babu Y (1986) The use of a single radial haemolysis technique for the measurement of antibodies to Newcastle disease virus. Indian Vet J 63: 982-984.

68. Gelb J, Cianci CG (1987) Detergent-treated Newcastle disease virus as an agar gel precipitin test antigen. Poult Sci 66: 845-853.

69. Beard CW (1980) Serologic Procedures. In: Hitchner SB, Domermuth CH, Purchase HG, Williams JE (eds.), Isolation and Identification of Avian Pathogens. American Association of Avian Pathologists: Kennett Square, PA, USA, pp: 129-135.

70. Brugh M, Beard CW, Wilkes WJ (1978) The influence of test conditions on Newcastle disease hemagglutination-inhibition titers. Avian Dis 22: 320-328.

71. OIE (2013) Newcastle disease. Epidemiology Diagnosis Prevention and Control.

72. Moerad B (1987) Indonesia: Disease Control. In: Copland JW (ed.), Newcastle Disease in Poultry: A New Food Pellet Vaccine. ACIAR Monograph No. 5: 73-76.

73. Alexander DJ, Manvell RJ, Banks J, Collins MS, Parsons G, et al. (1999) Experimental assessment of the pathogenicity of the Newcastle disease viruses from outbreaks in Great Britain in 1997 for chickens and turkeys and the protection afforded by vaccination. Avian Pathol 28: 501-512.

74. Guittet M, Le Coq H, Morin M, Jestin V, Bennejean G (1993) Distribution of Newcastle disease virus after challenge in tissues of vaccinated broilers. In: Proceedings of the Xth World Veterinary Poultry Association Congress, Sydney, p: 179.

75. Reeve P, Alexander DJ, Allan WH (1974) Derivation of an isolate of low virulence from the Essex '70 strain of Newcastle disease virus. Vet Rec 94: 38-41.

76. USMAN M (2002) Effects of vaccination of chickens against Newcastle disease with thermostable V4 and Lasota vaccines using different grains and their brans as vehicle.

77. Shim JB, So HH, Won HH, Mo I (2011) Characterization of avian paramyxovirus type 1 from migratory wild birds in chickens. J Avian Pathol 40: 565-572.

78. Xiao S, Paldurai A, Nayak B, Mirande A, Collins PL, et al. (2013) Complete genome sequence of a highly virulent Newcastle disease virus currently circulating in Mexico. Genome Announce 1: 01-02.

79. Cho S, Kwon H, Kim T, Kim JH, Yoo H, et al. (2008) Characterization of a Recombinant Newcastle Disease Virus Vaccine Strain. Clin Vaccine Immunol 15: 1572-1579.

80. Chukwudi OE, Chukwuemeka ED, Mary U (2012) Newcastle disease virus shedding among healthy commercial chickens and its epidemiological importance. Pakistan Vet J 32: 354-356.

81. Munir M, Zohari S, Abbas M, Berg M (2012b) Sequencing and analysis of the complete genome of Newcastle disease virus isolated from a commercial poultry farm in 2010. Arch Virol 157: 765-768.

82. Nadeem Y, Chaudhary TM, Shah MS, Ashraf A (2004) Oil adjuvanted Newcastle disease vaccine production using local viral isolates. Proceedings of 24th Pakistan Congress of Zoology. pp: 51-56.

83. Alexander DJ (2000) Newcastle disease and other avian paramyxoviruses. Rev Sci Tec. 19: 443-462.

84. Nolen RS (2003). Emergency declared: exotic Newcastle disease found in commercial poultry farms. J Am Vet Med Assoc 222: 411.

85. David E, Daniel JK (2003) Zoonosis update: Avian influenza and Newcastle disease. JAVMA 222: 1534-1540.

24

Update on Epidemiology, Diagnosis and Control Technique of Newcastle Disease

Nesradin Yune* and Nejash Abdela

School of Veterinary Medicine, College of Agriculture and Veterinary Medicine, Jimma University, Jimma, Ethiopia

Abstract

Newcastle disease is an acute, contagious viral disease of birds. It is one of the most important diseases which cause great economic loss in poultry industry. The virus that cause Newcastle disease is grouped under family Paramyxoviridae in the genus *Avulavirus* and species avian paramyxovirus type 1 (APMV-1) or Newcastle disease virus. Based on their virulence Newcastle disease virus can be divided in to viscerotropic, neurotropic, mesogenic and lentogenic strain. Although avian paramyxovirus type 1(APMV-1) can affect many species of birds including wild birds, Chickens are highly susceptible to the disease. The objectives of this paper were to highlight the epidemiology, diagnostic technique and control measures involved in Newcastle disease. Newcastle disease is currently distributed throughout the world including Central and South America, Asia, Middle East and Africa. APMV-1 can be transmitted by inhalation or ingestion, and birds shed these viruses in both feces and respiratory secretions. The virus can also be transmitted through direct contact with infected flock and indirect contact with contaminated materials. This disease can be diagnosed based history of disease outbreak, some pathognomic sign and laboratory test such as virus isolation, serological test and molecular technique. The latter has more important being its sensitive and rapid for diagnosis of the disease. Currently both live and killed vaccines are used in many countries to control and prevent the disease in chickens. Furthermore, strict biosecurity and separation infected once from health flock are also important to control and prevent spread of disease. Generally to make poultry free of this disease, good biosecurity and continual vaccination should be maintained.

Keywords: Newcastle disease; Avian paramyxovirus type 1; Diagnosis; Vaccination

Introduction

Newcastle disease is a highly contagious economically devastating viral disease of poultry [1]. The virus that cause Newcastle disease is grouped under family paramyxoviridae, genus *Avulavirus* and species Newcastle disease virus or avian paramyxovirus type 1 (APMV-1) [2,3]. The genus of this virus has RNA nucleotide, enveloped, single-stranded (SS) and has negative sense [4]. The avian paramyxovirus contain six structural protein matrix(M), RNA polymerase(L), phosphoprotin(P), nucleoprotein(NP), hemagglutinin neuraminidase(NH) and fusion(F) [5,6]. Protein V and W are additionally encoded by RNA editing of P protein [5]. Paramyxovirus type 1 can cause disease in birds of all types, sex and age [1].

Based on their virulence avia paramyxovirus (APMV-1) has been divided in to three or more pathotypes. Velogenic neurotropic strain typically associated with neurological and respiratory sign. Velogenic viscerotropic strain typically associated with gastrointestinal lesion. These two strains are more virulent. Mesogenic strain is moderate virulence while, lantogenic strains is the least virulence and used for vaccine preparation [3].

The disease was first observed in 1926 on the Indonesia island of Java then, later, it was found in various parts of the world [7]. Newcastle disease is endemic much of Asia, Africa and the Middle East, and some countries in Central and South America [3]. Newcastle disease can infect many species of birds, but the effects of the disease vary with different species. For example, ducks and gees are least sensitive and chickens are more sensitive [8]. Newcastle disease virus can be transmitted through direct contact with infected birds and secretion from mouth, noise and eyes of infected bird. Contaminated materials, feed and water can spread disease [9]. NCD can be diagnosed based on history of disease, sign and laboratory examination [10].

Only diagnosis based on clinical sign have not accurate because it resemble highly pathogenic avian flue [11]. Laboratory diagnosis for Newcastle disease includes virus isolation, serological and molecular test. Enzyme linked immune-sorbent assay(ELISA), virus neutralization test, and hemagglutination inhibition test, reverse-transcriptase polymerase chain reaction (RTPCR) and plaque neutralization test can be used for confirmation of the ND virus [10]. The clinical sign of Newcastle disease depends on strain of virus. Some virus strain attack respiratory system other affect nerve system or digestive system. The major clinical sign observed are loss of appetite, depression, weakness, greenish diarrhea, gasping, coughing, paralysis of wings and legs, corticoids and cyanosis of comb and wattle [12]. The effective way of controlling and preventing Newcastle disease is continual vaccination program using currently available vaccine. Implementing the effective biosecurity procedures is also very important to prevent the disease [13]. Despite, the huge economic impact of this disease there is scarcity of information. Therefore, the main objective of this review is to highlight the epidemiology, diagnostic technique and control measures involved in Newcastle disease.

General Information on Newcastle Disease

Newcastle disease is acute viral disease of many species of birds. NCD is economically the most important and cause loss in poultry industries

*Corresponding author: Nesradin Yune, School of Veterinary Medicine, College of Agriculture and Veterinary Medicine, Jimma University, Jimma, Ethiopia, E-mail: Nesradin.90@gmail.com

[14]. The virus that cause Newcastle disease is grouped under family paramyxoviridae, genus *Avulavirus* and species Newcastle disease virus or avian paramyxovirus type 1 (APMV-1) [2]. Although APMV-1 to APMV-12 serotype are there; APMV-1 is the most pathogenic serotype and is also referred to as Newcastle disease virus (NDV) [3]. Newcastle virus affect both wild and domestic avian species but their severity vary between different strains [15]. Newcastle disease found all over the world. Depending on its strain and clinical sign it causes NCD virus grouped in to four phenotypes [16,17]. Those are velogenic neurotropic NDV affects nerves and velogenic viscerotropic affect visceral organ, mesogenic cause moderate sever and lantogenic wich is the least sever of new castle virus [18].

Newcastle disease was first observed in 1926 in island of Java by Kranveld [19,20]. The disease has got its name from town Tyne, England and was named Ranikhet disease in Asia and India [21,22]. As studied by Spradbrow [23] and Alexander [24] the disease was observed in the same and subsequent year in other parts of Asia (India, Philippines, Korea). In 1930 it was also identified as the same virus cause different severity or cause different clinical sign [16].

Epidemiology

Distribution and transmission

Newcastle disease was distributed throughout the world. Newcastle disease is epizootics in Central and South America, Asia, and Africa while sporadic epizootics occur in Europe [25]. In in Europe Newcastle disease was reached in 1981 then spread rapidly throughout the world [26]. It is endemic in south East Asia and cause high economic loss in commercial poultry farm [27]. Newcastle disease can infect over 240 species of birds. When infected birds are introduced into susceptible flocks all birds will be infected within two to six days. The disease is transmitted through direct contact with infected or carriers birds. Transmission can also occur through contact with secretion and excretion of infected birds and contact with contaminated materials (Figure 1). Another important route of transmission is through air [9,8]. Fleas, rodent, insect and dog can also transmit NCD virus mechanical from infected faeces [28,29].

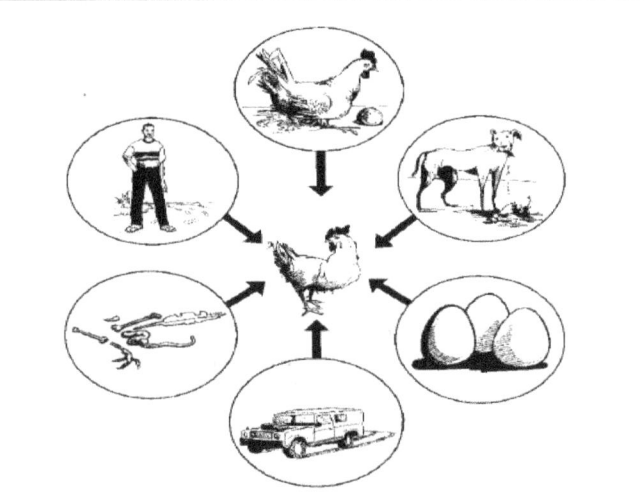

Figure 1: Newcastle disease can be transmitted from one village to another via people, vehicles, animals, baskets, hoes, cages and infected produce egg shells, feathers, bones, intestines, etc. [29].

Risk factor

Host risk factor: Newcastle disease can affect many species of birds. In addition to poultry, more than 230 species from more than one-half of the 50 orders of birds have been found to be susceptible to natural or experimental infections with avian paramyxoviruses. Chickens are mainly affected by Newcastle disease. Turkeys and pigeons, ducks [30,31], geese, as well as parrots and wild cormorants may also develop generalized disease, but clinical signs are rarely reported in geese and ducks [32,33]. In humans and rodents natural infection has been reported. NCD has less zoonotic importance and can cause conjunctivitis [33]. In all types of domestic poultry virulent strains of NCD virus have been found. High virulent serotype of NCD virus is not common for migratory wild birds [8].

In chicken mortality rate can reach 100%. The clinical sign observed during outbreak of NCD includes, depression, diarrhea, respiratory distress, cessation of egg production, nervous sign and death [16].

Pathogen risk factor: One of the major factors that determine pathogenicity of NCD virus is that it has ability to attach and penetrate host cells. To initiate viral infection two glycoproteins haemagglutinin neuraminidase (HN) and fusion protein (F) are required to expose as protrusions on the surface of the virion envelope [34]. Virus can survive for some weeks in all carcass of acutely infected bird or in egg and relatively stable and can be transmitted mechanically from infected material through movement of equipment and personnel. Virus is shade in all excretion and secretion. NCD virus is readily transmitted on fomites. This virus can survive for long period of time on eggshells and especially in feces, compared to an inorganic surface (filter paper) [3]. Isolate of NCD virus differs in there virulence strain and their tissue tropism in chickens [35] (Table 1).

Environmental risk factor: The environmental persistence of these viruses is highly variable, because it can be affected by many factors such as temperature, humidity, the suspending agent and exposure to light, as well as the technique used to detect the viruses. One study reported that APMV-1 survived for up to 7 days in summer in contaminated, uncleaned poultry houses, as long as 14 days in the spring, and 30 days during the winter. Another group reported virus isolation up to 16 days after depopulation of an unvaccinated flock. However, one study found that APMV-1 remained viable for up to 255 days in a henhouse, at ambient temperatures of -11°C (12°F) to 36°C (97°F). At 23-29°C (73-84°F), APMV-1 is reported to survive in contaminated litter for 10 to 14 days, and at 20°C (68°F) in soil for 22 days. Virus has also been recovered from earthworms for 4 to 18 days and from experimentally contaminated lake water for 11 to 19 days [3].

Diagnosis

Newcastle disease can be diagnosed based on history, clinical sign and laboratory test. Newcastle disease clinically resembles highly pathogenic avian influenza so during outbreak rapid and accurate diagnosis is important to control and prevent dissemination of disease [11]. Laboratory diagnosis for NCD includes virus isolation, serological (enzyme-linked immune sorbent assays (ELISA), immunodiffusion test, agar gel precipitation and molecular test (Reverse transcription-polymerase chain reaction (RT-PCR). Isolation of the NCD virus is definitive diagnosis of NCD [38].

Diagnosis based on clinical sign and lesion

The clinical sign of NCD is depends on age, immune status of the host, tissue tropism and virulence of virus strain. Sudden high

Types of Virulence Strain	Characteristics
Viscerotropic velogenic isolates	Cause severe fatal diseases characterized by hemorrhagic intestinal lesions
Neurotropic velogenic isolates	Cause acute disease characterized by nervous and Respiratory signs with high mortality
Mesogenic isolates	Cause mild disease with mortality confined to Young birds.
Lentogenic isolate	Cause mild or inapparent infection, coughing, gasping, sneezing and rales. Mortality is Negligible

Table 1: The four isolates group or pathotypes on the basis of virulence and tissue tropism in chickens [36,37].

mortality in a flock in the absence of premonitory clinical signs occurs when susceptible species are exposed to highly virulent strain. In susceptible flocks the mortality rate in fully can reach 100% [35]. The incubation period of NCD is usually about five days. In chicken's nerve, respiratory and digestive sign may occur. The major clinical sign observed in Newcastle disease are: greenish white diarrhea, with ruffled feathers; depression in the birds and a state of prostration, a condition known as torticollis (the head turned to one side (Figure 2) and other neurological sign like paralysis of leg and wing. NCD is acute disease can cause death within 2 to 3 days [39,40].

Necropsy lesions caused by velogenic APMV-1 viruses have mainly been characterized in poultry, especially chickens [3]. Viscerotropic velogenic and neurotropic velogenic strain cause hemorrhagic lesion particularly in mucosa of the proventriculus, small intestine and ceca. In respiratory tract gross lesions are not observed. Although less likely in older birds, haemorrhages of the thymus and bursa of fabriceus may also occur [41].

Laboratory diagnosis

Sample for laboratory diagnosis: The appropriate sample for diagnosis in Newcastle disease includes: tissue sample (trachea, lung, spleen, soft palate, colon, bursa and brain) witch are important for hisopathology and cloacal swabs, oro-nasal swabs and Serum sample [29]. Blood sample is usually collected from wing vein. When fresh sample is collected lung and spleen it should be wrapped in plastic and placed into cold box with ice. To do serological test haemolysed or contaminated samples should not be used because it will give unreal result [29].

Virus isolation: Virus is obligate intracellular parasite that requires living cell in order to replicate. Cultured cells, eggs and laboratory animals may be used for virus isolation. To diagnosis APM-1 infection virus isolation in embryonated eggs or cell cultures serves as important for viral isolation [42]. Cloacal and Tracheal swabs are a good sample for viral isolation of NCDV. Sample from fresh faeces may also used as an alternative. Collected sample should be transported at pH 7.0-7.4 in isotonic phosphate buffered saline (PBS), containing antimicrobial drugs and media protein. Higher concentrations of antibiotic should be used when collected sample is from feaces of suspected chickens [43].

Virus isolation in culture: centrifugation of sample from feces or tissue for 10 minute at temperature 25°C to obtain supernatanted sample and measure 0.2 ml of sample and inoculate in to allantoic cavity of embryonated SPF fowl egg of 9 -11 days' incubation then incubate for 4-7 days at 35-37°C. If the tests give positive result embroynated eggs will die. Finally all eggs remained of incubation should child to 4°C and do for haemagglutination test (HA) [43].

Serological test: In the absence of vaccination, the presence of specific antibodies against the ND virus is not necessarily that it was suffering from the disease at the time of sampling, but indicates that

the bird has been infected by the virus at some time. In practice, a high antibody titre is indicative of a recent infection. NDV may be employed as an antigen in a wide range of serological tests. Although numerous serological tests may be used to detect antibodies in serum they give little information on the infecting NDV strain. Two methods are used to measure antibody titres: the haemagglutination inhibition (HI) test, and the enzyme-linked immunosorbent assay (ELISA). The most commenaly used and show accurate result is haemagglutination inhibition (HI) test [41]. For both tests, it is necessary to collect blood samples from the chickens and should be taken from the wing veins [29].

Haemagglutination inhibition test: The haemagglutination inhibition (HI) test is used most widely in ND serology; its usefulness in diagnosis depends on the vaccinal immune status of the birds to be tested and on prevailing disease conditions. HI is done based on principle that the haemagglutinin on the viral envelope can bring about the clumping of red blood cells chicken and that this can be inhibited by specific antibodies [44]. Sera from species other than chicken red blood cells can also cause clumping (agglutination), so it should be removed by adsorption of the serum with chicken RBCs determining these properties. This is done by adding 0.5 ml of antisera to 0.025 ml of packed chicken RBCs, shaking gently and leaving for at least 30 minutes; the RBCs are then pelleted by centrifugation at 800 g for 2-5 minutes and the adsorbed sera are decanted. Any pretreatment of the sera is unnecessary as Chicken sera can rarely give nonspecific positive reactions in the HI test [37].

Enzyme linked immune sorbent assay: The ELISA works on the principle of recognition of anti-NDV antibodies, attached to a plate coated with viral antigen, by antibodies produced in another species against chicken antibodies [45]. Based on different strategies for detection of NCD antibodies, including, sandwich, indirect and blocking or competitive ELISAs using MAbs there are different commercial available ELISA kites. At least one kit uses a subunit antigen. Both ELISA and HI may measure antibodies to different antigens. ELISA test; depending on system used can detect antibodies to more than one antigen but, HI test is probably restricted to those directed against the HN protein. ELISAs are reproducible and have high specificity and sensitivity; they have been found to correlate well with the HI test [45].

Molecular technique: Molecular techniques such as polymerase chain reaction (PCR) and reverse transcription-polymerase chain reaction (RT-PCR) have been used for rapid and sensitive detection for Newcastle disease [46].

Polymerase chain reaction: The duplex PCR is done based on principle that it has the ability to amplify and differentiate multiple

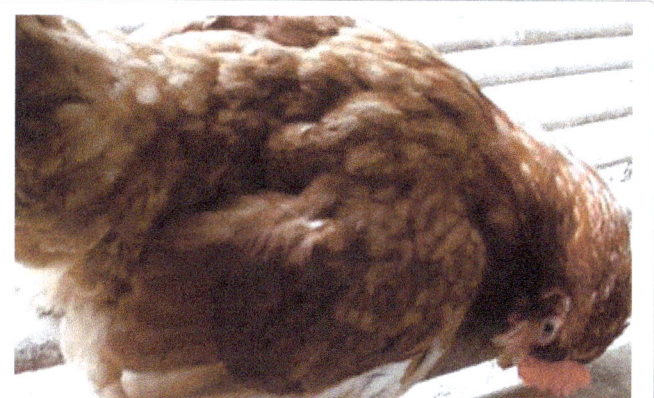

Figure 2: NDV infected layer chicken of 29 weeks of age showing nervous signs (twisted neck and paralysis) [40].

specific nucleic acids using polymerase enzymes [47,48]. However, those techniques can detect only one specific pathogen at a time [47]. PCR can detect virus following following the growth of virus in embryos in the laboratory and clinical specimens [49]. It has the potential to have high sensitivity and is now it is considered as the gold standard for nucleic acid detection [50]. However, PCR requires DNA as a template and the target viruses in this study have RNA as their nucleic acid. Therefore, RNA viruses require a reverse transcription step to produce single stranded complementary DNA (cDNA) through reverse transcriptase using a specific oligonucleotide primer and viral RNA as a template [50-52].

Reverse transcription-polymerase chain reaction: Molecular techniques like reverse transcription polymerase chain reaction (RT-PCR) have been frequently used all over the world to detect viruses from the field samples. Reverse transcription polymerase chain reaction (RT-PCR) is used to detect RNA virus which is negative and single stranded RNA virus. There are two different configurations of the RT-PCR assay. In the two step RT-PCR configuration, the cDNA is synthesized in a different tube before performing PCR assay. In contrast a one step RT-PCR firstly synthesises the cDNA. The reverse transcriptase is inactivated and the polymerase is activated simultaneously and the PCR reaction is carried out in a single tube [53]. This is rapidly becoming the assay of choice. Several important steps need to be considered in developing an RT-PCR protocol. The first aspect is the RNA extraction. This needs to be an efficient process that can extract RNA from the samples even when it's in low concentrations and eliminate contaminants that will degrade the RNA [53]. Another important aspect is the gene being targeted and the choice of primers. This can have a profound effect on the efficacy of the assay [54]. Poorly design primers can result in mispriming and the amplification of non-specific products or the formation of primer dimer [55].

Multiplex polymerase chain reaction: Multiplex PCR tests have been developed to allow simultaneous detection and differentiation of several avian viruses including NDV. These techniques have also been used experimentally to differentiate between velogenic, monogenic and lentogenic strains from chickens. It is applied simultaneously that required for avian infection including Newcastle disease for amplification and quantification of the virus. The primers that are specific for each virus are newly designated from the nucleoprotein gene of Newcastle disease virus. This technique helps mass amplification of the virus using common primers in the presence of fusion protein gene which increased the markedly sensitivity of the tests. At present, it should be noted that multiplexing RT-PCR assays aiming at broadening the range of virus detection frequently result in reduced sensitivity of the test compared with single target assays [56].

Control Techniques of New Castle Disease

Management strategies

The principal management procedures should include strict biosecurity measures which help in preventing the spread of infective material from house to house and from farm to farm [57]. Good biosecurity can protect poultry flocks from Newcastle disease. Avoid flocks not be to contact with domesticated poultry of unknown health status, any pet birds (particularly psittacines), and wild or feral birds (particularly cormorants, gulls and pigeons). Biosecurity measures include well ventilated houses, clean water supplies, minimizing travel on and off the facility, and disinfecting vehicles and equipment that enter the farm. Separation of infected from health flocks and proper disposal of died birds. Control of Pests such as insects and mice is also

important for control measures of NCD. All in/all out breeding (one age group per farm), with disinfection between groups, is also advisable [3].

Vaccination

Vaccination is the most important method of controls and prevention of new castle disease. Currently, both inactivated and live vaccines for NCD are available around the world [58,59]. There is also thermo stable vaccine which was specifically developed to be used in village chicken [60]. We can use varieties of route for administration of live vaccine and schedules from hatching till grow-out [13]. Killed virus oil emulsion vaccines are administered parentally prior to the onset of egg production. Lentogenic virus vaccines are generally recommended in drinking water, by eye drop, by aerosol or intranasally. A vaccine using a heat-tolerant V4 strain has been developed for feeding to village chickens in countries where these constitute a significant proportion of poultry production [33]. Although proper vaccination protects the birds from clinical disease but it does not prevent virus replication and shedding, which results in a source of infection [61].

Live vaccine: Live vaccines are relatively cheap, sold as freeze dried, easy to administer and can be used for mass vaccination. These have been divided in to mesogenic and lentogenic groups with their preferred mode of administration being eye drop, beak intranasal installation, or dipping for lentogenic vaccines while mesogenic vaccine requires intramuscular injection. Drinking water and aerosol administrations can also be used [41].

In most countries, Hitchner B1 and La Sota vaccines are used and are derived from the mesogenic strain of NDV [41]. Some mesogenic vaccines may cause disease; particularly in young birds, especially if there is a dual infection with exacerbating organisms. Because of heat liable the live vaccines are also have disadvantage under village management system where transport and cold storage facilities are often inadequate [62].

Inactivated vaccine: Inactivated vaccine can be used situations unsuited for live vaccine and induce high level of protective antibody over long period of time. These vaccines are produced from infective allantoic fluid of virulent NDV treated with B-propiolactone or formalin to kill the virus and then mixed with adjuvant. The vaccine can administered ether subcutaneous or intramuscular injection [41].

Vaccination program: Vaccination program affect the duration of immunity. One of the most important considerations affecting vaccination programs is the level of maternal immunity in young chickens, which may vary considerably from batch to batch, farm to farm, and among individual chickens. For this reason, one of several strategies is employed. Either the birds are not vaccinated until 2-4 weeks of age when most of them will be susceptible, or 1-day-old birds are vaccinated by conjunctival instillation or by the application of a coarse spray. This will establish active infection in some birds that will persist until maternal immunity has waned. Revaccination is then carried out 2-4 weeks later [37].

Conclusion

Newcastle disease (NCD) is one of the most important viral diseases in poultry industry which can affect several species of birds. NCD is characterized by acute mortality marked by hemorrhagic lesions, respiratory and apparent or unapparent. Today Newcastle disease virus is found in most countries of the world and its transmission is through air, direct contact with infected or carrier birds, contact with secretion and excretion of infected birds and infected materials. History, observable clinical sign and laboratory examinations are the important tools in diagnosis of NCD. Good biosecurity, separation of infected ones from health and appropriate vaccination should be practiced as control and prevention method of this disease.

Acknowledgments

We would like to acknowledge Jimma University for facility provision.

Conflict of Interest

Authors declare that they don't have any conflict of interest.

References

1. Iram N, Shah MS, Ismat F, Habib M, Iqbal M, et al. (2014) Heterologous expression, characterization and evaluation of the matrix protein from Newcastle disease virus as a target for antiviral therapies. Appl Microbiol Biotechnol. 98: 1691-1701.

2. Mayo MA (2002) A summary of taxonomic changes recently approved by ICTV. Arch Virol. 147: 1655-1663.

3. Center for food security and public health (CFSPH) (2016). IOWA State University College of Veterinary Medicine. Newcastle Disease Avian Paramyxovirus-1 Infection, Goos. Paramyxovirus infection, Ranikhet disease.

4. Alexander DJ, Senne DA (2008) Newcastle disease, other avian paramyxoviruses and pneumovirus infections. In: Saif YM, Fadly AM, Glisson JR, et al. eds. Iowa State University Press, USA, Dis. Poult.,12: 75-100.

5. Cattoli G, Susta L, Terregino C, Brown C (2011) Newcastle disease review of field recognition and current methods of laboratory detection. J Vet Diagn Invest. 23: 637-656.

6. Al-Habeeb MA, Mohamed MHA, Sharawi S (2013) Detection and characterization of Newcastle disease virus in clinical samples using real time RT-PCR and melting curve analysis based on matrix and fusion genes amplification. Vet World. 6: 239-243.

7. Ashraf A, Shah MS (2014) Newcastle Disease: Present status and future challenges for developing countries. African J Microbiol Res. 8: 411-416.

8. Caupa I, Alexander DJ (2009) Avian Influenza and Newcastle Disease. A Field and Laboratory Manual. Milan: Springer-Verlag.

9. Li X, Qiu Y, Yu A, Chai T, Zhang X, et al. (2009) Degenerate primers based RT-PCR for rapid detection and differentiation of airborne chicken Newcastle disease virus in chicken houses. J Virol Methods. 158: 1-5.

10. Chaka H, Goutard F, Gil P, Abolnik C, Almeida R, et al. (2013) Serological and molecular investigation of Newcastle disease in household chicken flocks and associated markets in Eastern Shewa zone, Ethiopia. Trop Anim Health Prod 45: 705-714.

11. Khan TA, Rue CA, Rehmani SF, Ahmad A, Wasilenko JL, et al. (2010) Phylogenetic and Biological Characterization of Newcastle Disease Virus Isolates from Pakistan. J Clin Microbiol. 48: 1892-1894.

12. Pazhanivel N, Balsubramaniam GA, George VT, Mohan B (2002) Study of natural outbreak of Newcastle disease in and around Namakkal. Indian Vet J. 79: 293-294.

13. Cho S, Kwon H, Kim T, Kim JH, Yoo H, et al. (2008) Characterization of a Recombinant Newcastle Disease Virus Vaccine Strain. Clin Vaccine Immunol. 15: 1572-1579.

14. Bulbule NR, Madale DS, Meshram CD, Pardeshi RB, Chawak MM (2015) Virulence of Newcastle disease virus and diagnostic challenges. Adv Anim Vet Sci. 3: 14-21.

15. Alexander DJ (1998) Newcastle disease and other avian paramyxoviruses. In: A Laboratory Manual for the Isolation and Identification of Avian Pathogens 4th edn. Edited by Swayne DE, Glisson JR, Jackwood MW, Pearson JE, Reed WM. American Association of Avian Pathologists: Kennet Square. pp. 156-163.

16. Alexander DJ, Bell JG, Alders RG (2004) A Technology Review: Newcastle Disease. With Special Emphasis on its Effect on Village Chickens. FAO Animal Production and health Paper, FAO. p: 161.

17. Engström B, Eriksson H, Fossum O, Jansson DS (2004) Compendium poultry diseases. 2nd edn. Uppsala: National Veterinary Institute.

18. Alexander DJ (2001) Gordon Memorial Lecture. Newcastle disease. Br Poult Sci. 42: 5-22.

19. Loretu K, Mkaria J (1981) Preliminary report on Newcastle disease pathotypes in Tanzania. Tanzania Vet Bull. 3: 63-66.

20. Arifin MA, Salim SH, Mel M, Abdul Karim MI, Hassan SS (2011) Optimization of Newcastle Disease Virus Production in T-flask. Proceedings of the 2nd International Conference on Biotechnology Engineering, ICBioE'11 May 17-19, Kuala Lumpur, Malaysia.

21. Doyle TM (1927) In: Rweyemamu MM, Palaya V, Win T, Sylla D (edn). Newcastle disease vaccines for Rural Africa, Pan African Veterinary Vaccine Center, Debre Zeit, Ethiopia, pp. 7-45.

22. Narayanan MS, Parthiban M, Sathiya P, Kumanan K (2010) Molecular detection of Newcastle disease virus using Flinders Molecular detection of Newcastle disease virus using Flinders Tehnology Associates-PCR Tehnology Associates-PCR. Vet Arhiv. 80: 51-60.

23. Spradbrow PB (1987) Newcastle Disease an overview. Newcastle disease in poultry, a new feed pellet vaccine, Canberra. Aust. Centre Int. Agric Res. 5: 12-18.

24. Alexander DJ (1988) Newcastle disease: Methods of spread. Newcastle disease. Boston, Kluwer Acad. Pub. pp: 1-10.

25. Naveen KA, Singh SD, Kataria JM, Barathidasan R, Dhama K (2013) Detection and differentiation of pigeon paramyxovirus serotype-1 (PPMV-1) isolates by RT-PCR and restriction enzyme analysis. Trop Anim Health Prod. 10: 01-06.

26. Mase M, Imai K, Sanada Y, Sanada N, Yuasa N, et al. (2002). Phylogenetic analysis of newcastle disease virus genotypes isolated in Japan. J Clin Microbiol. 40: 3826-3830.

27. Munir M, Zohari S, Abbas M, Berg M (2012) Sequencing and analysis of the complete genome of Newcastle disease virus isolated from a commercial poultry farm in 2010. Archive Virol. 157: 765-768.

28. Ullah S, Ashfaque M, Rahman SU, Akhtar M, Rehman A (2004) Newcastle disease virus in the intestinal contents of broilers and layers. Pak Vet J. 24: 28.

29. Alders R, Spradbrow P (2001) Controlling Newcastle disease in village chickens: a field manual. Australian Centre for International Agricultural Research (ACIAR).

30. Zhang S, Wang X, Zhao C, Liu D, Hu Y, et al. (2011) Phylogenetic and pathotypical analysis of two virulent newcastle disease viruses isolated from domestic ducks in China. J PLoS ONE. 6: 1-9.

31. Madadgar O, Karimi V, Nazaktabar A, Kazemimanesh M, Ghafari MM, et al. (2013) A study of Newcastle disease virus obtained from exotic caged birds in Tehran between 2009 and 2010. Avian Pathol. 42: 27-31.

32. Rima B, Alexander DJ, Billeter MA, Collins PL, Kingsbury DW, et al. (1995) Paramyxoviridae. In: Murphy FA, Fauquet CM, Bishop DH, Ghabrial AW, Jarvis GP, et al. (Eds.). Virus Taxonomy. Sixth report of the international committee in taxonomy of viruses. Springer-Verlag, Wien, pp: 268-274.

33. PLAN AVE (2010) Disease Strategy Newcastle disease.

34. De Leeuw OS, Koch G, Herzog L, Ravenshorst N, Peeters BP (2005) Virulence of Differentiation of pathogenicity of avian paramyxovirus serotypes 1. Offi J Eur Uni Avian Pathol. 31: 493-499.

35. Quinn PJ, Markey BK, Carter ME, Donnelly WJ, Leonard FC (2002) Veterinary Microbiology and Microbial Disease. 4th ed., Black well publishing company: Blackwell Science, London, UK, pp: 137-143.

36. Docherty, Douglas E (1999) Viral Diseases (Field Manual of Wildlife Diseases).

37. OIE (2012) Newcastle disease. In: Manual of Diagnostic Tests and Vaccines for Terrestrial Animals. Chapter 2.3.14.

38. Saif YM, Barnes HJ, Glisson JR, Fadly AM, McDougald LR, et al. (2005) Diseases of poultry, 11th edn, pp: 66-78.

39. Beard CW, Hanson RP (1984) Newcastle disease. In: Diseases of poultry.

40. Hasan AR, Ali MH, Siddique MP, Rahman MM, Islam MA (2012) Clinical and laboratory diagnoses of newcastle and infectious bursal diseases of chickens. Bangladesh J Vet Med. 8: 131-140.

41. Alexander DJ (2003) Newcastle disease, other Paramyxoviridae and Pneumovirus Infections. In; Diseases of Poultry. 11th edn. Iowa State press, Ames. pp: 63-100.

42. Aldous EW, Alexander DJ (2001) Detection and differentiation of Newcastle disease virus (avian paramyxovirus type 1). Avian Pathol 30: 117-128.

43. Office International des Epizootics (2009) Manual of Diagnostic Testsand Vaccines for Terrestrial Animals. Newcastle disease OIE Terrestrial Manual. OIE, Paris, France, pp. 576-589.

44. Alexander DJ, Bell JG, Alders RG (1995) Newcastle disease. State Vet J. 5: 21-21.

45. Brown J, Resurreccion RS, Dickson TG (1990) The relationship between the hemagglutination-inhibition test and the enzyme-linked immunosorbent assay for the detection of antibody to Newcastle disease. Avian Dis. 34: 585-587.

46. Hewson K, Noormohammadi AH, Devlin JM, Mardani K, Ignjatovic J (2009) Rapid detection and non-subjective characterisation of infectious bronchitis virus isolates using high-resolution melt curve analysis and a mathematical model. Archives Virol. 154: 649.

47. Bellau-Pujol S, Vabret A, Legrand L, Dina J, Gouarin S, et al. (2005) Development of three multiplex RT-PCR assays for the detection of 12 respiratory RNA viruses. J Virol Methods. 126: 53-63.

48. Albert B, Bray D, Hopkins K, Johnson A, Lewis J, et al. (2004) Essential biology, edited by cell 2nd. Garland Science.

49. Creelan JL, Graham DA, McCullough SJ (2002) Detection and Differentiation of pathogenicity of avian paramyxovirus Serotype 1 from field cases using one-step reverse transcriptase- Polymerase chain reaction. Avian Pathol. 31: 493-499.

50. Mackay IM, Arden KE, Nitsche A (2002) Real-time PCR in virology. Nucl Aci Res. 30: 1292-1305.

51. Mackay IM (2004) Real-time PCR in the microbiology laboratory. Clin Micro Infect. 10: 190-1212.

52. Turner P, McLennan A, Bates A, White M (2005) Molecular Biology, 3rd edn. Bios Instant Notes, edited by Hames BD, Taylor and Francis, Leeds, UK.

53. Pfaffl MW (2004) Quantification strategies in real-time PCR. A-Z of quantitative PCR. International University Line (IUL) La Jolla, CA, USA, Freising, Germany.

54. He Q, Marjamaki M, Soini H, Mertsola J, Viljanen M (1994) Primers are decisive for sensitivity of PCR. Bio Tech. 17: 82-87.

55. Abd-Elsalam KA (2003) Bioinformatic tools and guideline for PCR primer design. African J Biotechnol. 2: 91-95.

56. Tang Q, Wanga J, Bao J, Sun H, Sun Y, et al. (2012) A multiplex RT-PCR assay for detection and differentiation of avian H3, H5, and H9 subtype influenza viruses and Newcastle disease viruses. J Virol Methods. 181: 164-169.

57. Markos T, Abdela N (2016) Epidemiology and Economic Importance of Pullorum Disease in Poultry: A Review. Global Veterinaria 17: 228-237.

58. Shim JB, So HH, Won HH, Mo I (2011) Characterization of avian paramyxovirus type-1 from migratory wild birds in chickens. Avian Pathol. 40: 565-572.

59. Xiao S, Paldurai A, Nayak B, Mirande A, Collins PL, et al. (2013) Complete genome sequence of a highly virulent Newcastle disease virus currently circulating in Mexico. Genome Announc. 1: 01-02.

60. Spadbrow (1992) Newcastle disease in village chicken. Control with thermostable oral vaccine. Proceeding of an international workshop, Kuala lumpar, Malaysia. ACIAR, Canberra.

61. Chukwudi OE, Chukwuemeka ED, Mary U (2012) Newcastle disease virus shedding among healthy commercial chickens and its epidemiological importance. Pakistan Vet J. 32: 354-356.

62. Otim MO, Mukiibi GM, Christensen H, Bisgaard M (2005) Aflatoxicosis, infectious bursal disease and immune response to Newcastle disease vaccination in rural chicken. Avian Pathol. 34: 319-323.

25

Prevalence of Bovine Cysticercosis at Jijiga Municipal Abattoir, Ethiopia

Wolde Akalu Biruk*

Ministry of Agriculture and Rural Development, Ethiopia

Abstract

The study was made from November 2008 to April 2009 at the Ethiopia Somali region, Jijiga city. It was carried out with the objectives of providing base line data on the prevalence of *C. bovis*. A total of 400 carcasses of randomly selected bovine animals were used for the active abattoir survey. Of the 400 carcasses examined during the study period, 9 (2.25%) were infected with *C. bovis*. The distribution of organ infected with *C. bovis* were, tongue (55.5%) and heart (55.5%), shoulder muscle (33.3%), masseter muscle (22.2%), and liver (11.1%). Analysis of active abattoir survey revealed that there was no a significant difference (P>0.05) between sex and age of the animal. The viability test on all isolated cysts showed that 20% were viable. the tongue, shoulder muscle, masseter muscle and heart had the highest number of viable (60%), (60%), (50%) and (33.3%) cyst respectively. Meat inspection cannot totally prevent the consumer from being infected through row or under cocked meat/beef. Therefore, an effective control program has to include action intervening at various points of the life cycle of *T. saginata*. It requires an integrated approach among all stake holders: consumers, medical doctors and pharmacists, meat inspectors, veterinary practitioners and farmers.

Keywords: Prevalence; *C. bovis*; *T. saginata*; Jijiga

Introduction

Animal diseases are one of the most important constraints to increase productivity of food animals in all parts of the world. Parasitism is one of the major problems that affect the productivity of livestock worldwide. Among many parasitic problems of domestic animals, tapeworms are an economically important intestinal parasites found all over the world, which have infected human beings for thousands of years [1].

The nation's domestic meat consumption of about 45% comes from cattle, which generates export income mainly from the sale of live animals. In foreign trade, although the country is ideally placed to export live animals to the big markets of the Middle East and substantial markets of North and West Africa, export earning is relatively low. This is mainly due to the presence of a number of unimproved animal health problems, among which, *Taenia saginata* (*T. saginata*) or *Cysticercus bovis* (*C. bovis*) is one that remains a major public and animal health problem [2].

Transmission of the parasite occurs most commonly in the environment characterized by poor sanitation, primitive livestock husbandry practices and inadequate meat inspection management control police. Bovine cysticercosis is responsible for considerable amount of economic losses which can approach 30% when allowance is made for the loss in the carcass weight and the cost of freezing the infected meat. Generally the loss is determined by disease prevalence, grade of the animal infected, potential markets, prices of cattle treatment for detained carcass [3] and medical costs for infected human being [4]. The average annual loss due to taenicidal drugs for treatment in Ethiopia was estimated to be 4,937,583.21 Ethiopian birr [5,6].

Bovine *cysitcercosis* is widely distributed in Ethiopia and a number of individual reported the prevalence of bovine *cysitcercosis* in different parts of the country 2.25% reports of Tembo (3.2%) and (2.9% and 4.4%) prevalence Jimma in south-western Ethiopia (Megersa et al.; Tolosa et al.) and Ziway (3.0%) (Bedu et al.) in southern Ethiopia and (26.3%) (Abunna et al.) in Hawasa and in north-western Ethiopia (18.5%) (Kebede) [7-12].

On the other hand the contribution of *Cysticercus bovis* to organ condemnation in slaughtered cattle at different abattoir have been reported [12,13]. It is a great problem in developing country like Ethiopia due to the cultural habit eating raw meet as routine dish and holidays has promoted human taeniasis in Ethiopia. The above mentioned problems allow the parasite to continue its life cycle till to date and in the coming future (Ecker).

The objective of this particular research are:

• To determine the prevalence of bovine *cysticercosis* at Jijiga municipal abattoir

• To assess the viability of *Cysticercus bovis* cysts.

Materials and Methods

Study area

The study was conducted from November 2008 to April 2009 in Jijiga city. Jijiga which is the capital city of Ethiopia Somali region is found eastern part of Ethiopia 630 km away from Addis Ababa and 105 km of east of Harar city with population size of 105,634. Jijiga is situated at altitude of 1660 m.a.s.l, 9° 20° North Latitude and 45° 56° East Longitude. The climate of Jijiga is semi-arid type which is characterized by high temperature and low rain fall. The mean annual rain fall is about 543 mm and mean annual temperature is about 22°C.

Study population

Active abattoir survey: 400 presented for slaughter at Jijiga municipal abattoir were examined for the presence of *C. bovis* following routine meat inspection procedure as per the ministry of agriculture

*****Corresponding author:** Wolde Akalu Biruk, Ministry of Agriculture and Rural Development, Ethiopia, E-mail: birukakalu97@gmail.com

meat inspection procedure regulation.

Study design

The type of study was cross sectional type of study which was used to determine the prevalence cysticercosis in the abattoir.

Sample size

Active abattoir survey: To determine the sample size require for the abattoir i used the 50% prevalence as expected prevalence of cysticercosis because of no previous prevalence data recorded and the formula for sample size determination (Thrusfield)

$$n = \frac{1.96^2 \left(P_{exp} \left(1 - P_{exp} \right) \right)}{d^2}$$

where n=required sample size; P_{exp}=expected prevalence; d^2=desired absolute precision; By taking 50% expected prevalence and 5% desired absolute precision.

n=384

To increase my sample size 400 cattle were examined.

Study methodology

Active abattoir survey: During the study period 400 bovine carcasses were randomly examined for the presence of *C. bovis* following the customary meat inspection procedure stipulated in the ministry of agriculture (MOA) meat inspection regulation. cattle slaughtered were mainly old age, few young and emaciated.

The study animals were originated from Jijiga and around Jijiga city. prior to sampling each selected animals was given an identification number and data on each animal sex, age and breed were recorded. during meat inspection, identified animal and their respective organs were strictly examined separately to avoid mixing up of organs meat inspection was made in accordance with the procedure of Ethiopian ministry of agriculture meat inspection regulation for detection of *Cysticercus bovis*. Visual inspection and palpation followed by multiple incision of in each organ (heart, tongue, shoulder, liver and masseter) were made to examine the cysts of *T. saginata*.

Each organ, which is going to be inspected, was subjected to the following dissection procedure:

In the head two linear incision in to the external masseter muscle and one into the internal on each side of the lower jaw and parallel to it. In the tongue one longitudinal incision in to the underside; in shoulder, one deep incision into the triceps brachial muscle above the olecranon process; in the heart, incision in to both the ventricle and septum; further incision is made if necessary.

During the survey, detailed record were kept in each one or more number of cysts, either dead or live cysts was recorded. the information recorded was date, age, sex and the number of cysts (live or dead) in the inspection sites, when the cyst had a thick connective tissue and which contain caseous and calcified material they were assessed as dead. Cyst with translucent capsule through which the white scolex could be seen

were counted as live. Each caracass was aged based on the number of erupted permanent incisors teeth. The data were combined for analysis in to two age group, namely ≤ 6 years and >6 years.

Viability test: Any cyst that was found at meat inspection was removed with the surrounding tissue taken to Jijiga regional veterinary diagnostic and research laboratory. then, the cyst were incubated at 37°C in 40% Ox-bile solution dissolved in normal saline for 1-2 hours. The cyst was regarded as viable if the scolex evaginated during the incubation period. Examination was performed under microscope after pressing betwen two glasses for scolex whether it was *T. saginata* or other *metacestodes* based on the size of *cysticercus and* absence of hooks ontherostlum of the evaginated cyst [14].

Data management and analysis

From data collected in active abattoir survey the total number of *C. bovis* was determined. The relative frequency of *C. bovis* in various sites was calculated. Distribution of calcified and non calcified cyst and Viability of *C. bovis* cyst was assessed. the data were put in excel sheet and analyzed STATA analytical software version 12.

Results

Active abattoir survey

Among the 400 slaughtered cattle examined during this study period 342(85.5%) and 58(14.5%) were male and female animals respectively of this animal 9 (2.25%) were found to be infected with *C. bovis* under routine meat inspection.

The prevalence of *C. bovis* between different age groups animals is shown on Table 1. There was no significant difference among those age groups based on dental formulation. The percentage of infected carcass of male and female animals are presented in Table 2. There was no significant difference (P>0.05) among male and female animals slaughtered in the proportion of *C. bovis* infection (Tables 3-5).

Viability test

Viability test is presented in Table 6.

Discussion

During the abattoir survey conducted at Jijiga municipal abattoir the overall prevalence of bovine cysticercosis was indicated as 2.25% which is similar to the reports of Tembo (3.2%) and (2.9% and 4.4%) prevalence Jimma in south-western Ethiopia (Megersa et al.; Tolosa et al.) and Ziway (3.0%) (Bedu et al.) in southern Ethiopia, extremely different from (26.3%) (Abunna et al.) in Hawasa and in north-western Ethiopia (18.5%) (Kebede) [7-12].

However, large differences can also be found within a region. In two studies conducted in and around Addis Ababa in central Ethiopia, prevalence varied between 7.5% (Kebede, Tilahun and Hailu) and 89.4% (Tembo) [9,12]. Such differences in prevalence may be associated with the number of cattle examined, the sensitivity of the meat inspection procedures, which can be affected by the site and method of incision, abattoir facilities and management, the motivation and competency of the meat inspectors and the willingness of the owner to cooperate [11,15].

Age group	No. of carcass inspected	No. of infected carcass
>6 years	292 (73%)	7 (77.7%)
≤ 6 years	108 (27%)	2 (22.22%)
X²=0.1066	df=1	P=0.744

Table 1: Prevalence of bovine cysticercosis in different age groups.

Table 2: Prevalence of bovine cysticercosis in male and female animals.

Sex	No. of carcass inspected	No. of infected carcass
Female	58	2 (3.44%)
Male	342	7 (2.05%)
X²=0.4429	df=1	p=0.506

Age group	Heart	Tongue	Shoulder muscle	Masseter muscle	Liver
>6 years	4	4	1	1	0
≤ 6 years	1	2	2	1	1
Total	5 (55.5%)	6 (88.8%)	3 (33.5%)	2 (22.2%)	1 (11.1%)

Table 3: Distribution and frequency of *C. bovis* cyst infected cattle in relation with age and organ affected in positive animals.

	>6 years	≤ 6 years	Total
Total no. of animals examined	292	108	400
No. of cysticercus recovered	17	9	26
Heart	4	3	7 (26.92%)
Tongue	6	3	9 (34.01%)
Shoulder muscle	5	1	6 (23.07%)
Masseter muscle	1	2	3 (11/53%)
Liver	1	0	1 (3.84%)

Table 4: Infection with *C. bovis* in the organs of cattle with different age group during the study period.

Nature of the cyst	Heart	Tongue	Shoulder muscle	Masseter muscle	Liver
Calcified	4 (36.36%)	4 (36.36%)	1 (9.09%)	1 (9.09%)	1 (9.09%)
Non calcified	3	5	5	2	0
Total	7	9	6	3	1

Table 5: Distribution of calcified and non calcified cyst.

Infected organs	No. of cysts examined	No. of viable cysts	%Viable cysts
Heart	3	1	33.3%
Tongue	5	3	60%
Shoulder muscle	5	3	50%
Masseter muscle	2	1	50%
Liver	1	0	-

Table 6: Viability of *C. bovis* cyst in the laboratory study.

The geographical differences in the habit of raw meat consumption, environmental and personal hygiene, animal husbandry practices, proximity to waste water and accessibility of taenicides for treating animals might also contribute to differences in prevalence [15-17]. In this study it is found that sex and age has no association (p>0.05) with *C. bovis* prevalence in the selected cattle, it revealed that no significant risk factor for the infection of bovine cysticercosis among the animal slaughtered at Jijiga municipal abattoir. The organ wise prevalence of each organ in the abattoir survey (Jijiga) was found being in the tongue highly prevalent 6 (88.8%), heart 5 (55.5%), shoulder muscle 3 (33.5%), masseter muscle 2 (22.2%) and liver 1 (11.1%).

The most frequently affected organ was the tongue followed by heart and other organs which is similar were compared with Dawit, Viability test showed that tongue and shoulder muscle had the highest relative frequency proportion of viable cyst 3(60%) followed by masseter muscle and heart 1(50%) and 1 (33.3%) respectively [6]. The method of meat inspection, the ability of the meat inspector to identify the cases, different in management, sample size, sampling method and the number of cuts, and other factors can contribute for the variation of the prevalence of bovine cysticercosis.

Conclusion and Recommendation

T. saginata is a medically and economically important cestode parasite, while in cattle causes economic loss in the meat industry. In this study, the prevalence of bovine cysticercosis was relatively lower than the reports by different researchers in different parts of the country.

Among the potential risk factors, religion, occupation and consumption of raw meat were very risk factors for taeniasis. Based on the finding of the present study, the following are recommended.

- Farmers should be fully supported and informed of the life cycle of *T. saginata* and potential risk factors for cattle to become infected.

- There should be a public awareness about the health and economic significance the disease.

- Infected meat and meat products must undergo the process of freezing, boiling or distraction of the cysticerci based on the intensity of infection.

- Improvement in working condition of the inspectors with upgrading their skill and working conditions.

References

1. Thrusfield M (1995) Veterinary epidemiology. 2nd edn. Blackwell Science Ltd., UK, pp: 182-198.

2. Radostits OM, Blood DC, Gay CC, Hinchcliff KW, Constable PD (2007) Veterinary Medicine. Text book of the disease of cattle, sheep, goat. pig and horses. 10th edn. Saunders, Philadelphia, pp: 1581-1583.

3. Mekbib B, Abesha H, Tesfaye D (2013) Study on Zoonotic Metacestodes of Cattle Slaughtered at Bahir Dar Municipal Abattoir, Northwest Ethiopia. Global Veterinaria 10: 592-598.

4. Gruindle RG (1978) Economic loss resulting from bovine cysticercosis with special reference Botswana and Kenya. Trop Anim Health Prod 10: 127-140.

5. Fan PC (1997) Annual Economic loss caused by Taenia saginata taeniasis in East Asia. Parasitol Today 13: 194-135.

6. Dawit S (2004) Epidemiology of *T. saginata* taeniasis and Cysticercosis in North Gonder Zone. DVM Thesis, Faculty of Veterinary Medicine, Addis Ababa University, Debre Zeit, Ethiopia.

7. Fufa A (2006) Study on the prevalence of Bovine cysticercosis in Awassa Municipal Abattoir and Taenia saginata in Awassa town and its surrounding, Southern Ethiopia. MSc Thesis, Addis Ababa University, Debre Zeit, Ethiopia.

8. Tembo A (2001) Epidemiology of *T. saginata* taeniasis and cysticercosis in three selected agro-climatic zones in central Ethiopia. MSc Thesis, Faculty of Veterinary Medicine, Addis Ababa University, Debre Zeit, Ethiopia.

9. Megersa B, Tesfaye E, Regassa A, Abebe R, Abunna F (2010) Bovine cysticercosis in cattle slaughtered at jimma municipal Abattoir, South Western ethiopia: prevalence, cyst viability and its socio economic importance. Vet World 3: 257-262.

10. Tolosa T, Tigre W, Teka G, Dorny P (2009) Prevalence of bovine cysticercosis and hydatidosis in Jimma municipal abattoir, South West Ethiopia. Onderstepoort J Vet Res 76: 323-326.

11. Bedu H, Tafess K, Shelima B, Woldeyohannes D, Amare B (2011) Bovine cysticercosis in cattle slaughtered at Zeway municipal Abattoir: prevalence and its public health importance. J Vet Sci Technol 2: 108.

12. Abunna F, Tilahun G, Bersisa K, Megersa B, Regassa A (2008) Bovine cysticercosis in cattle slaughtered at Awassa municipal abattoir, Ethiopia: prevalence, cyst viability, distribution and its public health implication. Zoonoses and public health 55: 82-88.

13. Kebede N, Tilahun G, Hailu A (2009) Current Status of Bovine Cysticercosis of Slaughtered Cattle in Addis Ababa Abattoir, Ethiopia. Trop Anim Health Prod 41: 291-294.

14. Fekadu D (2003) A study on *cestodes* and *metacestodes* of sheep in sheno agricultural Research (SHARC), Northern shoa. DVM Thesis, Faculty of Veterinary Medicine, Addis Ababa University, Debre Zeit, Ethiopia.

15. Gracey FJ, Collins SD, Hucy RJ (1999) Meat Hygiene. 10th edn. Bailliere Tindall, 24-28 oval roads, London NW 17DX, UK, pp: 413-420.

16. Wanzala W, Onyango-Abuje JA, Kang`Ethe EK, Zessin KH, Kyule NM, et al. (2003) Analysis of Post-Mortem Diagnosis of Bovine Cysticercosis in Kenyan Cattle. J Vet Res 7: 1-9.

17. Kumar A, Tadesse G (2011) Bovine cysticercosis in Ethiopia: a review. Ethiop. Vet J 15: 15-35.

26

Prevalence and Antibiotic Resistance of *Salmonella* Species Isolated from Chicken Eggs by Standard Bacteriological Method

Kassahun Tessema[1], Hussen Bedu[1*], Mebrat Ejo[1] and Adem Hiko[2]

[1]*Department of Biomedical Sciences, Faculty of Veterinary Medicine, University of Gondar, Gondar, Ethiopia*

[2]*Department of Veterinary Epidemiology, Microbiology and Public Health, College of Veterinary Medicine, Haramaya University, Haramaya, Ethiopia*

Abstract

Salmonella have been found to be the major food borne disease in the world with a serious public health problem. The current study was carried out to detect and to determine the prevalence and antibiotic susceptibility of *Salmonella* isolated from fresh raw chicken eggs collected at Haramaya University Poultry Farm in Eastern Ethiopia. Among the total 384 chicken eggs, *Salmonella* spp. was detected from 2.9% (11/384) of egg samples using culture technique and was confirmed by biochemical test, nine *Salmonella* spp. (2.4%) were detected from egg shell and two (0.5%) from egg contents; predominantly occurred in floor house system. The prevalence of *Salmonella* in eggs on the bases of chicken breed sources was 2.9%, 3.8% and 2% for Bovans, Fayoumi and White leg horn, respectively. The prevalence difference did not show statistical significance (P>0.05) between the rate of detecting *Salmonella* spp. among the egg shell and egg contents, and similarly, non-significant analytical situation was observed in eggs sampled from different chicken breeds. Among the sample sources, egg samples examined from cage and floor house were found *Salmonella* positive with the prevalence of 2.3% and 3.3%, respectively. However, there was no statistically significant difference (P>0.05) in the prevalence of *Salmonella* among the two house systems. All identified isolates were tested for susceptibility to a six commonly used antimicrobials by disk diffusion technique. Out of the 11 isolates tested 8(72.7%) were resistant to one or more of the tested antimicrobials. The most common resistance observed was to tetracycline (72.7%), ampicillin (72.7%) and amoxicillin (63.6%). However, spectinomycin, kanamycin and chloramphenicol were effective against most of the *Salmonella* isolates.

Keywords: Antimicrobials; Eggs; Prevalence; Resistance; *Salmonella*

Introduction

Food borne diseases are among the most widespread global public health problems of recent times, and their implication for health and economy is increasingly recognized [1,2]. The majority of foodborne outbreaks are caused by *Salmonella, Listeria monocytogenes, Escherichia coli*, and *Campylobacter* strains [3]. Among these pathogens, *Salmonella* are considered the most prevalent foodborne pathogens worldwide [4,5] and has long been recognized as an important zoonotic pathogen of economic significance in animals and humans, predominantly in the developing countries. The important route of transmission of *Salmonella* organism from animals to man is via food products of animal origin which may be contaminated at the source or during handling [6]. Epidemiological studies show that chicken eggs and meat are two of the most important sources for consumer ingestion and contact of pathogens [7]. Chicken eggs in particular continue to be identified as leading food sources for human Salmonellosis [5,8].

The true incidence of salmonellosis in both humans and animals is difficult to evaluate in developing countries because of the lack of epidemiological surveillance systems [9,10]. The ubiquity of *Salmonella* isolates makes them a persistent contamination hazard to all raw foods [11]. Those of animal origin food products are often implicated in sporadic cases and outbreaks of human salmonellosis [12,13]. The distribution of *Salmonella* serotypes from poultry sources is geographically variable and changes over time, although several serotypes are consistently detected at a high incidence throughout much of the world. Many of the *Salmonella* serotypes that are most prevalent in humans are also common in poultry [14], suggesting a possible epidemiologic connection between the poultry and human reservoirs of *Salmonella. Salmonella* infection in chickens has important implication on public health worldwide [15]. Infected chickens can deposit *Salmonella* in either the yolk or albumen of developing eggs because of the colonization of different regions of the reproductive tract [16,17]. It is not yet clear as to which route is most important for *Salmonella* to contaminate the egg contents, which may be contaminated with *Salmonella*e by vertical transmission and/or horizontal transmission [18]. Although some authors claim horizontal transmission to be the most important way to contaminate eggs. Barrow and Lovell, most authors claim that vertical transmission is the most important route of egg contamination [19].

In recent years, *Salmonella* related diseases have been documented by several food related studies conducted in different parts of Ethiopia [9,20]. An increased in the resistance of *Salmonella* to commonly used antimicrobials has been also noted in both public health and veterinary sectors in Ethiopia [20]. Antimicrobial resistance is a natural consequence of infectious agents' adaptation to exposure to antimicrobials used in medicine, food animals, crop production and use of disinfectants in farms and households [21-23]. However, scarcity of surveillance data on the incidences of *Salmonella* species associated with eggs and its antimicrobial resistance pattern in the poultry farm is a major epidemiological issue. Despite some attempts to study prevalence of *Salmonella* in Ethiopia, mainly in meat and meat products, the status of the problem in eggs is still very much unknown.

*Corresponding author: Hussen Bedu, Department of Biomedical Sciences, Faculty of Veterinary Medicine, University of Gondar, Gondar, Ethiopia
E-mail: qaroo2016@gmail.com

Very little information is available at this time for *Salmonella* infection of egg in the country. However, studies made elsewhere indicated that eggs are important sources of *Salmonella* particularly among those raw consumers [24]. Therefore, this study was aimed to determine the prevalence and distribution of *Salmonella* spp. on chicken eggs by conventional culture methods and biochemical assays, and also to assess the antimicrobial resistance of the isolates.

Materials and Methods

Study site

The study was performed on egg samples collected in Haramaya University Poultry Farm located at Haramaya, Ethiopia. It is approximately 500 kilometres away from Addis Ababa, capital city of Ethiopia. Geographically the study site located at 41° 59'58" North latitude and 90°24'10" South longitudes. The elevation of this area is about 2000 meters above sea level and its mean annual temperatures ranges from 10°Cto 18°C with the relative humidity of 65 percent respectively. The area receives an annual rain fall of 800 millimetres within a bimodal distribution of the season's pattern peaking in mid-April and mid-August of the year. The farm serves mainly for people residing in and the surrounding of East Ethiopia. In the farm, three breeds of chicken (Bovans, Fayoumi and White leg horn) are used for the purpose of egg production and production of day old chicks, which distributed for consumers and farmers of the surroundings and to different regions of the country.

Study design and sampling

A Cross-sectional study was conducted to determine the prevalence, distribution and antimicrobial susceptibility of *Salmonella* in chicken eggs from three breeds of layer chickens. Simple random sampling technique was used to collect egg samples from Fayoumi, Bovansand White leg horn breeds of layer chickens in cage and floor housing systems

Egg sample collection

The sample size was calculated according to Thrusfield, using 95% confidence interval and 0.05 absolute precision by assuming expected prevalence of 50% [25]. In total, 384 freshly laid and unwashed chicken eggs were aseptically collected from the farm. The collected egg samples were transported to the laboratory of Veterinary Microbiology, College of Veterinary Medicine, Haramaya University under cold chain and analysed using microbiological protocols for *Salmonella* isolation and identification. Information on breed, coded ID number of egg and house was registered during collection of egg samples.

Culture method

Standard cultivation method recommended by the International Organization for Standardization (ISO 6579, 2002) was carried out for isolation and identification of *Salmonella* [26]. Each chicken eggshell were dipped in sterile peptone broth and swabbed with sterile cotton swabs and then added in Buffered Peptone Water (BPW). In addition, surface sterilized eggs were cracked with a sterile knife and each egg's content was mixed thoroughly and 25 gm of the mixed egg content was inoculated into 225 ml of peptone broth. The mixture then homogenized using a laboratory blender (Stomacher 400R, Seward, England) for 30 seconds. The pre-enriched samples, both from egg shells and egg contents, were incubated for overnight at 37°C. After the overnight incubation, 1 ml of the pre-enrichment broths was transferred aseptically into a tube containing 10 ml of

Muller-Kauffmann-tetrathionate(MK) broth and incubated at 37°C for overnight. Following incubation, a loopful of each enrichment broth culture streaked onto one plate of xylose lysine desoxycholate (XLD) agar and another plate on *Salmonella*-shigella (SS) agar and incubated at 37°C for 24 hr. The plates (XLD and SS agars) were examined for the presence of typical *Salmonella* colonies. Characteristic colony for *Salmonella* isolates were then transferred onto nutrient agar and incubated aerobically at 37°C for overnight.

Biochemical test

Each identified colonies with typical *Salmonella* morphology were confirmed biochemically by inoculating into lysine iron agar (LIA), triple sugar iron agar (TSI) slopes, urea agar base, tryptophan broth and methylered-vogesproskaur (MR-VP) medium with confirmation carried out following incubated at 37 °C for 18-48 hours, and interpreted with international organization for standardization (ISO 6579, 2002) [26].

Antimicrobial susceptibility test

Antibiotic sensitivity of the isolates was performed according to agar disc diffusion method on Mueller–Hinton Agar using National Committee for Clinical Laboratory Standard (NCCLS, 2002) guidelines [27]. The antibiotic discs (antibiotic concentration in mg) used were consisted of ampicillin (10 mg), tetracycline (30 mg), amoxicillin (20 mg), kanamycin (30 mg), chloramphenicol (30 mg) and spectinomycin (100 mg). Results were evaluated according to NCCLS of the reference zone diameter interpretive standards (millimeter) and minimal inhibitory concentration (MIC) breakpoints. Strains were evaluated as susceptible, intermediate and resistant. An isolate was defined as resistant if it was resistant to one or more of the antimicrobial drugs.

Data analysis

The raw data were entered and managed in Microsoft Excel work sheet; and descriptive statistic was utilized to summarize data. The prevalence was calculated for all data by dividing positive samples by total number of examined samples and multiplied by hundred. The association between the prevalence of *Salmonella* and associated factors (egg sample, breed and house) was assessed by Chi-square (χ^2). A statically significant association between variables is considered to exist if the computed p-value is less than 0.05.

Results

Prevalence

Salmonella spp. was isolated from 11 (2.9%) egg samples by conventional culture technique and all isolates were confirmed by biochemical test. Nine *Salmonella* spp. were identified from eggshells and 2 were recovered from egg content samples. Of the total egg samples examined, 3 (0.8%), 5 (1.3%) and 3 (0.8%) were found positive for *Salmonella* in eggs collected from Bovans, Fayoumi and White leg horn breeds of layer chickens, respectively (Table 2). Among the 11 chicken egg samples positive for *Salmonella*, 4 (1.0%) were collected from cage house system and 7 (1.9%) were received from floor house system (Table 2).

The specific prevalence of *Salmonella* detected from the total of 384

Samples	No positive	Prevalence (%)	χ^2	p-value
Eggshells	9	2.3	0.048	0.826
Egg contents	2	0.5		
Total	11	2.9		

Table 1: Prevalence of *Salmonella* by egg samples taken (n=384).

Source of Eggs	No of eggs examined	No of positive (%)	χ^2	p-value
Breeds				
Bovans	105	3 (2.9)	0.183	0.913
Fayoumi	132	5 (3.8)		
White leg horn	147	3 (2.0)		
House				
Cage	171	4 (2.3)	0.306	0.580
Floor	213	7 (3.3)		

Table 2: Association between Risk Factors.

egg samples examined for both egg shell and egg content were 2.3% and 0.5%, respectively (Table 1). Of the total egg samples examined, 9 egg shell samples found positive for *Salmonella*; 5 (2.3%) positive egg shell samples were obtained from floor house and 4 (2.3%) positive egg shell samples were obtained from cage house. From the total 384 egg contents examined only 2 (0.5%) were positive for *Salmonella*. There was slightly higher prevalence of *Salmonella* in egg shell than egg contents. On the other hand, the prevalence of *Salmonella* in the two houses of the farm is presented in Table 3. The prevalence of *Salmonella* in floor and cage houses was 3.3% and 2.3%, respectively. The result revealed that of 171 egg samples examined, 4 (2.3%) showed the presence of *Salmonella* while 7 out of 213 (3.3%) egg samples were found positive. The prevalence of *Salmonella* in cage house (2.3%) was slightly less than floor house (3.3%) in the studied farm.

Even though, there were different prevalence recorded in this study, the findings suggested that no statistically significant difference (χ^2=0.183, p-value=0.913) in the prevalence of *Salmonella* in eggs of Bovans (2.9%), Fayoumi (3.8%) and White leg horn (2%) breeds of layer chickens (Table 2). Similarly, there was no significant statistical variation (χ^2=0.306, p-value=0.580) in the prevalence of *Salmonella* in eggs among the sources from the two-house system, 3.3% in floor house and 2.3% in cage house of the farm.

Moreover, the study has also shown the prevalence of *Salmonella* between those egg shells and egg contents of the total sampled eggs, 2.9% in egg shell samples (2.3) and 0.5% in egg content samples. This result also indicated that there was no statistical significant difference (χ^2=0.048, p-value=0.826) in the prevalence of *Salmonella* in egg samples under classified egg shells and egg contents.

Antimicrobial susceptibility

Of the total 11 *Salmonella* isolates subjected to antimicrobial susceptibility test using six different antimicrobials, a total of 8 (72.7%) *Salmonella* isolates were found to be resistant to two or more (multidrug) antimicrobials tested. In relation to the total *Salmonella* isolates tested, 72.7%, 72.7% and 63.6% were found highly resistant to ampicillin, tetracycline and amoxacillin, respectively, while 36.4%, 27.3%, 18.2% and 9.0% were intermediate resistant to chloramphenicol, amoxicillin, ampicillin and kanamycin, respectively. Looking at individual antimicrobial drug, resistance to ampicillin and tetracycline was the most frequently observed, and followed by amoxacillin. In general, antimicrobial susceptibility test revealed that spectinomycin, kanamycin and chloramphenicol were the drugs indicated more active against *Salmonella* isolated from egg samples, while tetracycline, ampicillin and amoxacillin were less effective against *Salmonella* isolates.

Discussion

Eggs contaminated with micro-organisms play a significant role in poultry production pathology and in the spreading of diseases to humans [28]. The present study revealed an overall prevalence rate of 2.9% in the studied egg samples with the prevalence of *Salmonella* 2.3% from egg shells and 0.5% from egg contents, respectively. In this study, higher prevalence of *Salmonella* was obtained when compare with the prevalence reported by other studies, 0.8% from table eggs (EFSA) and 0.3% from poultry eggs in Dhaka [29,30]. The current finding is almost comparable with 3% prevalence observed in Belgium from egg shell and egg content samples examined in different housing system [31]. The prevalence of *Salmonella* in this study was however lower than 7.7% recorded in South India [32], 24.17% prevalence in Nigeria [33], 3.84% and 5.5% among the chicken eggs from poultry farm and marketing in North India [34], respectively and 8% *Salmonella* species isolated from chicken eggs of Dhaka city [35]. The variation in the prevalence of *Salmonella* in eggs may be due to lack of awareness of the status of *Salmonella* in chicken eggs and the unhygienic situation in the farm. Moreover, the management system in practice could also be the probable reason for the variation of the prevalence. Different authors reported that the presence of chickens of different ages in the farm, the presence of arthropod pests, wet and soiled litter in the farm [36], and the housing system and flock size could be important reasons for egg contamination with various micro-organisms. Chicken feeds and hatcheries also possible sources of *Salmonella* infections in the farm.

The result of this study showed a relatively higher prevalence of *Salmonella* in egg shells (2.3%) than 0.5% in egg contents. However, this difference was not statistically significant (p>0.05). The prevalence of *Salmonella* in egg shell (2.3%) in this study indicated relative agreement with 2.7% prevalence of *Salmonella* reported by Akhtar [37]. However, it is much lower than 10.5% prevalence reported by Loongyai et al. and 6.1% egg shell contamination [32,38]. Isolation of *Salmonella* from egg shell in this study may be due to contamination of eggshells at lay with faeces from intestinal carriers. De Buck et al. showed that infected birds produced the highest frequency of contaminated eggs in the first week post infection [39]. Chicken faeces, dust, litter and egg collector can also contaminate the egg shells. Smeltzer et al. indicated that eggs laid in wet, dirty nests or on the floor are more likely to be contaminated with microorganism [36]. Davies and Breslin also stated that farm environment, poor hygiene and disinfecting of materials are possible reasons of egg contamination in the farm. The findings of *Salmonella* prevalence in chicken egg contents was lower than the reports made by Suresh et al. [32] who reported 1.8% prevalence and also lower than Akhtar et al. who reports 8.33% prevalence [37]. The level of egg contents contamination in this study was slightly higher than the 0.017% prevalence reports (HKSAR) and no contamination of egg contents [38,40,41]. It is believed that the main source of egg content *Salmonella* contamination could be the infected ovary and/or oviduct. It is generally believed that the deposition of *Salmonella* inside eggs is thus most likely a consequence of reproductive tissue colonization in infected laying hens. Methner et al. also revealed that no correlation was found between the contamination of the eggshell and that of the egg contents [42]. In a study of naturally infected flocks, numerous

Antimicrobials	Number of antimicrobials tested isolates		
	Sensitive (%)	Intermediate (%)	Resistant (%)
Ampicillin	1 (9.1)	2 (18.2)	8 (72.7)
Tetracycline	3 (27.3)	0.0	8 (72.7)
Amoxicillin	1 (9.1)	3 (27.3)	7 (63.6)
Kanamycin	10 (91.0)	1 (9.0)	0.0
Chloramphenicol	7 (63.6)	4 (36.4)	0.0
Spectinomycin	11 (100)	0.0	0.0

Table 3: Percentage of antimicrobial sensitivity test among *Salmonella* isolated from raw chicken eggs.

Salmonella serotypes, such as *Salmonella enteritidis*, *S. typhimurium* and *S. hadar*, were isolated from eggshells, whereas only *S. enteritidis* was isolated from egg contents [43]. Other study also reported that one-day-old chicks orally infected with *S. pullorum* produced contaminated eggs frequently during the period of sexual maturity as a consequence of reproductive tract colonization [44].

In this study, the prevalence of *Salmonella* is not much house dependent even though there was a slight increase in the prevalence of *Salmonella* from egg sample in the floor housing system (3.3%) than cage housing system (2.3%). The difference was not statistically significant. This finding was supported by the prevalence result of 1.8% in floor house and 1.4% in cage house [31]. The slight increase of prevalence may be because of hygienic status, air quality and confinement of birds. In addition, dust originated from feed and faeces may contain large number of microorganisms. The study also indicated that *Salmonella* was isolated from egg shells collected from both floor and cage house systems, whereas *Salmonella* was detected in egg contents sampled from only floor house system. The positive egg contents in the floor house system may be due to cross contamination of eggs at time of laying. Contamination of eggs with *Salmonella* was believed to occur when the organism passed from the shells into its inner contents. Spark and Board, (1985) showed that the moisture content in newly laid eggs diminishes the ability of cuticle to protect the egg contents. With so-called bed wet eggs, drops of water penetrate the cuticle, change its structure and enable micro-organisms to enter the egg contents immediately after laying. According to Humphrey increased stress could play a role to induce some changes in the chemistry of the oviduct, which might create an environment that is more susceptible for *Salmonella* in floor house system [45]. Occurrence of *Salmonella* in eggs collected from Bovans, Fayoumi, and White leg horn chicken breeds were 2.9%, 3.8% and 2.0%, respectively. There was no statistical significant difference ($p > 0.05$) in the recovery rate of *Salmonella* from the eggs of the three breeds of layer chickens. This is presumably due to unequal exposure to the risk factors as the breeds were housed in different house system. Slightly higher prevalence was observed in eggs collected from Fayoumi chicken breed (3.8%). This difference might be due to Fayoumi breed was kept in the floor house system in which there is lower hygienic and high cross contamination between the flock eggs at laying than the cage house system.

Many of the isolates are resistant to multiple antimicrobial agents tested. The antimicrobial resistant recorded in this study is in consistent with 81% of tetracycline and 73% of ampicillin reported by Miko et al. [13]. High level of antimicrobial resistant *Salmonella* occurred in this study is probably an indication of their frequent usage both in the animal and public health sectors. The finding of this study shows slightly lower resistant than the study reported 93.1% for tetracycline and amoxicillin in Nigeria from *Salmonella* isolates in chicken eggs [33]. Alemayehu et al. also showed 52% of the *Salmonella* isolates from beef were resistant to at least three antibiotics from beef in Ethiopia, *Salmonella* isolates sensitivity to spectinomycin (100%) and kanamycin (91%) indicates the most active antimicrobial against *Salmonella* in poultry farms, which agrees with the report of an overall 2.9% spectinomycin resistance for *Salmonella* isolates from swine slaughtered in Addis Ababa abattoir [9,46]. Since the 1990s the frequency of antimicrobial drug resistance in zoonotic *Salmonella* and number of drugs to which the strains are resistant have increased, primarily as a consequence of antimicrobial use in food production may be associated with adverse consequences in several ways including treatment failures [47,48].

In the present study, the antimicrobial-resistant strains were found up to 72% of the total 11 *Salmonella* isolates tested, which is greater than those in previous studies of nonclinical isolates from dairy cattle. Most of these isolates are resistant to multiple antimicrobial agents tested, particularly for ampicillin, amoxicillin and tetracycline. Resistance to ampicillin, amoxicillin and tetracycline were widespread. This may be due to the widespread use of antibiotics included in feeds and in chickens. When compared to the resistant *Salmonella* isolates obtained from chickens in other studies, the prevalence of antimicrobial resistance in this study is much lower. 92% resistant to tetracycline *Salmonella* isolated from meat products in Ireland. The possible explanation could be the increased antimicrobial use in poultry farm and an association between resistance and virulence factors. Resistance rates to ampicillin, chloramphenicol, gentamycin, and trimethoprim of the isolates in the present study were low. However, it is important to note that these antibiotics are commonly used in veterinary medicine, and infections with these resistant *Salmonella* isolates could lower the efficiency of antibiotic treatment.

References

1. FAO (1999) Prospects for the future: emerging problems- chemical/biological. Conference on International Food Trade Beyond 2000: Science–based Decision, Harmonization, Equivalence and Mutual Recognition Melbourne, Australia, pp: 1-20.

2. Gomez TM, Motarjemi Y, Miyagawa S, Kaferstein FK, Stohr K (1997) Foodborne salmonellosis. World Health Stat 50: 81-89.

3. Velusamy V, Arshak K, Korostynska O, Oliwa K, Adley C (2010) An overview of foodborne pathogen detection: In the perspective of biosensors. Biotechnol Adv 28: 232-254.

4. Carrasco E, Morales-Rueda A, García-Gimeno RM (2012) Cross-contamination and recontamination by Salmonella in foods: a review. Food Res International 45: 545-556.

5. Finstad S, O'Bryan CA, Marcy JA, Crandall PG, Ricke SC (2012) Salmonella and broiler processing in the United States: Relationship to foodborne salmonellosis. Food Res International. 45: 789-794.

6. D'Aoust JY (1997) Salmonella Species. In: Doyle MP, Beuchat LR, Montville TJ (eds.). Food Microbiology Fundamentals and Frontiers, ASM Press, Washington DC, USA, pp: 129-158.

7. Luber P (2009) Cross-contamination versus undercooking of poultry meat or eggs-which risks need to be managed first? Int J Food Microbiol. 134: 21-28.

8. Mead G, Lammerding AM, Cox N, Doyle MP, Humbert F, et al. (2010) Scientific and technical factors affecting the setting of Salmonella criteria for raw poultry: Global perspective. J Food Prot 73: 1566-1590.

9. Ejeta G, Molla B, Alemayehu D, Muckle A (2004) Salmonella serotypes isolated from minced meat beef, mutton and pork in Addis Ababa, Ethiopia. Revue Med Vet. 155: 547-551.

10. Stevens A, Kabore Y, Perrier-Gros-Claude JD, Millemann Y, Brisabois A, et al. (2006) Prevalence and antibiotic-resistance of Salmonella isolated from beef sampled from the slaughterhouse and from retailers in Dakar (Senegal). Int J Food Microbiol 110: 178-186.

11. Bell C, Kyriakides A (2002) Salmonella: A Practical Approach to the Organism and Its Control in Foods. Wiley-Blackwell, Oxford.

12. Zhao S, White DG, Friedman SL, Glenn A, Blickenstaff K, et al. (2008) Antimicrobial resistance in Salmonella entericaserovar Heidelberg isolates from retail meats, including poultry, from 2002 to 2006. Appl Environ Microbiol. 74: 6656-6662.

13. Miko A, Pries K, Schroeter A, Helmuth R (2005) Molecular mechanisms of resistance in multidrug-resistant serovars of Salmonella enterica isolated from foods in Germany. J Anti Microb Chemother 56: 1025-1033.

14. Van Duijkeren E, Wannet WJB, Houwers DJ, VanPelt W (2001) Serotype and phage type Distribution of Salmonella strains Isolated from Humans, Cattle, Pigs, and Chickens in the Netherlands from 1984 to 2001. J Clin Microbiol 40: 3980-3985.

15. Humphrey TJ (1991) Infection by Salmonella Enteritidis in laying chickens y gallinas. Campylobalterolomestilas, Mexico. pp: 20-26.

16. Bichler LA, Nagaraja KV, Halvorson DA (1996) Salmonella enteritidis in eggs, cloacal swab specimens and internal organs of experimentally infected White Leghorn chickens. J Vet Res. 57: 489-495.

17. Gast RK, Guraya RJ, Guard-Bouldin PS, Holt, Moore RW (2007) Colonization of specific regions of the reproductive tract and deposition at different locations inside eggs laid by hens infected with Salmonella enteritidis or Salmonella heidelberg. Avian Dis. 51: 40-44.

18. Gantois I, Ducatelle R, Pasmans F, Haesebrouck F, Gast R, et al. (2009) Mechanisms of egg contamination bySalmonellaEnteritidis. FEMS Microbiol Rev. 33: 718-738.

19. Barrow PA, Lovell MA (1991) Experimental infection of egg-laying hens with Salmonella Enteritidis phage type 4. Avian Pathol 20: 335-348.

20. Molla B, Mesfin A (2003) A survey of Salmonella contamination in chicken carcass and giblets in central Ethiopia. Revue MédVét. 154: 267-270.

21. McEwen SA, Fedorka-Cray PJ (2002) Antimicrobial use and resistance in animals. Clin Infect Dis. 34: S93-S106.

22. Vidaver AK (2002) Uses of antimicrobials in plant agriculture. Antimicrob. Plant Agric. 34: S107-S110.

23. Wise R, Soulsby EJ (2002) Antibiotic resistance-an evolving problem. Vet Rec. 151: 371-372.

24. Jay JM (2000) Foodborne gastroenteritis caused by Salmonella and Shigella. In: Modern Food Microbiology. 6th edn. pp: 511-528.

25. Thrusfield M (2005) Veterinary Epidemiology. 3rd edn. UK: Blackwell Science, p: 233.

26. ISO (1998) Microbiology of Food and Animal Feeding Stuff-horizontal Method for the Detection of Salmonella, ISO 6579:2002, Geneva.

27. NCCLS (2002) Performance Standards for Antimicrobial Disk and Dilution Susceptibility Tests for Bacteria Isolated from Animals: Approved Standard. 3rd edn. NCCLS Document M31-A2. NCCLS, Wayne, PA, USA.

28. Hassan JO, Curtiss R (1997) Efficacy of a live avirulent Salmonella typhimurium vaccine in preventing colonization and invasion of laying hens by Salmonella typhimurium and Salmonella enteritidis. Avian Dis. 41: 783-791.

29. EFSA (2009) Special Measures to Reduce the Risk for Consumers through Salmonella in Table Eggs – e.g. cooling of table eggs. The EFSA J 957: 2-7.

30. Begum K, Reza TA, Haque M, Hossain A, Hussar FMK, et al. (2010) Isolate, Identification and Antibiotic Resistance Patterns of Salmonella Species from Chicken Eggs, Intestine and Environmental Samples. Bangladesh, Pharmaceutical Journal. 13: 0301-4606.

31. Devylder J, De Wulf J, Van Hoorebeke S, Pasmans F, Haesebrouck, et al. (2011) Horizontal transmission of Salmonella enteritidis in groups of experimentally infected laying hens housed in different housing systems. Poultry Sci. 90: 1-6.

32. Suresh T, Hatha AAM, Sreenivasan D, Sangaatha N, Lashmanaperumalsamy P (2006) Prevalence and Antimicrobial Resistance of Salmonella enteritidis and other Salmonellas in the Eggs and Egg-storing Trays from Retails Markets of Coimbatore, South India. Food Microbiol. 23: 294-299.

33. Ekundayo EU, Ezeake JC (2011) Prevalence and Antibiotic Sensitivity Profile of Salmonella Species in Eggs from Poultry Farms in Umudike, Abia State. J Animal Vet Adv 10: 206-209.

34. Singh S, Yadav AS, Singh SM, Bharti P (2010) Prevalence of Salmonella in Chicken Eggs Collected from Poultry Farms and Marketing Channels and Antimicrobial Resistance. Food Res International. 43: 2027-2030.

35. Ahmed MM, Rahman MM, Mahbub KR, Wahiduzzaman (2010) Characterization of Antibiotic Resistant Salmonella Species Isolated from Chicken Eggs of Dhaka City. J Scientific Res 3: 191-196.

36. Smeltzer T, Orange K, Peel B, Runge G (1979) Bacterial Penetration in Floor and Nest Box Eggs from Meat and Layer Birds. Aust Vet J. 55: 592-593.

37. Akhtar F (2008) Epidemiology and Immunoprophylaxis of Salmonella Enteritidis in Laying Hens in relation to Zoonosis. MSc Thesis, Department of microbiology, University of Agriculture, Faisalabd 12-14.

38. Loongyai W, Kiettisak P, Kangsukul N, Noppha R (2010) Detection of Salmonella in Eggs Shell and Egg Contents from Different Housing Systems for Laying Hens. World Academy of Science, Engineering and Technology 4: 232-234.

39. De Buck J, Van Immerseel F, Haesebrouck F, Ducatelle R (2004) Colonization of the Chicken Reproductive tract and egg Contamination by Salmonella. J Appl Microbiol. 97: 233-245.

40. HKSAR (2004) Salmonella in Eggs and Egg Products. Food and environmental, Hygiene Department, Queensway, Hong Kong. Pp: 1-20.

41. Sasaki Y, Sujiyama Y, Asai T, Noda Y, Katayama S, et al. (2011) Salmonella Prevalence in Commercial Raw Shell Eggs in Japan: A survey. Epidemiol Infect. 139: 1060-1064.

42. Methner U, Al-Shabibi S, Meyer H (1995) Experimental oral infection of Specific Pathogen-Free laying Hens and Cocks with Salmonella Enteritidis strains. Zoonoses Public health 42: 459-469.

43. Humphrey TJ, Whitehead A, Gawer A, Henley A, Rowe B (1991) Numbers of Salmonella enteritidis in the Contents of Naturally Contaminated Hen's Eggs. Epidemiol Infect. 106: 489-496.

44. Wigley P, Berchieri A, Page KL, Smith MH, Barrow PA (2001) Salmonella entericaserovarPullorum persists in Splenic Macrophages and in the Reproductive Tract during Persistent, Disease-Free Carriage in Chickens. Infect Immun. 69: 7873-7879.

45. Humphrey T (2004) Salmonella, Stress Response and Food Safety. Nature Reviews Microbiol. 2: 504-509.

46. Aragaw K (2005) Salmonella in Apparently Healthy Slaughtered Swine in Addis Ababa, Ethiopia.MSc thesis Addis Ababa University, Faculty of Veterinary Medicine, DebreZeit, Ethiopia.

47. Helms M, Vastrup P, Gerner-Smidt, Molbak K (2003) Short and long term mortality associated with foodborne bacterial gastrointestinal infections: registry based study. BMJ. 326: 1-5.

48. Beran H (1994) Hand book of Zoonoses Section A: bacterial, rickettsial, chlamydial and mycotic. USA CRC Press, pp: 289-300.

27

Novel Gene Mutations in Tunisian Isolate of Avian H9N2 Influenza Virus

Rim Aouini[1,2]*, Nacira Laamiri[1,2] and Abdeljelil Ghram[1]

[1]Laboratory of Epidemiology and Veterinary Microbiology, Pasteur Institute of Tunis, University Tunis El Manar, 13 Place Pasteur, Tunis- Belvedere, Tunisia
[2]Faculty of Sciences Bizerte, University of Carthage, Zarzouna Bizerte, Tunisia

Abstract

A new strain of H9N2 avian influenza virus (AIV) was isolated from suspected broiler flocks and characterized using RT-PCR and sequencing techniques which have shown new interesting mutations as compared to previously characterized Tunisian strains of major clinical importance. Reverse transcription-PCR, nucleotide sequencing, and GenBank BLAST database analyses of external and internal genes of the virus demonstrated that the new isolate, designated A/CK/TUN/145/12, has the ^{333}PSRSSR*GLF^{341} motif at the cleavage site of its hemagglutinin (HA), different from that described in the older Tunisian strains, which possess the motif ^{333}PARSSR*GLF^{34}, and others reported strains in the world. The presence of Leu at position 234 in the amino acid sequence of HA indicated the virus binding preference to the human cellular receptor α-2,6 sialic acid. Besides, such HA amino acid sequence showed two new mutations D280N and Y144S. The hemadsorption (HB) site of its neuraminidase (NA) did show three new mutations H441N, N342D and S331N in comparison to older Tunisian strains. Such mutations were reported for the highly pathogenic H5N2 subtype in Nigeria. Phylogenetic data allowed classification of the new Tunisian isolate in a new genetic group including the old Tunisian isolates.

Keywords: Characterization; Epidemiology; Phylogeny; Influenza virus

Abbreviations: AA: amino acid; AIV: Avian Influenza Virus; HA: Hemagglutinin; HB: Hemadsorption; HPAIV: High Pathogenic Avian Influenza Virus; LPAIV: Low Pathogenic Avian Influenza Virus; M: Matrix; NA: Neuraminidase; NP: Nucleoprotein; NS: Non Structural; PB2: Polymerase; PL: PDZ Ligand; RBS: Receptor Binding Site; RBD: RNA Binding Domain.

Introduction

The poultry sector is becoming an increasingly important agriculture sector, in Tunisia, This sector faces tough challenges due to viral infections in the region [1,2]. Influenza A viruses (IAV) belonging to the *Orthomyxoviridae* family, cause highly contagious respiratory diseases in chickens, leading to important economic losses related to mortality, severe egg drop and poor egg quality. The viral genome is a negative stranded RNA, made up of eight gene segments. These viruses have been divided into low pathogenic AI (LPAI) and high pathogenic AI (HPAI), on the basis of their capability to cause mild or severe disease in vulnerable birds, respectively. The subtypes H5, H7 and H9 cause respiratory and systemic diseases. The H9N2 subtype virus may infect chickens, turkeys, ducks and pigs and suspected to infect humans [3].

Phylogenetic analyses showed that avian H9N2 viruses are classified into three diverse groups: G1-like lineage, represented by G1 97, Y280-like lineage, represented by Y280 or A/Chicken/Beijing/1/94 (BJ 94) and Y439-like lineage, represented by A/Duck/Hong Kong/Y439/97 (Y439) [4]. Since 1998, a new common lineage of H9N2 viruses in eastern China is represented by the A/Chicken/Shanghai/F/98 lineage (F 98-like lineage) [5].

In Tunisia, where poultry industry is of great importance for its social and economic impacts, active surveillance of avian H9N2 virus and study of strain evolution is a great importance to effectively control the disease. The epizootiology of AIV in Tunisia is being documented. The disease has been reported since 2009 and the virus is still circulating causing severe economical losses. Thus, efforts are undertaken to better control the disease by isolating and typing AIV field strains that are very important not only for the study of emerging viruses and their evolution but also for adaptation of preventive measures.

Materials and Methods

Virus isolation

The H9N2 avian influenza virus was isolated and identified in 2012 during an avian influenza (AI) outbreak in the south of Tunisia. At least 10 cloacae and 10 trachea swab samples were collected from suspected chickens. Initial isolation was performed in 10-day-old specific-pathogen-free embryonated chicken eggs (ECE, inoculated via the allantoic route and incubated at 37°C for 72-96 h [6].

Hemagglutination inhibition test

Specific anti-H9N2 serum was prepared in chickens vaccinated with inactivated influenza vaccine (Nobilis H9N2-Intervet). Collected serum was titrated before its use in an inhibition hemagglutination test to confirm the identity of the isolated virus. The serum was heat treated at 56°C for 30 min and serially diluted in PBS (pH 7.4) in 96-well plate before adding an equal amount of 4HA units (25 μl) of A/Chicken/Tunisia/145/12 (H9N2) influenza virus in each well. After incubation for 30 min at room temperature, 25 μl of 1% chicken red blood cells were added to each well and the plate incubated for 30 min. A complete inhibition of hemagglutination indicates the identity of the virus tested (Table 1).

Viral nucleic acid extraction

Viral RNA was extracted using 200 μl of virus suspension following the Trizol method (Invitrogen, CA). The RNA was precipitated with

---

*Corresponding author: Rim Aouini, Laboratory of Epidemiology and Veterinary Microbiology, Institut Pasteur de Tunis, University of Tunis El Manar, 1002 Tunis-Belvedere, Tunisia, E-mail: rim_aouini@yahoo.fr

absolute ethanol, centrifuged and the final pellet suspended in 20 µl RNase-free water then stored at -80°C.

Viral RNA amplification

Two step RT-PCR techniques were carried out to amplify well defined regions of the six gene segments using segment-specific primers. The cDNA was synthesized using appropriate upstream primers with SuperScript™ II Reverse transcriptase (Invitrogen, CA) then amplified by PCR using a mixture made of 5 µl of cDNA, 2.5 µl of 10 × PCR buffer, 2.5 µl of 2.5 mM dNTPs, 0.5 µl Taq DNA polymerase (5 units/µl, Invitrogen), 1 µl of each primer (10 µM each) (Table 2) [7], 2 µl of 5 Mm MgCl$_2$ (Invitrogen, CA) and 17.5 µl RNase free water (BioBasic, CA). The PCR program was run as follows: 45°C for 30 min, 95°C for 10 min, 40 cycles of 95°C for 60 s, 58°C for 20 s (62°C for HA1, NA, PB2, and NS), 72°C for 1 min followed by 72°C for 10 min. The obtained PCR products were purified with QIA quick PCR purification kit (Qiagen).

Sequencing

The purified PCR products were then partially sequenced using Amersham ET Dye terminator kit and analyzed with ABI 3730 DNA sequencer (Perkin-Elmer Applied Biosystems).

Sequencing analyses

The Bio-Edit program 5.0.6 software and the ClustalW alignment algorithm (Version 1.83) were used to compare and align nucleotide sequences. Phylogenetic trees were constructed by MEGA5.01 program, version 3.65, with the neighbor-joining method using a grouping strength of 1000 bootstrap resembling. The Blast software and the Bio-Edit program were utilized to determine the sequence similarity between the Tunisian identified strains. The nucleotide sequences obtained were deposited in the GenBank data library under the accession numbers: KP058446, KP058447, KP271003, KP271004, KP271005 and KP772312. The amino acid residues were numbered

according to the HA sequences of Qu/HK/G1/97 (H9) with the GenBank accession number AF156378.

Results

Identification of AI virus isolate

The HA titer of the allantoic liquid of inoculated SPF embryonated chicken eggs was 512HA. The IH test allowed confirmation of the isolated virus as avian Influenza type A virus using a specific anti-H9N2 serum, showing a titer of 512 IH. The virus was further characterized using RT-PCR and sequencing.

Phylogenetic analysis of surface genes of H9N2 virus

To find out its genetic diversity, the isolated virus was amplified by RT-PCR and 6 out of its 8 gene segments were partially sequenced. These sequences were then aligned with different H9 viral sequences listed in the GenBank (Table 3).

The results showed that the viral HA gene was correlated to the Libyan and the Middle Eastern strains, especially A/Chicken/Libya/13VIR7225-5/2013, A/Chicken/Israel/1548/2006, A/Chicken/SaudiArabia582/2005, A/Chicken/Pakistan/47/2003. The HA and NA (neuraminidase) gene sequences showed high homology with Middle Eastern strains grouped in the G1 lineage, sharing the same ancestor with the isolate A/Quail/Hong Kong/G1/1997 (Table 4).

To study the evolutionary relationships between the new and the old Tunisian H9N2 isolates found in the Genbank (Table 3), phylogenetic analyses were carried out for the 6 considered viral gene segments (hemagglutinin (HA), neuraminidase (NA), polymerase (PB2), nucleoprotein (NP), matrix (M) and non structural (NS) genes) (Figures 1 and 2). The HA amino acid sequence of the newly identified strain A/Chicken/Tunisia/145/12 showed 95% to 99% concordance with that of other strains of the G1 lineage. Besides, the neuraminidase gene of this isolate (nucleotides 962 to 1372) clustered with the A/Qa/

Virus Name	Abbreviation	Host	HA titre	EID50/100 µl
A/Chicken/Tunisia/145/12	A/CK/TUN/145/12	Chicken	1/1024	10$^{6.75}$

Table 1: H9N2 virus isolated from infected chickens in Tunisia 2012.

Name	Sequence (5'- 3') a	Position	Expected products Size (pb)	Gene	Reference
AMF	CTTCTAACCGAGGTCGAAAC	7- 26	244	M	
AMR	AGGGCATTTTGGACAAAKCGTCTA	259-238		M	20
MF	CTCATGGAATGGCTAAAGACA	149-169	700	M	
MR	CGATCAADAATCCACAATATC	847-827		M	22
H9F	GAATCCAGATCTTTCCAGAC	426-445	384	HA	
H9R	CCATACCATGGGGCAATTAG	808-789		HA	23
NPF	CAGRTACTGGGCHATAAGRAC	1200-1220	326	NP	
NPR	GCA TTGTCTCCGAAGAAATAAG	1529-1510		NP	24
HAF1	GAATTGATTATTATTGGTCAGTA	710-732	550	HA	
HAR1	TCATCAATCT-TATTGTTGATCAT	1272-1249		HA	25
NAF	CTTGTTGGCGACACACCAAGRAA	961-983	410	NA	
NAR	GAGCCTGTTCCAT-AGGTACCTGA	1370-1348		NA	25
PB2F	TATTCAT-CRTCAATGATGTGGGA	1591-1613	540	PB2	
PB2R	GATGCTYAATGCTGGTCCATATC	2130-2108		PB2	25
NSF	AGCAAAAGCAGGGTGACAAA	1-20	890	NS	
NSR	AGTAGAAACAAGGGTGTTTT	890-871		NS	26

ªCodes for mixed bases positions: D=G/A/T, H=A/C/T, K=G/T, R=A/G, Y=C/T.

Table 2: Primer sequences as used in the RT-PCR.

References strains	Abbreviations	HA	NA	PB2	NP	M	NS
A/Chicken/Tunisia/145/12[a]	Ck/TUN/145/12	KP058446	KP058447	KP271005	KP271003	KP271004	KP772312
A/chicken/Tunisia/848/2011	Ck/TUN/848/11	JQ952591.1	JQ952595.1	-	-	-	-
A/turkey/Tunisia/2068/2010	Ck/TUN/2068/2010	JQ952589.1	JQ952593.1	-	-	-	-
A/chicken/Tunisia/2019/2010	Ck/TUN/2019/2010	JQ952588.1	JQ952592.1	-	-	-	-
A/chicken/Tunisia/345/2011	Ck/TUN/345/2011	JQ952590.1	JQ952594.1	-	-	-	-
A/migratory bird/Tunisia/51/2010	MB/TUN/51/10	JF323007.2	JF323009.2	JF323011.2	JF323013.2	JF323015.1	KF751661.1
A/chicken/Tunisia/12/2010	Ck/TUN/12/2010	JF323006.2	JF323008.2	JF323010.2	JF323012.2	JF323014.1	JF323016.1
A/chicken/Libya/13VIR7225-5/2013	CkLi13VIR7225513	KM244121.1	-	-	-	-	-
A/chicken/Israel/1548/2006	CkIs14806	FJ464729.1	-	-	-	FJ464611.1	-
A/chicken/Saudi Arabia/582/2005	AvSA58205	JX273556.1	-	-	-	-	-
A/avian/SaudiArabia/910135/2006	AvSA91013506	GU050287.1	-	GU050294.1	-	GU050288.1	GU050291.1
A/chicken/Pakistan/47/2003	CKPa4703	JX273552.1	-	-	-	-	-
A/chicken/Israel/182/2008	CkIs18208	GQ120549.1	-	-	-	-	-
A/chicken/Egypt/D4907A/2012	CkEgD4907A12	JX912984.1	-	-	-	KF881678.1	-
A/quail/UnitedArabEmirates/1819/2006	CkEmR181906	-	F188376.1	-	-	-	-
A/chicken/Dubai/339/2001	CkDu33901	-	KF188354.1	EF063556.1	-	-	EF063542.1
A/chicken/Dubai/383/2002	CkDu38302	-	EF063522.1	EF063557.1	-	-	EF063543.1
A/chicken/Dubai/339/2001	CkDu33901	-	EF063521.1	KF188349.1	-	-	EF063542.1
A/Hong Kong/1074/1997	QuHKG197	AF156378	GU053180.1	AJ289872.1	AF255743.1	-	-

[a]Viruses whose HA, NA, PB2, NP, M and NS genes were sequenced in the present study; N.D, not done; b, - No sequence data available

Table 3: Abbreviations used and GenBank accession numbers for H9N2 Avian Influenza virus isolates included in the phylogenetic analyses.

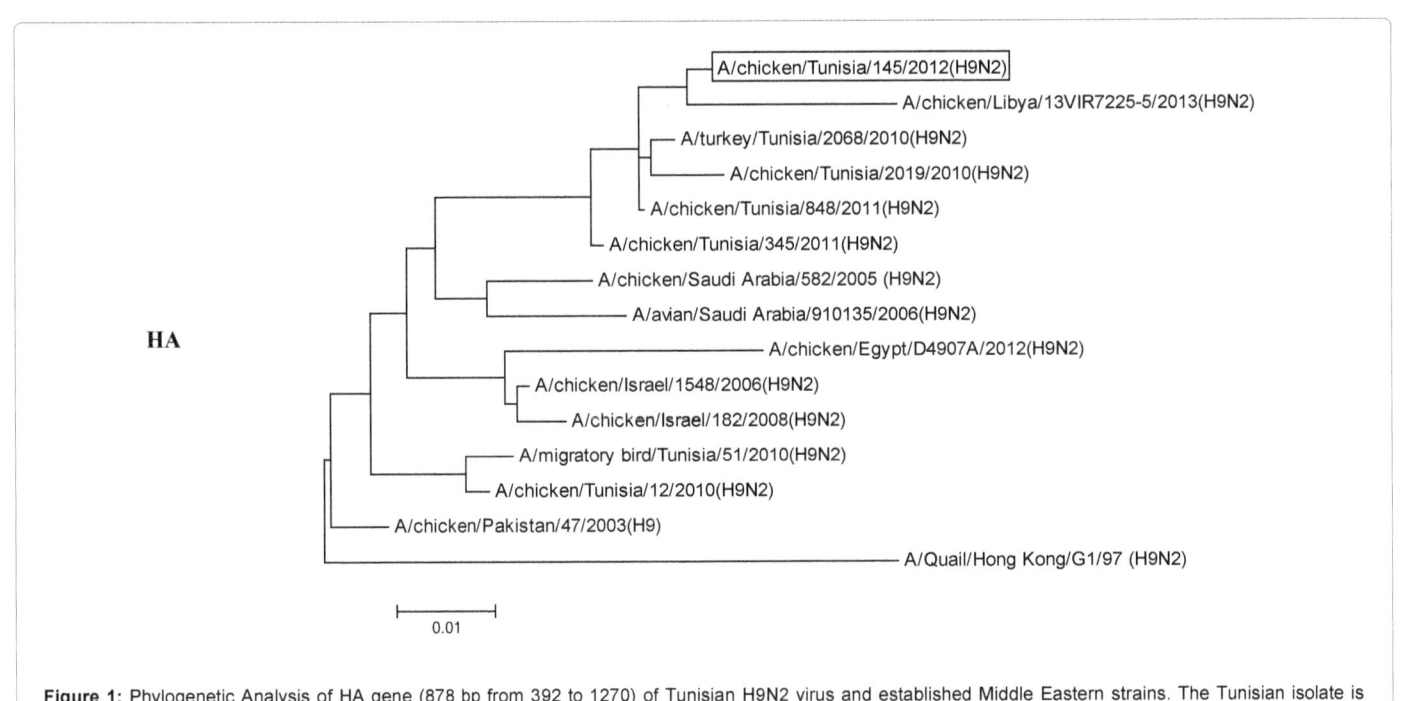

Figure 1: Phylogenetic Analysis of HA gene (878 bp from 392 to 1270) of Tunisian H9N2 virus and established Middle Eastern strains. The Tunisian isolate is framed.

HK/G1/97 lineage, as did isolates from Dubai, Hong Kong and United Arab Emirates.

Phylogenetic analyses of internal genes

Four internal genes (PB2, NP, M and NS) of the Tunisian H9N2 strain showed more than 91% nucleotide similarity with those of the Middle-Eastern strains isolated in 1997 and 2011 (Table 4). Phylogenetic studies of PB2 gene, using a 540- base-long nucleotide sequence (nucleotides 1591 to 2130) that codes the PB2 protein region between positions 530 and 710, showed a close similarity between the A/Ck/TUN/145/12 and the old Tunisian strains which have close

relationship with the Middle Eastern isolates (more than 93% identity) (Figure 3).

Analysis of NP gene of A/Ck/TUN/145/12 allowed its classification in the same genetic group as the old Tunisian genotypes (Figure 4), showing a percentage of similarity of 98 to 97% with A/Hong Kong/1074/99 (H9N2) and A/chicken/China/27402/1997 (H5N1), respectively (Table 4).

The matrix gene (regions of the overlapping reading frames of M1-M2, nucleotides 7 to 845) of A/Ck/TUN/145/12 strain (Figure 5)

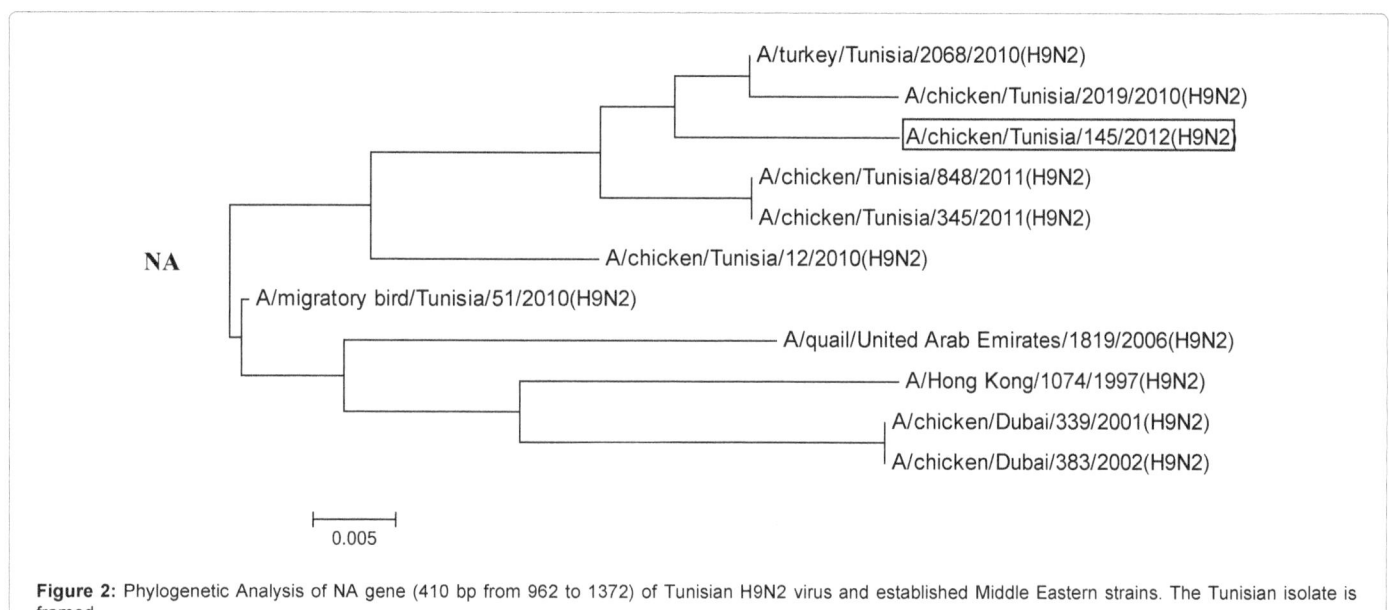

Figure 2: Phylogenetic Analysis of NA gene (410 bp from 962 to 1372) of Tunisian H9N2 virus and established Middle Eastern strains. The Tunisian isolate is framed.

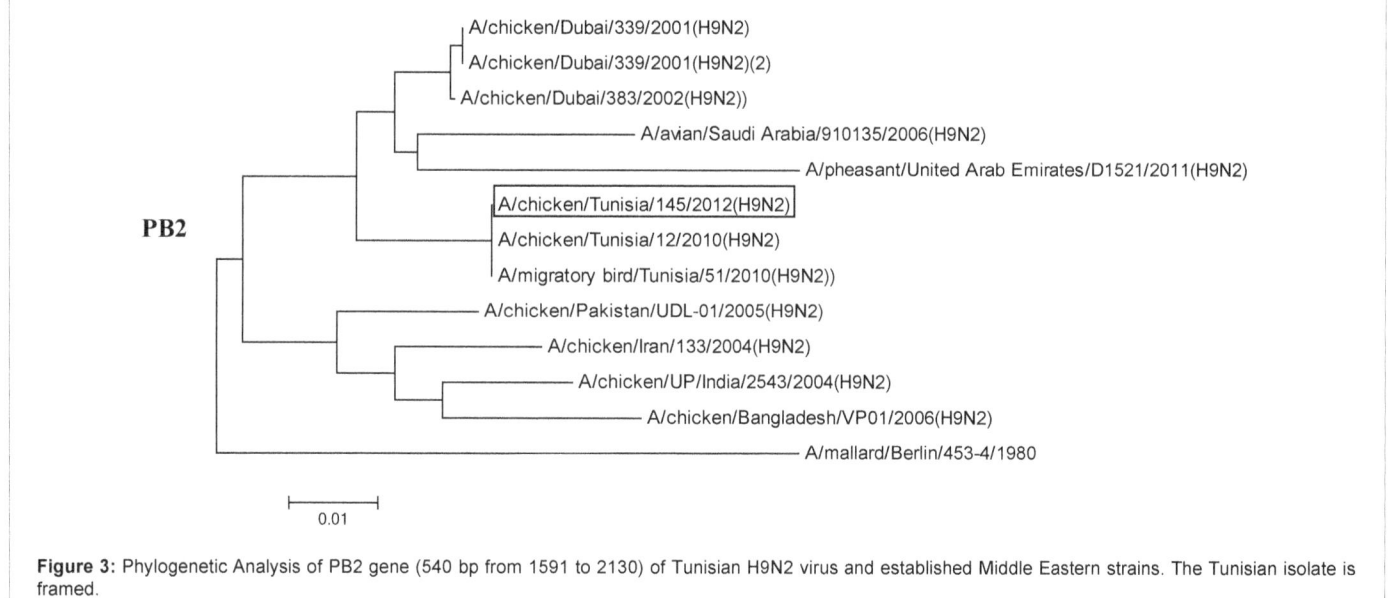

Figure 3: Phylogenetic Analysis of PB2 gene (540 bp from 1591 to 2130) of Tunisian H9N2 virus and established Middle Eastern strains. The Tunisian isolate is framed.

showed a close relationship with that of Middle Eastern isolates (96% to 98% similarity) and full identity with the Tunisian isolates previously identified. It has also demonstrated 96.93% and 96% similarities with other subtypes like A/Ck/KHNC/100/04 (H7N3) and A/Environment/Hong Kong/258/1997 (H5N1) strains, respectively.

The NS gene (nucleotides 1591 to 2130) of Ck/TUN/145/12 strain demonstrated an evidence of a reassortment with other viral subtypes, showing 96% similarity with that of A/mallard/Sweden/3240/2003(H8N4) strain (Figure 6).

Genetic characteristics of surface glycoproteins

Hemagglutinin: The molecular determinants of pathogenicity and virulence of influenza virus are the HA1/HA2 connecting (cleavage site) polypeptide sequence, the specific amino acid (aa) residues at the receptor binding site (RBS), and the presence or absence of glycosylation sites around the receptor binding site.

The HA cleavage site motif of the sequence of our isolate A/Ck/TUN/145/12 was ^{333}PSRSSR* GLF^{341}. Interestingly, this motif is different from that of other Tunisian H9N2 and Asian H9N2 viruses including those described in Libya, Israel, Pakistan, Saudi Arabia and Egypt which have the motif ^{333} PARSSR* GLF^{341}, meaning that our Tunisian isolate carries amino acid substitution in the cleavage site at position A334S.

Residues at positions 110, 161, 163, 191, 198, 234, 235 and 236 are known to be the major components of the receptor binding site of HA molecule [6]. Our isolate showed conservation of residues P110, W161, T163, H191, A198 and I235 in the receptor binding pocket in comparison with those of the old Tunisian isolates and other isolates from all over the world. However, the left edge (amino acid residues at

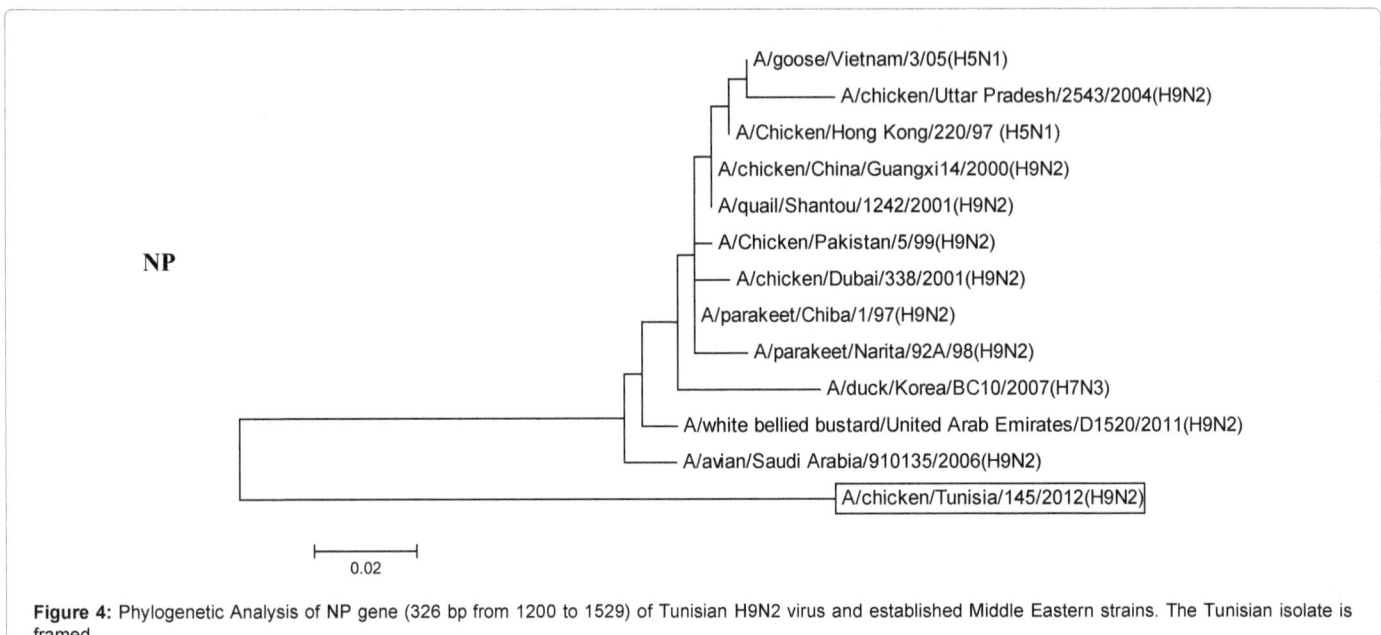

Figure 4: Phylogenetic Analysis of NP gene (326 bp from 1200 to 1529) of Tunisian H9N2 virus and established Middle Eastern strains. The Tunisian isolate is framed.

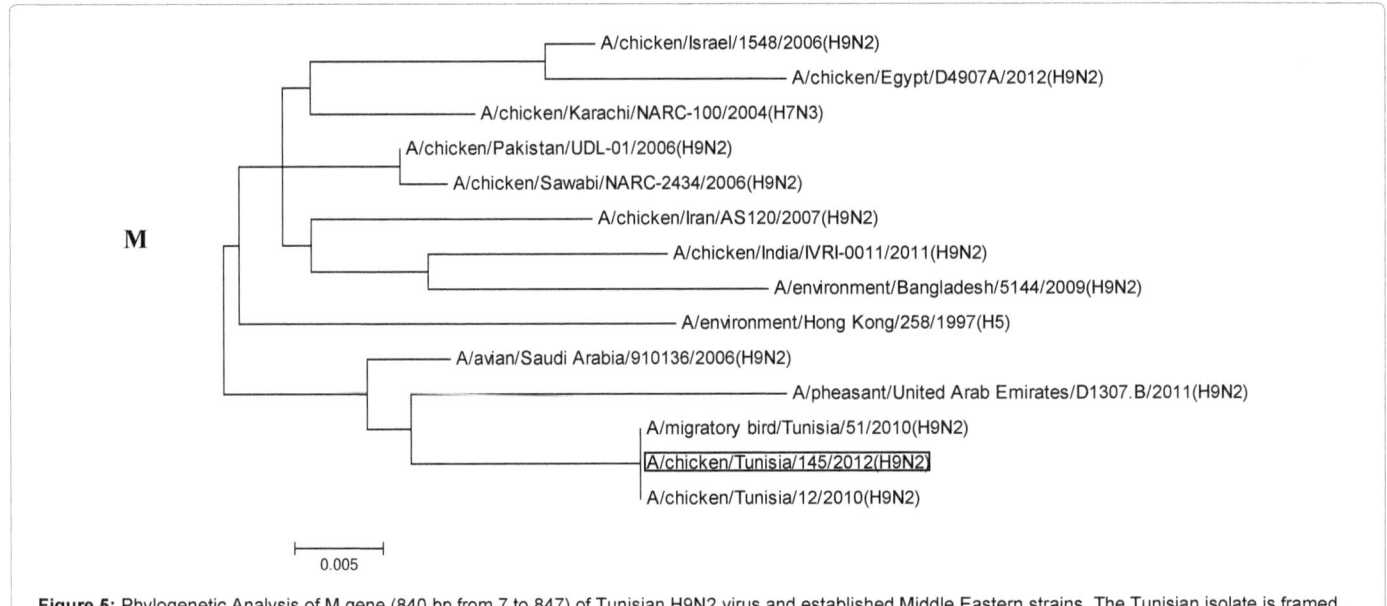

Figure 5: Phylogenetic Analysis of M gene (840 bp from 7 to 847) of Tunisian H9N2 virus and established Middle Eastern strains. The Tunisian isolate is framed.

positions 232-236) of the binding pocket motif was: NGLIG and the A/CK/TUN/145/12 H9N2 strain carried the amino acid substitutions (Y144S) and (D280N). The Y144 and D280 residues are shown to be engaged in both receptor binding and ligand interaction. Receptor mutations at this position (Y144S) showed dramatic impact on binding affinity and functionality [8].

Analysis of HA protein sequences indicated that the Tunisian H9N2 isolate has many potential glycosylation sites with an N-X-T/S motif (X can be any amino acid except Proline). In fact, X could be an S (Serine) at position 298-300 (NST) or any other substitutions as indicated in Table 5.

HB site of Neuraminidase: The HB site of neuraminidase is situated on the NA surface, far from the enzymatic site. Analysis of

the neuraminidase and the framework sites of NA protein showed mutations in aa residues in the 3 loops that interact directly with the sialic acid. In the loop carrying amino acids at positions 367-370-372, three S (Serine) were substituted by KLA, respectively; the new substitutions H441N, N342D and S331N were also found. On the other hand, the framework site contained R371, A372, N402, and E425 (Table 6). The Tunisian isolate presented the same mutations found in previously characterized Tunisian strains except for the three new mutations (H441N, N342D and S331N).

Molecular characteristics of internal proteins: The novel Tunisian H9N2 strain has shown the same PB2, M, NP and NS protein sequences as the Tunisian isolates previously identified showing the same described mutations [9].

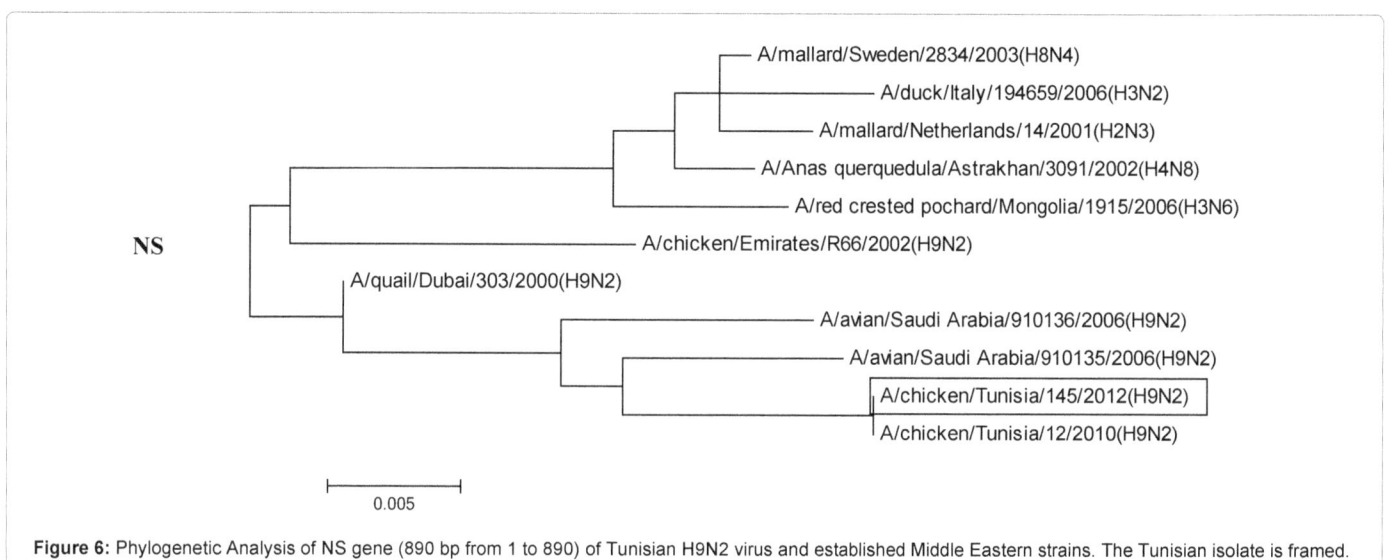

Figure 6: Phylogenetic Analysis of NS gene (890 bp from 1 to 890) of Tunisian H9N2 virus and established Middle Eastern strains. The Tunisian isolate is framed.

Gene	Nucleotide similarity	%	Lineage
PB2	A/chicken/Tunisia/12/2010(H9N2) A/chicken/Dubai/338/2001(H9N2) A/chicken/Dubai/383/2002 (H9N2) A/quail/Dubai/303/2000(H9N2) A/chicken/Pakistan/UDL-01/2005(H9N2) A/chicken/Iran/68/2006(H9N2) A/environment/Bangladesh/8463/2010(H9N2)	100 98 97 96 95 94 93	G1
HA	A/chicken/Tunisia/848/2011(H9N2) A/chicken/Libya/13VIR7225-5/2013(H9N2) A/avian/Libya/RV35D/2006 (H9N2) A/chicken/Israel/1548/2006 (H9N2) A/chicken/Pakistan/47/2003 (H9N2)	99 98 97 96 95	G1
NP	A/chicken/Tunisia/12/2010(H9N2) A/Hong Kong/1074/99(H9N2) A/chicken/China/27402/1997(H5N1)	100 98 97	G1
NA	A/chicken/Tunisia/2019/2010(H9N2) A/chicken/Tunisia/848/2011(H9N2) A/chicken/Tunisia/12/2010(H9N2) A/migratory bird/Tunisia/51/2010 (H9N2) A/quail/United Arab Emirates/1819/2006 (H9N2) A/white bellied bustard/United Arab Emirates/D1520/2011 A/quail/Shantou/1912/2001 A/Hong Kong/1074/1997(H9N2) A/quail/Shantou/308/2003 (H9N2) A/chicken/Iran/450/2001(H9N2)	99 98 96 95 94 93 92 92 91 91	G1
M	A/migratory bird/Tunisia/51/2010(H9N2) A/chicken/Tunisia/12/2010(H9N2) A/avian/Saudi Arabia/910135/2006(H9N2) A/chicken/Karachi/NARC-100/2004(H7N3) A/chicken/India/IVRI-0011/2011(H9N2)	100 100 98 97 96	G1
NS	A/chicken/Tunisia/12/2010(H9N2) A/avian/Saudi Arabia/910135/2006(H9N2) A/chicken/Emirates/R66/2002(H9N2) A/mallard/Sweden/3240/2003(H8N4)	100 98 97 96	G1

Table 4: Similarity indices of the Tunisian H9N2 (A/CK/TUN/145/12) genes at the nucleotide levels.

Virus	RBS 110	RBS 161	RBS 163	RBS 191	RBS 198	RBS 202	RBS 203	Left-edge of Binding pocket 232-236	Connecting peptide aa sequence 152 333	Glycosylation site at position 338 168
A/Ck/TUN/145/12	P	W	T	H	A	L	Y	N G L I G	P S R S S R	+
A/Ck/TUN/12/2010	P	W	T	H	A	L	Y	N G L I G	P A R S S R	+
A/Ck/TUN/345/2011	P	W	T	H	A	L	Y	N G L I G	P A R S S R	+
A/Tu/TUN/2068/2010	P	W	T	H	A	L	Y	N G L I G	P A R S S R	+
A/Av/Libya/13VIR7225-5/2013	P	W	T	H	A	L	Y	N G L I G	P S K S S R	+
A/Ck/Israel/1548/2006	P	W	T	H	T	L	Y	N G L I G	P A R S S R	+
A/Av/SA/582/2005	P	W	T	H	T	L	Y	N G L I G	P A R S S R	+
A/Av/SA/910135/2006	P	W	T	H	A	L	Y	N G L I G	P A R S S R	+
A/Qu/HK/G1/97	P	W	T	H	E	L	Y	N D L Q G	P A R S S R	+
A/CK/TUN/848/2011	P	W	T	H	A	L	Y	N G L I G	P A R S S R	+
A/CK/TUN/51/2010	P	W	T	H	A	L	Y	N G Q I G	P A R S S R	+
A/Ck/Pak/47/2003	P	W	T	H	A	L	Y	N G L I G	P A R S S R	+
A/Ck/Is/182/2008	P	W	T	H	T	L	Y	N G L I G	P A R S S R	+
A/Ck/Eg/D4907A/2012	P	W	T	H	A	L	Y	N G L I G	P A R S S R	+

-/+ absence or presence of the glycosylation site.

Table 5: Analysis of the amino acid sequences of the HA protein of the Tunisian isolate A/Ck/TUN/145/12 in comparison with old Tunisian and reference strains.

Virus	Neuraminidase active site (HB) 366. 373	Framework Site NA 399. 406	Framework Site NA 431. 433	Framework Site NA 425
A/Ck/TUN/145/2012	IKKDLRAG	DSDNWSGY	PKE	E
A/Ck/TUN/2019/2010	IKKDLRAG	DSDNWSGY	PKE	E
A/Tu/TUN/2068/2010	IKKDLRAG	DSDNWSGY	PKE	E
A/Ck/TUN/848/2011	IKKDLRAG	DRDDWSGY	PKE	E
A/Ck/TUN/345/2011	IKKDLRAG	DRDDWSGY	PKE	E
A/Ck/TUN/12/2010	IKKDLRAG	DSDNWSGY	-	-
A/MB/TUN/51/2010	IKKDLRAG	DSDNWSGY	PQE	E
A/Ck/Du/339/2001	IKKDLRAG	DS - - - - - -	PQE	E
A/Ck /Du/338/2002	IKKDLRAG	DSDNWSGY	PQE	-
A/Ck/Em/1819/2006	IKEDLRAG	DSDNWSGY	PQE	E
A/Ck/HK/1074/1997	IKKDSRAG	DSDNWSGY	PQE	E

(-)=gap

Table 6: Analysis of the amino acid sequences of the NA protein of the Tunisian isolate in comparison with older Tunisian and reference strains.

Discussion

The study of the six genes of Tunisian H9N2 subtype of avian influenza reported, for the first time, new mutations that are not found in previously described Tunisian strains. Considering the sequences and the phylogeny analyses of Middle Eastern and older Tunisian viruses, it appeared that they are closely related and represent a single sub-lineage, the G1-like lineage, indicating similar origin. It might reflect geographical parameters responsible of virus restriction in these areas.

The genetic data of H9N2 subtype circulating in Tunisian poultry farms are presented. The results revealed that H9N2 virus infection is well established in many endemic areas of the country and allowed the characterization of our strain from a flock in southern of Tunisia. Thus, understanding the genetic and the biological characteristics of circulating H9N2 virus can give more comprehensive vision on the biology and the ecology of H9N2 virus, and the capacity of migratory birds to disperse AI viruses. Although infected birds might be able to spread the virus over short distances, during periods of cold weather, experiments in which birds are subjected to physiologic stresses associated with migration are needed to determine their capacity to spread virus over long distances. Indirect estimations of virus dispersal derived from knowledge of bird migrations could also provide complementary information related to the spread of avian influenza viruses [10].

The Blast analysis (NCBI) of the nucleotide sequences of HA and NA genes showed that A/Ck/TUN/145/12 is the closest strain (more than 92% identity) to the Middle Eastern isolates belonging to the G1-like lineage of H9N2 subtype.

The results of phylogenetic analyses were totally in accordance with blast data, and confirmed that our isolate fall, along the Middle Eastern isolates, into one cluster in relation to the G1 lineage; a result that may indicate that both strains have the same origin.

Based on the deduced amino acid sequences, the HA1-HA2 connecting peptides of the Tunisian H9N2 isolate did not harbor multiple basic amino acids with the motif PSRSSR/GL which is not exactly as found for the newly isolated H9 viruses in Middle East, having the motif PARSSR/GL [11,12]. A new substitution of Alanine, a non polar amino acid, by Serine, a polar amino acid, at position 334 is noticed. The biological significance and the role of such substitution are not yet known. This may reveal the LPAI nature of H9N2 strain, despite a motif identical to the RX RYK-R required for the highly pathogenic H5 and H7 subtypes [13]; noting that such new mutation was also found in highly pathogenic H5N2 subtype in Nigeria [14].

These genetic results indicated that our H9N2 virus may have the capacity to acquire basic amino acids in HA connecting peptide sequence, required to become highly pathogenic through the addition of a single basic amino acid. Moreover, A/Ck/TUN/145/12 possesses a Leu (L) at position 234 in its HA1 portion; the receptor binding site (RBS) residue being essential for the transmission of the H9N2 viruses in ferrets [13,15,16]. Besides, Q234L substitution, found in G1 lineage isolated in Hong Kong, was shown to allow H9N2 viruses to infect non ciliated cells and to grow more efficiently in human airway epithelial cell cultures, resulting in the increase of the severity of human infection [13].

Antigenic and phylogenetic analyses of the Tunisian isolate demonstrated that its surface glycoproteins are related to those of A/Qa/HK/G1/97 lineage, with the highest homology with A/chicken/Libya/13VIR7225-5/2013(H9N2) (98%), A/chicken/Israel/1548/2006 (96%) and A/chicken/Pakistan/47/2003 (H9N2) (95%) viruses. The two new mutations D280N and Y144S in HA gene and their significance are not yet known.

Three new mutations H441N, N342D and S331N are found in NA gene. The N342D mutation was found in the NA gene of H1N1 and H3N2 avian influenza viruses in Japan [14,15]. This may indicate the capacity of H9N2 virus to pass to humans. Besides, a potential additional glycosylation site was discovered at position 331 of NA gene in A/CK/TUN/145/2012 (S331N mutation); such mutation was also detected in H5N2 Nigerian isolate in 2007 [12]. The significance of H441N mutation is not known, yet. Therefore, all these new mutations may contribute to the change of a low pathogenic to a high pathogenic avian influenza H9N2 virus.

The Q432K substitution in NA gene is similar to that observed in other identified Tunisian strains. But, the biological meaning of this mutation is not known. All other mutations found in previous Tunisian strains are absent in A/CK/TUN/145/2012 isolate.

The E627K mutation in PB2 gene contributes to higher polymerase activity of influenza virus [4]. The PB2 E627K mutation has shown, *in vitro*, a promoting effect on virus growth in mammalian but not in avian cells [16].

The M1 protein showed a V15I substitution in all H9N2 lineages [17]. When the complete genome phenotypes of high-pathogenic strains were compared to those of low pathogenic ones, 5 amino acid differences were found and correlated with high-pathogenic strain phenotype. One of these changes was seen in M1 (V15I) of our strain, a change that has also been found in PR34 but not in Brevig18 strains [18].

Recently, NS1 protein of avian influenza A viral was shown to be a type I interferon (IFN) antagonist which plays a major role in viral pathogenesis [19]. Molecular analysis demonstrated that our isolates contain a NS1 protein with 230aa in length, typical of H9N2 viruses. In its RNA- binding domain of NS1, A/Ck/TUN/145/2012 isolate has incorporated R38 and K41 amino acids, which are shown to be critical for RNA binding. Similarly, amino acid residues P31, D34, R35, G45, R46, T49 and D55 also mediate NS1-dsRNA interaction and residue D55 is situated within the third alpha- helix (residues 54-70) of the dsRNA-binding domain RBD (residues 1-73) of NS1 [20]. However, NS1 D55G may stabilize the coiled-coiled helical structure. The old Ck/TUN/12/2010 Tunisian strain showed an Asp (N) at position 217 which is also found in our A/CK/TUN/145/12 strain but differs from other H9N2 strains, showing a K at this position. The biological significance of this substitution is not known yet. However, the Ck/TUN/145/2012 isolate didn't show the five amino acid deletion

(80TIAS84) already described for avian strains isolated in 2001 in Hong Kong; their significance being still not understood [21]. Finally, our H9N2 Tunisian strain showed a PL motif "GSEV" as previously found in Tunisian strains isolated in 2010; the biological signification of this motif is not yet known [22]. Interestingly, the E227G mutation in NS1 introduces an S70I mutation into nuclear export protein.

Acknowledgements

This work was supported by the Institut Pasteur de Tunis and the Ministry of Higher Education and Scientific Research (LR11IP03).

Disclosure

There is no conflict of interest.

References

1. Bourogâa H, Hellal I, Hassen J, Fathallah I, Ghram A (2012) S1 gene sequence analysis of new variant isolates of avian infectious bronchitis virus in Tunisia. Vet Med Res Rep 3: 41-48.

2. Tombari W, Paul M, Bettaieb J, Larbi I, Nsiri J, et al. (2013) Risk factors and characteristics of low pathogenic avian influenza virus isolated from commercial poultry in Tunisia. PloS one 8: e53524.

3. Kang N, Chen M, Bi FY, Chen MM, Tan Y (2016) First Positive Detection of H9 Subtype of Avian Influenza Virus Nucleic Acid in Aerosol Samples from Live Poultry Markets in Guangxi, South of China. Chin Med J 129: 1371-1373.

4. Zhang H, Li X, Guo J, Li L, Chang C, et al. (2014) The PB2 E627K mutation contributes to the high polymerase activity and enhanced replication of H7N9 influenza virus. Journal General Virology 95: 779-786.

5. Xie Z, Pang YS, Liu J, Deng X, Tang X, et al. (2006) A multiplex RT-PCR for detection of type A influenza virus and differentiation of avian H5, H7, and H9 hemagglutinin subtypes. Mol. Cell. Probes 20: 245-249.

6. Tombari W, Nsiri J, Larbi I, Guerin JL, Ghram A (2011) Genetic evolution of low pathogenicity H9N2 avian influenza viruses in Tunisia: acquisition of new mutations. Virol J 8: 467.

7. Amir B, Wernery U, Ilyushina N, Webster RG (2007) Characterization of avian H9N2 influenza viruses from United Arab Emirates 2000-2003. Virology 361: 45-55.

8. Lundström L, Kuhn B, Beck J, Borroni E, Wettstein JG, et al. (2009) Mutagenesis and molecular modeling of the orthosteric binding site of the mGlu2 receptor determining interactions of the group II receptor antagonist H-HYDIA. Chem Med Chem 4: 1086-1094.

9. Homayounimehr AR, Dadras H, Shoushtari A, Pourbakhsh SA (2010) Sequenceand phylogenetic analysis of the haemagglutinin genes of H9N2 avian influenza viruses isolated from commercial chickens in Iran. Trop Anim Health Prod 42: 1291-1297.

10. Kilpatrick AM, Chmura AA, Gibbons DW, Fleischer RC, Marra PP, et al. (2006) Predicting the global spread of H5N1 avian influenza. Proc Natl Acad Sci 103: 19368-19373.

11. Gaidet N, Cattoli G, Hammoumi S, Newman SH, Hagemeijer W, et al. (2009) Evidence of Infection by H5N2 Highly Pathogenic Avian Influenza Viruses in Healthy Wild Waterfowl. Plos Medicine 4: e1000127.

12. Haghighat Jahromi M, Asasi K, Nili H, Dadras H, Shooshtari AH (2008) Coinfection of avian influenza virus (H9N2 subtype) with infectious bronchitis live vaccine. Arch Virol 153: 651-655.

13. Wan H, Sorrell EM, Song H, Hossain MJ, Ramirez-Nieto G, et al. (2008) Replication and transmission of H9N2 influenza viruses in ferrets: evaluation of pandemic potential. PLoS ONE 3: e2923.

14. Dapat IC, Dapat C, Baranovich T, Suzuki Y, Kondo H, et al. (2012). Genetic Characterization of Human Influenza Viruses in the Pandemic (2009–2010) and Post-Pandemic (2010–2011) Periods in Japan. PloS one 7: e36455.

15. Dapat C, Suzuki Y, Kon M, Tamura T, Saito R, et al. (2010) Phylogenetic Analysis of an Off-Seasonal Influenza Virus A (H3N2) in Niigata, Japan. Jpn J Infect Dis 64: 237-241.

16. De Jong RM, Stockhofe-Zurwieden N, de Boer-Luijtze EA, Ruiter SJ, de Leeuw OS (2013) Rapid emergence of a virulent PB2 E627K variant during adaptation of highly pathogenic avian influenza H7N7 virus to mice. Virol J 10: 276.

17. Jakhesara SJ, Bhatt VD, Patel NV, Prajapati KS, Joshi GC (2014). Isolation and characterization of H9N2 influenza virus isolates from poultry respiratory disease outbreak. Springer Plus 3: 196.

18. Perdue ML, García M, Senne Fraire M (1997) Virulence-associated sequence duplication at the hemagglutinin cleavage site of avian influenza viruses. Virus Res 49: 173-186.

19. Basler CF, Reid AH, Dybing JK, Janczewski TA, Fanning TG (2001) Sequence of the 1918 pandemic influenza virus nonstructural gene (NS) segment and characterization of recombinant viruses bearing the 1918 NS genes. Proc Natl Acad Sci 98: 2746-2751.

20. Wang W, Riedel K, Lynch P, Chien CY, Montelione GT, et al. (1999) RNA binding by the novel helical domain of the influenza virus NS1 protein requires its dimer structure and a small number of specific basic amino acids. RNA 5: 195-205.

21. Long JX, Peng DX, Liu YL, Wu YT, Liu XF (2008) Virulence of H5N1 avian influenza virus enhanced by a 15-nucleotide deletion in the viral nonstructural gene. Virus Genes 36: 471-480.

22. Agustin P, Digard P (2002) The influenza virus nucleoprotein: a multifunctional RNA-binding protein pivotal to virus replication. J Gen Virol 83: 723-734.

28

Abundance Detection and Molecular Characterization of *Toxoplasma gondii* by SAG1 Gene in Rodents and Cattle of Golestan Province, Northeast of Iran

Javid Sadraie and Ehsan Shariat Bahadory*

Medical University of Tarbiat Modaress, Tehran, Iran

Abstract

Background: *Toxoplasma* parasite is from Toxoplasmatidea family that initially was seen in *ctinodactylus gondii* rodent. *Toxoplasma* parasites that extracted from different rodents are same in immunologic and morphologic characteristics but have differences in pathogenicity and genotypes in mice. The rodents and cattle are most reservoir hosts in environment that by attention of human environment vicinity to cattle and rodent's environment causes *Toxoplasma* dispersion in that area. The aim of this study was Molecular detection of *Toxoplasma gondii* in rodents and cattle of Golestan province, northeast of Iran.

Materials and methods: In this study we collected 285 mice and 185 cattle tissues from Golestan forest and extracted brains of rodents and hearts tissues of cattle to obtain DNA from these tissues. We divided these rodents to 4 groups and then detected the positive samples by PCR method.

Results: In this study we found 68 samples of these rodents were positive for SAG1 gene. 38 samples were *Ratus ratus*, 10 samples were *Ratus norvegicus*, 10 samples were *Mus musculus* and 10 samples were *Rombumys opimus*. Also 81 samples of cattle hearts were positive for SAG1 gene.

Conclusion and discussion: in this study we found that the different types of rodents were responsible to spread of toxoplasmosis, also SAG1 gene was very useful marker to detect toxoplasmosis in rodents of northeast area of Iran. Also in this area the numbers of toxoplasmosis cattle were in very high range.

Keywords: Toxoplasmosis; SAG1 gene; PCR; Golestan forest; Rodents; Cattle

Introduction

Toxoplasma gondii is an intracellular parasite that infected many hosts in Iran, including human, rodents, cats and domestic animals. Because domestic and feral cats are the natural definitive host, they play an important role in disseminating of toxoplasmosis [1-5]. Rodents are very important reservoir in dissemination of toxoplasmosis in Iran. The brain of rodents and the heart of cattle are the most important tissues that can infect by toxoplasmosis. Toxoplasmosis infection causes tissue cysts in these organs of rodents and cattle. The major gene that extracted from these organs to detect toxoplasmosis is SAG1 gene [5-10].

Toxoplasmosis infection pathway is eating of infected tissues from rodents by cats or uncooked meats from domestic animals to human, then laying Oocysts from cats in environments to dissemination of infection to human or domestic animals. The major disease of this parasite in human is encephalitis or brain disorders [11-13]. Primary routes of acute human *T. gondii* infection include ingestion of tissue cysts in undercooked, contaminated meat, congenital infection through the placenta, and ingestion of Oocysts from soil, water, or cat litter. Oocysts are shed in cat feces and can remain viable in soil and water samples for months to years. The infected rodents are the main food for cats, and this cycle is the important cause of spreading toxoplasmosis infection. My purpose was the abundance detection of toxoplasmosis in rodents and cattle of Golestan province using SAG1 gene in brain and heart tissues [14-18].

Materials and Methods

Different regions of Golestan province have different climate and are notably heterogeneous. Northern parts are located in the arid and semi-arid climate, southern parts show a mountainous climate, and central and southern west parts have a moderate Mediterranean climate (Weather Centre Hashem). 185 cattle were collected from 20 villages of 5 towns locating in different climates of Golestan province. Also rodents were collected from Golestan forest. This study was done on March to September 2016. Because of this study was based on molecular detection; we did not use other examinations for example histopathology examinations.

Preparation of samples

We collected 285 mice from Golestan forest and 185 cattle hearts from 20 villages. Then brains and hearts of mice and cattle were removed. These organs were fixed in 95% Ethanol, and preserved in 4°C until DNA extraction. These rodents divided in 4 groups: (*Rattus rattus*, *Rattus norvegicus*, *Mus musculus* and *Rombomys opimus*) (Table 1).

DNA extraction

To extraction genomic DNA, we cut approximately 3 g of brain and heart tissues by DNG/proteinase K method from Sinacolon company and eluted into 50 µl DDH2O according to the manufacturer's

***Corresponding author:** Ehsan Shariat Bahadory, PhD of Medical Parasitology, Medical University of Tarbiat Modaress, Tehran, Iran
E-mail: ehsanshariat63@gmail.com

Rodents type	Numbers
Rattus rattus	130
Rattus norvegicus	45
Mus musculus	60
Rombomys opimus	50

Table 1: The total samples of rodents divided in 4 groups [14-18].

Materials	Volume	Final concentration
Master Mix	7.5 µl	2X
DNA Sample	2 µl	10-100 ng/µl
Work Primer	1 µl	20 pmol
Distilled water	4.5 µl	-
Total	15.0 µl	-

Table 2: PCR substrates [14-18].

Rodents type	Numbers	Numbers of positive
Rattus rattus	130	38
Rattus norvegicus	45	10
Mus musculus	60	10
Rombomys opimus	50	10

Table 3: Total samples and positive samples for SAG1 gene [14-18].

recommendations. A PCR targeting the *T. gondii* SAG1 gene was performed to detect possible infection with T. gondii. DNA samples giving positive SAG1 amplification were then used for genetic characterization.

We cut 3 g of tissue into small places and placed the samples into a 1.5 ml sterile tube. Then added 180 µl (microliter) lyse buffer (pepsin) to homogenization and 400 microliter (DNG/proteinase K) and then homogenized the samples. If the sample size was larger than 3 g we should increase the amount of lyse buffer proportionally.

Added 20 µl proteinase K to the samples. Then mixed immediately by shaking for 20 seconds. Then incubated at 60°C for 1 hour to lyse samples. If tissue was difficult to lyse, we increased the incubation time to 2-3 hours. Then inverted the samples every 10-15 minutes. Then we added 300 microliter isopropanol to DNA precipitation. After 5-10 minutes we washed the tubes by 70% ethanol and finally we eluted the DNA by DDH20. The eluted DNA preserved in -20°C freezer until using PCR method to detection of infection. The purification of DNA was done with Nanodrop instrument.

PCR analysis for *T. gondii* SAG1 gene

To genetically identify the presence of KI-1 Tachyzoites in visceral organs, PCR analysis was performed to detect *Toxoplasma* SAG1 gene as a diagnostic gene. DNA extraction was performed using the DNeasy®Tissue kit (DNG Sinacolon). The primers were designed by BLAST method from NCBI site and produced by Pishgam Company.

Primer sequences were:

5´- GCTGTAACATTGAGCTCCTTGASTTCCTG-3´ for forward and

5´- CCGGAACAGTACTGATTGTTGTCTTGAG-3´ for reverse

Amplification of the SAG1 gene was completed in the following conditions: 1 cycle of 5 min at 95°C for initial denaturation followed by 30 cycles of 1 min at 95°C, 1 min at 62°C, and 3 min at 74°C. The best annealing temperature was 62°C. Amplification was performed using a DNA thermal cycler (Eppendorf instrument). PCR amplification products were examined in 1.5% agarose gels and confirmed by staining with Safe stain and visualized under Gel Doc using UV. The statistical surveys were done with SPSS 18 software (Table 2).

Results

In this study we found 68 samples of these rodents were positive for SAG1 gene. 38 samples were *Ratus ratus*, 10 samples were *Ratus norvegicus*, 10 samples were *Mus musculus* and 10 samples were *Rombumys opimus*. The samples were positive in 1180 bp location. Also 81 heart samples of cattle were positive for SAG1 gene. *Toxoplasma gondii* SAG1 gene after NCBI blast, complete cds (Table 3; Figures 1 and 2).

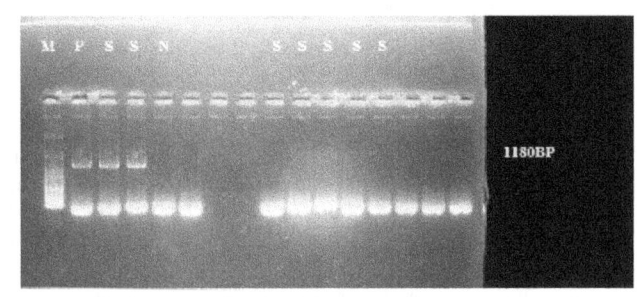

Figure 1: PCR conclusion for SAG1 gene. P: Positive control. M: Size marker. S: Sample. N: Negative control [14-18].

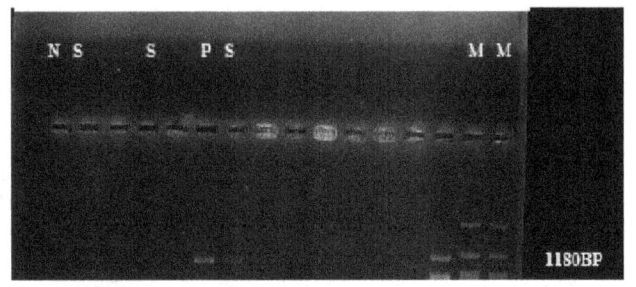

Figure 2: PCR conclusion for SAG1 gene. P: Positive control. M: Size marker. S: Sample. N: Negative control [14-18].

Origin:

1 acaatgtgca cctgtaggaa gctgtagtca ctgctgattc tcactgttct cggcaagggc

61 cgacgaccgg agtacagttt ttgtgggcag agccgttgtg cagctttccg ttgttctcgg

121 ttgtgtcaca tgtgtcattg tcgtgtaaac acacggttgt atgtcggttt cgctgcacca

181 cttcattatt tcttctggtt ttttgacgag tatgtttccg aaggcagtga gacgcgccgt

241 cacggcaggg gtgtttgccg cgcccacact gatgtcgttc ttgcgatgtg gcgttatggc

301 atcggatccc cctcttgttg ccaatcaagt tgtcacctgc ccagataaaa aatcgacagc

361 cgcggtcatt ctcacaccga cggagaacca cttcactctc aagtgcccta aaacagcgct

421 cacagagcct cccactcttg cgtactcacc caacaggcaa atctgcccag cgggtactac

481 aagtagctgt acatcaaagg ctgtaacatt gagctccttg attcctgaag cagaagatag

541 ctggtggacg ggggattctg ctagtctcga cacggcaggc atcaaactca cagttccaat

601 cgagaagttc cccgtgacaa cgcagacgtt tgtggtcggt tgcatcaagg gagacgacgc

661 acagagttgt atggtcacag tgacagtaca agccagagcc tcatcggtcg tcaataatgt

721 cgcaaggtgc tcctacggtg cagacagcac tcttggtcct gtcaagttgt ctgcggaagg

781 acccactaca atgaccctcg tgtgcgggaa agatggagtc aaagttcctc aagacaacaa

841 tcagtactgt tccgggacga cgctgactgg ttgcaacgag aaatcgttca aagatatttt

901 gccaaaatta actgagaacc cgtggcaggg taacgcttcg agtgataagg gtgccacgct

961 aacgatcaag aaggaagcat ttccagccga gtcaaaaagc gtcattattg gatgcacagg

1021 gggatcgcct gagaagcatc actgtaccgt gaaactggag tttgccgggg ctgcagggtc

1081 agcaaaatcg gctgcgggaa cagccagtca cgtttccatt cttgccatgg tgatcggact

1141 tattggctct atcgcagctt gtgtcgcgtg agtgattacc gttgtgc

These results showed that positive samples in 1180 bp location by SAG1 gene. These results obtained from GelDock instrument. Primer designation was done by BLAST software from NCBI site. In 130 samples from *Rattus rattus* 38 samples were positive, in 45 samples from *Rattus norvegicus* 10 samples were positives, in 60 samples from *Mus musculus* 10 samples were positive and finally in 50 samples from *Rombomys opimus* 10 samples were positives. Also 81 samples of heart tissues of cattle were positive for toxoplasmosis.

Figure 3 showed that 1=*Rattus rattus*, 2=*Rattus norvegicus*, 3=*Mus musculus* and 4=*Rombomys opimus*. Series 1 (blue) were total sample and series 2 (red) were positive samples. Positive samples bands detected on 1180 bp region [14-18]. These results obtained from GelDock instrument (Figure 4). Figure 5 showed that in the 185 heart tissues of cattle, 85 samples were positive for *Toxoplasma* SAG1 gene.

Discussion

Regarding to free living of rodents, cattle and also presence of them in large number in rural areas, obtaining data about *T. gondii* dynamic in rodents and cattle' population of rural area is critical for the establishment of monitoring programs [19-21]. My purpose of this study was abundance detection of toxoplasmosis in rodents and cattle of Golestan province using SAG1 gene. Toxoplasmosis is a zoonosis infection between rodents, cats, human and domestic animals. Rodents are main reservoir host for toxoplasmosis to infect feral cats and uncooked meat of domestic animals such as cattle or sheep can transfer toxoplasmosis to human. In both ways the human can plague with toxoplasmosis. In Golestan province, the population of rodents is higher than cattle but both animals have same role in spreading of toxoplasmosis. Climate characteristic of Golestan province is optimum for dissemination of toxoplasmosis. Prevalence of 40% *T. gondii* antibodies in stray cats in Sari, Northern Iran, has been reported by Sharif et al. They also survey anti *T. gondii* antibodies with latex agglutination test (LAT) on 100 serum samples collected from stray cats in five urban areas of Sari. Sari is located near Golestan province in North Iran and has humid climate which has been introduced suitable for *T. gondii* growth [22-25]. A study in Tabriz by Jamali clarified 36/2% *T. gondii* infection of cats by using dye test that differed with our methods. In this study most positive sampled has been belonged to Azadshahr villages and also Gorgan villages. Compare to Bandar-Turkmen,

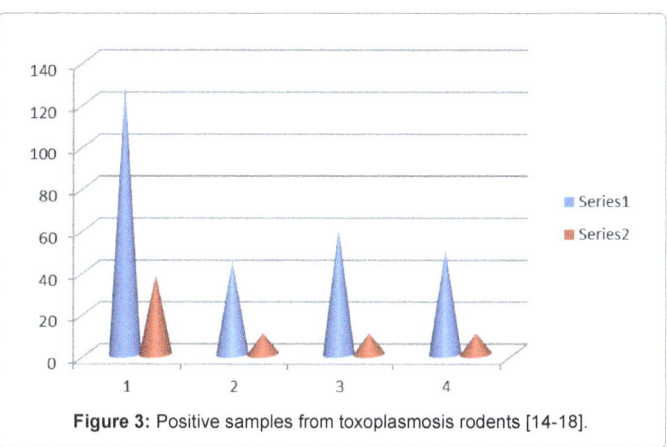
Figure 3: Positive samples from toxoplasmosis rodents [14-18].

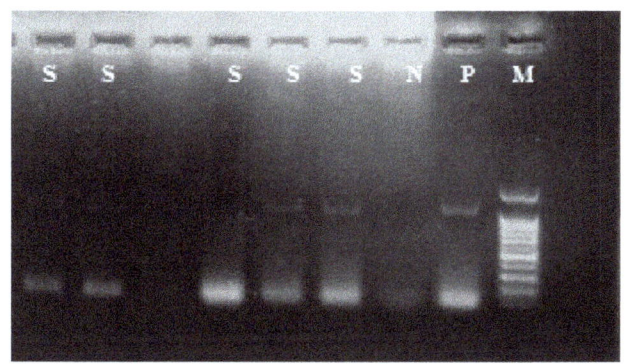
Figure 4: Positive samples of cattle heart tissues. M: Size marker. S: Samples. N: Negative control. P: Positive control.

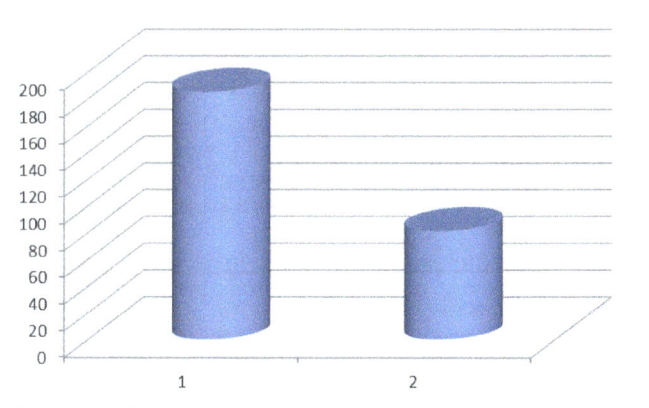
Figure 5: 1=Total heart samples of cattle. 2=Number of positives for toxoplasmosis cattle [14-18].

Gonbad and Aghghala that have semi-arid and arid climates, these two regions have humid climate. So detection of higher positive sample in Azadshahr villages and also Gorgan villages can be due to more suitable condition for growth of *T. gondii* oocyst in these areas. Also Mostafavi et al. reported highest prevalence of human toxoplasmosis, 70%, in humid regions of North Iran. Prevalence of *Toxoplasma gondii* antibodies in cats from Urmia, Northwest of Iran. In Sari by contrast, differences in *T. gondii* infection were detected between male stray cats and female stray cats. In 2013, Cong detected house sparrows toxoplasmosis in China, Khademvatan detected birds toxoplasmosis in southwest of Iran and Ortega found pigs toxoplasmosis in Mexico [22-26]. Most of the studies didn't reported significant different in *T. gondii* infection of two sexes and the role of sexuality in *T. gondii* exposure is not clear. In recent years had not any studies in rodents toxoplasmosis in Golestan area. In 2011, Hong did very important study in genotyping of cat's toxoplasmosis. In 2011, Dubey done a study in genotyping of zoonosis toxoplasmosis in USA. In 2012, Selseleh did a study in genotyping of Tehran rodent's toxoplasmosis by SAG1 gene. In 2012, Habibi did very important study in detection of sheep toxoplasmosis by SAG1 gene. In 2013, Ling jang did immense study in detection of rodent toxoplasmosis by SAG1 gene in china. In 2013, Cabral did a study in detection of rodent toxoplasmosis in Brazil. In 2014, Barros et al. had found genetic characteristics of *Toxoplasma gondii* from doves in Brazil. In 2014, Yan et al. found genetic characteristics of *Toxoplasma gondii* from rodents in china. In 2014, Gjerede et al. had found genetic characteristics of *Toxoplasma gondii* from muscles of Lutra in Norway. In 2014, Chen et al. detected *Toxoplasma gondii* from HIV positive people in China [26-30]. In recent years have not perform any studies to detect rodents and cattle toxoplasmosis at the same time in Golestan area. This study showed important role of rodents and cattle in dissemination of toxoplasmosis in humid area. In this study we showed that the SAG1 gene was very important marker to detection of abundance of zoonotic toxoplasmosis and brain or heart tissue was main tissues to follow SAG1 gene from Tachyzoites of *Toxoplasma* parasite, also the rodents and cattle were very important reservoirs in dissemination of toxoplasmosis to human in Golestan area, northeast of Iran [26-30].

Conclusion

In this study we concluded: The northeast of Iran was very important region for following toxoplasmosis infection, specifically in animals such as rodents and cattle. In other study that had done four month after this surveillance, we found that the dominant genotype of *Toxoplasma gondii* in that area was genotype using PCR-RFLP by HaeII restriction enzyme.

Acknowledgements

The current research was funded by Tarbiat Modaress University.

References

1. Evers F, Garcia JL, Navarro IT, Zulpo DL, Nino BS, et al. (2013) Diagnosis and isolation of Toxoplasma gondii in horses from Brazilian slaughterhouses. Rev Bras Parasitol Vet 22: 58-63.

2. Quan JH, Zhou W, Cha GH, Choi IW, Shin DW, et al. (2013) Kinetics of IL-23 and IL-12 secretion in response to Toxoplasma gondii antigens from THP-1 monocytic cells. Korean J Parasitol 51: 85-92.

3. Dubey JP, Hill D, Zarlenga D, Choudhary S, Ferreira LR, et al. (2013) Isolation and characterization of new genetic types of Toxoplasma gondii and prevalence of Trichinella murrelli from black bear (Ursus americanus). Vet Parasitol 196: 24-30.

4. Assmar M, Yassaei F, Terhovanesian A, Esmaeili AR, Nahrevanian H, et al. (2004) Prenatal Diagnosis of Congenital Toxoplasmosis Validity of PCR Using Amniotic Fluid against Indirect Fluorescent antibody assay in mothers. Iranian J Public Health 33: 1-4.

5. Pena HF, Vitaliano SN, Beltrame MA, Pereira FE, Gennari SM, et al. (2013) PCR-RFLP genotyping of Toxoplasma gondii from chickens from Espírito Santo state, Southeast region, Brazil: new genotypes and a new SAG3 marker allele. Vet Parasitol 192: 111-117.

6. Quan JH, Kim TY, Choi UI, Lee YH (2008) Genotyping of a Korean isolate of Toxoplasma gondii by multilocus PCR-RFLP and microsatellite analysis. Korean J Parasitol 46: 105-108.

7. Hong SH, Jeong YI, Kim JY, Cho SH, Lee WJ, et al. (2013) Prevalence of Toxoplasma gondii infection in household cats in Korea and risk factors. Korean J Parasitol 51: 357-361.

8. Dubey JP, Randall AR, Choudhary S, Ferreira LR, Verma SK, et al. (2013) Occurrence, isolation, and genetic characterization of Toxoplasma gondii from white-tailed deer (Odocoileus virginianus) in New Jersey. J Parasitol 99: 763-769.

9. Selseleh M, Modarressi MH, Mohebali M, Shojaee S, Eshragian MR, et al. (2012) Real-time RT-PCR on SAG1 and BAG1 gene expression during stage conversion in immunosuppressed mice infected with Toxoplasma gondii Tehran strain. Korean J Parasitol 50: 199-205.

10. Habibi G, Imani A, Gholami M, Hablolvarid M, Behroozikhah A, et al. (2012) Detection and Identification of Toxoplasma gondii Type One Infection in Sheep Aborted Fetuses in Qazvin Province of Iran. Iran J Parasitol 7: 64-72.

11. Selseleh MM, Keshavarz H, Mohebali M, Shojaee S, Modarressi M, et al. (2012) Production and Evaluation of Toxoplasma gondii Recombinant Surface Antigen 1 (SAG1) for Serodiagnosis of Acute and Chronic Toxoplasma Infection in Human Sera. Iran J Parasitol 7: 1-9.

12. Lim H, Lee SE, Jung BK, Kim MK, Lee MY, et al. (2012) Serologic survey of toxoplasmosis in Seoul and Jeju-do, and a brief review of its seroprevalence in Korea. Korean J Parasitol 50: 287-293.

13. Lee SE, Hong SH, Lee SH, Jeong YI, Lim SJ, et al. (2012) Detection of ocular Toxoplasma gondii infection in chronic irregular recurrent uveitis by PCR. Korean J Parasitol 50: 229-231.

14. El Behairy AM, Choudhary S, Ferreira LR, Kwok OC, Hilali M, et al. (2013) Genetic characterization of viable Toxoplasma gondii isolates from stray dogs from Giza, Egypt. Vet Parasitol 193: 25-29.

15. Edwards JF, Dubey JP (2013) Toxoplasma gondii abortion storm in sheep on a Texas farm and isolation of mouse virulent atypical genotype T. gondii from an aborted lamb from a chronically infected ewe. Vet Parasitol 192: 129-136.

16. Dubey JP, Choudhary S, Kwok OC, Ferreira LR, Oliveira S, et al. (2013) Isolation and genetic characterization of Toxoplasma gondii from mute swan (Cygnus olor) from the USA. Vet Parasitol 195: 42-46.

17. Herrmann DC, Wibbelt G, Götz M, Conraths FJ, Schares G (2013) Genetic characterisation of Toxoplasma gondii isolates from European beavers (Castor fiber) and European wildcats (Felis silvestris silvestris). Vet Parasitol 191: 108-111.

18. Lilly EL, Wortham CD (2013) High prevalence of Toxoplasma gondii oocyst shedding in stray and pet cats (Felis catus) in Virginia, United States. Parasit Vectors 6: 266.

19. Zhang XX, Lou ZZ, Huang SY, Zhou DH, Jia WZ, et al. (2013) Genetic characterization of Toxoplasma gondii from Qinghai vole, Plateau pika and Tibetan ground-tit on the Qinghai-Tibet Plateau, China. Parasit Vectors 6: 291.

20. Cabral AD, Gama AR, Sodré MM, Savani ES, Galvão-Dias MA, et al. (2013) First isolation and genotyping of Toxoplasma gondii from bats (Mammalia: Chiroptera). Vet Parasitol 193: 100-104.

21. Mancianti F, Nardoni S, D'Ascenzi C, Pedonese F, Mugnaini L, et al. (2013) Seroprevalence, detection of DNA in blood and milk, and genotyping of Toxoplasma gondii in a goat population in Italy. Biomed Res Int 2013: 905326.

22. Ortega-Pacheco A, Acosta Viana KY, Guzmán-Marín E, Segura-Correa JC, Alvarez-Fleites M, et al. (2013) Prevalence and risk factors of Toxoplasma gondii in fattening pigs farm from Yucatan, Mexico. Biomed Res Int 2013: 231497.

23. Galván-Ramírez ML, Sánchez-Orozco LV, Rodríguez LR, Rodríguez S, Roig-Melo E, et al. (2013) Seroepidemiology of Toxoplasma gondii infection in drivers involved in road traffic accidents in the metropolitan area of Guadalajara, Jalisco, Mexico. Parasit Vectors 6: 294.

24. Shichao X, Chen Z, Lei H, Tongyao W, Liusong N, et al. (2013) DNA Detection of Toxoplasma gondii witha Magnetic Molecular Beacon Probe via CdTe@Ni Quantum Dots as Energy Donor. J Nanomater 2013: 473703.

25. Cong W, Huang SY, Zhou DH, Zhang XX, Zhang NZ, et al. (2013) Prevalence and genetic characterization of Toxoplasma gondii in house sparrows (Passer domesticus) in Lanzhou, China. Korean J Parasitol 51: 363-367.

26. Khademvatan S, Saki J, Yousefi E, Abdizadeh R (2013) Detection and genotyping of Toxoplasma gondii strains isolated from birds in the southwest of Iran. Br Poult Sci 54: 76-80.

27. Barros LD, Taroda A, Zulpo DL, Cunha IA, Sammi AS, et al. (2014) Genetic characterization of Toxoplasma gondii isolates from eared doves (Zenaida auriculata) in Brazil. Rev Bras Parasitol Vet 23: 443-448.

28. Yan C, Liang LJ, Zhang BB, Lou ZL, Zhang HF, et al. (2014) Prevalence and genotyping of Toxoplasma gondii in naturally-infected synanthropic rats (Rattus norvegicus) and mice (Mus musculus) in eastern China. Parasit Vectors 7: 591.

29. Gjerde B, Josefsen TD (2014) Molecular characterisation of Sarcocystis lutrae n. sp. and Toxoplasma gondii from the musculature of two Eurasian otters (Lutra lutra) in Norway. Parasitol Res 114: 873-886.

30. Chen LJ, Jia YX, Leng L, Luo M, Gao J, et al. (2014) Comparation of Toxoplasma gondii separated from HIV-positive people and RH strain GRA6 gene. Zhongguo Xue Xi Chong Bing Fang Zhi Za Zhi 26: 434-436.

29

Major Dermatological Disorders of Carthorses in Selected Towns of Central Ethiopia

Yidnekachew Tadesse[2] and Fanos Tadesse Woldemariyam[1*]

[1]College of Veterinary Medicine and Agriculture, Addis Ababa University, Addis Ababa, Ethiopia

[2]Horo Guduru Zone Livestock and Fisheries Office, Ethiopia

Abstract

The study was conducted between November 2007 and June 2008 to provide base line information concerning causes and major skin disorders of carthorses in selected towns of Central Ethiopia. Physical clinical examination and laboratory tests were used in the Investigation. The overall prevalence of dermatological disorders in carthorses was found to be 93.3%. This has no statistically significant difference (p>0.05) among the study sites. The major dermatological disorders identified were wounds (67.2%), infectious skin diseases (10%), tumor (2.5%), ectoparasites (7.3%) and mixed disorders (6.4%). The majority of the horses (82.6%) had dermatological disorders in more than one site. Laceration, erosion, puncture, avulsion, mixed and complicated wound types were identified. The major causes of wounds were improper harnessing, shoeing, beating, road accidents and multifactorial causes. Harness inflicted wounds were detected on lips, chest, back, girth and base of the tail. There was no statistically significant difference (p>0.05) in the occurrence of harness related wounds among the study sites. The ectoparasites identified were louse (2.7%), ticks (4.7%) and mange mite (1.78%). The infectious skin disorders detected in the study were dermatophilosis (0.6%), dermatophytosis (2.5%) and epizootic lymphangitis (6.9%). Most of the skin disorders were afflicted by improper management of working horses. Education of cart owners on proper management with regular veterinary care was recommended to alleviate the prevailing dermatological disorders in the study sites. In addition, the infectious causes should be objectively researched.

Keywords: Carthorses; Central Ethiopia; Prevalence; Skin disorder

Introduction

There are about 115.2 million domestic equids (horses, donkey and mule) in the world of which 44.3 million are donkeys, 57.6 million horses and 13.3 million mules. Ethiopia shares approximately half of Africa's equine population; according to UN Food and Agriculture Organization there are over 7 million donkeys, mules and horses in Ethiopia, including 1.9 million horses [1].

In a country where there is less developed transport and communication services and road network insufficiently developed, the natural choice rests on the use of human labor and pack animals as a mode of transport, as it has been the case in some parts of the world. This remains true in the Ethiopian context. The mountainous nature of the land has made the travel time consuming and difficult, which has resulted the back of animals to remain as the only means of transport for Ethiopian terrain for centuries [2]. Horses have a prominent position in the agricultural systems as draft, pack and riding animals. In many towns of Ethiopia horse pulled carts are used as a major means of transportation and as a source of income for cart owners [3,4]. In other words, the use of equines in door to door transport service provides urban dwellers with the opportunity of income generation [5,6].

Despite their invaluable contributions, equines in Ethiopia are the most neglected animals, accorded low social status, particularly the male working equines. Horses involved in pulling carts often work continuously for 6 to 7 hours per day, carrying 3 to 4 persons (195-260 kg) in single trip [7]. They are provided with wheat bran and cereal straw by moistening with water and grasses where season provide on access during the night and allowed to graze pasture and road side in the town fringe during the day. Feed shortage and disease are the major constraints to the productivity and work performance of carthorses. They are brutally treated, made to work overtime without adequate feed

or health care. The increasing human population, demand for transport of goods to and from far, remote areas, and construction activities around the town are making cart horses high demanded animal [8].

There are several causes of health problem in carthorses which are actively participating in the transport sector. The causes of this health problem emanates from infectious diseases, parasite infestation, mechanical damage, lack of adequate feed and some others. So the outcome that arises from these causes in combination or alone could affect the entire body systems or a single tissue, organ or system which has great impact on the performance expected from the animal. Of these dermatological (skin) problems is among the major ones.

Skin is the largest organ of the body which serves as an inclosing barrier and providing environmental protection, regulating temperature, providing pigment and vitamin D, sensory perception, etc. Anatomically it consists of epidermis, basement membrane zone, dermis, appendageal system and subcutaneous muscles and fat. The skin is affected by a wide variety of diseases and reacts to disease in a limited number of ways. Thus, many diseases can appear similar and cause similar presenting signs yet have vastly different etiologies. Some skin diseases have predictable clinical features, whereas others can have a variety clinical forms.

***Corresponding author:** Fanos Tadesse Woldemariyam, College of Veterinary Medicine and Agriculture, Addis Ababa University, Addis Ababa, Ethiopia, E-mail: fanos.tadesse@aau.edu.et

In Ethiopia, though few reports indicated that external injuries and epizootic lymphangitis (Endebu, 1996; SPANA, 2003) are major health problems of working horses, there have been no formal researches conducted to elucidate general dermatological disorders of carthorses. Therefore, the objectives of this study were:

- To provide base line information concerning the major skin disorders of carthorses in selected districts of Ethiopia.

- To indicate factors influencing the occurrence and distribution of skin disorders of carthorses.

Materials and Methods

Study area

The study was conducted in three selected towns of central Ethiopia namely Debre Berhan, Debre Zeit, and Adama. These places were previously selected as working area by the mobile clinic of the society for the protection of Animals Abroad (SPANA) Ethiopia based on their high equine population, poor welfare condition and low economic status of carthorse owners. These areas were a working site of SPANA Ethiopia and believed to be vaccinated and dewormed.

Debre Brehan: It is a town located in Amhara Regional State, in the central highlands of Ethiopia, 130 km north east of Addis Ababa, at 9°36' N and 39°38' E, with an altitude of 2780 meter above sea level. The average annual rainfall is 950 mm and the average monthly minimum and maximum air temperature ranges from 17.6°C in August to 22.5°C in June. The mean relative humidity is 68.2%. There are 714 carthorses and 357 carts in the town [9].

Debre Zeit: The town is 45 km south east of Addis Ababa, located 9°E at an altitude of 1850 m above sea level. The rainfall is bimodal. It receives the annual rainfall of 1151.6 mm with a mean maximum and minimum temperature of 30.7°C and 8.5°C respectively, and a mean relative humidity of 61.3% [10]. There are 1170 carthorses and 585 carts in the town [11].

Adama: The town is located in Eastern shoa zone of Oromia Regional State, 100 km southeast of Addis Ababa at 8°32'N and 39°17'E. It has an altitude of 1622 meter above sea level in the Great Rift Valley and receives annual rainfall ranging from 400 mm to 800 mm and a temperature of 13.9°C [10]. There are 1579 carthorses and 790 carts in the town [12].

In all the three sites the means of transportation include vehicle and horse drawn carts. Horse drawn carts are preferably used on roads inaccessible to taxi and because of relatively low charges. However, there is great competition between horse drawn carts and Bajaj (a three wheel motor bike).

Target population and sampling strategy

The total population of carthorses in the present study areas was 3423. Simple random sampling method was employed on each study sites irrespective of owner's primary complaint, age, body condition score, coat color

and/or any other parameters of horses. Discussion was made with the owners to know about the causes of dermatological disorder in their respective areas.

Sample size determination

The sample size was determined according to Thrusfield [13]. Simple random sampling for an infinite population with 95% confidence level, 5% derived absolute precision and 50% expected prevalence, since there was no previous information on the prevalence of major skin disorders in present study areas. Accordingly, 74 horses in Debre Brehan, 123 horses in Debre Zeit and 163 horses in Adama were selected.

$$n = \frac{1.96^2 \cdot Pexp (1 - Pexp)}{d^2}$$

$$Nadj = \frac{Nxn}{N+n}$$

Nadj : adjacent population

N: required sample size

P: prevalence

d: desired absolute precision

Pexp: expected prevalence

Study methodology

Physical examination of skin: Physical examination of skin included inspection at a distance to get general idea of the distribution and the extent of the disease. Then the skin was closely examined by sight and touch. Examination was undertaken from cranial to caudal body parts; from the head region to the tail including mucous membranes and mucoutaneous junctions. Age, body condition score, skin elasticity, skin thickness, type of hair coat, type and cause of dermatological disorders and body sites affected were recorded for all horses in each site.

Laboratory examination: Laboratory examination was employed where infectious and parasitic disorders were suspected during physical examination. Samples were taken by skin scrapings, hair plucking, collection of crusts and pus material from abscessed parts. Then, the samples were labeled and laboratory results for isolation of causative agents in cases where necessary were recorded.

Data analysis: The collected data were entered to computer using excel soft ware data. Data were listed in a format i.e., rows for horses identification number and sites of study, and columns for physical and laboratory examination results. SPSS 13.0 for windows was used to analyze the descriptive statistics. In the analysis confidence level was held at 95% and P<0.05 was set for significance.

Results

Physical and laboratory examination

The overall prevalence rate of dermatological disorder in the study sites was 93.3% (Table 1). Up on physical and laboratory examination wounds (67.7%), infectious diseases (10%), parasitic infestations (7.2%), skin tumor (2.5%) and other disorders (6.4%) were found among the major dermatological disorder of horses in the study site (Table 2). About 82.6% of the horses had dermatological disorders in more than one site (Table 3). There was no statistically significant difference in

Study site	Count	Percentage
DebreBrehan	67	90.50%
DebreZeit	117	95.10%
Adama	152	93.30%
Total	336	93.30%

Table 1: Overall prevalence of dermatological disorder in study sites.

Dermatological disorders	Percentage
Wounds	242 (67.7%)
Infectious diseases	36 (10%)
Parasitic infestations	26 (7.2%)
Skin tumor	9 (2.5%)
Other skin disorders	23 (6.4%)
Total	360 (100%)

Table 2: Type of dermatological disorders identified in the study sites.

Study site	Number of body sites affected			
	One body site (%)	Two body sites (%)	Multiple body sites (%)	Total (%)
Debre Brehan	16(23.88%)	23(34.32%)	28(41.79%)	67(19 .94%)
Debre Ziet	22(18.8%)	32(27.35%)	63(53.84%)	117(34.82%)
Adama	23(15.03%)	36(23.68%)	93(61.18%)	152(45.23%)
Total	61(18.15%)	91(27.08%)	184(54.76%)	336(100%)

Table 3: Distribution of dermatological disorders on body parts.

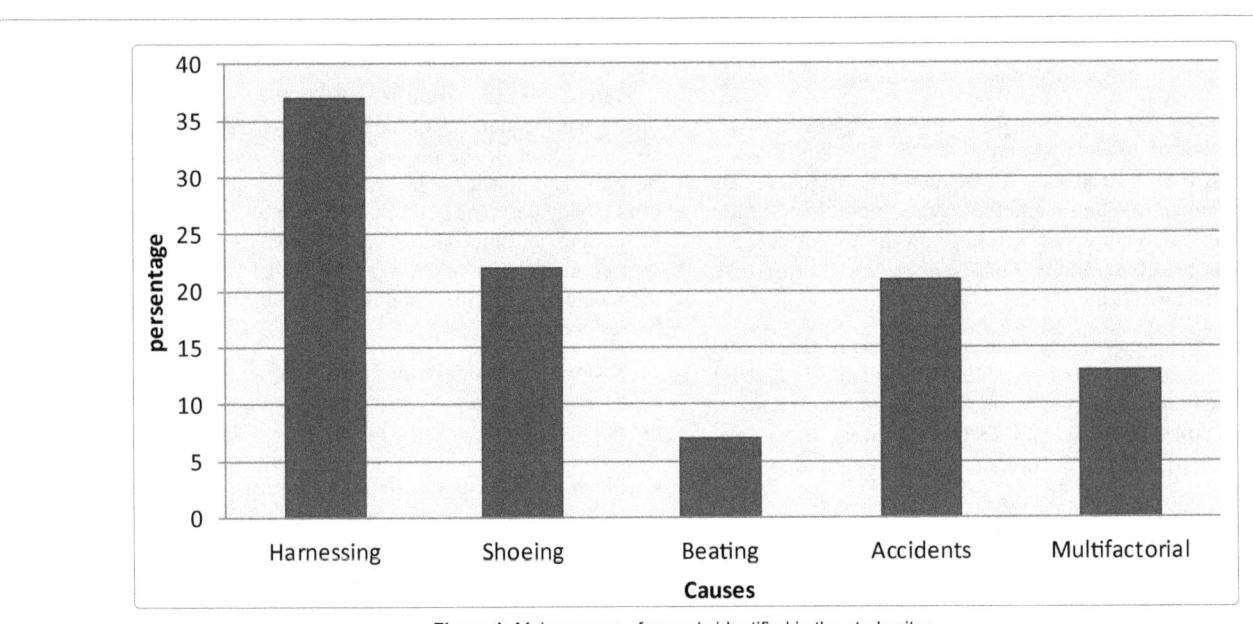

Figure 1: Major causes of wounds identified in the study sites.

Study site	Wound type						
	Erosion	Puncture	Laceration	Avulsion	Mixed	Complicated	Total
Debre- Berhan	0(0.0%)	7(15.9%)	17(38.6%)	1(2.3%)	10(22.7)	9(20.5%)	44(100%)
Debre- Zeit	1(1.1%)	29(31.87%)	28(30.8%)	4(4.4%)	15(16.48)	14(15.4%)	91(100%)
Adama	5(4.67%)	15(14.02%)	47(43.3%)	4(3.47%)	20(18.69%)	16(14.95%)	107(100%)
Total	6(2.48%)	51(21.07%)	92(38%)	9(3.72%)	45(18.6%)	39(16.1%)	242(100%)

Table 4: Type of wounds identified in the study sites.

the prevalence rate and type of disorders identified with respect to the study sites as well as the body parts affected by dermatological disorder (p>0.05).

The type of wounds identified were Laceration, erosion, puncture, avulsion, mixed and complicated wound types where Laceration and puncture takes about 60% of the share of wounds type in the three study sites (Table 4). The major causes of wounds were improper harnessing, shoeing, beating, road accidents and multifactorial causes (a combination of improper harnessing, shoeing, beating and road accident) (Figure 1).

Discussion

In the present study it is showed that the extremely high prevalence different types of dermatological disorders in carthorses with multiple body part appearance taking the largest share. The overall prevalence dermatological disorder in carthorses was found to be 93.3% which is in agreement with the finding of Biffa and Woldemeskel; Demsasha and Denka in different parts of Ethiopia [7,14]. The major dermatological disorders identified were wounds, infections skin diseases, tumor and ecto-parasites. Of these disorders wounds took the largest share (67.7%) of the dermatological disorders in the study site. This finding clearly indicated the magnitude of the problem in working horses. These dermatological disorders inevitably decrease the performance and effective working life of horses. This is comparable with the findings of Tamirat et al. (58.6%) in Wolaita Soddo and Abreha et al (30.3%) in Tigray which showed wounds are the major dermatological problems followed by infectious skin diseases, tumor and ecto-parasites [15,16].

The majority of the wounds identified were severe type where a wide area of the skin were removed. Most of these wound that affect the skin of the horses were due to mis-management and ill treatment of horses where poorly fitted harness with rigid and rough edges, improper shoeing and beating were the prevailing mal-practice in all the study sites. This is in agreement with the findings of Tamirat et al. and Abreha et al. in wolaita and Tigray, Ethiopa [15,16]. Our finding agrees with explanation of Pearson and her colleagues who stated that harness related problems were raised from incorrect size, inappropriate fitness, too narrow or too thin, made of unsuitable synthetic materials, poor paddle, poor design and synthetic rope to tried be fitted to the animal.

The dermatological disorders were found in one, two or multiple body parts of the horses in three study areas where the multiple body part occurrence was in higher proportion (54.76%) similar to our finding Biffa and Woldemeskel also found the multiple occurrence of wounds in different equine species.

Conclusions and Recommendation

The present study revealed higher prevalence of dermatological disorders in cart horses of the study sites. The major disorders were wounds, ecto-parasites, infectious skin diseases and tumors. Most of the wounds were afflicted by improper management of working horses. Based on the above concluding remark the following points are forwarded:

- There should be better or modern utilization harnessing system in carthorses
- Appropriate management system should develop in order to avoid the occurrence of wound.
- Develop regular deworming programme towards the control of ectoparasites.
- The infectious cases should be objectively researched.
- Develop better skill or awareness of animal welfare towards cart owners and drivers.

References

1. ANON (2010) FAOSTAT. FAO Statistics Division. Accessed January 13, 2017.

2. Hassen K (2000) Preliminary Study on socio- economic importance, Health Problems and other Management Constraints Horse in Mid and Highland area of North Gonder. DVM Thesis. FVM, AAU, Debre-Zeit, Ethiopia.

3. Endebu B (1996) Epidemiology of Epizootic Lymphangitis in Ethiopia. Retrospective Analysis, Cross Sectional Study and Treatment Trial at Debre-Zeit and Akaki Towns. DVM Thesis. FVM, AAU, Debre-Zeit, Ethiopia.

4. SPANA Ethiopia, Consultant Document (2003) Welfare of Carthorses Baseline Survey. Society for the Protection of Animals Abroad (SPANA), Ethiopia.

5. Wilson RT (1991) Equine in Ethiopia. In: Fielding D, Pearson RA (eds.), Donkey, Mule and Horse in Tropical Agricultural Development Proceeding Colloquium Held 3-6 September 1990. Centre for Tropical Veterinary Medicine, University of Edinburgh, Scotland, pp: 33-47.

6. Agajie T, Tamirat D, Pearson A, Temesgen T (2000) Socio-economic circumstances of Donkeys, Use and Management in the Rural and Urban Areas of Central Part of Ethiopia. Proceedings of the workshop on promoting the peri-urban livelihood through better donkey welfare. Debrezeit, Ethiopia, pp: 16-28.

7. Biffa D, Woldemeskel M (2006) Causes and Factors Associated with Occurrence of External injuries in working equines in Ethiopia. Intern J Appl Rev Vet Med 4: 1-4.

8. Mengistu A (2003) The Genetic Resources Perspective of Equines in Ethiopia and their contribution to the Rural Livelihood. Proceedings of the 11th annual conference of Ethiopia society of animal production (ESAP). Addis Ababa, Ethiopia, pp: 18-85.

9. Debre-brehan Municipality (2007) Debre-brehan Municipality (Office). Unpublished.

10. NMSA (2000) National Metrology Service Agency. Addis Ababa, Ethiopia.

11. DebreZeit Municipality (2007) DebreZeit Municipality (Office), Unpublished.

12. Adama Municipality (2007) Adama Municipality (Office), Unpublished.

13. Thrusfield M (1995) Veterinary Epidemiology. 3rd edn. Black Well Publishing, p: 339.

14. Demsasha T, Tamiru BD (2015) Injuries are the Predominant Cause of Deviation in the Health of Working Equines in and Around Gondar Town, North West Ethiopia. External J Vet Adv 5: 1071-1078.

15. Tamirat H, Mulisa M, Ayalew N, Teka F (2015) Assessment on Working Donkey Welfare Issue in Wolaita Soddo Zuria District, Southern Ethiopia. Global Veterinaria 14: 867-875.

16. Abreha T, Yohannes T, Habtamu T, Kalab G, Hagos Y (2015) Survey of Common Skin Problem of Working Equines in and Around Mekelle, North Ethiopia. Acad J Anim Dis 4: 30-38.

30

Infectious Coryza in Jimma Backyard Chicken Farms: Clinical and Bacteriological Investigation

Iyasu Angani Dereja* and Dagnachew Hailemichael
Animal Products, Veterinary Drug and Feed Quality Assessment Center, Addis Ababa, Ethiopia

Abstract

A cross sectional study on infectious coryza was conducted in Jimma, Ethiopia, from November 2011 to April 2012 with the objectives of determining the prevalence of infectious coryza, and associated factors. A total of 456 specimens from chicken were processed and the overall infection prevalence was 22.4%. From animal related risk factors considered, breed and age were found to be risk factors. Isolation of the agent, *Avibacterium paragallinarum*, in exotic and cross breeds were highly statistically significant compared to local breeds (odds ratio=3.890, P-value=0.000 and odds ratio=2.282, P-value=0.010, respectively). The highest incidence was observed January to April. Swab specimens revealed more infection (27.1%) than fecal samples (18.9%) suggesting the disease is more respiratory than it is digestive or systemic. Though clinically ill ones, there were numerous chickens with the infection without showing any sign of the disease. Based on these findings, keeping the genetic potential of the local breed poultry while upgrading their productive potential is recommended as a best method to control the infection.

Keywords: *Avibacterium paragallinarum*; Backyard; Infectious coryza; Isolation; Jimma

Abbreviations: *A. paragallinarum*: *Avibacterium paragallinarum*; CI: Confidence interval; DF: Degree of freedom; IC: Infectious coryza; JUCAVM: Jimma University College of Agriculture and Veterinary Medicine; NAD: Nicotinamide adenine dinucleotide; OR: Odds ratio; SPSS: Statistical package for social science; URT: Upper respiratory tract.

Introduction

Chicken production promises considerable potential to improve livelihood of rapidly increasing populations of developing countries. For many poor people in these countries, chickens are the only type of livestock they can afford to keep, which are relatively risk free [1]. With an estimated 60% of the total chicken population in East Africa, Ethiopia has an around 45 million heads. Of the national flock, the local breeds represent 98% [2].

Despite this huge population of poultry, the industry in the country remains highly undeveloped due to many constraints of which one is diseases. Although it is understood that diseases cause great losses, many of them are unstudied. Infectious coryza is one of such poultry catastrophes. Because many countries having trade relation with it have reported losses, it is rational argument that studies should be conducted to determine the status of the infection in Ethiopia. This study was therefore, conducted in the city of Jimma with the objectives of: Determining the prevalence of the disease in the study area, using clinical and bacteriological inquiries; and

Showing associated factors in the study area.

Literature Review

Infectious coryza

Infectious coryza is a disease caused by a bacterium *Avibacterium paragallinarum* (previously *Haemophilus paragallinarum)*. It is an acute to chronic respiratory disease of chickens. However, there are some experts that believe the disease also has digestive system or systemic nature. It is mainly observed in pullets and layers, and occasionally broilers [3-5].

The disease was named infectious coryza because it was infectious and affected primarily the nasal passage. The clinical syndromes have been described in the early times as roup, contagious catarrh, cold and uncomplicated coryza. Infectious coryza is characterized by conjunctivitis, catarrhal inflammation of the URT (upper respiratory tract), sneezing, swelling of the face under the eyes, and reduction in egg production.

Etiology

Avibacterium paragallinarum is a causative agent for Infectious coryza (IC). It was previously known as *Haemophilus paragallinarum*. It is from the genus *Haemophilus*, which is a member of the family Pasteurellaceae. The family is known for its pleomorphic, gram negative, non-motile, bacilli and coccobacilli organisms that are able to reduce nitrates and utilize carbohydrates. As many species in the genus, *A. paragallinarum* is catalase negative microaerophilic rod [3,6].

Epidemiology

The disease occurrence is worldwide. It was reported from Argentina, Australia, Germany, India, Indonesia, Japan, Malaysia, Mexico, Morocco, Pakistan, Taiwan, Thailand, the Americas and Uganda [7-11]. Chickens of all age group are susceptible, yet susceptibility increases with age. Some studies show that susceptibility increases four weeks post hatching. Thus, multiage farms tend to preserve the disease [3,12].

*Corresponding author: Iyasu Angani Dereja, Animal Products, Veterinary Drug and Feed Quality Assessment Center, Addis Ababa, Ethiopia
E-mail: iyasuangani@uopeople.edu

Physicochemical property

The *Haemophilus* group of bacteria is a heterogeneous group of small, gram negative, aerobic, bacilli, non-motile, non-spore forming and which require enriched media which include V-factor/ nicotinamide adenine dinucleotide (NAD). However, there are some isolates of *A. paragallinarum* that do not need NAD. Some scholars prefer in other hand 5% sheep blood agar as the most universally used isolation medium for *A. paragallinarum*. The bacterium doesn't grow on standard media used in antimicrobial sensitivity testing; it grows with supplement Muller Hinton agar which is capable of supporting the growth of *A. paragallinarum*. The minimal and maximal temperatures for the growth of the bacterium are 37 and 38°C. It is able to produce acid from maltose, mannitol, sorbitol and sucrose [4,13,14].

Serological variations

Two classification systems applied to *A. paragallinarum* are the "Page" and the "Kume" methods. Based on the first method, which employed the use of the plate agglutination method, three different serotypes termed A, B and C was detected. On the other hand, the Kume method is based on hemagglutination. Accordingly, three different serogroups I, II and III consisting of seven serovars (HA-1 to HA-7) were detected. Kume's serogroups I, II and III correspond to Page's serovars A, C and B respectively. This subsequently led towards the proposal to alter the Kume scheme nomenclature concluding with the nine currently recognized serovars [15-17]. Studies indicated that A and C are the pathogenic serovars of the bacterium whereas B is not clearly understood regarding its pathogenicity. Yet, Yamaguchi et al. [18] reported that the serovar is pathogenic, in Argentina [10,19,20].

Transmission

Bird to bird is the most recognized transmission way of the disease. However, contaminated feed and water is also mode of blowout, most probably in case of outbreaks in flocks. It spreads mainly through clinically affected and carrier birds. Birds that have recovered from field infection are said to be immune to reinfection at least for a year. Bird to bird transmission is via respiratory rout or by contact with contaminated drinking water [5,12,21-24].

Pathogenesis

The initial step in the pathogenesis of infectious coryza is adherence to and colonization of the nasal mucosa. A polysaccharide capsule of *A. paragallinarum* mediates its attachment to the cilia of the nasal mucosa. The lipopolysaccharide (LPS) in the cell wall and hyaluronic acid component of these capsules are believed to contribute to pathogenesis although these interactions of the host have not been clearly defined. A belief from other scholars is that endotoxin play a role in the pathogenesis. Still, virulence factures haven't been fully identified. Some others still believe that outer membrane proteins of the agent are of potential as virulence determinants. Studies report that secreted proteins of *A. paragallinarum* are lethal for chicken embryo [12,25-27].

Incubation period, clinical signs, and morbidity and mortality

The incubation period of IC varies 24 to 48 hours after experimental inoculation of the organism. However, it may depend on particular exposure from 24 hours by intrasinusal inoculation to 14 days by air born transmission [9,28]. A characteristic swelling of the infraorbital region, oculonasal discharge, swollen wattles, diarrhea and inappetence are common clinical signs. Losses are due to decreased feed consumption which impacts meat and egg yield. Some other unusual clinical presentations are arthritis and septicemia.

In the mildest form, depression, nasal discharge and occasional slight facial swelling may be the only signs. In the sever form, there is a server swelling of one or both infraorbital tissues with edema of the surrounding tissues, which may close one or both eyes. This edema may extend to the wattles and the inter-mandibular spaces. The swelling usually subsides in 10-40 days. Still, it may persist for months in complicated cases [3,12]. Clinically, IC is usually characterized by high morbidity rates. Losses due to persistent mortality are culling where up to 5%. Affected flocks may suffer an egg drop of up to 10%, and to 100% in more serious situations [29-32].

Post mortem lesions and histopathology

Whereas lesions may be limited to the infraorbital sinuses in acute cases, other complicated signs may be observed in chronic ones. The lesions may include yellowish sinus exudate, conjunctivitis, thracheitis, and bronchitis. Upon postmortem, affected birds show increased mucus and necrotic debris in the trachea. There is also infraorbital swelling escorted by congestion of mucus membrane of the nasal cavity and sinuses. Sometimes, there may be lung edema and opacity, and congealing of the abdominal air sacs. Upon histological examination of the URT, there are usually lesions ranging from necrosis of the respiratory epithelium to marked hypoplasia and squamous metaplasia of the sinuses [3,12,23,33].

Diagnostic techniques

Although the history and the clinical signs can be suggestive, they are neither confirmative nor pathognomonic. In a certain study [34], 46% of chickens which finally found to be positive to many other diseases showed signs similar to that of IC. Therefore, laboratory investigations including bacteriology are required to demonstrate the presence of the causative agent [35]. Chocolate agar or blood agar inoculated with a streak of *Staphylococcus aurous*, incubated at 37°C for 2-3 days in moist atmosphere, is used for isolation.

Prevention and control

Prevention is the only sound method of control. Improved management aspects including hygiene, housing, flock structure and young chick care and others are most economical and effective means of prevention. Hygienic measures include frequent turning and changing of poultry liter, frequent clearing of feeders and drinkers, and regular disinfection of poultry houses. Whereas, housing measures include ventilation, quarantine of new entries, and proper spacing. Replacements should be raised on the same farm or obtained from clean flocks. Segregation of birds by age is also another remarkable measure that can be applied especially in outbreak cases [12,34].

Bacterins are available to prevent and control the disease. Early vaccination is also useful method of prevention. All replacement birds on endemic farms should be vaccinated [19,25]. A killed vaccine containing serovars A and C have been developed. Yet, outbreaks have been reported in vaccinated flocks in several countries, suggesting the existing new serotypes [3,16,34,36,37].

Treatment

Because early treatment is necessary, water medication is recommended. Many drugs have bacteriostatic effect on the organism. Erythromycin, Tetracycline, Fluoroquinolones, Sulphadimetoxine, and Sulphamethazine can be used as treatment medication. Although treatment may result in improvement, the disease may recur when medication is discontinued [3,12,21-24,38].

Materials and Methods

The study area

The study was conducted from November 2011 to April 2012 in Jimma town, which is located about 375 Km from Addis Ababa, the capital city of Ethiopia. It is positioned at latitude of about 7°13' to 8°56'N and longitudes of about 35°52' to 37°37' E. The area receives a mean annual rainfall of about 1530 milliliters with bimodal rainfall. The minimum and maximum annual temperatures are 7°C and 30°C, respectively. Jimma has a livestock population of about 4,540,311 of which 1,139,735 (25.10%) are poultry.

The study population

The study elements were backyard chickens from selected kebeles of Jimma town. The study was carried out on all ages of both sexes from three breeds (Pure local, cross, and pure exotic) and two management systems (backyard extensive and backyard intensive).

Study design

The study was cross-sectional experimental to isolate *A. paragallinarum* both in clinically ill and non-clinical backyard chickens in the study area. It was conducted in five randomly selected kebeles of Jimma town.

Sampling and sample size determination

The households with backyard chicken production were selected by simple random sampling technique until the desired sample size was met. The sample size was determined using the formula of Thrusfield [35]. Based on this formula and considering 95% confidence level, 5% desired absolute precision and 50% expected prevalence, the sample size was 384. Yet, to increase the accuracy of representation, it has been increased to 456.

$$n = \frac{(1.96)^2 p_{exp}(1 - p_e xp)}{d^2}$$

Where n=Required sample size, P_{exp}=Expected prevalence and d=Desired absolute precision.

The study sample was comprised of 86 male and 370 female chickens of which 147 were local, 143 cross and 136 exotic breeds. 184 of the chickens were young and the rest 272 were adult (all chickens whose age are six or less were taken as young, whereas older as adult). 217 chickens from backyard extensive management system and 239 from backyard intensive management system were considered. Of this, 238 were reared for egg, 85 for meat and the rest 133 for dual reason.

Study methodology

Sample collection and transportation: Data were collected from the owners on their management system, production purpose, and age of the poultry. The data so generated was then recorded on the data recording sheet. The health status of the sampled chicken was recorded as clinically ill or healthy by general physical observation. From each study element, two types of specimens (swab from trachea and infraorbital sinus, and fecal sample from rectum) were collected for isolation of *A. paragallinarum*.

Sterile gloves, cotton and bottles were employed for the collection.

The bottles were then labeled with chicken identities, specimen type, date of sampling, and other notes. The pack was then transported on the date it was collected to the JUCAVM microbiology laboratory using an ice box.

Sample processing: The specimens collected were diluted with distilled water prior to isolation. Then the dilutions were cultured on a blood agar plate in which 5% sheep blood was added, and *Staphylococcus aureus* was streak on. After being incubated at 37°C for 28 hours with 5% CO_2, the plates have been sub cultured. The bacterial colonies showing satellite growth were taken as culture positive and cells from discrete colonies were picked up for Graham's and Giemsa's stains [39].

The inocula which both found gram negative and bipolar on Giemsa's stain were taken for oxidase and catalase tests while those failed even in one of the two staining techniques were rejected. Oxidase and catalase tests were done as recommendation of Salle [40]. The IC positive plates were negative for both tests. Sugar fermentation tests for sucrose, lactose and mannitol were conducted on those slides, as recommended by Gordan and Jordan [24].

Data management and analysis: The data collected on the study were processed using computer software. While Microsoft excel 2010 was used for data entry, analysis was performed using statistical data social science (SPSS) version 17. To summarize the data, descriptive statistics such as percentage were used. The strength of association of potential risk factors (explanatory variables) to presence of infectious coryza infection (response variable) was determined by binary logistic regression using SPSS-17. For all tests p-values less than 0.05 were considered statistically significant.

Results

The causative agent of Infectious coryza, *A. paragallinarum*, was isolated from 22.4% (95% CI 18.57%, 26.23%) of the study samples. The prevalence in swab samples (27.1%) was 1.72 times more than the prevalence in fecal samples (18.9), which was statistically significant (Table 1).

The explanatory variables considered in this study were grouped as animal related (age, sex and breed), season and others (breeding purpose, management system and clinical illness). From animal related risk factors, breed and age were found to be risk factors for isolation of the etiology (Table 2). Isolation of the agent in exotic (32.4%) and cross (23.1%) breeds was highly statistically significant as compared to its local (12.2%) equivalent (OR=3.890, P=0.000 and OR=2.282, p=0.010, respectively). Younger chickens were more resistant than adults (OR=2.169, p=0.002). Males (30.2%) were more susceptible than females (20.5%). However not statistically significant (OR=1.529, p=0.163).

The study showed that there is considerable difference on the incidence of the infection on the different months of the study period. Minimum and maximum percentages were 8.8% on November and 39.7% on March, respectively (Table 3).

Other factors considered in the study were management system, breeding system and clinical sickness. The result revealed that all these factors have no significant association with isolation of *A. paragallinarum* (Table 4). No outbreak occurred during the study although there were numerous chicken showing sign of coryza. Still,

Sample type	Prevalence (%)	95% CI of prevalence	P-value	OR	95% CI of OR
Fecal (n=264)	18.9	18.80-18.99			
Swab (n=192)	27.1	26.97-27.22	0.018	1.72	1.09-2.71
Total (n=22.4)	22.4	18.57-26.23			

Table 1: Prevalence of isolation of *A. paragallinarum* in backyard chickens of Jimma town.

Factor	Category	Prevalence (%)	P-value	OR	95% CI of OR
Breed	Local	12.2			
	Cross	23.1	0.010	2.282	1.22-4.267
	Exotic	32.4	0.000	3.89	2.067-7.32
Sex	Female	20.5			
	Male	30.2	0.168	1.529	0.842-2.779
Age	Young	15.2			
	Adult	27.2	0.002	2.169	1.328-3.544

Table 2: Isolation of *A. paragallinarum* based on animal related risk factors.

Month	Positive (%)	DF	x²-value	p-value
November (n=57)	8.8			
December (n=95)	12.6			
January (n=114)	21.9	5	25.178	0.000
February (n=17)	29.4			
March (n=73)	39.7			
April (n=17)	29.4			

Table 3: Occurrence of *A. paragallinarum* infection based on the time of investigation.

Factor	Category	Prevalence (%)	P-value	OR	95% CI of OR
Management	Intensive	19.7			
	Extensive	25.3	0.236	1.312	0.837-2.058
Purpose	Dual	22.6			
	Meat	29.4	0.531	1.246	0.625-2.484
	Egg	19.7			
Clinical illness	Yes	32.1			
	No	21.7	0.661	1.224	

Table 4: Association of poultry management system, breeding purpose and clinical illness with isolation of isolation of *A. paragallinarum*.

clinically ill birds were more likely to develop IC (32.1%) than clinically healthy ones (21.75%).

Discussion

Infectious coryza is highly infectious poultry disease caused by *A. paragallinarum* and is seen in many countries all over the world. Although there are numerous reports from neighboring countries, no evidence of previous study on the infection found in the country. As such, focus was given to its incidence and associated factors to its occurrence in the study area.

In this study, *A. paragallinarum*, causative agent of IC was isolated from backyard poultry farms of Jimma. It showed a total isolation prevalence of 22.4%, which agrees with the report of Byarugaba et al. [41] where they found a seroprevalence of 22% in Uganda, but higher than the findings of Mustefa and Ali [42] 8.3%, Rahman et al. [43] 0.59% and Islam et al. [44] 0.37% occurrences in Bangladesh. These differences might have been arisen from factors such as agroecology; the tropical climate is favorable to proliferation of the microorganism [3,45]. The result of the present study was in line with this general fact. Disease complications are much more complicated in the study country, which help the microorganism to invade the immunity of chickens [15]. Moreover, chicken vaccination is not practiced strictly in the community; this might have increased the chance of infection

of the chickens. In addition, the present work was conducted from November to April, which comprises the windy season of the year in the country which favors transmission of the agent [46].

The this result however, is much lesser than the report of Byarugaba et al. [7] in which they investigated 40.5% coryza cases and the works of Sakamato et al. [47] who reported antibody prevalence level of 80% for serovar A and 60% for serovar C on ELISA. This variation might be due to the fact that their work was on disease outbreak and may also be due to the laboratory techniques employed; unlike the present study, they used antibody detection technique where there are numerous false positives due to cross protections [48].

Infectious coryza is a known respiratory disease but it is not limited to the respiratory system. It sometimes takes systemic form and even cause diarrhea [49], which indicates that it has digestive system significance too. In the present study, the bacterium was isolated on both fecal and swab samples.

Naturally male chickens are more susceptible too *A. paragallinarum* than females [38]. The present study result was in line with this fat in that the prevalence was 30.2% in males and 20.5% in females. Normally a male chicken reaches numerous females than a female chicken reaches males or females reach each other. That might be why males are more vulnerable than females.

Age wise, the disease was more common in adult birds. This is because, as the poultry gets older, the bursa of fabricius, where B lymphocytes are produced, shrinks; this weakens the humeral immunity of the hosts which intern becomes favorable to the disease causing microorganism [50]. This result agrees with the study conducted in Thailand by Thitisak et al. [50] which showed that higher proportion of infected chickens were below two months and above six months.

In this study, there was a strong association between the isolation of *A. paragallinarum* and season of the investigation in the study area. The highest incidence was observed during the months of January to April. This agrees with the report of Thitisak et al. [50] who reported the occurrence of infection during the windy months of the year. The months are in the hottest season of the year in the study area and they are also in the windy months which facilitate ease of transmission of the microorganism [51]. In addition, this is the time in which the popular holidays "Genna" and "Fasica" are celebrated and poultry are marketed more than any other time whole over the country. These active market times may contribute for the infection transmission.

Per this study, management system and breeding purpose couldn't affect the occurrence of the disease in the study populations. This might be due to irregularity of the management system in the study area. In the country, chickens are usually raised by children and females; they usually have not well proposed purpose by raising the chickens. Thus, this condition might have contributed for the difficulty to know the effect of the management on the disease's incidence.

The isolation of *A. paragallinarum* was higher in clinically ill birds (32.1%) than clinically healthy ones (21.7%). The greater percentage of infection on the clinically ill birds might be from immunosuppression due to complications. This indicated that not only sick ones, but also members recovered from the clinical coryza cases may harbor the disease without showing any clinical signs [12].

Conclusion and Recommendations

In summary, isolation of *A. paragallinarum* confirmed the presence of infectious coryza in Ethiopia. The infection was highly prevalent in the study area. The animal related factors such as breed, age and sex were observed affecting the occurrence of the infection. The disease is highly contagious and once entered the flock, it's usually a risk for the whole farm. The disease has significant economic importance which is too risky to farms, which is usually observed by drop in egg production and body condition. This intern affects the poor, which mainly comprises women and children, aggravating its effect on food security of the country.

In general, the disease may be one of the economic risks to the country unless appropriate measures are taken with the right time. But immediate and cooperated responses can reduce its effect. Thus, the following are recommended based on this conclusion:

- Public awareness creation should be performed using various intervention techniques;

- The genetic potential of indigenous chickens ought to be kept while upgrading their productivity;

- Strict biosecurity measures must be practiced in poultry farms; and

- Further researches should be done concerning the disease and associated factors as it pertains to economic and social lives in developing countries.

Conflict of Interest Statement

The authors declare that there is no conflict of interest.

References

1. Tadelle D (2011) Livestock exchange: why chicken research for development? ILRI, Addis Ababa, Ethiopia.

2. Pagani P, Abebe W (2008) Review of new features of Ethiopian poultry sector biosecurity implications. FAO, Addis Ababa.

3. Aiello E, Amstutz HE, Anderson DA, Armour IS, Ieffcott LB, et al. (1998) The Merck veterinary manual. 8th edn., Merck and Co Inc., New Jersey, USA.

4. Saif Y (2003) Poultry diseases. 8th edn. Blackwell, Low state, USA.

5. McMullin P (2004) The poultry site, Infectious Coryza.

6. Baron E, Peterson L, Fingold S (1994) Diagnostic microbiology. 9th edn. Mosby.

7. Byarugaba D, Minga U, Gwakisa P, Katunguka E, Bisgaard M, et al. (2006) Occurrence, isolation and characterization of *Avibacterium paragallinarum* from poultry farms in Uganda. Proceedings of the 11th international symposium on veterinary epidemiology and economics.

8. Hinz K (1973) Differentiation of Haemophilus strains isolated from chickens. IV. Studies on the dissociation of Haemophilus paragallinarum. Avian Pathol 5: 51-66.

9. Kume K, Sawata A, Nakase Y (1978) Haemophilus infections in chickens. 1. Characterization of Haemophilus paragallinarum isolates from chickens affected with coryza. Japanese J Vet Sci 40: 65-73

10. Thornton A, Blackall P (1984) Serological classification of Australian isolates of Haemophilus paragallinarum. Aust Vet J 61: 251-253.

11. Ziani ZB, Iritani Y (1992) Serotyping of Haemophilus paragallinarum isolated in Malysia. J Vet Med Sci 54: 363-365.

12. Songer J, Post K (2005) Veterinary microbiology: bacterial and fungal agents of animal diseases. Aust Vet J 84: 438.

13. Blackall P (2011) An update on the diagnosis and prevention of fowl cholera and infectious coryza. Clinical Microbiology Reviews 93: 1522-1533.

14. Poernomo S, Sutarma S, Rafiee M, Blackall P (2000) Characterization of isolates of Haemophilus paragallinarum from Indonesia. Aust Vet J 78: 759-762.

15. Blackall P (1999) Infectious coryza: overview of the disease and new diagnostic options. Clinical Microbiol Rev 12: 627-632.

16. Kume K, Sawata A, Nagaki T, Matsumoto M (1983) Serological classification of Haemophilus paragallinarum with a haemagllutinin system. J Clin Microbial 17: 958-964.

17. Roodt Y (2009) Towards unraveling the genome of Avibacterium paragallinarum. University of free state, Bleomfontein, South Africa.

18. Yamaguchi T, Blackall P, Yakigami Y, Iritani Y, Hayashi Y (1990) Pathogenicity and serovar-specific haemagglutinating antigens of Haemophilus paragallinarum serovar B strains. Avian Dis 34: 964-968.

19. Page L (1962) Haemophilus infection in chickens: characteristics of 12 Haemophilus isolates recovered from diseased chickens. Amer J Vet Res 23: 85-95.

20. Kume K, Sawata A, Nakase Y (1980) Immunologic relationships between Page's and Sawata's serotype strains of Haemophilus paragallinarum. Amer J Vet Res 41: 757-760.

21. Chukiatsirin K, Chansiripornchai N (2008) An outbreak of infectious coryza in a layer farm. J Thai vet Med Assoc 58: 98-107.

22. Chukiatsiri K, Sasipreeyajan J, Neramitmansuk W, Chansiripornchai N (2009) Efficacy of autogenous killed vaccine of Avibacterium paragallinarum. Avian Dis 53: 382-386.

23. Abd El-Ghany W (2011) Evaluation of autogenous Avibacterium paragallinarum bacterins in chickens. Int J Poult Sci 10: 56-61.

24. Gordan R, Jordan F (1982) Poultry diseases. 2nd edn. London.

25. Neramitmansuk W, Neramitmansuk P, Tantichareunyod T, Trongwongsa L

(1995) The study of local strain infectious coryza vaccine in chicken. J Thai Vet Med Assoc 46: 53-60.

26. Iritani Y, Katagri K, Arita H (1980) Purification and properties of Haemophilus paragallinarum haemagllutinin. Amer J Vet Res 41: 2114-2118.

27. Marquez V, Marquez A, Caballero J, Lugo G, Cruz C, et al (2008) Secreted proteins of Avibacterium paragallinarum are lethal for chicken embryo. Anim Biodivers Emerg Dis 1149: 380-383.

28. Quinn P, Markey B, Carter M, Donnelly W, Leonard F (2002) Vet Microbiol Microb Dis. Wiley-Blackwell.

29. Satary G, Rao P (2006) Veterinary pathology. 7th edn. JS Offset Printers, Delhi, USA.

30. Vagas E, Terzolo H (2004) Epizootiology, prevention and control of infectious coryza. Vet Mex, p:35.

31. Bland M, Bickford A, Charlton B, Cooper G, Sommer F, et al. (2002) Case report: a sever infectious coryza infection in multi age layer complex in central California. Proceedings of the XXVII convention annual ANECA and 51st western poultry diseases conference. Puerto Vallarta (Jalisco), Mexico.

32. Chukiatsirin K, Chotinun S, Chansiripornchai N (2010) An outbreak of Avibacterium paragallinarum serovar B in a Thai layer farm. Thai J Vet Med 40: 441-444.

33. Welcham D, King S, Wragg P (2010) Infectious coryza in chickens in Great Britain. Vet. Record 167: 912-913.

34. Sonajya E, Swan S (2004) Small scale poultry production technical guide. FAO, Rome, Italy.

35. Sandoval V, Terzolo H, Blackall P (1994) Complicated infectious coryza outbreaks in Argentina. Avian Dis. 38: 672-678.

36. Hobb R, Tseng H, Downess J, Terry T, Blackall P, et al. (2002) Molecular analysis of a haemagglutinin of Haemophilus paragallinarum. Microbiology 184: 2171-2179.

37. Rimler R, Davis R, Page R, Kleven S (1978) Infectious coryza: preventing complicated coryza with Haemophilus gallinarum and Mycoplasma gallisepticum bacterins. Avian Dis 22: 140-150.

38. Jacobs A, Vanderberg K, Malo A (2003) Efficacy of new tetravalent coryza vaccine against emerging variant type B strains. Avian Pathol 32: 265-269.

39. Thrusfield M (2005) Veterinary epidemiology. 3rd edn. Blackwell, Berlin, Germany.

40. Salle A (2002) Fundamental principles of microbiology. 21st edn. TMH Publishing Company Ltd., New Delhi, India.

41. Byarugaba D, Minga U, Gwakisa P, Katunguka E, Bisgaard M, et al. (2007) Investigation of occurrence of Avibacterium paragallinarum infections in Uganda. Avian Diseases 51: 534-539.

42. Mustefa M, Ali S (2005) Prevalence of infectious diseases in local and fayoumi breeds of rural poultry (Gallus domesticus). Punjab Univ J Zool 20: 177-180.

43. Rahman M, Rahman A, Islam M (2009) Bacterial disease of poultry prevailing in Bangladesh. Res J Poult Sci 1: 1-6.

44. Islam M, Das B, Hossain K, Lucky N, Mostafa M (2003) A study on occurrence of poultry diseases in Sylhet region of Bangladesh. Int J Poult Sci 2: 354-356.

45. Azage T, Birhanu G, Hoekstra D (2010) Livestock impact supply and service provision in Ethiopia: challenges and opportunities for market oriented development. ILRI.

46. Shewantasew M (2010) Assessment of biosecurity situation and practices in live poultry markets of Addis Ababa. Jimma, Ethiopia.

47. Sakamato R, Sakai T, Ushijima T, Imamura T, Kino Y, et al. (2012) Development of an Enzyme-linked immunosorbent assay for the measurement of antibodies against infectious coryza vaccine. Avian Dis 56: 65-72.

48. Bragg R, Rensburg P, Heerden E, Albertyn J (2004) The testing and modification of a commercially available transport medium for transportation of pure cultures of Haemophilus paragallinarum for serotyping. Onderstepoort J Vet Res 71: 93-98.

49. Bragg R (2005) Effects of virulence of different serovars of Haemophilus paragallinarum on perceived vaccine efficacy. Onderstepoort J Vet Res 72: 1-6.

50. Davison F, Kaspers P, Schat K (2008) Avian immunology, London.

51. Thitisak W, Janviriyansopak O, Morrisur S, Srihakim S, Krueder R (1988) Causes of death foundation on epidemiological study of native chickens in Thai villages. Proceedings of the 5th international symposium on veterinary epidemiology and economics.

31

Occurrence of Mastitis at Cow and Udder Quarter Level in the Agro-Pastoral District of Soroti, Uganda

Zirintunda G[1]*, Ekou J[1], Omadang L[1,2], Mawadri P[1,2], Etiang P and Akullo J[1]

[1]*Department of Animal Production and Management, Faculty of Agriculture and Animal Sciences, Busitema University, Soroti, Uganda*
[2]*National Livestock Resources Research Institute, National Agricultural Research Organization, Tororo, Uganda*

Abstract

A cross sectional study was carried in Aloet Parish, Soroti district-Uganda to assess and quantify the prevalence of mastitis of lactating cows at cow level in the villages and udder quarter level for cows brought for sale at the Soroti livestock market. The objective was to acquire an empirical basis for stakeholders' awareness in the small holder pastoral zones.

Both clinical and subclinical mastitis were quantified at the village level and only SCM was considered at the market level. In the villages and the market SCM was tested using California Mastitis Test (CMT). In the villages of Aloet, 4 (12.5%) of the crosses and 60 (22.4%) Small East African zebu had mastitis. Overall, SCM and CM were at 50 (16.7%) and 14 (4.7%) occurrence and SCM was responsible for 78% of all the mastitis. Predisposing factors to mastitis among the pastoralists in communal grazing systems in Aloet were possibly habits such as stripping of teats using rough abrasion of fingers during milking coupled with none usage of milking salves. In the market, the right fore (RF) had a 34.2% (27/79) SCM and 1.25% (1/80) blind quarters. Right hind (RH) had a 30.8% (24/78) SCM and 2.5% (2/80) blind quarters. The left fore (LF) had a 36.6% (27/78) SCM and 2.5% (2/80) blind quarters. The left hind (LH) had a 31.4% (22/70) SCM and 12.5% blind quarters. The quarter prevalence rates were higher for the fore quarters than for the hind quarters. For all the quarters SCM prevalence was at 32.8% (100/305) and 4.9% (15/320) were blind. Bovine mastitis is an escalating hindrance to the upcoming dairy industry in agro-pastoral areas and requires urgent measures, SCM is possibly confounded by poor performance of local breeds and poor feeding management.

Keywords: Clinical; Subclinical; Mastitis; Prevalence

Abbreviations: SCM: Subclinical Mastitis; CM: Clinical Mastitis; SCC: Somatic Cell Count; RH: Right Hind; RF: Right Fore; LH: Left Hind; LF: Left Fore; -: Negative; +: Mild gel; ++: Real gel; +++: Clumps and High Viscosity gel; T: Traces of gel; B: Blocked teat.

Introduction

Mastitis affects dairy animals and their production [1-3]; it leads to pathological changes in the milk and the glandular tissue [4]. Bovine mastitis can be categorized as clinical (CM) or subclinical mastitis (SCM) where the former manifests changes in the appearance of milk with obvious signs of inflammation of the udder whereas the later doesn't show obvious signs but its effects on can be detected by subjecting the milk to tests [5]. The disease causes losses of reduced production and the milk acquires undesirable components like ions and enzymes while decreasing in casein which leads to an undesired taste [6,7]. Mastitis reduces milk quantity and quality [8,9] and may cause death of the cow [10]. The etiological agent for mastitis produce toxins that damage milk producing tissue and ducts [9]. SCM is difficult to diagnose because the milk appear normal, however, it is the most prevalent compared to the CM [11,12]. SCM and CM are wide spread in small scale dairy sector in sub-Saharan Africa [13]. SCM is thought to be more economically important because it persists longer in the herd causing production losses [14-18]. Although more quarters may be affected in SCM, it is usually one quarter affected in CM except when caused by *Mycoplasma spp* [19,20]. CM and SCM affect not only production but even the reproductive performance of lactating animals [21,22]. Mastitis associated losses are estimated at more than $200 per cow per year [23]; bovine mastitis affects farmers' economy and may continue to be a problem even after meticulous control methods [2].

The major causing agents of mastitis are *Staphylococcus aureus*, *Streptococcus dysagalactiae*, coagulase-negative staphylococcus, *Arcanobacterium pyogenes*, *E. coli*, *Staphylococcus simulans*, *Staphylococcus hycus*, *Staphylococcus chromogenes*, *Klebsiella spp*, *Pseudomonas spp* and *Mycoplasma spp* [24-30]. However any bacterial and mycotic organism that can opportunistically invade the udder may cause mastitis. Mammary epithelial cells play a key role in the onset of the process of defense therefore mastitis with regard to *E. coli* and *S. aureus* [31]. Infections may be contagious or environmental but contaminated teat dips, udder towels, laborers, skin lesions teat trauma and flies have been implicated as sources of infection [12,32]. The major risk factors are water scarcity. Detection of SCM is best done by examining of milk for somatic cell counts (SCC) using the California Mastitis Test (CMT) or automated methods. Normal milk should have below 200,000 SCC/ml, milk showing traces of viscosity has 200,000-400,000 SCC/ml, milk showing a mild gel has 500,000-1,500,000 SCC/ml, milk that shows a real gel has 2,000,000-5,000,000 SCC/ml and the milk which shows clumps with very high viscosity has over 5,000,000 SCC/ml [33]. The agro-pastoral communities depend on livestock especially cattle of low milk production capacities, milk is gathered from many animals and sold to the neighborhoods or taken to the dairies for processing. Milk production is a way of boosting the household economy and taxes for

*Corresponding author: Zirintunda G, Faculty of Agriculture and Animal Sciences, Department of Animal Production and Management, Busitema University P.O. Box 203, Soroti, Uganda
E-mail: gzerald777@gmail.com

the local governments however farmers have inadvertently not done any intervention on mastitis. The farmers and therefore the government are suffering losses because there is no clear basis for sensitization. The study also affirms whether the communities are at risk; since bacterial contamination leading to mastitis provides mechanisms for spread of milk transmissible zoonoses [34].

Materials and Methods

This was a cross-sectional study carried out in the Aloet Parish, Soroti Sub County of Soroti district. The purpose was to cover the Soroti livestock market and the surrounding villages. The study was divided into two sections: one considering the herds in the villages of Aloet parish and the second considering the lactating cows brought to the cattle market. At villages level, 300 cows were randomly selected and tested for mastitis. Clinical mastitis was observed by the signs of obvious inflammation of an udder quarter or more than one and visible changes in milk for example presence of blood or pus in the milk. SCM was detected using the CMT test. For the villages of Aloet, the details of the quarters and the grades of SCM were not included. In the Soroti livestock market, 10 lactating animals were tested for SCM at udder quarter levels weekly for 8 weeks making a total of 80 cows and the results were graded as Negative (–) meaning those with no observable reactions observed, Traces (T); were some trace of viscosity were seen, Mild (+) were a mild gel was formed, severe (++) were real gels were formed and very severe (+++) were clumps with high viscosity were seen [33]. Only the severe and the very severe grades were assumed to be SCM during the calculation of the percentage SCM infection.

Results

From the villages of aloet parish

A total of 300 cows were examined and tested, 32 were crosses and 268 were the East African zebu (locals). Among the crosses 4 (12.5%) had mastitis and among the locals 60 (22.4%) had mastitis. SCM and CM were at (50)16.7% and (14) 4.7% prevalence, SCM was over 78% of the observed mastitis in the area as shown in Table 1 below.

SCM at udder-quarter level in the soroti livestock market

The RF had a 34.2% (27/79) SCM and 1.25% (1/80) blind quarters. The RH had a 30.8% (24/78) SCM and 2.5% (2/80) blind quarters. The LF had a 36.6% (27/78) SCM and 2.5% (2/80) blind quarters. The LH had a 31.4% (22/70) SCM and 12.5% blind quarters. For all the quarters, SCM was at 32.8% (100/305) and 4.9% (15/320) were blind as shown in Tables 2 and 3 below.

Discussion

From the villages of aloet parish

Local cows had higher prevalence of mastitis (22.4%) compared to the crosses (12.5%), this was possibly a statistical challenge because

we had more locals than crosses during the study. This is contrary to the findings of Sharma and Maiti [35] who found a higher prevalence of Mastitis in Holstein-Jersey crosses compared to the local Zebu although Rahman et al. [36] found no significant difference of mastitis prevalence between Holstein-Friesian and Zebu. The findings are almost in agreement with Biffa et al. [37] who found Mastitis more prevalent in local Zebu than Jersey although the prevalence in Friesians was more than in local Zebu. However, farmers tend to offer crosses better conditions and care because they consider them not only more productive but also more susceptible to diseases. SCM was 16.7% prevalent while CM was 4.7% prevalent, it agrees with the findings of Joshi and Gokhale [16] who found SCM between 10% and 50% in the dairy farms of India. However, this prevalence was low because the study was done in a dry season which is usually cleaner. The prevalence of SCM was much lower than the 51.8% observed by Tripura et al. [38] in Bangladesh and the 37.2% observed by Byarugaba et al. [7] in the small holder dairy farming systems in Uganda. SCM was responsible for 78% of mastitis in the area, this agrees with the studies of Byarugaba et al. [39] in North Kyadondo county-Kampala district of Uganda; Kassa et al. [11] in the Ethiopian Central Highlands; Kivaria et al. [12] in the small holder dairy cows in Tanzania; Mdegela et al. [40] in Kibaha and Morogoro districts of Eastern Tanzania. Challenges of tick control could be responsible for the high mastitis prevalence [2]. However the high prevalence of mastitis was possibly because of the low hygiene standards in the communal grazing systems; such systems are associated with primitive tendencies of having no dry cow therapy, not using milking salve and inadvertent transfer of bacteria from one cow to another by the milkers. The farmers usually have rough hands because of the garden work and these bruise the teats and sometimes maneuvers in overgrown grasses and thickets leads to the trauma of teats predisposing them to mastitis. The primitive tendencies of rough dragging away of suckling calves leads to wounds on teats culminating into mastitis [41] ; this is method used in Soroti and is possibly one of the causes for the observed mastitis. The high prevalence of SCM compared to CM was also possibly because the farmers have no idea about this condition which only requires testing; this is in agreement with Karimuribo et al. [42], Sharma et al. [2] and Kivaria [5].

SCM per quarter in the lactating cows in soroti livestock market

SCM was highest in LF quarter followed by RF, LH and RH; this agrees with Khanal and Pandit, [43] and Tripura et al. [39] who found the LF with the highest prevalence. Possibly shorter duration of increase and decline milk phases predisposes to SCM because Tancin et al. [44] found a shorter duration in the fore quarters compared to the hind quarters. Possibly the fore quarters easily touch the ground during sitting and the hind quarters are in the groins for animals with small

Village	No.sampled	SCM	%	CM	%	x^2	OR	P- value
Teso college West	46	10	21.7	04	8.7	3.033	3.02(10.79, 14.32)	0.09
Teso college East	34	08	23.5	02	5.9	2.6606	4.8 (0.86, 50.40)	0.08
Arabaka	34	09	26.5	00	00	10.3729	-	0.002
Ogolo	29	05	17.2	02	6.9	1.4622	2.8 (0.41, 31.57)	0.42
Aloet akum	36	04	11.1	03	8.3	0.1582	1.4(0.2, 10.09)	0.69
Abalang	31	03	9.7	02	6.5	0.2175	1.5 (0.16, 19.77)	0.64
Arapai Agric	31	04	13	01	3.2	1.9579	4.4(0.40, 225.75)	0.35
Akaikai	29	04	13.8	00	00	4.2963	-	0.11
Aloet central	30	03	10	00	00	3.1579	-	0.08
Total	300	50	16.7	14	4.7	19.3363	3.3 (1.8, 6.3)	< 0.001

Table 1: Prevalence of SCM and CM in Aloet parish.

Variable	Quarters	Percentage grades of mastitis (%)					
		Negative (-)	Mild gel (+)	Real gel (++)	High viscosity (clumps) (+++)	Blind quarters (B)	Traces (T)
Week 1	RF	20	10	40	0	0	30
	RH	20	50	20	0	0	10
	LF	30	20	40	0	0	10
	LH	30	10	30	0	20	10
Week 2	RF	50	30	0	20	0	0
	RH	70	10	10	10	0	0
	LF	50	20	10	10	0	10
	LH	50	10	10	10	20	0
Week 3	RF	50	30	0	10	10	0
	RH	60	10	20	0	0	10
	LF	50	10	40	0	0	0
	LH	40	40	10	10	0	0
Week 4	RF	40	20	10	30	0	0
	RH	30	30	20	20	0	0
	LF	30	20	20	10	10	10
	LH	30	10	20	20	10	10
Week 5	RF	20	10	20	50	0	0
	RH	10	10	40	0	20	20
	LF	10	20	20	40	10	0
	LH	10	0	20	40	20	10
Week 6	RF	80	10	0	0	0	10
	RH	80	10	0	0	0	10
	LF	100	0	0	0	0	0
	LH	80	0	0	0	20	0
Week 7	RF	50	10	10	30	0	0
	RH	50	0	20	30	0	0
	LF	20	30	20	30	0	0
	LH	30	20	0	30	10	10
Week 8	RF	30	20	30	20	0	0
	RH	50	10	20	20	0	0
	LF	50	20	10	20	0	0
	LH	60	0	10	30	0	0

-: Negative test; T: Traces; +: Mild gel; ++: Real gel; +++: Presence of clumps and high viscosity and B: Blind quarter.

Table 2: Grades of mastitis at the udder quarter level among the lactating animals brought to the Soroti livestock market.

Quarter	CMT Result					
	-	T	+	++	+++	B
RF	34	04	14	11	16	01
RH	37	05	12	12	12	02
LF	34	03	14	16	11	02
LH	33	04	11	08	14	10

Table 3: Quantifying of grades of mastitis at the udder quarter level among the lactating animals brought to the Soroti livestock market.

udders. The LF being the most affected is associated with side that cows prefer when declining to sit on the ground. However the findings don't absolutely agree with the work of Lancelot et al. [45] in dairy herds in Britany of France; Barkema et al. [46] and Saini et al. [47] in Punjab who found the hindquarters most affected by SCM. The overall SCM for all the quarters was at 32.8% which is higher than 30.15% found in the dairy livestock of Lamjung by Khanal & Pandit [43] and 26.7% found by Giannechini et al. [48] in West Littoral region in Uruguay. However the observed overall quarter prevalence was lower than 51.6% observed by Kivaria et al. [49] in Dar-es-Salaam region of Tanzania. The prevalence would have been much higher than observed if it was rainy season [36]; however it was a dry season with few flies and fair sanitation.

The trend of blindness of quarters was highest in LH, the LF and RH had an equal percentage and RF had the smallest percentage. Possibly the LH structure predisposes it to blindness, this partly agrees with Weiss et al. [50] who states that the rear teats are shorter and thicker than the front teats, and this is what predisposes them to infection [51]. The trend possibly is related to trend of untreated mastitis, predisposition to trauma and genetic predisposition. However the real cause of the trend is not explicitly known. The overall quarter blindness of 4.9% is lower than 8% that was observed by Khan and Mohammad [52] in Faisalabad, Pakistan. Bovine mastitis is an escalating hindrance to the upcoming dairy industry as seen in Aloet parish, it is perhaps the greatest bottleneck to the transition from subsistence to commercial dairy farming. SCM is possibly confounded by poor performance of local breeds and poor feeding management. Therefore more farmer education and routine testing are needed in order to enable the farmers to maximize production.

Acknowledgement

We are thankful to the following people for the support in the collection of data; Nyode I, Ongora M, Okello G, Okot S, Atima S, Operemo SP, Etimu I, Aruki I, Obete G, Katumba S, Kahandi J, Oyesigye P, Kisembo G, Nancha M, Buwembo L, Isabirye A, Pithuwa J, Nagudi N and Nakiwendo B. The Farmers of Aloet parish were cooperative in this study and the leadership of the Soroti cattle market were so supportive by allowing us to use their lactating animals.

Competing Interests

The authors declare that they have no competing interests whatsoever.

Funding

The research was partly facilitated by Busitema University

References

1. Tiwari JG, Babra C, Tiwari HK, Williams V, De Wet S, et al. (2013) Trends in Therapeutic and Prevention strategies for Management of Bovine Mastitis: An over view. J Vaccines Vacc 4: 176.

2. Sharma N, Rho GJ, Hong YH, Kang TY, Lee HK, et al. (2012) Bovine Mastitis: An Asian perspective. Asian J Anim Vet Adv 7: 454-476.

3. Elango A, Doraisamy KA, Rajarajan G, Kumaresan G (2010) Bacteriology of sub-clinical mastitis and anti-biogram of isolates recovered from cross-bred cows. Indian J Anim Res 44: 280-284.

4. Radostits OM, Gay CC, Blood DC, Hinchkliff KW (2000) A Text Book of Veterinary Medicine 9th Edn. W.B. Saunders, New York, pp: 563-618.

5. Kivaria FM (2006) Epidemiological studies on bovine mastitis in smallholder dairy herds in the Dar es Salaam region, Tanzania. Doctoral thesis, Utrecht University, The Netherlands.

6. Hogeveen H (2005) Mastitis in dairy production, current knowledge and future solutions. Wageningen Academic Publishers. ISBN 978-90-76998-70-1 pp:744.

7. Byarugaba DK, Nakavuma JL, Vaarst M, Laker C (2008) Mastitis occurrence & constraints to mastitis controlin small holder dairy farming systems in Uganda. Livestock Res Rural Dev 20: 1.

8. Halasa T, Nielen M, De Ross APW, Van Hoorne R, De Jong G, et al. (2009) Production loss due to new subclinical mastitis in Dutch Dairy cows estimated with a test-day model. J Dairy Sci 92: 599-606.

9. Jones GM, Bailey TL (2009) Understanding the basics of mastitis. Virginia cooperation extension publication 404-233. Accessed on 4th August 2015.

10. Urech E, Puhan Z, Schallibaum M (1999) Changes in milk protein fraction as affected by subclinical mastitis. J Dairy Sci 82: 2402-2411.

11. Kassa T, Wirtu G, Tegegne A (1999) Survey of Mastitis in dairy herds in the Ethiopian Central highlands. Ethiop J Sci 22: 291-301.

12. Kivaria FM, Noordhuizen JP, Kapaga AM (2004) Risk indicators associated with subclinical mastitis in small holder dairy cows in Tanzania. Trop Anim Health Prod 36: 581-592.

13. FAO (2014) Impact of mastitis in small scale dairy production systems. Animal production &Health working paper. No.13, Rome.

14. Godkin A, Leslie K, Martin W (1990) Mastitis in bulk tank milk culture in Ontario. Highlights 132: 13-16.

15. Kader MA, Samad MA, Saha S (2003) Influence of host level factors on prevalence and economics of subclinical mastitis in dairy cows in Bangladesh. Indian J of Dairy Sci 56: 235-2240.

16. Joshi S, Gokhale S (2006) Status of mastitis as an emerging disease in improved and peri-urban dairy farms in India. Ann NY Acad Sci 1081: 74-83.

17. Halasa T, Huips K, Østras O, Hogeveen H (2007) Economic effects of bovine mastitis and mastitis management: a review. Vet Q 29: 18-31.

18. Seeger H, Fourichon C, Beaudeau F (2003) Production effects related to mastitis and mastitis economics in dairy cattle herds. Vet Res 34: 475-491.

19. Contreras A (2012) Detecting Mycoplasma mastitis. Michigan Dairy Review. Accessed on 14th September 2016.

20. Brand T, Kersling KW (1999) Mycoplasma mastitis in Dairy cattle. Iowa State University Veterinarian 61: 4.

21. Barker AR, Schrick FN, Lewis MJ, Dowlen HH, Oliver SP (1998) Influence of clinical mastitis during early lactation on reproductive performance of Jersey cows. J Dairy Sci 81: 1285-1290.

22. Schrick FN, Hockett ME, Saxton AM, Lewis MJ, Dowlen H, et al. (2001) Influence of subclinical mastitis during early lactation on reproductive parameters. J Dairy Sci 84: 1407-1412.

23. Schroeder JW (2012) Bovine mastitis and milking management (Mastitis control programs). North Dakota State University (NDSU). External Service, AS1129 (Revised).

24. Waage S, Mørk T, Røros A, Aasland D, Hunshamar A, et al. (1999) Bacteria Associated with clinical mastitis in Dairy heifers. J Dairy Sci 82: 712-719.

25. Barkema HW, Schukken YH, Lam TJGM, Beiboer ML, Wilmink H, et al. (1998) Incidence of clinical mastitis in Dairy Herds grouped in three categories by Bulk milk somatic cell counts. J Dairy Sci 81: 411-419.

26. Busato A, Trachsel P, Schallibaum M, Blum JW (2000) Udder health & risk factors for subclinical mastitis in organic dairy farms in Switzerland. Prev Vet Med 44: 205-220.

27. Kivaria FM, Noordhuzen JP (2006) A retrospective study of the aetiology & temporal distribution of bovine clinical mastitis in small holder dairy herds in the Dar es Salaam region of Tanzania. Vet J 173: 617-22.

28. Thorberg BM, Daielsson-Tham ML, Emmanuelson U, Waller KP (2009) Bovine subclinical mastitis caused by different types of coagulase-negative Staphylococci. J Dairy Sci 92: 4962-4970.

29. Plozza K, Llevaart JJ, Potts G, Barkema HW (2011) Subclinical mastitis and associated risk factors on dairy farms in New South Wales. Aust Vet J 89: 41-46.

30. Oliveira L, Hulland C, Ruegg PL (2012) Characterization of clinical mastitis occurring in cows on 50 large dairy herds in Wisconsin. J Dairy Sci 96: 7538-7549.

31. Gilbert FB, Cunha P, Jensen K, Glass EJ, Foucres G, et al. (2013) Differential Response of bovine mammary epithelial cells to Staphylococcus aureus or Escherichia coli agonists of the innate immune system. Vet Res 44: 40.

32. Ohnstad I, Mein GA, Baines JR, Rasmussen MD, Farnsworth R (2007) Addressing teat condition problems. National Mastitis Council, Annual meeting proceedings.

33. Varatanovic N, Podzo M, Mutevelic T, Podzo K, Cengic B, et al. (2010) Use of California Mastitis Test, Somatic Cells Counts and bacteriological findings in diagnostics of subclinical mastitis. Biotech Anim Husbandry 26: 65-74.

34. Sharma N, Singh NK, Bhadwal MS (2011) Relationship of Somatic cell count and mastitis: An overview. Asian-Aust J Animal Sci 24: 429-438.

35. Sharma N, Maiti SK (2010) Incidence, etiology and antibiogram of sub clinical mastitis in cows in Durg, Chhattisgarh. Indian J Vet Res 19: 45-54.

36. Rahman MA, Bhuiyan MMU, Kamal MM, Shamsuddin M (2009) Prevalence & risk factors of mastitis in dairy cows. The Bangladesh Veterinarian 26: 54-60.

37. Biffa D, Debela E, Beyene F (2005) Prevalence and risk factors of mastitis in lactating dairy cows in Southern-Ethiopia. Int J Applied Res Vet Med. 3: 189-198.

38. Tripura TK, Sarker SC, Roy SK, Parvin MS, Rahman AKMA, et al. (2014) Prevalence of subclinical mastitis in lactating cows & efficacy of intramammary infusion therapy. Bangladesh J Vet Med 12: 55-61.

39. Byarugaba DK, Khaitoa ML, Opuda A (1998) Bovine mastitis North Kyadondo county of Kampala district. Uganda Vet Journal 4: 139-146.

40. Mdegela RH, Kasiluka LJM, Kapaga AM, Karimuribo ED, Turuka AFM, et al. (2004) Prevalence and determinants of mastitis and milk borne zoonoses in small holder dairy farming sector in Kibaha and Morogoro districts in Eastern Tanzania. J Vet Med B Infect Dis Vet Public Health 51:123-128.

41. Hameed S, Arshad M, Ashraf M, Avais M, Shahid M.A (2012) Cross-sectional epidemiological studies on mastitis cattle and buffaloes of Tehsil Burewala, Pakistan. J Anim Plant Sci 22: 371-376.

42. Karimuribo ED, Fitzpatrick JL, Bell CE, Swai ES, Kambarage DM, et al. (2006) Clinical & Subclinical Mastitis in small holder dairy farms in Tanzania: risk, intervention& knowledge transfer. Prev Vet Med 74: 84-98.

43. Khanal T, Pandit A (2013) Assessment of subclinical mastitis and its associated risk factors in dairy livestock of Lamjung, Nepal. Int J Infect Microbiol 2: 49-54.

44. Tancin V, Ipema B, Hogewerf P, Macuhowa J (2006) Sources of variation in milk flow characteristics at udder & quarter level. J Dairy Sci 89: 978-988.

45. Lancelot R, Faye B, Lescourret F (1997) Factors affecting the distribution of clinical mastitis among udder quarters in French dairy cows. Vet Res 28: 45-53.

46. Barkema HW, Schukken YH, Lam TJGM, Galligan DT, Beiboer ML, et al. (1997) Estimation of interdependence among quarters of the bovine udder with subclinical mastitis & implications for analysis. J Dairy Sci 80: 1592-1599.

47. Saini SS, Sharma JK, Kwatra MS (1994) Prevalence and etiology of subclinical mastitis among cross bred cows and buffaloes in Punjab. Indian J Dairy Sci 47: 103-106.

48. Gianneechini R, Concha C, Rivero R, Delucci I, Lopez JM (2002) Occurrence of clinical and subclinical mastitis in dairy herds in the West Littoral Region in Uruguay. Acta Vet Scand 43: 221-230.

49. Kivaria FM, Noordhuzen JP, Nielen M (2006) Interpretation of California Mastitis Test scores using staphylococcus aureus culture results for screening of subclinical mastitis in low yielding small holder dairy cows in the Dar es Salaam region of Tanzania. Prev Vet Med 78: 274-285.

50. Weiss D, Weinfurtner M, Bruckmaier RM (2004) Teat Anatomy & its relationship with quarter & udder milk flow characteristics in Dairy cows. J Dairy Sci 87: 3280-3289.

51. Zadok RN, Allore HG, Barkema HW, Sampimon OC, Wellenberg GJ, et al. (2001) Cow and quarter level risk factors for Streptococcus uberis and Staphylococcus aureus mastitis. J Dairy Sci 84: 2649-2663.

52. Khan AZ, Muhammad G (2005) Quarter wise comparative prevalence of mastitis in buffaloes and cross bred cows. Pakistan Vet J 25: 1.

32

Prevalence of Bovine Trypanosomosis in Dembecha Woreda Amhara Region, Northwest Ethiopia

Demelash Mekonnen, Amare Eshetu and Tesfaheywet Zeryehun*

College of Veterinary Medicine, Haramaya University, PO Box 301, Dire Dawa, Ethiopia

Abstract

This study was conducted in Dembecha Woreda of Amhara region, Northwest Ethiopia. The study was carried out on 384 indigenous cattle kept in mixed crop-livestock production system to estimate the prevalence of bovine trypanosomosis and associated risk factors. The study employed parasitological survey (buffy coat examination) and hematological study (packed cell volume [PCV] and thin blood smear). In the present study, the overall prevalence of trypanosomosis was 8.6% (33/384). *Trypanosoma congolense* (54.54%) and *Trypanosome vivax* (45.45%) were the only two species of *Trypanosomas* encountered in the study area. Among the risk factors, sex and age were found to have no significant association with the prevalence of trypanosomosis ($p>0.05$), but body condition and coat color of animals were found to have a significant association ($p<0.05$) with prevalence of trypanosomosis in the studied animals. In this study infected animals were with mean PCV value of $22.94 \pm 2.70\%$ which is significantly lower ($p<0.05$) than that of the non-infected animals ($27.24 \pm 5.02\%$). The study concluded that Trypanosomosis being an economically important disease in cattle the 8.6% prevalence entail that more attention should be given to be adapting on integrated disease control strategy including the vector as well as the parasites.

Keywords: Cattle; Packed cell volume; *Trypanosoma congolense*; *Trypanosoma vivax*; Dembecha district

Introduction

Trypanosomosis is an economically important disease of domestic animals in many part of the world particularly in sub Saharan Africa [1,2]. The disease is among factors that limit the expected outcome from animal production in tropical Africa.

In countries like Ethiopia trypanosomosis is among the major setback to cattle production with direct and indirect economic loss. It is a serious constraint to agricultural production in extensive area of the tsetse infested Ethiopian low land [3]. It's highly prevalent in most arable and fertile land South West and North West part of the country. In Ethiopia an aggregated annual economic losses from animal death through direct mortality and reduced productivity and reproductive performance where estimated at 150 million US dollars [4].

Bovine trypanosomosis is a parasitic disease caused by protozoan parasite in the genus *Trypanosoma* [3]. They are obligatory parasites which are microscopic, elongated, unicellular, usually having two hosts, the invertebrate and vertebrate hosts. The three most important *Trypanosomas* species affecting cattle are *Trypanosoma vivax* (sub genus duttenelle); *T. congelense* (sub genus nannomonas) and *T. brucie* (sub genus trypanozoon). The problem of Africa animal trypanosomosis is associated with the disease with the presence of tsetse flies [5]. The disease is mostly associated with the occurrence of tsetse fly between 14° N and 29° South. *T. vivax* is the only species of tsetse transmitted Trypanosomas established in area free of tsetse flies [6]. Tsetse flies inhibit wide range of habitats in African continent including Ethiopia. Currently a wide area of the country is infested with tsetse flies including *Glossina tachinoides*, *Glossina pallidip*, *Glossina morsitans* and *Glossina longipennis* [7].

Trypanosomosis is argued to be the single most important constraints to animal agriculture in the sub humid and non-forested portion of humid zone of Africa. The disease has caused direct and indirect economic impact on livestock production. The indirect impact is related to the opportunity cost of land and other resources currently not used for livestock production owning prevention and control strategies of tsetse flies. The annual losses in meat production alone with estimated at 5 billion US dollars [8]. Economic losses due to trypanosomosis are estimated 2 billion US dollars per year. Approximately 30% of the 150 million cattle in the life are at risk of the infection. Thus, if control of trypanosomosis could be achieved there could be potential even at the current low rate of production to increase meat supply of continent by the approximately 16% and milk supply by 17% of current production level [9].

In West Gojjam Zone of Amhara regional state trypanosomiasis is among the most important disease of cattle [10-12]. But little has been done with regard to systematic investigation of the diseases and the associated risk factors in this area. The study aims to estimate the prevalence of bovine trypanosomosis in Dembecha Woreda of West Gojjam Zone in Amhara regional state, North West Ethiopia.

Materials and Methods

Study area

The current study was carried out in Dembecha Woreda of Gojjam Zone in Amhara Regional State, North-western Ethiopia. It is located about 370 km North West of the capital of Ethiopia, Addis Ababa, and 220 km South East of Bahair Dar, the capital of Amhara region. West Gojjam zone is located at 10°30′ North, Latitude and 37°29′ East longitude [12]. The climate alternate with long summer rainfall

---

***Corresponding author:** Tesfaheywet Zeryehun, College of Veterinary Medicine, Haramaya University, PO Box 301, Dire Dawa, Ethiopia E-mail: tesfahiwotzerihun@yahoo.com

between June-September and winter dry season between December-March with a mean annual rainfall 1200-1600 mm. The mean temperature of the study area is between 10-20°C and altitude ranges from 1400-2300 m.a.s.l. The mean agricultural activities currently practice includes irrigation (modern to traditional), animal production and crop production (mixed farming) activities holds 90% of the total agricultural activities. The major agricultural production seasonally harvested includes sorgum, wheat, teff, maize and other legume groups [13].

Study design, study population and sample size determination

The study was carried out on 384 local indigenous Zebu which are kept under mixed farming system. The study was conducted to assess the status of vector born trypanosomosis in each district of the Dembecha Woreda. Animals were selected from the study population using simple random sampling technique and purposive sampling was the method followed to select the two study peasant associations (PA`s). During sampling the age, sex, breed, coat color and clinical signs were recorded. The required sample size was determined using the procedure described by Thrusfield [14] using 50% expected prevalence of bovine *Trypanosomas* in the area and 5% desired absolute precision and at 95% confident level. Accordingly, the total sample was determined to be 384. Classification of the body condition of animal was made by previously described method [15] with scale ranging from 1 (emaciated) to 5 (obese). The age of the animals was grouped as young (1-3 years) and adults (≥ 3 years) according to method followed by Bitew et al. [16].

Parasitological study

Packed Cell Volume (PCV) determination: Blood samples were collected by puncturing the ear vein with a lancet which was then transferred into a heparinized capillary tubes. Using appropriate procedure in the laboratory the tubes were centrifuged at 12,000 rpm for 5 minute. The centrifuged capillary blood was then red with a haematocrit reader and the reading was recorded in percentage. Animals with PCV ≤ 24% were considered to be anaemic [17].

Buffy coat technique: The buffy coat was recovered by centrifugation of the blood collected in heparinized microhaematocrit capillary tubes at 12,000 rpm for 5 minute. Since *Trypanosomas* are found in the Buffy coat layer, the capillary tube was cut 1 mm below and 3 mm above the Buffy coat. The Buffy coat was then placed onto a glass slide, and covered with cover slip and was examined for movement of parasite under x40 objective and x10 eye piece [18]. Identification of the *Trypanosoma* species was done based on morphological descriptions as well as movement in wet film preparations [19].

Thin blood smear: A small drop of blood collected using a micro hematocrit capillary tube was placed on a glass slide, air dried and fixed in methyl alcohol for 2 minute and later it was stained with Giemsa stain (1:10 solution) for 30 minute. The excess stain was washed with distilled water and the slide was air dried and examined under the microscope (x100) oil immersion objective lens [20].

Data analysis: The data collected was entered in MS-Excel spreadsheets and hematological data was analyzed using statistical packages for social sciences (SPSS) version 20 software program. The association between prevalence of *Trypanosoma* infection and risk factors such as age, sex, breed, body conditions and coat color of animals was done using Pearson's chi-square (χ^2). Statistical significance was held at P-values less than 0.05 in all analysis.

Results

Parasitological finding

The current study on vector born trypanosomosis in Dembecha of west Amhara region revealed an overall prevalence of 8.6% (33/384). The result of the presents study was lower than the finding of previous reports including 14.2% in Arbaminch [21], 23.36% [22] from Bahir Dar and 14.68% [23] from Abay Basin, in Northwest Ethiopia respectively. But the present finding was higher than the prevalence of 2.66% [24] and 2.10% [25] reported from West Tigray from North Ethiopia and West Gojam from Northwest Ethiopia respectively. It was also observed that the finding of the present study was in close agreement with the finding of Adane and Gezahegn [26] who reported prevalence of 8.2% in areas bordering the Blue Nile in Degen, Basoliben and Machakel districts. The discrepancies in the different study areas may be attributed to the geographic area which differs in the population of vectors as well as the various control activities in different areas. For example there were ongoing tse-tse control project activities in 2011 and 2013 northern parts of Ethiopia which has led the prevalence to go down as low as 2.10- 2.66% [24,25].

In the present study out of 384 animals examined 18 (4.7%) were infected with *T. congolense* and 15 (3.9%) were infected with *T. vivax*. Hence, *T. congolense* was the predominant species (54.54%) followed by *T. vivax* (45.45%) with no mixed infection at all. Such a high ratio of *T. congolense* may suggest that the major cyclical vectors of Glossina species (*G. tachinoide*, *G. morsitans* and other species) are more efficient transmitters of *T. congolense* than *T. vivax* [27]. The transmission of *T. congolense* is cyclical; it requires the presence of tsetse flies whereas *T. vivax* is more rapidly transmitted via mechanically by biting flies than tsetse fly. The current finding is in agreement with the study conducted by Shimelis et al. [11] (Table 1).

Prevalence of trypanosomiasis with associated risk factors

In the current study, the association of prevalence with the various risk factors including age, breed, body conditions and coat color were computed (Table 2). Accordingly, the prevalence of Trypanosomosis, although in significant (p=0.235) it was higher in adults cattle above 3 years old than young ones below 3 years of age. A relatively higher prevalence of Trypanosomosis in adults than young cattle has been previous reported in the country [21,25]. The effect of the maternal antibodies which could afford protection to young animals might have contributed to the lower prevalence of *Trypanosoma* in these animals [28].

With regard to sex of animals, the prevalence of Trypanosomosis was not significantly different (p.0.05) in female and male animals. Similar finds were reported from various parts of the country [24-26] and this might be due to the management of animals where both male and female are allowed to graze in the field which consequently lead to similar exposure to the biting flies. In animals with poor body condition, the prevalence of Trypanosomosis was significantly higher (p=0.000) than medium and good body condition cattle apparasitaemic for bovine Trypanosomosis. Similar observations were recorded from studies conducted elsewhere [21,24,25,29,30]. This might entail that

Species	No. positive	Prevalence (%)
T. vivax	15	3.9
T. congolense	18	4.7
Total	33	8.6

Table 1: Overall prevalence of *Trypanosoma* species.

the disease is responsible to reduce the body condition of animals or trypanosomosis infection occurs in animals with poor body conditions which are likely to have poor immunity against the disease.

The present study revealed that prevalence of Trypanosomosis was significantly different (P=0.001) among animals with different coat color, where the prevalence is higher in animals with black coat color. The finding agreed to the observation that Glossina species prefers black surfaces as its strongest landing response [31].

Hematological examination

Cattle with mean PCV values ≤ 24% were considered anaemic [32]. In the current study, 48.48% of the parasitemic cattle were anaemic (Table 3). Furthermore, the mean PCV of parasetemic animals (22.94 ± 2.70%) was significantly lower (p=0.000) than the aparastiemic animals (27.24 ± 5.02%) (Table 4). These lowered PCV of parasitemic animals was previously reported in similar studies elsewhere [21,30,33,34]. The finding of aparasitemic animals with mean PCV values of ≤ 24% might

be due to the inadequacy of the technique used for detection or delayed recovery of anaemic situation after recent treatment with trypannocidal drugs or factors other than trypanosomosis such as compound effects of poor nutrition and blood feeding helminth infections such as haemonchosis and bunostomosis [35,36].

Conclusion

Trypanosomiasis is a serious, fatal disease of all domestic and wild animals including human beings. The prevalence of trypanosomiasis in cattle in the present study was 8.6%, and the infection was due to T. congolense and T. vivax. Although the prevalence seems low, owing to the economic importance of the disease serious attention should be given to reduce the prevalence and bring the disease under control.

Acknowledgements

The authors would like to thank the Bahir Dar Regional Laboratory for the provision of laboratory materials and consumables. More over all the animal owners involved in the study are duly acknowledged for their unreserved willingness and cooperation.

Risk factor		Total examined	No. positive	Prevalence	χ² (p- value)
Age					
	≤ 3	63	3	4.80%	1.409 (0.235)
	>3	321	30	9.30%	
Sex					
	Male	245	19	7.80%	0.606 (0.436)
	Female	139	14	10.10%	
Body condition					
	Poor	88	22	25%	39.46 (0.000)
	Medium	284	10	3.50%	
	Good	12	1	8.30%	
Coat color					
	Black	112	19	17%	14.134 (0.001)
	Red	207	11	5.30%	
	White	65	3	4.60%	

Table 2: Prevalence of *Trypanosoma* species based on coat color.

PCV	No Examined	No. Infected (%)	Prevalence (%)	P-value
Anaemic (PCV ≤ 24)	292	16 (48.48%)	5.47	15.048 (0.000)
Normal (PCV>24)	92	17 (51.51)	18.4	
Total	384	33 (100)	-8.6	

Table 3: Prevalence of bovine Trypanosomosis based on PCV value.

Infection status	No of animals	Mean PCV (Mean ± SD)	t-test	p-value
Parasitemic	33	22.94 ± 2.70	4.86	0
Aparasitemic	351	27.24 ± 5.02		

Table 4: Mean PCV value of parasitemic and aparasitemic animal in cattle.

References

1. Aulak, GS, Singla LD, Singh J (2005) Bovine trypanosomosis due to Trypanosoma evansi: Clinical, haematobiochemical and therapeutic studies. In: New Horizons in Animal Sciences, Sobti RC and Sharma VL (eds), Vishal Publishing and Co., Jalandhar, pp: 137-144.

2. Sharma A, Singla LD, Tuli A, Kaur P, Bal MS (2015) Detection and assessment of risk factors associated with natural concurrent infection of Trypanosoma evansi and Anaplasma marginale in dairy animals by duplex PCR in eastern Punjab. Trop Ani Helth Prod 47: 251-257.

3. Slingenbergh J (1992) Tsetse control and agricultural development in Ethiopia. World Ani Rev 70: 30-36.

4. Admasu B (2002) Welcome address; Animal health and poverty reduction strategies. In: Prov. 16th Animal Conference of Ethiopia the Ethiopia Veterinary Association (EVA), held 56, pp: 117-137.

5. Uilenberg G (1998) A field guide for diagnosis treatment and prevention of African animals trypanosomosis. FAO, Rome, pp: 43-89.

6. Stephen LE (1986) Trypanosomosis; a veterinary prospect. Pergamma Press, UK, p: 551.

7. MOA (Ministry of agriculture) (1995) Federal democratic republic of this ruminant livestock development strategy, Ethiopia. p: 28.

8. Murray M, Gray AR (1986) The current situation on animal trypanosomosis in Africa. Preventive Veterinary Medicine 2: 23-30.

9. Dehaan C, Bekure S (1999) Animal health service in Sub-Saharan Africa, initial experience with new approaches. Washington DC, World Bank.

10. Cherenet T, Sani RA, Speybroeck N, Panandam JM, Nadzr S (2004) Seasonal prevalence of bovine trypanosomosis in tsetse infected zone and tsetse free zone of Amhara region, North West Ethiopia. J Vet Res 71: 307-314.

11. Shimelis D, Aran KS, Getachew A (2005) Epidemiology of tsetse transmitte trypanosomosis in Abay (Blue Nile) basin of North West Ethiopia. In: proceedings of the 28th meeting of the International Scientific Council for Trypanosomosis.

12. Sinishaw A (2004) Prevalence of trypanomiasis of cattle in three Woreda of Amhara Region. MSc Thesis FVM, AAU, Debre Zeit, Ethiopia.

13. Amhara Regional Agriculture and Rural Development Office (ARARDO) (2010) Woreda livestock palpation data for Debre Elias, Dembecha and Jabitehenan of Amhara Regional Agriculture and Rural Development Office.

14. Thrusfield M (2005) Veterinary Epidemiology. 3rd edn. Blackwell Science Ltd, UK, pp: 233-250.

15. Nicholson MJ, Butterworth MH (1986) A guide to condition scoring of zebu cattle. ILCA, Addis Ababa, Ethiopia.

16. Bitew M, Amedie Y, Abebe A, Tolosa T (2011) Prevalence of bovine Trypanosomosis in selected areas of Jabi Tehenan district, West Gojam of Amhara regional state, Northwestern Ethiopia. Afr J Agri Res 6: 140-144.

17. Murray M, Murray PK, McIntyre WIM (1977) An improved parasitological technique for the diagnosis of African trypanosomisis. Transaction Royal Soc Trop Med Hyg 71: 325-326.

18. Paris J, Murray M, Mcodimba F (1982) A comparative evaluation of the parasitological technique currently available for the diagnosis of African Trypanosomosis in cattle, Act Trop 39: 307-316.

19. Woo PTK (1996) The hematological centrifugation technique for the detection of Trypanosomas. Canadian J 47: 921-923.

20. OIE 2008 Trypanosomosis (tsetse-transmitted): Terrestrial Manual. Office International des. Epizooties (OIE), Paris, France.

21. Abraham Z, Tesfaheywet Z (2012) Prevalence of Bovine Trypanosomosis in Selected District of Arba Minch, Snnpr, Southern Ethiopia. Global Vet 8: 168-173.

22. Solomon WM (2003) Amhara project plan and estimate on survey of tsetse and trypanosomosis of domestic animal in Amhara region, Bahir Dar, Ethiopia, p: 5.

23. Shimelis D (2004) Epidemiology of bovine trypanosomosis in the Abay basin area of North West Ethiopia. MSc Thesis, Addis Ababa, FVM, Debre Zeit.

24. Abebayehu T, Berhanu M, Rahmeto R, Solomon M (2011) Mechanically transmitted Bovine Trypanosomosis in Tselamity wereda, Western Tigray, Northern Ethiopia. J Agri 6: 10-13.

25. Ayana M, Tesfaheywet Z, Getnet F (2012) A cross-sectional study on the prevalence of bovine Trypanosomosis in Amhara region, Northwest Ethiopia. Lives Res Rural Develop 24: 1-8.

26. Adane M, Gezahagne M (2001) Bovine trypanosomosis in three districts of East Gojam Zone boardering the Blue Nile River in Ethiopia. J Infect Dev Countries 1: 131-325.

27. Langridger WP (1976) Tsetse and trypanosomosis survey of Ethiopia. Ministry of oversee Department, UK, pp: 1-40.

28. Fimmen HO, Mehlitz D, Horchiner F, Korb E (1992) Colostral antibodies and Trypanosoma congolense infection in calves. Trypanotolerance research application. GTZ, Germany 116, pp: 173-187.

29. Mussa A (2002) Prevalence of Bovine Trypanosomosis in Goro wereda, Southwest Ethiopia. DVM Thesis, FVM, AAU, Debre Zeit, Ethlopia.

30. Nigatu SD (2004) Epidemiology of bovine trypanosomosis in the Abbay Basin areas of Northwest Ethiopia. MSc Thesis, FVM, AAU, Debre Zeit, Ethiopia.

31. Leak SGA (1999) Tsetse biology and ecology. Their role in the epidemiology and control of trypanosomosis. Wallingford, UK: CABI publishing in association with the ILRI, pp: 152-210.

32. Van den Bossche P, Shumba W, Makhambera P (2000) The distribution and epidemiology of bovine trypanosomosis in Malawi. Vet Parasitol 88: 163-176.

33. Dinka H, Abebe G (2005) Small ruminant trypanosomosis in the southwest of Ethiopia. Small Rum Res 57: 239-243.

34. Sinishaw A, Abebe G, Desquesnes M, Yoni W (2006) Biting flies and Trypanosoma vivax infections in three highland districts bordering Lake Tana, Ethiopia. Vet Parasitol 142: 35-46.

35. Afework YS, Clausen PH, Abebe G, Tilahun G, Mehlitz D (2000) A prevalence of multiple drug-resistant T. congolense population in village cattle of Mekele district, North-West Ethiopia. Act Trop 76: 231-138.

36. Van den Bossche P, Rowlands GJ (2001) The relationship between the parasitological prevalence of trypanosomal infection in cattle and herd average packed cell volume. Act Trop 78: 163-170.

33

Tick Prevalence and Associated Udder Damage and Mastitis on Cattle in Jimma Town, Southwestern Ethiopia

Sena Meskela[1]* and Abebaw Gashaw[2]

[1]*Akaki Woreda Livestock and Fisheries Development, Ethiopia*
[2]*College of Agriculture and Veterinary Medicine, Jimma University, Ethiopia*

Abstract

A cross-sectional survey was conducted to determine tick prevalence and their association with mastitis on 390 cattle at three communal grazing sites and two dairy farms from October 2008 to April 2009 in Jimma town. Ticks were collected from half body parts and udder and teats were examined on lactating cows and heifers to identify tick lesions and mastitis. Of total 3015 ticks in number collected, 3 genera and 5 species of ticks had been identified: *Amblyomma cohaerens* (44.94%), *Amblyomma variegatum* (31.11%), *Boophilus decoloratus* (18.97%), *Rhipicephalus evertsi evertsi* (3.08%) and *Amblyomma gemma* (1.9%). There was a significant variation with predilection site of tick species. *A. variegatum*, *A. gemma* and *R. evertsi evertsi* had a significance variation with age of the animal. *B. decoloratus* and *R. evertsi evertsi* had significance variation with breed of cattle. Udder, Brisket and Perineum were the predominant predilection sites for the tick species collected. *R. evertsi evertsi* was the only species prefer Ano-vulva region. Result on the immature ticks (larvae and nymphs) shows that, 63.47% *Amblyomma*, 35.75% *Boophilus* and 0.77% *Rhipicephalus* genera. Neck, Dewlap, Udder and Perineum were the main predilection sites of ticks on which the immature ticks were collected. Although (123) 31.6% of the sampled cattle had some degree of udder and teat damage, out of those cows and heifers with udder and teat damage (30) 24.39% was positive for mastitis. The tick species found on cattle with udder and teat damage were *Amblyomma cohaerens* (46.51%), *Amblyomma variegatum* (40.62%), *Boophilus decoloratus* (11.88%) and *Amblyomma gemma* (0.99%). There was a significance variation between study sites and breed of cattle on animals with mastitis. Tick infestations associated udder lesions, and mastitis is major problems in cattle and deserves further attention owning to their potential impact on milk production affecting food security.

Keywords: Cattle; Ticks; Mastitis; Udder damage; Jimma; Ethiopia

Introduction

Tick infestation and tick-borne diseases (TBDs) are important conditions affecting livestock health and productivity in Ethiopia. Ticks are responsible for direct damage to livestock through their feeding habits. The damage is manifested as hide damage, damage to udders, teats and scrotum, myiasis due to infestation of damaged sites by maggots and secondary microbial infections. They transmit a variety of infective organisms mechanically or cyclically to animals and man. Most of the diseases transmitted by ticks are of major economically importance. Moreover, they inflict great havoc by continual loss of blood and creating different grade of lesions on the skin [1,2].

Mastitis usually occurs in response primarily to intramammary bacterial infection, but also to intramammary mycoplasmal, fungal or algal infections. Mechanical trauma, thermal trauma, and chemical insult predispose the gland to intramammary infection. Occurrence of mastitis depends on the interaction of host, agent, and environmental factors. Mammary tissue damage reduces the number and activity of epithelial cells and consequently contributes to decreased milk production [3].

Ticks also affect production in various ways. They can affect growth rate, milk production, fertility and the value of hides, cause udder damage, and mortality. Among this, mastitis is one of the most complex diseases of cows that mostly predisposed by different tick species under different management system and breed [4].

In Ethiopia, the studies so far conducted in the country indicated that the most important ticks belong to genera *Amblyomma*, *Boophilus*, *Hyalomma* and *Rhipicephalus*. These ticks are important transmitter of diseases and can damage hides and skins and interfere with meat and milk production.

Ticks are one of the dominant ectoparasite of cattle that cause cow's and heifer's udder to swollen and harden which leads the culling and decrease in milk production. Relevant data on the population dynamics of ticks on cattle (exotic and local) and mastitis (hardening and swelling of udder) due to tick's species is essential for the development of effective tick, and tick borne disease control strategies.

Therefore, the objectives of this study are to identify the tick species with its predilection site, determine the prevalence of tick species and to see the effect of tick on udder and teat and its association with mastitis on cattle in Jimma town, southwestern Ethiopia.

Significance of the study

The study result is useful for strengthen the tick control program like using acaricides, tick resistant breed, chemotherapy and chemoprophylaxis (for TBDs), traditional tick control and management. It also opens the future further study on the effect of ticks on mammary gland on other parts of the country. The result also used for local program in improving production quality and access to control service.

*Corresponding author: Sena Meskela, Akaki Woreda Livestock and Fisheries Development, Ethiopia, E-mail: senameskela62@gmail.com

Materials and Methods

Study area

The survey was conducted in Jimma town by selecting three grazing sites where cattle's of Jimma town grazing together and dairy farms. The sites were, Seto, Kito, Jiren and two dairy farms in the town. Jimma town is found in Oromia Regional State 357 km from Addis Ababa. The altitude of the area varies between 1600-2110 above sea level. The total area of the town cover is 4626 hectare. The mean annual rainfall is ranging from 1420-1800 mms. The area has 12°C-28°C an average range of temperature. The human population of the town was estimated approximately 150, 000. Jimma town has 18354 cattle, 1846 goat, 3310 sheep, 1400 horses, 250 donkeys, and 65 mule populations [5].

Study population

Study animal: A total of 390 cattle (local and cross) was selected by systematic random sampling technique for ticks collection and identification from eight half- body regions of cattle: Udder, brisket, perineum, thigh, anovulva, ear, abdomen and neck, for the tick survey in Jimma town, during study period (from November 2008 to April 2009).

The animals was identified by their own breed and categorized into age, and site. The animal's management system in all study sites of Seto, Kito and Jiren was more traditional in which they graze a natural pasture during day time (extensive management) and of a two dairy farms, i.e., a cross breed is feed and watered in house and graze outside together some times (semi-intensive).

Study design: The study type is a cross-sectional study which is describing and quantifying the distribution of tick species tick borne disease and mastitis.

Sample size and sampling method: Ticks was collected from 390 cattle selected based on the availability of ticks on their body purposeful sampling technique from three selected sites and two dairy farms of Jimma town. The sample size was determined using the formula given by Thrusfield, by assuming the expected prevalence of 50% tick infestation, confidence interval 95% and at 5% absolute precision and minimum sample size value [6].

Therefore, 390 cattle sample size employed. Then adult ticks were collected from eight different half- body parts of cattle. Cattle grazing in group from three sites and two dairy farms were selected randomly in every study days per week. After that adult Ixodid ticks were collected from eight half-body regions of the animal body into separate sample bottle. All the collected adult ticks were identified to species level using stereomicroscope at JUCAVM Veterinary parasitology and pathology laboratory within one week of the collection.

Study methodology

Tick collection and identification: Tick samples were collected early in the morning. The samples were preserved in 70% alcohol and identified according to their species, sex, and developmental stage. Collection is done by hand picking method after examine the presence of the tick on different body parts of the animal. Udder, brisket, perineum, thigh, anovulva, ear, abdomen and neck were the body part where ticks were collected. Ticks were identified, counted and recorded by species, sex. All ticks was counted and kept in pre-labeled by time, date of collection, predilection site of ticks, ages of the animals, and breed of animals in universal Bottles containing 70% alcohol until identification was done under stereomicroscope according to Walker et al. and Morel [7,8].

A total of 100 thin blood smears was made during study period. The smears were dried, fixed with methanol alcohol for 5 minutes, stained with Giemsa solution in phosphate buffered saline (pH 7.2) for 30 minutes and examined under oil immersion compound microscope for tick borne diseases [9,10].

The presence of tick and lesions on the udder was first observed visually and then palpation of the hardening and swelling of udder later checked for mastitis with California mastitis test (CMT). Finally, the number of cows and heifers having this problem were registered from all study sites and ticks collected and identified from those affected animals.

Data analysis: Data was entered to Microsoft Excel data base system and using SPSS 16.00 version software computer program. Chi-Square test was employed to determine the association between tick species with age, breed and predilection site of the animals. Descriptive statistic was used to summarize the data generated from the study and the prevalence of mastitis was calculated using percentage values and chi-square test used to calculate the association of the disease with breed, age and site of study.

Results

A total of 3015 tick species collected, 3 genera and 5 species of ticks had been identified. 78.73% (*Amblyomma*), 19.16% (*Boophilus*) and 3.11% (*Rhipicephalus*) genera were encountered (Table 1). Among the five species identified *Amblyomma cohaerens* (44.94%), *Amblyomma variegatum* (31.11%), *Boophilus decoloratus* (18.97%), *Rhipicephalus evertsi evertsi* (3.08%) and *Amblyomma gemma* (1.90%) contained. *A cohaerens* was the most abundant and followed by *A. variegatum* and *B. decoloratus*. The least one was *A. gemma* (Table 2). There was a highly significance variation of all tick species with predilection sites (p<0.000). *A. variegatum* (p<0.005), *A. gemma (p<0.001) Rh. e evertsi* (p<0.010) had a significance variation with age of the animal. *B. decoloratus* (p<0.001) and *Rh. e evertsi* (p<0.027) had significance variation with breed of cattle. Udder, Brisket and Perineum were the most sites where the tick species collected. *Rh. e evertsi* was the only species prefer Anovulva region (Graph 1).

Data on the immature ticks (larvae and nymphs) shows that, 63.47% (*Amblyomma*), 35.75% (*Boophilus*) and 0.77% (*Rhipicephalus*) genera. Neck, Dewlap, Udder and Perineum were the sites on which the immature ticks were collected.

No	Genus	Total tick	Prevalence %
1	*Amblyomma*	2350	78.73%
2	*Boophilus*	572	19.16%
3	*Rhipicephalus*	93	3.11%

Table 1: Prevalence of tick genera collected on cattle in Jimma town.

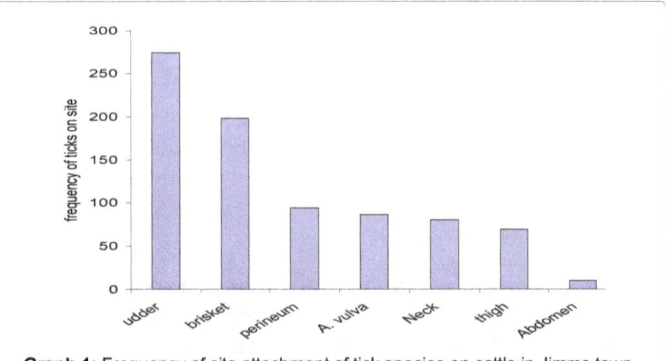

Graph 1: Frequency of site attachment of tick species on cattle in Jimma town.

No	Tick species	Total ticks	Prevalence	Predilection sites
1	*Amblyomma cohaerens*	1355	44.94%	Udder, Brisket, Perineum, thigh Anovulva and Abdomen
2	*Amblyomma variegatum*	938	31.11%	Udder, Brisket, Perineum, thigh, Anovulva and Abdomen
3	*Boophilus decoloratus*	572	18.97%	Udder, Brisket, Perineum, thigh, Anovulva and Abdomen
4	*Rhipicephalus e. evertsi*	93	3.08%	Anovulva
5	*Amblyomma gemma*	57	1.90%	Udder, Brisket, Perineum, thigh, Anovulva and ear

Table 2: Percentage distribution of tick species infesting cattle at Jimma town with predilection site encountered.

From 100 thin blood smear slide observed, 1 (1%) *Babesia Bigemina* parasite was identified. From a total of 123 udder of cows and heifers observed and examined during the study period, 30 (24.39%) of cows and heifers was positive to mastitis due to tick species. Tick species found were *Amblyomma cohaerens* (46.51%), *Amblyomma variegatum* (40.62%), *Boophilus decoloratus* (11.88%) and *Amblyomma gemma* (0.99%). There was a significance variation between study sites (X^2=9.576, p>0.023) and breed (X^2=15.682, p>0.000) of cattle udder examined.

Amblyomma cohaerens was the most abundant tick species found in the western Ethiopia and recorded on the first in this study. Although, generally observed in low numbers as compared to the previous findings. The species was collected from Udder, Brisket, Perineum, Anovulva and Abdomen. There was a significance difference between the predilection sites (p<0.000) and found in high count on udder of cattle than other body parts.

Amblyomma variegatum was the second most abundant tick species found. This tick was found through all the study time and sites next to *Amblyomma cohaerens*. It was also collected from the animal body where of the *Amblyomma cohaerens* collected but in less count than it. The p-value of predilection site (p<0.000) was also the same as *A. cohaerens*, but there was a significance difference on age group (p<0.005). It increases on older animals. *Boophilus decoloratus* was the third abundant tick species next to *Amblyomma variegatum* encountered in Jimma town. The species was observed on all body parts collected. But, it is mainly collected from neck of the cattle.

Rhipicephalus evertsi evertsi was the only species found from the genera *Rhipicephalus* in Jimma town. The tick was counted in small number and only collected from Anovulva (under the tail and around the vulva), which was the favorable site and specific to it. Predilection site (p<0.000), age (p<0.010) and breed (p<0.027) had significance variation when compared with the species. *Amblyomma gemma* was the least species found in the study area. Only 0.99% from the total tick species collected and identified. It was collected from Brisket, Udder, Thigh, Anovulva, Ear and Perineum in least count. There was a significance variation between the species and age of the cattle (p<0.001).

During the period of observation, 772 immature ticks were collected. The immature ticks were identified into genera and *Amblyomma* 490 (63.47%), *Boophilus* 276 (35.75%) and *Rhipicephalus* 6 (0.77%) were found. Dewlap, Neck and udder were the major sites on the body of cattle where mainly the larvae and nymphs collected. In the prevalence of tick borne disease, 100 thin smear blood samples were made and examined under compound microscope. From examined slides only 1(1%) of *Babesia* parasite was observed. The parasite was *Babesia bigemina*.

The study done on the mastitis due to tick species infestation on the udder showed 30 positive cases (swelling, hardening, pyogenic swelling and teat closure and deformity). Ticks develop resistance to back dip. Out of 123 udders of cows and heifers examined during the study period, 21 cows and 9 heifers of both breeds were with the disease (Table 4). This case was highly observed on cross breeds, which is highly significant (p<0.000) and also on dairy farms cows and heifers (p<0.023). The new own result on this Harding and swelling of udder and teat (mastitis) due to ticks was, the observation of the case on heifers. From this, the only cross breed heifers were positive to the case and most of them were JUCAVM heifers. This swelling and hardening of udder and teat will make the heifer's teats partially or fully will be closed during they give birth. The ticks also make the heifers to leave for longer time without giving birth. The tick loads on all positive cases from half body part of the cattle's were 10-20/udder. The tick species frequently encountered were 46.51% (*Amblyomma cohaerens*), 40.62% (*Amblyomma variegatum*), 11.88% (*Boophilus decoloratus)* and 0.99% (*Amblyomma gemma*) in decreasing order (Graph 2 and Table 3).

Discussion

In the present study five species of the three genera were found. These are *Amblyomma cohaerens*, *Amblyomma variegatum*, *Boophilus decoloratus*, *Rhipicephalus evertsi evertsi* and *Amblyomma gemma*. The climatic factor, vegetation, and the grazing of cattle together in group increase the prevalence and the presence of similar tick species distribution in the area [10]. This result was consistent with previous tick species survey in western part of the country and Jimma zone [8,11-14].

Amblyomma cohaerens was the most abundant tick from all tick species surveyed (44.94%). The present observation (survey) supports the previous findings [11-14]. *A. cohaerens* was the most abundant in western, Ethiopia, where the climate is humid for much of the year it is the most abundant tick on cattle [15]. It also predominates in areas of broad leaved forest [12]. This species was collected mainly from udder; this is due to its long mouth and behavior of the tick.

Amblyomma variegatum was the second most abundant tick species (31.11%). The *A. variegatum* distribution is similar to that of *Boophilus decoloratus* and it is more wide spread throughout the western zone

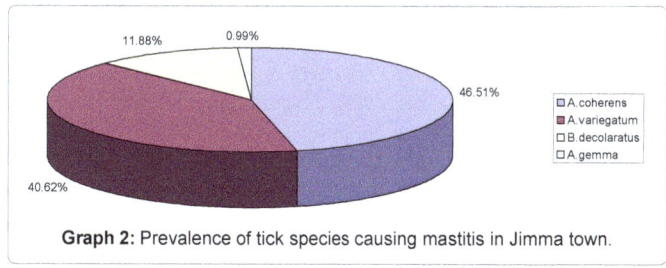

Graph 2: Prevalence of tick species causing mastitis in Jimma town.

Swelling/Harding of udder and teat	No of examined	Prevalence (%)
Present	30	24.39
Absent	93	75.61

Table 3: Prevalence of mastitis (udder and teat injuries) that influenced by tick on cow and heifer at Jimma town.

Risk factors	No examined	Positive	Prevalence (%)	X²	p-value
Site					
JUCAVM	22	11	8.943	9.576	0.023
Seto	46	9	7.317		
Kito	45	8	6.504		
Jiren	10	2	1.623		
Age					
Cow	75	21	17.07	1.358	0.171
Heifer	48	9	7.317		
Breed					
Cross	52	22	17.886	15.682	0.000
Local	71	8	6.504		

Table 4: Prevalence of mastitis (udder and teat swelling/harding) by site, age and breed in Jimma town.

but less abundant than *Amblyomma cohaerens* [11,12]. It is also the most widely distributed cattle tick in Ethiopia, but its abundance varies greatly [15]. In the present survey *Amblyomma variegatum* was increase or collected more than *Boophilus decoloratus*. This is due to the change in behavior of the tick and climatic condition. Its presence for long time on the animal body also increases the distribution on cattle. This species was collected more on larger animals or cows; this was due to the large size of the animals and physiological condition of cows.

This species has a great economic importance on cattle, because it has an association with heart water (cowdriosis) and dermatophilosis. Its long mouth also causes the deep penetration to skin tissue which predispose to secondary bacterial complication. It is one of the main tick species that lead the cow and heifers to mastitis case. This effect is due to its long mouth, strong attachment and longevity on the udder.

Boophilus decoloratus was the third tick species encountered (18.97%). Climatic factors and cattle raising practices associated with different breeds have a direct influence on the biology and ecology of *B. decoloratus*. No significant increase in tick population was observed during the short rains, *Boophilus decoloratus* peak population occur in May, June and July(maximum) and September and October is moderate [16]. This species has also a great economic importance on cattle, because it transmits *Babesia bigemina* and *Anaplasma marginale* on cattle. On this study it was the third abundant species next to *Amblyomma variegatum*. This result supports the seasonal finding of Abebaw and Pegram et al. [11,16]. This species collection was high on cross breed than local this was due to the blood level of the animals i.e., cross breed are more susceptible than local.

Rhipicephalus evertsi evertsi was the fourth common and abundant tick species (3.08%). *Rh. e. evertsi*, never numerous, appears to occupy a wide range of climatic and ecological condition, in coincide with the previous reports [11]. The present finding supports the previous finding of Abebaw [13]. This species prefer the site Anovulva, because of its short mouth can feed on soft or thin area, the high body temperature of the animal on the site, and also the needs to protect from external manual and climatic effect make it specific to the site.

Amblyomma gemma was the fifth species encountered during the study period (1.90%). It was the least species encountered during the study period, which supports the previous findings [12,14].

On immature ticks collection *Amblyomma genera* (63.42%) had been more than *Boophilus* (35.75%) and *Rhipicephalus* (0.77%). This result supports the previous finding of Yitbarek [14]. But, the dominant predilection site of these immature ticks collected was Neck, Udder, Dewlap and Perineum. This is due to the immature stage preferred to

attach the soft areas, because of the mouth parts of the ticks and the penetration by hypostome is not as such possible.

The preference of *Amblyomma* species (*Amblyomma cohaerens* and *Amblyomma variegatum*) to the udder (46.51% and 40.62%) respectively signifies their importance in causing udder and/or teat deformation in Jimma town. The prevalence of mastitis 30 cases (24.39%) of cows and heifers in Jimma town is due to the species *Amblyomma cohaerens* and *Amblyomma variegatum* effect on the udder. The 46.51% of the ticks collected from the udder was *Amblyomma cohaerens* this is due to high abundance in the area, the finding of 40.62% *Amblyomma variegatum* presence on udder is due to its long mouth, site preference, longevity on the site and its resistance to acaricide makes it the dominant causative agent of udder disease. The present result greatly support the Alekaw, which is 35.8% culling of cows due to useless udder and teat closure [17].

There is a great significance variation between cross and local breeds (p<0.000) of the town cattle. This finding also supports the previous findings of Demelash et al. [18]. The other significance variation present was the sites of study. JUCAVM dairy farm cattle are highly affected than other site, this is due to the breed and management system (which increase on semi-intensive cross than extensive local cattle) of ticks population. In JUCAVM farm the ticks *Amblyomma variegatum* was highly becoming resistant to acaricide sprayed weekly, for this the cattle in the farm were highly infected with the ticks and they resist the tick infestation, even the heifers waited for long time without giving the calf. Therefore, since the ticks were endemic to this area and the control of these ticks is become difficult, the strategic tick control and application acaricides of the *Amblyomma* sites is essential.

In general, the distribution limits of ticks are not fixed and constant, but are determined by a complex interaction of factors such as climate, host density, host susceptibility and grazing habits [19]. It follows that update studies of the present kind are necessary for the continuous understanding of the dynamic of tick population and the effect of the species on cattle (mastitis and TBDs). Such understanding ultimately leads to application of improved control strategies.

Conclusion and Recommendation

Available information on tick species, tick population dynamics and its effect on udder and disease transmission are essential to asses the losses encountered due to ticks. The survey of tick species is the main factor that exerts a major quantities influence on mastitis and the transmission of TBD. Therefore, this study of cattle tick species survey and its association with mastitis on cattle was done in Jimma town to provide this basic information. The tick species identified in the study area were *Amblyomma cohaerens*, *Amblyomma variegatum*, *Boophilus decoloratus*, *Rhipicephalus evertsi evertsi* and *Amblyomma gemma*. Among the species identified *A. cohaerens*, *A. variegatum* and *B. decoloratus* were the most abundant in the area. These species has a great economic importance on the cattle especially due to their mechanical effect on animal body and as a vector of disease transmission in Jimma town. JUCAVM dairy farm is highly at risk to udder infection; in this farm *Amblyomma variegatum* causes a great damage on udder and teats. This species also increase in number on wet condition and rainfall. Generally, the presence of these species on the study area needs a strong strategic, threshold, tick resistant cattle and management control programs. *Boophilus decoloratus* is also observed next to *Amblyomma variegatum*, this species transmitting the disease called *Babesiosis*. To control this species the seasonal observation and application of acaricides on immature stages and adults are essential. Depend on the above conclusion the following recommendations are forwarded:

- Controlling tick species should be by observing the life cycle with these influencing factors on the area is essential.

- Spraying of acaricides especially to udder area is essential to control *Amblyomma* species, strategic control and proper follow up of mammary gland infection should be given attention to heifers of JUCAVM dairy farm.

- Cross and exotic breed cattle in the town also need the threshold and strategic control program.

- Strategic tick control application of acaricides based on tick population,

- integrated tick control (biological, chemical and ecological control methods combined with short interval pasture rotation and burning), and

- Extension work (educating animal owners on the problems of tick especially on mastitis, and the different control methods, which can be available in the area) is more essential.

- TBDs in the town, needs a further investigation to control the *Babesia* parasite and other parasites with the tick *Boophilus decolaratus.*

References

1. Abebaw G (2004) Seasonal dynamics of ticks (*Amblyomma cohaerens* and *Boophilus decoloratus)* and development of a management plan for tick and tick born diseases control on cattle in Jimma zone, Southwestern Ethiopia. Institute of Agronomy and Animal Production in the Tropics. Georg-August-University Göttingen.

2. Salih DA, Hussein AM, Singla LD (2015) Diagnostic Approaches for tick-borne haemoparasitic diseases in livestock. J Vet Med Anim Health 7: 45-56.

3. Zhao X, Lacasse P (2007) Mammary tissue damage during bovine mastitis: Causes and control. J Anim Sc. 86: 57-65.

4. Mekonnen S, Hussein I, Bedane B (2001) The distribution of ixodid ticks (Acari: Ixodidae) on domestic animals in central Ethiopia. Onderstepoort J Vet Res 68: 243-251.

5. BPEDORS (2000) Physical and socio economical profile of 180 District of Oromia Region. Bureau of Planning and Economic Development of Oromia Regional state, Physical Planning Development. Addis Ababa, Ethiopia, pp: 248-251.

6. Thrusfield M (1995) Veterinary Epidemiology. 2nd edn. Black Well Science Ltd., UK, pp: 182-198.

7. Walker AR, Bouattour A, Camicas JJ, Estrada-Pena A, Horak IG, et al. (2003) Ticks of domestic animals in Africa: a guide to identification of species. Bioscience Report, Edinburgh, Scotland, UK, pp: 1-1221.

8. Morel P (1989) Manual of tropical veterinary parasitology. Tick-borne Diseases of livestock in Africa. CAB International, UK, pp: 299-460.

9. Gupta SS, Singla LD (2012) Diagnostic trends in parasitic diseases of animals. In: Veterinary Diagnostics: Current Trends. Gupta RP, Garg SR, Nehra V, Lather D (eds.), Satish Serial Publishing House, Delhi, pp: 81-112.

10. Singh AP, Singla LD, Singh A (2000) A study on the effect of macroclimatic factors on the seasonal population dynamics of Boophilus micropus (Canes, 1888) infesting the cross breed cattle of Ludhiana district. Int J Anim Sci 15: 29-31.

11. Pegram RG, Hoogstral, HH, Wassef HV (1981) Ticks of Ethiopia distribution, ecology and host relationships of tick species infesting livestock. Bull Entomol Res 71: 339-359.

12. De Castro JJ (1994) Tick survey, Ethiopia. A survey of the tick species in western Ethiopia. Technical Report. FAO, Rome.

13. Abebaw G (1996) Epizootology of tick and tick borne diseases in Jimma Zone Southwestern Ethiopia, MSc Thesis, Institute of Agronomy and Animal Production in the Tropics. Georg-August-University Göttingen.

14. Yitbarek G (2004) Tick species infesting livestock in Jimma area, southwest Ethiopia. DVM Thesis, Faculty of Veterinary Medicine, Ababa University, Debre Zeit, Ethiopia.

15. Pegram RG, Tatchell RJ, Decastro JJ, Chizyuka HGB, Creck MJ, et al. (2002) Tick control: New Concept.

16. Abebaw G (2004) Seasonal dynamics and host preference of *Boophilus decoloratus* (Koch, 1944) on naturally infested cattle in Jimma zone, south western Ethiopia. Ethiopia Vet J 18: 19-28.

17. Alekaw S (2000) Distribution of ticks and tick-borne diseases at Metekel Ranch. Ethiopian Vet J 4: 3.

18. Demelash B, Etana D, Fekadu B (2005) Prevalence and Risk Factors of Mastitis in Lactating Dairy Cows in Southern Ethiopia. J Appl Res Vet Med 3: 3.

19. Tatchell RJ, Easton E (1986) Ticks (Acari Ixodoidae), ecological studies in Tanzania. Bull Entomol Res 76: 229-246.

34

Occurrence and Distribution of Varroa Mite and Antivarroa Effect of Propolis in Walmara District of Oromia Special Zone Around Finfine, Ethiopia

Ebisa Mezgabu[1], Eyob Hirpa[1]*, Dasselegn Begna[2], Lama Yimer[1], Abdisa Bayan[3] and Misganu Chali[4]

[1]School of Veterinary Medicine, Wollega University College of Medical and Health Science, PO Box 395, Nekemte, Ethiopia
[2]Holeta Research Institute, Bee Research Center, Holota, Ethiopia
[3]Gudeya Bila Veterinary Clinic, Ethiopia
[4]Haru District Jeto Veterinary Clinic, Ethiopia

Abstract

A cross-sectional study was carried out from November, 2014 to April, 2015 aimed to assess the occurrence, infestation rate and associated risk factors of Varroa mite on Honeybees; investigation of the effect of propolis on varroa mites in Walmara District. Purposive sampling was used in Peasant Association; twelve apiaries and sixty four hives were randomly selected for inspection. Interviews, direct observation and experimental set up were the main data collection techniques used to gather the information. The results revealed the whole (384) bee colonies examined for Varroa mites were Positive with varies infestation range 4%-53% in brood and 4%-36% in adult Honeybees. The highest Adult infestation rate 18.20 ± 7.99% of Varroa mites was observed in Tullu Harbu, while the lowest infestation rate (14.25 ± 5.12%) was observed Wajitu Harbu. on other side The highest Brood infestation rate (22.76 ± 9.64) % of Varroa mites was observed in Nano Suba, while the lowest infestation rate 13.73 ± 5.88% was observed Wajitu Harbu. Infestation levels showed significant relationship with colony type (p=0.006). Weak colony type is highly infested than strong colony, However, associated risk factors including age, sex, educational status, duration of experience of Beekeepers, and site and hive type were not showed statistical significance with Varroa mite infestation (P>0.05). Effect of Propolis against Varroa Mite has been investigated and showed lethal effect. Propolis extracted with 70% ethanol was found to be highly toxic, at 20% (w/v) of propolis resulting in 94.44% mortality with a brief contact time of 5 sec. The study showed that whole bee colonies examined were co-existed with the mites and lethal effect of propolis on Varroa mites. Therefore, improved management system and further research to use propolis extract as a treatment option was recommended.

Keywords: Honeybee; Infestation; Propolis; Varroamites; Walmara

Introduction

Most Honeybee researchers consider the ectoparasitic mite *Varroa destructor* (*V. destructor*) to be the most damaging enemy of the Honeybee. It has been recently identified as one of the major factor responsible for colony losses worldwide [1]. No other pathogen has had such a large impact on beekeeping or Honeybee research through the history of apiculture. The mite weakens the Honeybees immunity and their susceptibility to other environmental stressors and vectors lethal Honeybee viruses [2].

Varroa mite was originated from South-East Asia and was originally confined to the Eastern Honeybee *Apis cerana* (*A. cerana*). After a shift to the new host the Western Honeybee, *Apis mellifera* (*A. mellifera*), during the first half of the last century, the parasite has become widespread across most continents. The mite is spread by foraging and swarming bees and Varroa females are transported on adult bees to brood cells for reproduction. Shortly after leaving the brood cell on a young bee, the mites preferentially infest nurse bees for transport back to the brood cells. This may be an adaptive strategy for the Varroa females to increase their reproductive success [3].

The mite feeds on the bee by injuring the cuticle of the pupae and sucking substantial amounts of haemolymph. The haemolymph is an insect's equivalent to blood, distributing nutrients throughout the bee, including immune components which form one of the primary lines of defense against invading microorganisms [4].

The threat of Honeybee infestation by *V. destructor* forces Beekeepers in many parts of the world to treat their colonies with acaricides, which are associated with drawbacks. The most serious drawbacks are the buildup of residues in bee products [5] and the development of resistant mite strains. The problems associated with the use of acaricides provide considerable incentive to develop new treatment strategies and screening for potential acaricides that minimize these problems. Natural products having components with various modes of action might provide effective solution to the problem of varroosis [6]. One of such natural products is propolis, a complex mixture of several compounds collected by honeybees from plants, mixed with wax and used in the construction and protection of the beehive [7].

Propolis is a natural remedy that has been used extensively since antiquity. The Egyptians, who knew very well the anti-putrefactive properties of propolis, used it for embalming [7]. It was recognized for its medicinal properties by Greek and Roman physicians, such as Aristotle, Dioscorides, Pliny and Galen. The drug was used as an

*Corresponding author: Eyob Hirpa, Assistant Professor, School of Veterinary Medicine, Wollega University, PO Box 395, Wollega, Ethiopia
E-mail: eyobresearch@gmail.com

antiseptic and healing in the treatment of wounds and as a mouth wash, and its use in the Middle Ages perpetuated among Arab doctors [8]. Also, it was widely used in the form of ointment and cream in the treatment of wounds in battle field, because of their healing effect. This healing property of propolis is known as "Balm of Gilead," is also mentioned in the Holy Bible [9].

From the pharmacological point of view, propolis has been used as solid; in an ointment based on Vaseline, lanolin, olive oil or butter, and in the form of alcoholic extract and hydro alcoholic solution. The proportion propolis/carrier may vary, in order to obtain bacteriostatic or bactericidal results. In Dentistry, there are studies investigating the pharmacological activity of propolis some situations, such as gingivitis, periodontitis, oral ulcers, pulp mummification in dogs' teeth and dental plaque and caries in rats [10]. Also, it has been used in dressings of pre and post-surgical treatment, oral candididosis, oral herpes viruses and oral hygiene. The global interest in propolis research increased considerably in relation to its various biological properties [11].

Literature on the acaricidal or insecticidal action of propolis is very limited. It has been assumed that components of nectar, pollen and propolis may adversely affect the development of *V. destructor* in the hive of some bee populations. Some authors proposed that some flavonoid components of propolis have insecticidal or at least insect static (inhibition of insect larval development) effects [12,13].

Even though our country is rich with different floras and climate which are conducive for Beekeeping, honey and other hive product production is limited due to many problems like pests infestation of honey bee colonies. Of these pests, Varroa mite causes huge impact. This impact can be solved by using a natural product, propolis.

Therefore, the study was designed with the following objectives:

- To assess the occurrence and infestation rate of Varroa mite in Walmara District and

- To investigate the effect of propolis on varroa mites.

Materials and Methods

Study area

The study was conducted in central high land of Ethiopia, in Oromia special zone around Finfine in Walmara District from November, 2014 to April, 2015. Walmara District is located at 25 kms to the West of Addis Ababa (8.5°-9.5°N and 38.4°-39.2°E) with altitude of 2000-3380 meters above sea level. It has annual rain fall and temperature ranging from 334-1350 mm and 5°C-27°C respectively. Walmara District has number of livestock on the basis of species as 188221 cattle, 108652 sheep, 15420 goats, 365294 poultry, 8062 horses, 229 Mules and 1853 traditional, 870 transitional 843 modern bee hives with the estimated human population of 83,784 and the district has large forest, shrubs and herbs. It is bordered by Burayu town to the East, Ejere District to the west, Sululta District to the North and Sebeta Hawas District from the south and its weather condition is classified as 39% Woinadegaand 61% dega respectively (Walmara District Livestock and Agricultural Office 2014).

Study populations

Study populations included honeybee colonies found in the selected Peasant Associations of Walmara District and respondents (Beekeepers).

Study design

A cross sectional study was conducted in Beekeeping potential areas of Walmara District. Prior to the actual survey, information was gathered from secondary data from reports of the District's Agricultural Development Office and informal consultation with key informants.

Sample size determination and sampling technique

The total number of Bee colonies sample needed for the study were calculated by the rule of thumb, where there is no information for an area, it is possible to take 50% expected prevalence. The Z value of 1.96 is used at 95% CI and margin of error is 5% (n=sample size, P=proportion, D=margin of error [14]. Accordingly, the sample size (n) of the study is calculated as follows,

$$n = \frac{1.96^2(p)(1-p)}{d^2}$$

Where n=sample size; p=Expected prevalence; d=Desired level of precision (5%); n=384

Study methodology

Questionnaire survey and sampling procedure: Potential beekeeping Peasant Associations were identified in Walmara District according to the information gathered from Holeta Bee Research Center and secondary data from reports of the District's Agricultural Development Office and informal consultation with key informants Based on the information obtained from secondary data and informal survey, a structured questionnaire was developed and pre-tested for its consistency and applicability to the objectives of the study.

Based on this information, six Honeybee colonies potential Peasant Associations administrations including: Gole Liban, Nano Suba, Wajitu Harbu, Dawaf Lafto, Gebarobi and Tullu Harbu were selected out of thirty four Kebeles administrations in the district. Per selected Peasant Associations Administration, twelve model beekeepers, a total of seventy two respondents were selected by using purposive sampling technique and interviewed. Simultaneously, samples of broods and adults of Honeybees from the hive of each of the seventy two selected model Beekeepers randomly. Therefore, seventy two apiaries were sampled from the selected Peasant Associations, sixty four from each of the six Peasant Associations with a total of 384. Of the 384 colonies 129, 127, 128 were from traditional, transitional and modern hives respectively. One colony was counted as one sample. These colonies were sampled by using random sampling method by taking adult honey bee and brood samples from each colony the sample was taken to HBRC Laboratory for the diagnosis purpose. Sampling was carried out during the night to prevent bee sting and colony disturbance.

Adult and brood of honey bee sample collection: Samples of approximately 200-300 worker bees were taken from the brood chamber of the hive to determine the phoretic Varroa mite infestation rate on adult bees. The bees from each sample, which were 250 in number counted and then washed in soapy water to dislodge the mites. Using a strainer the mites were separated from the bees and were counted to calculate the proportion of mites per bee. Similarly, Samples of brood were collected by selecting an area of 5 × 5 cm in the middle of a worker comb. The cells were scratched and all stages of Varroa females in each cell were counted [15].

Propolis collection, preparation and extraction: Propolis sample used in the experiment was obtained by scraping off from frames of honey comb sampled from Gole Liben Peasant Association. Then, the collected propolis was weighed and frozen sample was homogenized using a coffee mill. The homogenate powder was then extracted in 70% ethanol. For effective extraction, the propolis powder was suspended in the corresponding ethanol solution in a ratio of 1:9 (w/v) [16]. The suspension was extracted in a rotary evaporator at 60°C for 2 hours. The suspension was then cooled at room temperature for 1 hour and suction filtered. The filtrate was dried in an incubator at 40°C to weight constancy, which was achieved in two weeks' time. The 70% ethanol extract was used in 55% ethanol in the bioassay to reduce the effect of strong ethanol solution on the experimental organisms. The concentrations used in the bioassay were 5%, 7.5%, 10%, 15%, 20% (w/v). However, the acaricide residue analysis of propolis was not performed. These activities were carried out in Holeta Bee Research Center Laboratory.

Varroa mite collection for experiment: Varroa Mites used for the experiment were collected from infested colonies of Holeta Bee Research Center apiary according to Garedew et al. [17]. The combs containing broods and infested with Varroa mites were taken and brought to. Then, cells were uncapped and broods were removed from the cells and mites were collected from it. In order to avoid starvation of the mites, they were kept in a Petri dish on bee larvae or pupae. Collection of mites was done from both the larval and pupal stage of healthy brood.

Bioassay: Treatment of the mites was done in Holeta Bee Research Center Laboratory, by applying 250 μL of a given concentration of propolis on a 3 cm × 3 cm tissue paper in a Petri dish and by immediately placing six mites per experiment on the wetted tissue paper. To observe the effect of contact time of propolis on the activity of *V. destructor*, the following treatment times were used: 5, 10, 20, 30, 40, 60, 75 and 90 seconds. The treatment was stopped after the allocated time by removing the mites with the tissue paper from the Petri dish and immediately placing them on a pad of paper towel for 1 minute to blot the excess fluid from the surfaces. They were then transferred to a clean Petri dish and their activity was observed under a dissecting lens every five minutes for the first hour, every 10 minutes for the next one hour and every 30 minutes for the next two hours. All treatments were done at room temperature. Control experiments for each experimental group were done by treating the mites with distilled water at the corresponding times. An individual was considered inactivated if it showed no leg movement or movement of any body part when gently prodded with a probe. If it showed movement it was counted as alive, irrespective of whether it was partially paralyzed or normal. If the inactivation lasted more than four hours after the treatment time, the mites were considered dead. Each treatment was repeated three times and the mean values, and in some cases the Mean ± Standard deviation values, were used in the presentation of results [17].

Data management and analysis

Collected data were stored in Microsoft Office Excel 2007 and analyzed by SPSS software version 20 for presentation of the results.

Results

Adult and brood of honey bees diagnosis result

This study showed that all the sampled Peasant Associations were tested positive to varroa mites. A two hundred fifty Bees per colony were examined through adult bee colonies and an infestation rate of 15.73 ± 6.903 (ranging from 4-36) varroa mites were recovered (Table 1). Although there was no much difference infestation rates between Peasant Associations, the result revealed Tullu Harbu, Geba Robi,

Sample type	Sample No	Prevalence	Infestation Rate(Range)
Brood	384	100%	18. 07 ± 7.03 (4-53)
Adult	384	100%	15.73 ± 6.903 (4-36)

Table 1: Prevalence and infestation rate in different sample type.

Kebeles	Sample type	Colonies sampled	Average infestation rate
TulluHarbu	Brood	64	19.41 ± 6.59 (5 to 33)
	Adult	64	18.20 ± 7.99 (4 to 36)
GebaRobi	Brood	64	20.69 ± 9.57 (5 to 33)
	Adult	64	16.52 ± 7.35 (5 to 35)
Nano Suba	Brood	64	22.76 ± 9.64 (8 to 53)
	Adult	64	15.02 ± 7.18 (5 to 33)
DawafLafto	Brood	64	17.94 ± 6.79 (6 to 36)
	Adult	64	15.22 ± 6.89(6 to 36)
GoleLiben	Brood	64	13.91 ± 5.74) (5 to 30)
	Adult	64	15.15 ± 6.00 (6 to 34)
Wajituarbu	Brood	64	13.73 ± 5.88 (4 to 34)
	Adult	64	14.25 ± 5.12 (6 to 27)

Table 2: Infestation rate at different peasant association.

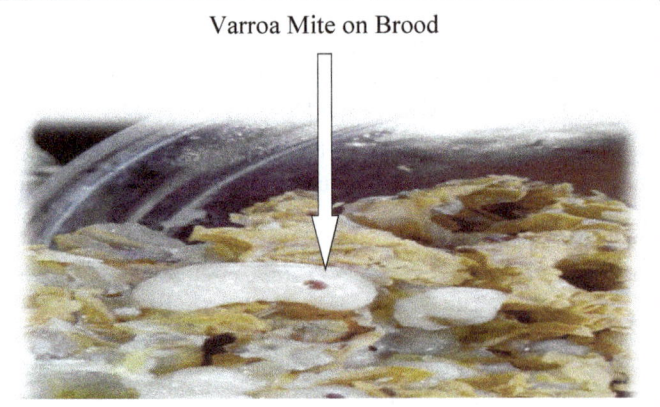

Varroa Mite on Brood

Figure 1: Brood infested with Varroa mite.

Dawaf Lafto, Gole Liben, Nano Suba, and Wajitu Harbu with 18.20 ± 7.99, 16.52 ± 7.35, 15.22 ± 6.89, 15.15 ± 6.00, 15.02 ± 7.18 and 14.25 ± 5.12 from the highest to the lowest respectively (Table 2). Therefore, overall varroa mite prevalence in Walmara District was 100%. In the similar way, all of the bee colonies diagnosed for adults were also diagnosed for brood, and found positive with Varroa mites (Figure 1). This also revealed that all the sampled Peasant Associations were infested with these mites and Brood bee shows high infestation rate than Adult bee even though it's not statically significant (P>0.05). The highest infestation rate was recorded in Nano Suba (22.76 ± 9.64) while lowest was recorded in Wajitu Harbu (13.73 ± 5.88) This indicated that Nano Suba and WajituHarbu Peasant Associations were found with highest and lowest varroa mite infestation rates respectively (Table 2). Regarding associated risk factors and Varro mite infestation, there is no statistically significant variation for type of Hive, type of sample and Peasant association (P>0.05) except Colony type showed Significant variation, Thus weak colony was highly infested than Strong colony (X^2=78, P=0.006).

Anti varroa effect of propolis result

The control solution of 55% propolis extract with distilled water, at different concentrations (5%, 7.5%,10%, 15% and 20%), at specified times (5, 10, 20, 30, 40, 60, 75, and 90 seconds) had no effect at all. The experiment result revealed that 20% (W/V) propolis concentration

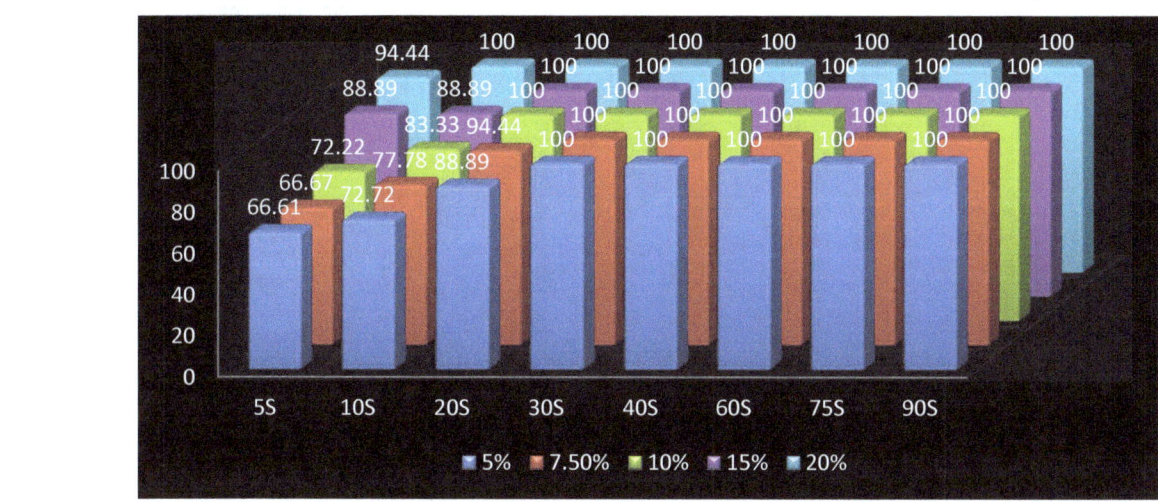

Figure 2: Average effect of propolis at different concentrations, at different times (in seconds).

were highly toxic for mite. It narcotized 100% within ten seconds and the lowest effect at 10 second was 72.72% in 5% (W/V) concentration. All propolis concentration type inactivate the whole Mite (100%) at greater than or equal to thirty second Contact time (Tables 3 and 4; Figure 2).

Questionnaire survey result

Among interviewed beekeepers, 69 (95.8%) were male and 3 (4.2%) were females and their educational status were, 21 (29.2%), illiterate, 35 (48.6%), elementary, 14 (19.4%), high school and 2 (2.8%) high level. About 69.4% (50/72) interviewed Beekeepers were did not have awareness of a Varroa Mite. Similarly, among the 22 Beekeepers who knew this mite, only 6 (27.27%) know the damage caused by it. There were no significant variation between risk factor such as, sex, educational status, Peasant Association and duration of experience with awareness of varroa mite and damage of Varroa mite (P>0.05).

Discussion

This study revealed that all sampled areas of the Walmara District were tested positive to varroa mites with infestation rate of 15.73 ± 6.9% Varroa mites per colonies were recorded. The finding agreed with the result 100% prevalence with average of 15 ± 7.45% infestation rate in Tigray Region, Ethiopia [18], 92% in Tanzania [19], 83% in Kenya [20] and similar results were also reported in South Jordan [21] and in Sudan Shambat apiary [22]. However, the present finding is higher than previous report 2.33 ± 0.83% (mean and standard deviation) for adult bees and 5.06 ± 2.47% for brood in Brazil [23]. This finding showed tremendous infestation behaviour of mites (Varroaspp) since they were not obstructed by variations in colony type, Hive type, and vegetation type of an area. Even though high varroa mite infestation was seen in this finding in Brood than Adult it was statistically insignificant (P>0.05). Although, there is no mechanism explaining why the varroa leaves an adult bee to invade brood cells, it is known that the number of varroas on brood is related to the season of the year and availability of brood in the hive [24,25]. According to Boot et al. [26], the mite enters a brood cell immediately after abandoning the body of an adult bee. Varroas moving on the comb have never been observed, showing that the mite does not look for a specific brood cell to invade. It is known that, to complete their reproductive cycle, adult Varroa females abandon adult bees and invade worker and drone brood cells [23].

Propolis Concentration (w/v)%	Average effect of propolis at different times (in seconds)							
	5 S	10 S	20 S	30 S	40 S	60 S	75 S	90 S
5%	66.61	72.72	88.89	100	100	100	100	100
7.50%	66.67	77.78	94.44	100	100	100	100	100
10%	72.22	83.33	100	100	100	100	100	100
15%	88.89	88.89	100	100	100	100	100	100
20%	94.44	100	100	100	100	100	100	100

Table 3: Anti Varroa effect of propolis trials average at different times (in seconds).

On the other hand, it is not certain how and when these mites invaded the honeybee colonies in the districts where mites were found. About 69.4% (50/72) interviewed beekeepers were did not have awareness of a Varroa mite. However, some of the beekeepers interviewed at different peasant association on Same District, reported that, they were familiar with the pest "Varroa mite" on its presence in honeybee broods they had no prior knowledge on its name "Varroa mite" or its impacts on honeybees. Similarly, among the 22(30.6%) Beekeepers who knew this mite, only 6 (27.27%) know the damage caused by it. In this study the majority (95.8%) of beekeepers were found to be males. This finding is in line with the study of Beyene and Verschuur [27] who noted beekeeping as the activity of men in Wonchi District of South West Shewa Zone. The limited number of female participation recorded in this study might be due to the fact that, even though all of the beekeeping activities or a part of it was carried out by females was reported as the activity of men. From the total respondents, 68% of them were attended elementary school to high school which is advantageous for easily grasping of any trainings in general and Beekeeping trainings in particular and apply it into practice to enhance production and productivity of honey and other hive products. However, 29.2% of respondents were illiterate.

Treatment of mites with propolis causes narcosis and death. The narcotic effect of propolis on different animals has already been mentioned in the literature [28,29]. The control experiment performed by using distilled water at different times (5, 10, 20, 30, 40, 60, 75, and 90 seconds did not shown any effect on the Varroa mites. This finding is Agree with the report of (30) in study of Varroacidal effect of propolis, noted that, contact with water had no effect at all. This may be due to the absence of components of propolis which cause mortality to varroa mites. The present experimental finding revealed

Propolis Concentration (w/v %)	Repeatability	Percentage of inactivated mite at different seconds							
		5	10	20	30	40	60	75	90
5%	Control	0	0	0	0	0	0	0	0
	A	50	83.33	83.33	100	100	100	100	100
	B	66.67	66.67	100	100	100	100	100	100
	C	66.67	66.67	83.33	100	100	100	100	100
7.5%	Control	0	0	0	0	0	0	0	0
	A	66.67	83.33	100	100	100	100	100	100
	B	66.67	66.67	83.33	100	100	100	100	100
	C	66.67	83.33	100	100	100	100	100	100
10%	Control	0	0	0	0	0	0	0	0
	A	66.67	83.33	100	100	100	100	100	100
	B	66.67	83.33	100	100	100	100	100	100
	C	83.33	83.33	100	100	100	100	100	100
15%	Control	0	0	0	0	0	0	0	0
	A	83.33	83.33	100	100	100	100	100	100
	B	100	100	100	100	100	100	100	100
	C	83.33	83.33	100	100	100	100	100	100
20%	Control	0	0	0	0	0	0	0	0
	A	100	100	100	100	100	100	100	100
	B	83.33	100	100	100	100	100	100	100
	C	100	100	100	100	100	100	100	100

Table 4: Percentage of inactivated mites at different concentrations, at different seconds.

that 20% (W/V) propolis concentration were highly toxic for mite it narcotize 100% within ten seconds. This finding is higher than previous research work reported by Garedew et al. [17] 55% narcotizing rate in twenty seconds. The death of mites in higher amount might be due to Propolis Extraction procedural difference and Acaracide residue in our propolis. Similarly, the narcotizing effect of propolis extracts increases as its concentration increases with the duration of increment of time of contact. This result agrees with the result of Garedew et al. [17], reported that the varroacidal action of propolis increases with increasing concentration and contact of time. In the similar way, the increment of mortality of mites with increment of concentration may be related with the increment of composition of propolis which causes the death of these mites.

Conclusion and Recommendations

Depending upon the evidence obtained from this study, majority of Beekeepers did not know the damage come with Varroa mite infestation. However, Varroa mite has infested both adult and brood of Honeybee colonies found in selected Peasant Associations of Walmara District. Based on this fact, this pest was one of the most series threats of honey bees which cause reduction in honey production and other hive products that were used. This study justifies the report which noted the presence of Varroa mites in the country at different times. On the other hand, the investigation observed, by conducting experiment that showed the effect of propolis on this mite can be a solution for the treatment of it without fearing of drug residues in honey and other products.

Therefore, depending upon the above facts, the following recommendations were forwarded:

- Varroa mite (*V. destructor*) which was one of the most threat of Beekeeping activity was found in the District and all the concerned bodies including governmental and non-governmental organizations should participate in the awareness creation for Beekeepers which focuses on prevention and control of this mite.

- Researchers should participate to conduct the effect of propolis on Varroa mites for the treatment of Varroosis and that can be used as commercial raw materials which are not known in our country for income diversification which can increase the economy of Beekeepers and the Country in general.

Competing Interests

The authors declare that they have no competing interests.

Authors' Contributions

Dasalegn Begna initiated the research, Ebisa Mezgebu conducted the data Collection and Eyob Hirpa performed the data analysis and drafted the manuscript. The four authors edited and approved the final manuscript.

Acknowledgements

The authors would like thank the University of Wollega for funding this study. We are also grateful to the Oromia regional State, the western Shoa Walmera district and Holeta bee research institute for facilitating this study. Last but not least, we extend our thanks to all the data collectors and Supervisors.

References

1. Nazzi F, Brown SP, Annoscia D, Del Piccolo F, Di Prisco G, et al. (2012) Synergistic Parasite-Pathogen Interactions Mediated by Host Immunity Can Drive the Collapse of Honeybee Colonies. PLoS Pathog 8: e1002735.

2. Boecking O, Genersch E (2008) Varroosis–the ongoing crisis in bee keeping. J Verbrauch Lebensm 3: 221-228.

3. Rosenkranz P, Aumeier P, Ziegelmann B (2010) Biology and control of Varroa destructor. J Invertebr Pathol 103: S96-S119.

4. Genersch E (2010) Honey bee pathology: current threats to honey bees and beekeeping. Appl Microbiol Biotechnol 87: 87-97.

5. Wallner K (1999) Varroacides and their residues in bee products. Apidologie 30: 235-248.

6. Imdorf A, Bogdanov S, Ibaez Ochoa R, Calderone NW (1999) Use of essential oils for the control of *Varroa jacobsoni* Oud. in honey bee colonies. Apidologie 30: 209-228.

7. Ghisalberti EL (1979) Propolis: a review. Bee world 60: 59-84.

8. Castaldo S, Capasso F (2002) Propolis, an old remedy used in modern medicine. Fitoterapia 73: S1-S6.

9. Park YK, Alencar SM, Moura FF, Ikegaki FFM (1999) Atividade biológica da própolis. Revista OESP–Alimentação 27: 46-53.

10. Geraldini CAC, Salgado EGC, de Mello Rode S (2010) Ação de diferentes soluções de própolis na superfície dentinária-avaliação ultra-estrutural. Brazilian Dental Science 3: 28-32.

11. Auricchio MT, Bugno A, Almodóvar AAB, Pereira TC (2006) Avaliação da atividade antimicrobiana de preparações de própolis comercializadas na cidade de São Paulo. Revista do Instituto Adolfo Lutz (Impresso) 65: 209-212.

12. König B, Dustmann JH (1988) Baumharze, Bienen und antivirale Chemotherapie. Naturwissenschaftliche Rundschau 41: 43-53.

13. Walmara District Livestock and Agricultural Office (2014) Walmara District. Oromia Special Zone around Finfine, Ethiopia.

14. Thrusfield M (2007) Veterinary Epidemiology. 3rd edn. Blackwell science Ltd., UK, pp: 182-198.

15. Fries I, Aarhus A, Hansen H, Korpela S (1991) Comparison of diagnostic methods for detection of low infestation levels of Varroa jacobsoni in honey-bee (Apis mellifera) colonies. Exp Appl Acarol 10: 279-287.

16. Strehl E, Volpert R, Elstner EF (1994) Biochemical activities of propolis-extracts III. Inhibition of dihydrofolate reductase. Z Naturforsch 49: 39-43.

17. Garedew A, Lamprecht I, Schmolz E, Schricker B (2002) The varroacidal action of propolis: a laboratory assay. Apidologie 33: 41-50.

18. Begna D (2015) Occurrences and Distributions of Honeybee (Apis mellifera Jemenetica) Varroa Mite (Varroa destructor) in Tigray Region, Ethiopia. J Fisheries Livest Prod 3: 126.

19. Mumbi CT, Mwakatobe AR, Mpinga IH, Richard A, Machumu R (2014) Parasitic mite, Varroa species (Parasitiformes: Varroidae) infesting the colonies of African honeybees, Apis mellifera scutellata (Hymenoptera: Apididae) in Tanzania. J Entomol Zool Stud 2: 188-196.

20. Muli E, Patch H, Frazier M, Frazier J, Torto B, et al. (2014) Evaluation of the distribution and impacts of parasites, pathogens, and pesticides on honey bee (Apis mellifera) populations in East Africa. PloS one 9: e94459.

21. Al-Chzawi AAMA, Zaitoun ST, Shannag HK (2009) Incidence and geographical distribution of Honeybee (Apis mellifera L.) pests in Jordan. In Annales de la Société Entomologique de France 45: 305-308.

22. El-Niweiri MAA, El-Sarrag MSA, Satti AA (2008) Survey of diseases and parasites of honeybees (Apis mellifera L.) in Sudan. SJBS Series B: Biol Sci 14: 141-159.

23. Eguaras M, Marcangeli J, Oppedisano M, Fernández N (1994) Seasonal changes in Varroa jacobsoni reproduction in temperate climates of Argentina. Bee Sci 3: 120-123.

24. Moretto G, Leonidas JDM (2003) Infestation and distribution of the mite Varroa destructor in colonies of Africanized bees. Braz J Biol 63: 83-86.

25. Boot WJ, Sisselaar DJ, Calis JN, Beetsma J (1994) Factors affecting invasion of Varroa jacobsoni (Acari: Varroidae) into honeybee, Apis mellifera (Hymenoptera: Apidae), brood cells. Bulletin of Entomological Research 84: 3-10.

26. Boot WJ, Beetsma J, Calis JN (1994) Behaviour of Varroa mites invading honey bee brood cells. Experimental & applied acarology 18: 371-379.

27. Beyene T, Verschuur M (2014) Assessment of constraints and opportunities of honey production in Wonchi District South West Shewa Zone of Oromia, Ethiopia. American Journal of Research Communication 2: 342-353.

28. Prokopovich NN, Flis ZA, Frankovskaya ZI, Kope'eva EP (1956) An anaesthetizing substance for use in stomatology. Vrachebnoe Delo 1: 41-44.

29. Prokopovich NN (1957) Propolis a new anaesthetic. Vrachebnoe Delo 10: 1077-1080.

35

Evaluation Commonly Used Anthelmintics Efficacy in Gastrointestinal Nematodes through Fecal Egg Count Reduction Test in Adaberga Dairy Farm, West Shewa Zone, Central Ethiopia

Anmaw Shite[1]*, Bemrew Admassu[1], Tadesse Guadu[2] and Yosef Malede[1]

[1]Faculty of Veterinary Medicine, Unit of Biomedical Sciences, University of Gondar, PO Box: 196, Gondar, Ethiopia
[2]Faculty of Veterinary Medicine, Department of Veterinary Epidemiology and Public Health, University of Gondar, PO Box: 196, Gondar, Ethiopia

Abstract

This study was conducted in Adaberga dairy farm West Showa Zone, from November, 2014 to April 2015 to evaluate commonly used anthelmintics efficacy against gastrointestinal nematodes. An experimental study design and purposive sampling procedure were employed to select 36 naturally infected jersey breed cattle from source population. And study populations were randomly allocated into three groups, twelve in each; the first group was treated with albendazole, the second with tetraclozan and the last group was left untreated (control). Fecal samples were collected from each cow before and after treatment and modified McMaster method was used to count eggs. Third stage larvae (L3) were recovered from the fecal cultures by the Baerman technique to identify gastrointestinal nematodes. The efficacy of each anthelmintic was determined by Fecal Egg Count Reduction Test (FECRT). SPSS Windows version 16.0 was used for data analysis. Descriptive statistics (means, standard error of mean and reduction percentages) were calculated to manage data. Means were compared among groups through analysis of variance (ANOVA) and difference between treatments was compared using least square method of multiple comparisons. The percentage reduction in mean fecal egg count, after 10 days of treatment, for Albendazole and tetraclozan were 95.51% and 98.18% respectively. There was no statistically significant difference (p=0.262) among the egg count of control, albendazole treated and tetraclozan treated groups before treatment. Statistically egg counts were not different (p=0.85) between treatment groups but there were strict differences (p=0.00) between treatment and control groups on the post-treatment. Generally, these findings indicate that albendazole and tetraclozan are effective against gastrointestinal nematodes in the study area. But, appropriate use of these anthelmintics is credible to prevent future occurrence of resistance.

Keywords: Anthelmintics; Efficacy; Gastrointestinal nematodes

Introduction

In Western Oromiya region of Ethiopia, agriculture is the mainstay of the smallholder farmers. Mixed crop-livestock production system is largely practiced in this part of the country [1]. Cattle production is an important component and they are kept under traditional management within this farming system. The animals depend mostly on grazing natural pastures for feed sources with scanty supplements and minimum health care interventions [2].

Livestock diseases are one of the major production constraints frequently observed in the region among which helminthes parasites are the biggest causes of production losses. In general, Gastrointestinal (GI) nematode parasites remain one of the most prevalent and important diseases affecting large ruminants worldwide. They are responsible for both direct and indirect major losses [3]. Losses occur through mortalities, reduced production due to subclinical parasitism and direct costs associated with control [4].

Globally, parasitic and other endemic diseases continue to be a major constraint on profitable livestock production. They are rarely associated with high mortality and easily identifiable clinical signs and their effects are usually characterized by lower outputs of animal products, by- products, manure and traction all contributing to production and productivity losses. However, parasitic diseases are repeatedly identified by livestock owners, particularly small ruminant producers, as constraints to animals reaching their full production potential. It is generally accepted that the cost of control of most parasitic and endemic diseases is the responsibility of the animal owner [5].

Ruminants are prone to infection with helminthes parasite throughout the world inflicting heavy economic losses in ruminant industry due to high mortality in addition to reduction in productivity [6]. Parasitic worms infect livestock and crops, affecting food production with a resultant economic impact and they are also important in the infection of domestic pets. Indeed, the companion animal market is a major economic consideration for animal health companies undertaking drug discovery programs [7].

Therapeutics are concerned with the application of drug in the treatment of the disease such details as the choice of drug, the route of administration, the form in which the drug is applied and the frequency of administration. Most of the anthelmintics used for ruminant are identical, with exception, and vary with dose only. The control of parasitic helminths in domestic animals relies largely on the use of anthelmintic drugs [8]. Therapeutic efficacy and anthelmintic drug resistance will allow detection of changing patterns of parasite susceptibility and timely revision of national and global parasite treatment policies [9].

Most of the nematodes of domestic animals possess the capacity to develop resistance to anthelmintic drugs. Resistance to antiparasitic

---

*Corresponding author: Anmaw Shite, Faculty of Veterinary Medicine, Unit of Biomedical Sciences, University of Gondar, PO Box: 196, Gondar, Ethiopia
E-mail: anmawvet@gmail.com

drugs in ruminant is rapidly increasing, particularly in warm and humid climatic regions, probably due to frequent dosing and adoption of common management, nutritional, and therapeutic strategies [10].

In livestock production throughout the world, the use of antiparasitic drugs to control internal and external parasites is a widespread practice. The number of domestically available broad spectrum anthelmintic drugs has increased since 1960s. Several anthelmintics with different modes of action are available in the market for the control of helminthosis. Currently, failure of anthelmintics efficacy due to anthelmintic resistance in ruminant becoming a wide-spread threat all over the world. Resistance to anthelmintics has become a major problem in veterinary medicine, and threatens both agricultural income and animal welfare [11].

Gastrointestinal helminth infections are very common in many parts of Ethiopia and their control is almost exclusively based on anthelmintic treatment [12]. In Ethiopia, the use of anthelmintics has been practiced for a long time, taking a considerable share in drug costs spent by the country in the control of animal diseases. Smuggling and misuse of veterinary drugs involving anthelmintics is a widespread practice in the country. Despite the high use of common specific anthelmentic substances in Ethiopia there are scarce reports on the efficacy of theses anthelmintics against economically important parasites [13].

The prevalence and impact of helminth parasites as well as their sensitivity to the commonly used anthelmintics have been studied in small ruminants in many parts of the country [13-15]. On the other hand, no systematic surveys have been carried out to evaluate anthelmintic efficacy in cattle. Therefore, the objectives of this study were; to evaluate the current efficacy of commonly used antheliminthic drugs against GIT nematodes of cattle, and isolate and identify resistant worms.

Materials and Methods

Study area

The study was conducted from November 2014 to April 2015 in Adaberga dairy farm; Central Ethiopia, West Showa Zone of Oromia Regional State, located around 72 km west of Addis Ababa. The area lies at longitude 38° 30' E and latitude 9° 3' N and includes highland and midland agro-ecologies with an altitude of at about 2600 meters above sea level. The site is characterized by cool sub-tropical climate with mean maximum and minimum temperatures of 26°C and 10°C, respectively with mean relative humidity of 59%. The mean annual rainfall ranges from 800 to 1400 milliliters [16].

Study animals and treatments

Total 36 naturally infected female jersey breed cows of four to five years of age with uniform size and weight were used for the study. The cows which have been bred in Adaberga dairy farm were purposively selected to evaluate commonly used anthelmintic efficacy against gastrointestinal nematodes. Animals which have not been treated in the previous 8 to 12 weeks were considered for the study and grouped into control and treatment groups. A control (untreated) group had been used to allow for monitoring of natural changes in egg

counts during the test period. The quality of the drug were evaluated by Ethiopian veterinary drug authority for the presence of required active ingredient, and then Animals were treated with the respective anthelmintic dosage as per the recommendations of the manufacturers according to the weight of animal (Table 1).

Generally each animal under the study was identified by ear tag and were randomly allocated into three groups (twelve in each). The first group was treated with albendazole, the second with tetraclozan and the last group was left untreated (control).

The history of the farms indicated that all animals received regular treatments with anthelmintics twice a year at the beginning and end of the long rainy season in June and November, respectively. Additionally, farmers also experienced to treat with anthelmintics based on individual animal exhibiting clinical parasitism. However, this treatment regimen could lack precision in determining the appropriate dosages. The records available indicated that the types and sources of anthelmintics used on the farms included mainly albendazole 2500 mg as well as tetraclozan (Tetraclozan QK Cattle) for cattle were all available on the local markets.

Study design and methodology

An experimental study design was conducted from November 2014 to April 2015 to investigate the commonly used anthelmintics efficacy in GIT nematodes through fecal egg count reduction test in naturally infected cattle of governmental dairy farm (Adaberga dairy farm) in Adaberga district.

Sampling technique

Purposive sampling technique was used as sampling technique to select the experimental study animals based on their age, size and body weight uniformity as well as egg count whereby animals were selected in Adaberga dairy farm and randomly allocated into three groups.

Sampling procedures and laboratory investigation

Faecal samples were collected from each cows for pre-screening of animals for sufficient egg counts, a minimum of 5 gm of faeces was collected from each animal directly from the rectum using rubber glove. The same procedure was followed at the post-treatment sampling. Samples were placed in individually sealed containers and labeled with specific identification mark then returned rapidly to the Holeta livestock research center parasitology laboratory (Addis Ababa) for egg counts. The post-treatment collection of faecal samples from the experimental cows was 10 days after treatment according to Coles et al. [17]. Waiting for at least 10 days after the treatment allows worms that had been impacted but not removed by the drug to reach full egg production again. If the second set of samples is collected more than 10 days after treatment, worms that infected the animals after they were treated would have a chance to mature and start producing eggs [18].

Fecal egg counts and faecal egg count reduction test

For the process of Fecal egg counts modified McMaster method was used according to FAO [5]. The most commonly used field

Generic name	Trade name	Manufacturer	Route of administration	Recommended dose
Albendazole	Albentong 2500	Chongqing fantong animal pharmaceutical co., Ltd, China	Bolus/oral	1 bolus/350 kg or 7.14 mg/kg
Tetraclozan	Tetraclozan QK Cattle	Chengdu QiankumVet Pharma China	Bolus/oral	1 bolus/150 kg or 22.7 mg/kg

Table 1: Detail information about anthelmintic used in the treatment.

detection method for anthelmintic resistance is the Fecal Egg Count Reduction Test (FECRT). This method can be adapted for use as a screening agent for Veterinarians and producers to identify less than desired clearance of the parasites after anthelmintic treatment [19]. The procedure compares the pre-treatment parasite level with the parasite levels after treatment. The efficacy of each anthelmintic was determined by comparing the fecal egg count reduction percentage from a group of animals before and after treatment.

The differences between the two tests were then calculated and reported as a reduction percent. Arithmetic means of pre-treatment and post-treatment fecal egg counts of control and treated groups were used to calculate the percentage efficacy using the following formula according to Coles et al. [17]: FECRT%=(T1-T2)/T1 × 100 where T1 is pre-treatment egg count and T2 is post- treatment egg count. The 95% confidence limits were calculated by using a software program RESO [20]. Anthelmintic resistance was declared to exist when the FECR% was less than 95% and the lower 95% confidence limit for the reduction was less than 90%. If only one of the two criteria was met, resistance was suspected [17].

The FECRT detects clinical cure rather than the total elimination of the parasites [17]. However, there is no direct relationship between the FECRT and the number of resistant worms Whether or not to continue using a drug once a FECRT indicates that a substantial population of resistant worms may be present depends on the situation [21].

Larval identification

About 10 gm faecal samples from each cow were collected on each sampling day (before and after treatment) and composite faecal cultures were made for each group. Small amount of water was added to moisten, and the samples left for 14 days at room temperature in a Petri dish [22], adding small amounts of water as necessary. Third stage larvae (L3) were recovered from the cultures by the Baerman technique and identified according to Hansen et al. [23].

Data management and analysis

While collecting fecal samples from study animals, all data were recorded with pre-designed format and entered in to computer using Microsoft excel spread sheet. All data were analyzed using Statistical Package for Social Sciences (SPSS) version 16 statistical software. Descriptive statistics (means, standard error of means and reduction percentages) were calculated. pre-treatment and post-treatment faecal egg counts were transformed to the natural logarithm and means were

compared among groups through analysis of variance (ANOVA) and difference between treatments was compared using least square method of multiple comparisons Arithmetic means of pre-treatment and post-treatment fecal egg counts of control and treated groups were used to calculate the percentage efficacy of anthelimentics by using fecal egg count reduction test (Table 2).

Results

Mean faecal egg counts and percent reduction after treatment

The reduction in mean fecal EPG, after 10 days of post treatment, for Albendazole and tetraclozan were 95.51% and 98.18% respectively. The pre-treatment, post-treatment egg count mean, standard error of mean and the percent reduction in the fecal egg counts are present in Table 3.

There was no statistically significant difference (p=0.262) between the egg count of control and treated groups as well as between the two treated groups, albendazole treated and tetraclozan treated, before treatment.

Statistically post-treatment egg counts and percentage reduction of the drugs were not different (p=0.85) between treatment groups but there were strict differences (p=0.00) in net egg count between treatment and control groups on the post-treatment.

Survivor parasite after treatment

Fecal cultures were conducted parallel to fecal egg count to differentiate strongly type of eggs both in before and after treatments in each group. In Albendazole treated animals the percentage reductions for *Haemonchus* and *Trichuris* were 92.85% and 90.47% respectively and for other parasites 100%. The only survivor parasite in Tetraclozan treated group was *Trichuris* with percentage reduction of 90.65 (Table 4).

Discussion

The result showed that the mean FECR value of Albendazole and tetraclozan were 95.51 and 98.18 percent with the lower 95% confidence interval of 94.29 and 96.4 respectively. Consequently, FECR test indicated that the anthelmintic resistance was not found for any of the tested anthelmintic drugs. Both albendazole and tetraclozan had good drug efficacy in gastrointestinal nematodes in Adaberga dairy farm. As per World Association for the Advancement of Veterinary Parasitology (WAAVP) guidelines Coles et al. [17], Resistance is considered if the percentage reduction in egg counts is less than 95 percent and /or the lower 95 percent confidence level is less than 90 percent. If only one of the two criteria is met, resistance is suspected.

Group	Anthelmintics	Pre-treatment coproculture	Post-treatment coproculture
1	Albendazole	*Trichuris, ascaris, Haemonchus, bunostomum, nematodirus*	*Haemonchus, trichuris,*
2	Tetraclozan	*Trichuris, ascaris, Haemonchus, bunostomum, nematodirus*	*Trichuris*
3	Untreated control	*Trichuris, ascaris, Haemonchus, bunostomum, nematodirus*	*Trichuris, ascaris, Haemonchus, bunostomum, nematodirus*

Table 2: Larval composition (L3) of faecal cultures from experimental animals before and after treatments with anthelmintics.

AH	Mean FEC ± SEM		Reduction (%)			95% Confidence interval	
	Pre treatment	Post treatment	Mean ± SEM	Minimum	Maximum	Lower	Upper
ALB	650.00 ± 104.76	29.17 ± 14.38	95.51 ± 1.46	85.00	100.00	94.29	100
TR	683.33 ± 92.34	12.50 ± 8.97	98.18 ± 1.02	88.24	100.00	96.40	100
NRX	808.33 ± 110.75	835.42 ± 106.09	NA	NA	NA	NA	NA

AH: Anthelmintics; ALB: Albendazole; TR: Tetraclozan; NRX: Untreated control; FEC: Faecal Egg Count; SEM: Standard Error of the Mean; NA: Not Applicable.

Table 3: Mean faecal egg count and percent reduction after treatment of cattle using different anthelmintics.

Group	Anthelmintics	Survived parasite
1	Albendazole	*Haemonchus, trichuris,*
2	Tetraclozan	*Trichuris*
3	Untreated control	*Trichuris, ascaris, Haemonchus, bunostomum, nematodirus*

Table 4: Survivor parasite after treatment with anthelmintics.

The result of FECR test showed that the efficacy of albendazole in this finding was similar with the studies done by Demeler et al. [24] in Germany on monitoring the efficacy of ivermectin and albendazole against gastro intestinal nematodes of cattle North Europe.

Though, anthelmintic resistance is widely accepted in small ruminants based upon the general assumption that cattle are usually less frequently dosed than small ruminants, there are anthelmintic resistance in gastrointestinal nematodes of cattle according to the study done by Gasbarre et al. [19] in US on the identification of cattle nematode parasites resistant to multiple classes of anthelmintics in a commercial cattle population in the US.

Most research works regarding to anthelmintic resistance and drug efficacy for GIT nematodes in Ethiopia and most other world have been concerned in small ruminants. The finding of this study is in contrast with that of Bersisa and Abebe [25] observations who reported the presence of resistance in nematodes of small ruminants owned by Hawassa and Haromaya Universities. The disagreement with my report may be highly depending on species difference, drug usage strategies, quality of the available drug and under dosing the anthelmintic drugs.

Conclusion and Recommendations

In general the current finding indicated that both albendazole and tetraclozan were found to be effective in gastrointestinal nematodes in Adaberga dairy farm. Tetraclozan was more efficient than albendazole against gastrointestinal nematodes.

A possible approach could be Targeted selective treatment, only a part of the animal group is treated with anthelmintics, contrary to the current manner to treat the whole group to prevent future existing resistance. To prevent future development of anthelmintic resistance in this area, the following practices were recommended:

- Producers should use drugs to treat their animals from reliable source.

- Frequent and unnecessary anthelmintic treatments should be avoided,

- Optimizing strategic deworming.

- Avoid under dosing of animals

- Further studies, are needed to determine the anthelmintic resistance status of the different species of gastrointestinal nematodes in cattle in different areas of Ethiopia.

Conflict of Interests

The authors declare that there is no conflict of interests regarding the publication of this paper.

Acknowledgements

The authors are very much indebted to Sebeta Laboratory (Addis Ababa) for their maximum cooperation for providing research facilities.

References

1. Gizaw S, Getachew T, Edea Z, Mirkena T, Duguma G, et al. (2013) Characterization of indigenous breeding strategies of the sheep farming communities of Ethiopia: A basis for designing community-based breeding programs. ICARDA working paper, Aleppo, Syria.

2. Edea Z, Haile A, Tibbo M, Sharma AK, Sölkner J, et al. (2012) Sheep production systems and breeding practices of smallholders in western and south-western Ethiopia: Implications for designing community-based breeding strategies. Livestock Research for Rural Development 24: 117.

3. Hoste H, Torres-Acosta JF, Aguilar-Caballero AJ (2008) Nutrition-parasite interactions in goats: is immunoregulation involved in the control of gastrointestinal nematodes? Parasite Immunol 30: 79-88.

4. Miller JE, Horohov DW (2006) Immunological aspects of nematode parasite control in sheep. J Anim Sci 84 Suppl: E124-132.

5. FAO (2004) Guidelines resistance management and integrated parasite control in ruminants. Animal Production and Health Division Agriculture Department Food and Agriculture Organization of the United Nations Rome.

6. Hamad KK, Iqbal, Z, Sindhu Z, Muhammad G (2013) Antinematicidal Activity of *Nicotiana tabacum* L. Leaf Extracts to Control Benzimidazole-Resistant *Haemonchus contortus* in Sheep. Pak Vet J 33: 85- 90.

7. Holden-Dye L, Walker JR (2007) Anthelmintic drugs. Sci Int 45: 34-37.

8. Daykin PW, Brander GC, Hoare EW, Pugh DM (1971) Veterinary applied pharmacology and therapeutics. 2nd edn, Bailliére Tindall, London.

9. World Health Organization (2010) Global report on antimalarial drug efficacy and drug resistance 2000-2010.

10. Jackson F (1993) Anthelmintic resistance--the state of play. Br Vet J 149: 123-138.

11. Wolstenholme AJ, Fairweather I, Prichard R, von Samson-Himmelstjerna G, Sangster NC (2004) Drug resistance in veterinary helminths. Trends Parasitol 20: 469-476.

12. Getachew T, Urgessa F, Yacob HT (2013) Field investigation of anthelmintic efficacy and risk factors for anthelmintic drug resistance in sheep at Bedelle District of Oromia Region. Ethiopia Veterinary Journal 17: 37-49.

13. Kumsa B, Abebe G (2009) Multiple anthelmintic resistance on a goat farm in Hawassa (Southern Ethiopia). Trop Anim Health Prod 41: 655-662.

14. Sissay MM, Asefa A, Uggla A, Waller PJ (2006) Anthelmintic resistance of nematode parasites of small ruminants in eastern Ethiopia: exploitation of refugia to restore anthelmintic efficacy. Vet Parasitol 135: 337-346.

15. Lidetu D (2009) A survey on the occurrence of anthelmintic resistance in nematodes of sheep and goats found in different agro-ecologies in Ethiopia. Eth J Anim Prod 9: 159-175.

16. NMA (2011) National Meteorological Agency of Ethiopia. Annual climate bulletin for the year 2011.

17. Coles GC, Bauer C, Borgsteede FH, Geerts S, Klei TR, et al. (1992) World Association for the Advancement of Veterinary Parasitology (W.A.A.V.P.) methods for the detection of anthelmintic resistance in nematodes of veterinary importance. Vet Parasitol 44: 35-44.

18. Taylor MA, Hunt KR, Goodyear KL (2002) Anthelmintic resistance detection methods. Vet Parasitol 103: 183-194.

19. Gasbarre LC, Smith LL, Lichtenfels JR, Pilitt PA (2014) The identification of cattle nematode parasites resistant to multiple classes of anthelmintics in a commercial cattle population in the US. Vet Parasitol 166: 281-285.

20. Anonymous (1990) Faecal egg count or worm counts reduction test analysis (RESO), CSIRO, Australia.

21. Petersson K, Zajac A, Burdett H (2014) Improving Small Ruminant Parasite Control. Trop Med Int Health 12: 567-571.

22. Waghorn TS, Leathwick DM, Rhodes AP, Lawrence KE, Jackson R, et al. (2006) Prevalence of anthelmintic resistance on sheep farms in New Zealand. NZ Vet J 54: 271-277.

23. Hansen J, Perry B (1994) The epidemiology, diagnosis and control of helminth parasites of ruminants: A hand book. 2nd edn, Nairobi, Kenya: ILRAD (International Laboratory for Research on Animal Diseases).

24. Demeler J, Van Zeveren AM, Kleinschmidt N, Vercruysse J, Höglund J, et al. (2009) Monitoring the efficacy of ivermectin and albendazole against gastro intestinal nematodes of cattle in Northern Europe. Vet Parasitol 160: 109-115.

25. Kumsa B, Wossene A (2006) Efficacy of Albendazole and Tetramisole anthelmintics against *Haemonchus contortus* in experimentally infected Lambs. Intern J Appl Res Vet Med 4: 94-99.

36

Bovine Mastitis: Prevalence, Isolation of Bacterial Species Involved and its Antimicrobial Susceptibility Test around Debrezeit, Ethiopia

Tesfaye Belachew*

Assela Regional Animal Health Diagnostic Laboratory, Assela, Oromiya, Ethiopia

Abstract

A total of 300 local zebu lactating cows of small holders farmers around Debrezeit were examined to determine the prevalence of mastitis with associated risk factor, isolate bacterial pathogens involved and its antimicrobial susceptibility profiles. Clinical prevalence was determined through examination of abnormalities of milk and udder and California Mastitis Test (CMT) were used for determining subclinical mastitis. Bacterial culture and Agar disc diffusion was used for isolation and antibiotic susceptibility test. Based on the result out of 18 (6%) positive samples, 2 (0.7%) were clinical and the other 16 (5.3%) were sub-clinical mastitis. Among the potential risk factors considered, there was significant difference (P<0.05) between semi-intensive and extensive farming system. All positive samples were positive for aerobic bacteria. The bacterial species isolated were CNS and *Micrococcus* species 22.2%, *Staphylococcus aureus* 16% *Staphylococcus epidermis* and *Mycoplasma* species 11.1%, *Enterococcus* species, *Streptococcus agalactiae* and *Staphylococcus hycus* were 5.65%. Comparing the overall efficacy of antimicrobials on isolate kanamycin was the most effective antibiotic where 85.7% of the total isolate were found to be susceptible.

Keywords: Antimicrobial susceptibility; Bacterial pathogen; CMT; Bovine mastitis; Subclinical mastitis

Abbreviations: AWARDO: Ada Woreda Agriculture and Rural Development Office; DARC: Debrezeit Agricultural Research Center; CMT: California Mastitis Test; CNS: Coagulase Negative Staphylococci; FAO: Food and Agricultural Organization; masl: Meter above Sea Level; NVI: National Veterinary Institute; NMC: National Mastitis Council; MOARD: Ministry of Agriculture and Rural Development.

Introduction

Mastitis is the resulted from injurious agents including pathogenic microorganisms, trauma and chemical irritants [1]. According to Quinn et al. [2] over 130 different microorganisms have been isolated from bovine mastitic milk samples, of which almost all are bacteria. The most common pathogen comprises contagious bacteria mainly *S. aureus* and *S. agalactiae* and environmental bacteria mainly coli forms and some species of streptococci that are commonly present in the environment [1,3].

Mastitis infection is spread to teats between milking with organism being transferred up in to udder during milking process itself. *Streptococcus uberis* is the bacteria causing the majority of the problems, due to its resistance to treatment and chronic infections result in high cell count [4,5].

Mastitis causes milk unsuitable for human consumption or provide a mechanism for the spread of diseases like tuberculosis, Streptococcal intoxication, colibacillosis, Streptococcal sore throat and Brucellosis to human [1]. Public hazards associated with the consumption of antibiotic contaminated milk and products cause allergic responses, changes in intestinal flora and development of antibiotic resistant pathogenic bacteria [6].

Besides, mastitis has been recorded as one of the major disease of economic importance in dairy industry worldwide. It causes greater economic loss: much of the losses are related to production lose from inflammation of the infected quarters [4,5]. Owing to the heavy financial implication involved and the inevitable existence of latent infection, mastitis is obviously an important factor that limits dairy production. Evidence to date shows that affected dairy cows may lose 15% of their production and the affected quarter a 30% reduction in productivity. To these gross losses could be added losses associated with its keeping quality and manifesting processes. The disease is also responsible for high percentage of the cows being culled from the dairy herd. Change in milk quality, the possibility of permanent blindness to one or more quarter or even entire udder and death of the cow can resulted from the disease interims of economic loss, it is undoubtedly the most important disease which the dairy industry has to embark upon [1].

In Ethiopia, cows represent the largest proportion of cattle population. According to the food and agriculture organization [7], 42% of the total cattle heads for the private holding are milking cows. Milk produced from these animals provides important dietary sources for the majority of urban and per urban population. However, milk production often doesn't satisfy the country's requirement due to multitude of factors contributing disease of the mammary glands known as mastitis which is among the leading various factors contributing to reduced milk production [8]. According to Lema et al. [9], of the major diseases of cross bred cows in Addis Ababa milk shed, clinical mastitis was the second most frequent disease next to reproductive diseases in which 171 cows out of 556 were found to be affected with mastitis.

The control of mastitis in dairy herds is accomplished in part with the aid of antibiotic; however, it is not the entire answer to the problem. In addition, indiscriminate uses of drugs which are widely used in the country have potential effect on the development of resistant bacteria. Due to complexity of problem of mastitis in Ethiopia the application

***Corresponding author:** Tesfaye Belachew, Assela Regional Animal Health Diagnostic Laboratory, Assela, Oromiya, Ethiopia
E-mail: teyobeku@gmail.com

of single preventive and control measure is impractical [10]. Hence scrutinizing the degree of the problem of mastitis in dairy cows, assessments of associated risk factors in relation to the type of mastitis, isolation of bacterial causes and testing for antibiotic susceptibility are the core for looking strategic treatment, control and prevention of the disease so as save economic loss from milk, milk product and culling. Based on the above motive the objectives of the study is to determine the prevalence of Bovine mastitis and associated risk factors, isolate and identify the major mastitis causes bacterial and conduct *in-vitro* antimicrobial susceptibility test of isolates in small holders privately owned Dairy farm around Debre Zeit.

Materials and Methods

Study methodology

Study design and population: Across sectional study was conducted to determine the prevalence of both clinical and subclinical mastitis after a total 300 cow's milk samples were collected by simple random sampling from local indigenous lactating cows that are kept by small holder farmers around Debrezeit town under extensive and semi intensive husbandry system.

Data collection: A structured questioner was developed and all information relating to the study objectives were recorded. Data which was recorded includes type of dairy husbandry system, breed, age, parity and location stage, udder and milk abnormalities (injury, blindness, swelling, milk clots, abnormal secretion etc.) were also recorded during sample collection.

Clinical inspection of udder: The udder was examined through visual inspection and palpation to detect possible fibrosis, consistency of mammary quarters, swelling of super mammary lymph nodes, disproportional symmetry of teats, blindness, discoloration of milk, presence of clots, flakes of blood and watery secretions, increased temperature, pain and disturbance of function [1,2].

Detection of mastitis: Mastitis was detected using the CMT and result of clinical inspection of udder. Equal quantity of milk and CMT reagent was added to the cup on a white paddle and gentle swirling was applied to the mixture in horizontal plane. The result of the test was indicated on the basis of gel formation [11]. The interpretation (grades) of CMT was evocated the result grade as for normal 0 and 1, 2, 3, for positive [2].

Microbial investigation of mastitis

Milk sample collection: Milk was collected before the cow treated with either intra-mammary or systemic antimicrobial agent. For good collection of sample the teats were wiped thoroughly with 70% ethyl alcohol, paying particular attention to the test orifice and removed the first stripe of milk. The sterile collection bottle will be kept in the crook of the little finger so that the lid does not become contaminated. The milk sample was kept refrigeration from the time of collection to the time of bacteriological examination [2].

Direct Microscopy: The milk sample was centrifuged and stained smears from the deposit. A gram-stain is used routinely. Zehil Nelson staining was done when bacteria such as *Mycobacterium bovis* are suspected [2].

Culture: The bacteriological culture was formed following the standard microbiological technique and microbiological procedures for the diagnosis of bovine mastitis infection [2,6]. A loop full of milks streaked on 7% sheep blood agar plates are checked for growth after 24, 48 and up to 72 hours to rule out slow growing microorganisms such as *Corynebacterium* species sample was considered negative if there is no growth after 72 hours. For primary identification, colony size, shape color hemolytic characteristic, gram reactions were considered. These colonies were sub cultured to get pure colonies to nutrient agar, MacConkey agar, Edwards medium etc. other biochemical Estes.

Characterizations of isolated mastitis causing bacteria was done by different methods, biochemical tests such as catalase, oxidase, coagulase, sugar fermentation test, oxidation fermentation test and indole test. The procedures adapted from Quinn et al. [2] for the identified pathogens were used.

Antimicrobial sensitively testing: Selected bacterial isolates were tested for sensitivity to different antimicrobials. Using *in vitro* disk diffusion (Kirby-Baur) method as described in [2]. Cultured broth was cross-checked with McFarland to Mueller Hinton agar and disc application. After measuring the zone of inhabitation, it was classified as sensitive, intermediate and resistant according to national committee for clinical laboratory standard (NCCLS) [2].

Statistical analysis

SPSS version 20 was used to analyze the collected data. The association among and between the considered risk factors were tested by using Chi square (χ^2) and Odds ratio (OR). The level of significance was also expressed using P-value less than 0.05.

Results and Discussion

Prevalence of clinical and sub clinical mastitis

A total 300 indigenous zebu lactating cows from small holder dairy farm around Debrezeit were examined to determine the prevalence of bovine mastitis. Out of 300 examined cows there was high prevalence of sub clinical mastitis 16(5.3%) than clinical 2(0.7%) as shown in Table 1. A total of 1200 quarters were examined and 72(6%) were CMT positive whereas 33(11.1%) were found blind teats (Table 2).

Prevalence of mastitis using multivariate risk factors

The prevalence of mastitis using multivariate risk factors was shown in Table 3. Those cows with different lactation stage and farming system revealed significant difference (p<0.05) in prevalence of mastitis (p>0.05). The prevalence of both clinical and sub-clinical mastitis by risk factors were insignificance (P>0.05) with treatment history, lactation stage and parity however, there was significance difference between semi intensive and extensive farming system (P<0.05). The proportions of sub-clinical mastitis were higher than clinical one within all current considered risk factors Table 4.

A total of 18 cows that were positive both clinically and sub clinically, all samples were collected and cultured. From 18 cultured samples, 18(100%) samples were positive for aerobic bacteria. The isolated bacterial species and were presented below in Table 5. Coagulase Negative *Staphylococcus* (CNS) and *Micrococcus* species were

Number of cows examined	Clinical mastitis	Sub-clinical mastitis	Total
	Positive No. (%)	Positive No. (%)	
300	2(0.7%)	16(5.3%)	18(0.4%)

Table 1: Prevalence of clinical and sub clinical bovine mastitis at Cow level using CMT.

Quarter	CMT Positive No (%)	CMT Negative No (%)	Blind No (%)
Left Back	28(2.33)	1172(97.7)	11(1.2)
Left Front	24(2)	1176(98)	3(0)
Right back	12(1)	1188(98.7)	17(1.2)
Right Front	8(0.67)	1192(99.3)	2(0.8)
Over all	72(6)	1128(94)	33(11.1)

Table 2: Quarter level of prevalence of mastitis and blind teats.

Risk factor	No of cow Examined	Positive No (%)	x^2	p-value
Location stage Early Mid Late	108 128 64	7 (6.4) 3(16.7) 8 (44.4)	7.873	0.020
Age (yr) 3.5-6 6-9 9-13	134 133 33	8(44.5) 6(33.3) 4(22.2)	1.85	0.229
Parity 1-3 3-6 6-9	138 84 78	6(33.3) 5(27.8) 7(38.9)	1.892	0.388
Farm system Extensive Semi intensive	293 7	14(77.7) 4(22.2)	39.953	0.000
History treatment Treated Untreated	187 113	10(55.6) 8(44.4)	0.338	0.561

Table 3: The prevalence of mastitis within the considered risk factors.

Risk factors		Type of mastitis positive		x^2	p-value
		Clinical No (%)	Sub clinical No (%)		
Treatment history Treated	114	1(50)	9(56.2)	0.367	0.832
Untreated	186	1(50)	7(43.8)		
Location stage Early	108	1(50)	6(37.5)		
Mid	128	0(0)	3(18.8)	8.129	0.089
Late	64	1(50)	7(43.8)		
Age (year) 3.5-6	134	1(50)	(57.8)		
6-9	133	1(50)	62(54.9)	4.145	0.387
9-13	33	0(0)	35(53.0)		
Parity 1-3	138	1(50)	6(37.5)		
3-6	84	1(50)	4(25)	1.892	0.388
6-9	78	0(0)	6(37.5)		
Farm system Extensive	293	2(100)	12(75)	45.622	0.000
Semi intensive	7	0(0)	4(25)		

Table 4: Prevalence of clinical and sub clinical mastitis in different risk factor.

isolated with high prevalence (22.2%), *Staphylococcus aureus* 16.7%, *Staphylococcus intermedius* and *Mycoplasma* species were 11.1%, and *Streptococcus agalactiae*, *Enterococcus* species and *Staphylococcus hycus* were 5.6%.

From the tested bacterial isolate using selected antimicrobial agent all are susceptible for kanamycin and except one isolate of CNS. CNS shows intermediate (50%) for both Chloramphinacol and Kanamycin as shown in Table 6.

Discussion

In this study, the overall bovine mastitis prevalence is 6%. The prevalence is very less compared to the others study finding done on

mastitis elsewhere in Ethiopia such as 52.27% by Abunna et al. [12], 34.9% by Biffa et al. [13], 74.7% by Zeryehun et al. [14] and Ashenafi [15] who reported 75% prevalence. This might be due to management system the farmers have practiced in the study area. Farmers have maximum of cow 2-3 and they release their cows to open grazing land this system decreases the chance of transmission of contagious mastitis between cows [1]. Up on taking history on the cows' production of milk, they only give less than 1.5 liter/day. Local Zebu breed are low in milk production and resistant to mastitis [16]. Higher yielding cows have been found more susceptible to mastitis owing to position of teats, udder, and anatomy of teat cannel making them prone to injury, and due to fewer efficacies of pathogenic cells in higher yielding cows associated to dilution [1,17].

The clinical mastitis prevalence in this study was 0.7% which was comparable with that of Gizat [18], who reported 0% in local Zebu lactating cows in and around Bahir Dar. However, the present finding was lower than that of Tesfaye [19], who reported 7.3% in Adama, and Adugna [20], who reported 5.7% in Dire Dawa and Haramaya University Dairy farm. Most of the time when comparing clinical and sub-clinical mastitis, clinical mastitis is lower than that of sub-clinical mastitis and this is because of treatment of clinical mastitis is commonly practiced [19].

In Ethiopia, the sub-clinical mastitis received little attention and efforts have been concentrated on the treatment of clinical cases while the high economic loss could come from sub-clinical mastitis [21]. The present finding of prevalence of sub-clinical mastitis was 5.3% which is comparable with that of Tesfaye [19] who reported 7.3% in Adama and less than that of Adugna [20] who reported 18.9% in Dire Dawa and Haramaya University Dairy farm and Gizat [18] who reported 17% in and around Bahir Dar on the local Zebu lactating cows. In the present study, as well in other conducted studies, over whelming cases of mastitis were sub-clinical compared to clinical mastitis [22,23].

Dairy farms in the study area usually complain about the decrease in milk yield irrespective of adequate feed provision and deworming practice. The high prevalence of sub-clinical mastitis may be due to attributed to improper milking hygiene, poor house hygiene, lack of post milking teat dipping and practicing of milk by contact labors use of lubricant, absence of order in milking cows of different ages. Moreover, its occurrence was high in dairy farms without noticeable in farm treatment as Radostitis et al. [1] and Quinn et al. [2] provide the same reasoning.

The prevalence of mastitis which was not significantly influenced by considered potential risk factor (P>0.05) are age, parities, and treatment history. But lactation stage and farming system are significantly the potential risk factors. This could be due to as lactation stage increases chance of cows exposed to the mastitis increases because daily contact of cows while milking and in farming system with no care milking management.

From total examined 1200 quarters 72(6%) quarter were CMT positive and 33 (11.1%) blind teats. Blindness of the teat could be due to failure to detect the disease in early stage attributable to lack of strip cup examination and skill milker's to establish a prompt treatment. Generally, it indicates a poor treatment regime and husbandry [6].

Analysis of the bacteriological examination of the milk samples was made to isolate and identify the main etiological agents involved in the disease process. The organisms were identified on the bases of their culture, staining characteristics and biochemical reactions. The result of bacteriological analysis in the present study showed that Coagulase Negative Staphylococcus and Micrococcus species were predominant pathogens which were 22.2% of all the isolated bacterial species. The high isolation rate of CNS in the study could be associated with it characteristics of chronicity. The CNS isolated was all found from sub-clinical mastitis. However, CNS was isolated from bovine and other dairy animals' mastitic milk samples which indicated that they could be pathogenic even causes more mastitis than S. aureus [24]. According to Pyorolla, over 30% sub-clinical and nearly 20% of acute cases of mastitis were usually due to CNS which is in agreement with the present result (22.2%). The isolated Micrococcus species (22.2%) was comparable with the finding of Amen et al. who reported 26.67% in different parts of Ethiopia and it was higher than the findings of Tarekegn [6], Gizat [18] and Mekonnen et al. [25] who reported 8.15, 5.2 and 10.2% respectively.

The isolation rate of S. aureus 16.7% in the present study is the second next to CNS and Micrococcus species and closely comparable with the findings of Gizat [18]. Bishi [24] and Hussein [21] reported 17.8% and 9% in Addis Ababa respectively. However, the present finding is lower than that of Workineh et al. [22] and Kerro and Tereke

No.	Isolates Frequency	No (%)
1.	*Staphylococcus aureus* 3	16.7%
2.	Micrococcus Species 4	22.2%
2.	*Staphylococcus hycus* 1	5.6%
4	*Staphylococcus intermedius* 2	11.1%
5.	*Streptococcus agalactiae* 1	5.6%
6.	*Mycoplasma species* 2	11.1%
7.	Coagulase Negative *Staphylococcus* 4	22.2%
8.	*Enterococcus* species 1	5.6%
Total	18	100%

Table 5: Isolated bacteria species from CMT Positive milk sample.

Bacteria isolates	N	C_{30}			AP_{10}			TE_{30}			AX_{10}			K_{30}		
		S	I	R	S	I	R	S	I	R	S	I	R	S	I	R
S. aureus	2	1(50%)	1(50%)			2(100%)	-	-	-	2(100%)	1(50%)	1(50%)	-	2(100%)	-	-
S. intermedius	1	1(100%)	-	-	1(100%)	-	-	-	1(100%)	-	1(100%)	-	-	1(100%)	-	-
Micrococcus Sp.	2	1(50%)	1(50%)	-	1(50%)	1(50%	-	2(100%)	-	-	2(100%)	-	-	2(100%)	-	-
CNS	2	-	1(50%)	1(50%)	-	-	-	2(100%)	-	-	2(100%)	-	-	-	2(100%)	-
S. hycus	1	-	1(100%)	-	1(100%)	1(100%)	-	-	-	-	-	-	1(100%)	1(100%)	-	-
Enterococci	1	1(100%)	-	-	-	-	-	-	-	-	1(100%)	-	-	1(100%)	-	-
S. agalactae	1	-	1(100%)	-	1(100%)	-	-	1(100%)	-	-	1(100%)	-	-	-	1(100%)	-

Keys: N: Number of observations; AX: Amoxicillin; C: Chloramphnicol; I: Intermediate K: Kanamycin, R: Resistance, S: Susceptible, TE: Tetracycline

Table 6: Antibiotic sensitivity testing.

[10] where *S. aureus* account 39.2 and 40.5% isolates respectively in Addis Ababa and Sothern Ethiopia. The relatively high prevalence of *S. aureus* in this study could be associated with total absence of dry cow therapy and post milking teat dipping, the invariable hold milking practice and low culling rate of chronically infected cows. Culling was usually due to feed shortage, ageing and reproductive problem. *Staphylococcus intermidus* and *Staphylococcus hycus* were found in the rate of 11.1 and 5.6% respectively.

Streptococcus agalactiae was found 5.6% and this bacterial species was lower isolate in the study area and this could be due to management system in the study area. Environmental Streptococci may be due to poor housing facilities which predispose to the accumulation of feces on cows which could increase the rate of exposure of the teats and udder to the pathogens. *Mycoplasma* species was found with rate of 11.1% in the study farms. Mycoplasmas are group of very small organisms that can be cultured from multiple body sites of both sick and healthy cattle. Some common Mycoplasma include *M. bovis* most commonly cultured from the udder [26]. The organisms were isolated from clinical infected cows which agree with the finding of Thomas [26]. In milk samples obtained from individual cows, a negative Mycoplasma culture usually means that the organism is not present. However, intermittent shedding of organism has been reported, so false negative cultures may rarely occur [27].

When comparing the overall efficacy of antimicrobials on isolates, kanamycin was the most effective antibiotic where 85.7% of the total isolate were found to be susceptible. The drug was not used in the study area for the treatment of animals. *S. aureus* was 100% resistant to Tetracycline. The development of antibiotic resistance nearly always has followed the continuous and under dosage use of the antimicrobial agents [2].

The dominant pathogens in the study area were CNS and Micrococcus species. CNS isolate were 100% susceptible to Tetracycline, Amoxicillin and Kanamycin however intermediate to Chloramphenicol and Ampicillin (50%) which is in agreement with the report by Bishi [24].

In this study *S. aureus* was the most susceptible to Kanamycin and Ampicillin and intermediate to Chloramphenicol, and Amoxicillin 100 and 50% respectively. A report of Bishi [24] indicated that Tetracycline was not effective in *S. aureus*.

Micrococcus species were 100% susceptible to Tetracycline, Amoxicillin and Kanamycin. This might be due to non-drug treatment with Amoxicillin and Kanamycin in the study areas [28]. *Staphylococcus hycus*, *Staphylococcus intermidius* and Enterococci species were also 100% susceptible to Ampicillin, Tetracycline and Kanamycin.

Acknowledgements

First and foremost, I like to thank the heavenly father God for giving my strength and patience during my all life and study program. I would like to express my deep sincerely appreciation and thanks to Dr. Henok Ayalew, for his intellectual guidance, close supervision and devotion of time in criticizing this paper.

Conflict of Interest

I declare that this paper presents the work carried out by myself and does not incorporate with the acknowledgement of any material and finance.

References

1. Radostits OM, Gay CC, Blood DC, Hinchllif KW (2007) Mastitis. In: Veterinary Medicine. 9th edn. Haracourt Ltd, London, pp: 603-700.

2. Quinn PJ, Carter ME, Markey BK, Carter GR (2002) Clinical Veterinary Microbiology. Harcourt Publishers, Virginia, USA, pp: 331-344.

3. Bhatt VD, Patel MS, Joshi CG, Kunjadia A (2011) Identification and antibiogram of microbes associated with bovine mastitis. Anim Biotechnol 22: 163-169.

4. Erskine RJ (2001) Mastitis control in dairy farms. In: Herd Health, Food Animal Production Medicine. 3rd edn, Radostits OM (eds.). WB Saunders Company, Philadelphia, Pennsylvania, USA, pp: 397-432.

5. Behiry AE, Schlenker G, Szabo I, Roesler U (2012) In vitro susceptibility of Staphylococcus aureus strains isolated from cows with subclinical mastitis to different antimicrobial agents. J Vet Sci 13: 153-161.

6. Kassa T, Wirtu G, Tegegne A (1999) Survey of mastitis in dairy herds in the Ethiopian central highlands. SINET: Ethiopian J Sci 22: 291-301.

7. Akam DN, Dodd FH, Quick AJ (1989). Milking, milk production hygiene and udder health. Vol 78. Food & Agricultural Organization.

8. Fekadu K (1995) Survey on the prevalence of bovine mastitis and the predominant causative agents in Chaffa valley. In: Proceedings of the 9th Conference of Ethiopian Veterinary Association: Addis Ababa, Ethiopia, pp: 101-111.

9. Lema M, Kassa T, Tegegne A (2001) Clinically manifested major health problems of crossbred dairy herds in urban and periurban production systems in the central highlands of Ethiopia. Trop Anim Health Prod 33: 85-93.

10. Kerro O (1997) A study on bovine mastitis in some selected areas of southern Ethiopia. DVM Thesis, Faculty of Veterinary Medicine, Addis Ababa University, Debre Zeit, Ethiopia.

11. Smith M, Sherman D (1994) Goat medicine. 1st edn. Williams and Wilkins Awaverly Company, USA, pp: 465-487.

12. Abunna F, Fufa G, Megersa B, Regassa A (2013) Bovine Mastitis: Prevalence, Risk Factors and Bacterial Isolation in Small-Holder Dairy Farms in Addis Ababa City, Ethiopia. Glob Vet 10: 647-652.

13. Biffa D, Debela E, Beyene F (2005) Prevalence and risk factors of mastitis in lactating dairy cows in Southern Ethiopia. International J Appl Res Vet Med 3: 189-198.

14. Zeryehun T, Aya T, Bayecha R (2013) Study on prevalence, bacterial pathogens and associated risk factors of bovine mastitis in small holder dairy farms in and around Addis Ababa, Ethiopia. J Anim Plant Sci 23: 50-55.

15. Ashenafi G (2008) Prevalence of bovine mastitis, identification of the causative agent and drug sensitivity test in and around kombolcha. DVM. Thesis, FVM, Haramaya University, Ethiopia 17: 41-46.

16. Almaw G, Molla B (2000) Prevalence and etiology of mastitis in camels (Camelus dromedarius) in eastern Ethiopia. Journal of Camel Practice and Research 7: 97-100.

17. Schalm W, Carrlole FJ (1971) Bovine mastitis. Led and Teliger, Philadelphia, USA, pp: 1-21.

18. Gizat A (2004) A cross sectional study of Bovine mastitis in and around Bahir Dar and Antibiotics resistance patterns for major pathogens. MSc Thesis, Faculty of Veterinary Medicine, Addis Ababa University, Debrezeit, Ethiopia.

19. Tesfaye A (2007) Small scale dairy farming practice and cross-sectional study of mastitis in Nazareth, East Shoa, Ethiopia. MSc Thesis, Faculty of Veterinary Medicine, Addis Ababa University, Ethiopia.

20. Adugna B (2008) Cross sectional study of mastitis in Dire Dawa and Haramaya University dairy farms, prevalence isolation and identification of pathogens and Antimicrobial sensitivity testing, Eastern Ethiopia. DVM Thesis, FVM Haramaya University, Ethiopia.

21. Hussein N (1999) Cross-sectional and longitudinal study of bovine mastitis in urban and peri-urban dairy systems in the Addis Ababa region, Ethiopia. Doctoral Dissertation, MSc Thesis, Free University of Berlin, Germany and Addis Ababa University, Ethiopia, Joint programme.

22. Workineh S, Bayleyegn M, Mekonnen H, Potgieter LND (2002) Prevalence and aetiology of mastitis in cows from two major Ethiopian dairies. Trop Anim Health Prod 34: 19-25.

23. Dego OK, Tareke F (2003) Bovine mastitis in selected areas of southern Ethiopia. Trop Anim Health Prod 35: 197-205.

24. Bishi AS (1998) Cross-sectional and longitudinal prospective study of bovine clinical and subclinical mastitis in periurban and urban dairy production systems in the Addis Ababa region, Ethiopia.

Bovine Mastitis: Prevalence, Isolation of Bacterial Species Involved and its Antimicrobial Susceptibility Test around...

191

25. Mekonnen H, Workineh S, Bayleyegn M, Moges A, Tadele K (2005) Antimicrobial susceptibility profiles of mastitis isolates from cows in three major Ethiopian dairies. Revue Med Vet 156: 391-394.

26. Thomas CB (1998) Bovine Mycoplasmas: A practitioner's orientation to host and agent interaction. In: Proceeding of WI Vet Med Assoc. 84th Ann Conf WI. Vet. Med. Assoc., Madison WI, USA, pp: 55.

27. Jasper DE (1980) Bovine mycoplasmal mastitis. Adv Vet Sci Comp Med 25: 121-157.

28. Bramely AJ, Cullor JS, Erskine RJ, Fox LK, Harmon RJ, et al. (1996) Current concepts of bovine mastitis. National Mastitis Council Inc., Arlington, VA, USA.

37

Prevalence of Bovine Trypanosomosis and Apparent Density of Tsetse Flies in Eastern Part of Dangur District, North Western Ethiopia

Endalu Mulatu[1], Kumela Lelisa[2] and Delesa Damena[3]*

[1]Mettu University, Bedelle College of Agriculture and Forestry, Mettu, Oromia, Ethiopia
[2]National Institute for Control and Eradication of Tsetse and Trypanosomosis, Addis Ababa, Ethiopia
[3]National Animal Health Diagnostic and Investigation Center, Sebeta, Oromia, Ethiopia

Abstract

Trypanosomosis is a parasitic disease that causes serious economic losses in livestock, in sub-Saharan African countries. A cross sectional study was conducted from October 2011 to March 2012 in the eastern part of Dangur district, Benishangul-Gumuz regional state, Ethiopia to determine the prevalence of bovine trypanosomosis and apparent density of tsetse flies. For prevalence study, a total of 543 blood samples were collected from randomly selected animals. Packed Cell Volume (PCV) was determined and samples were examined for the presence of trypanosomes using the buffy coat technique. In total, 46 (8.5%) of the samples were tested positive for trypanosomes. The majority of the infections were caused by *Trypanosoma congolense* (95.7%), and the remaining was caused by *Trypanosoma vivax*. The difference between prevalence of trypanosomes among study sites was statistically significant ($p<0.05$). The mean PCV value of parasitemic animals (22.6%) was significantly lower ($p<0.05$) than that of aparasitemic animals (27.0%). A total of 528 tsetse flies were caught by deploying 78 monopyramidal traps. Of these tsetse flies, 71.8% were Glossina tachinoides and the remaining were *G. morsitans submorsitans*. The overall apparent density of tsetse flies was 3.4 flies per trap per day (F/T/D). In conclusion, this study revealed that trypanosomes and their vectors are prevalent and pose a huge threat to cattle production in the area. Therefore, proper intervention strategies should be put in place and implemented to minimize the burden of the disease.

Keywords: Tsetse; Apparent density; Cattle; Dangur; Prevalence; Trypanosomosis

Introduction

Trypanosomosis is a disease complex caused by several species of blood and tissue dwelling protozoan parasites of the genus Trypanosoma [1-3]. It is a disease of domestic livestock that causes a significant negative impact on food and economic growth in many tropical and subtropical countries of the world including sub-Saharan Africa [4]. The course of the disease may run from an acute and rapidly fatal to a chronic long lasting one depending on the vector-parasite-host interactions. It is characterized mainly by intermittent fever, progressive anaemia and loss of condition of susceptible hosts which if untreated leads to high mortality rates [5,6].

The disease is distributed over approximately 10 million km² of Sub Saharan Africa between latitudes 14°N and 29°S which directly coincide with distributions of tsetse flies [2,7]. In Ethiopia, the most important tsetse born trypanosomes inflicting economic losses in domestic livestock are *T. congolense, T. vivax, and T. brucei* [8]. The distribution of tsetse flies is determined principally by climate and influenced by altitude, vegetation and presence of suitable hosts [9]. Five species of, tsetse flies, *G. m. submorsitans, G. pallidipes, G. tachinoides, G. f. fuscipes* and *G. longipennis* have been recorded in Ethiopia. Tsetse infested areas lie in lowlands and in the valleys of Abay (Blue Nile), Baro, Akobo, Didessa, Ghibe and Omo Rivers. The infestation is confined to the southern and western regions of Ethiopia between 33°-38°E and 5°-12° N which amounts to about 200,000 km². Out of the nine administrative regions of Ethiopia, five (Amhara, Benishangul-Gumuz, Gambella, Oromia and Southern Nations and Nationalities and People Regional State (SNNPRS) are infested with more than one species of tsetse fly [8].

Although few studies were conducted in Northwestern Ethiopia, no study was conducted in Dangur district. Owing to the fact that, tsetse and trypanosomosis fronts in many places in Ethiopia are unstable

and tsetse animal interface is constantly moving [10], studies on the epidemiology of trypanosomosis are crucial to plan and implement evidence based interventions. Aiming at filling the information gap in Dangur district, this study was conducted to determine the prevalence of trypanosomosis, identify trypanosome and tsetse species in cattle in the study areas.

Materials and Methods

Study area description

The study was conducted in 5 Kebeles (lowest administrative units in Ethiopia): Kitili, Burji, Gublak, Ipupuwa and Beles 2 of Dangur district, located 563 kms west of Addis Ababa in the Benishangul-Gumuz administrative region. Mixed agriculture is the mainstay of the livelihood of the society where crop and livestock production play integral roles. The district (Figure 1) is situated at 11°18' N and 36°14' E with a total area of 838,700 hectares. It has an elevation that varies from 800 to 2000 meters above sea levels (masl) and has 70% plains, 8% valley and 22% mountainous topographic feature. The average annual low and high temperatures are 30°C and 38°C respectively and the mean annual rainfall ranges from 900 to 1400 ml. The dominant vegetations in the

---

Corresponding author: Delesa Damena, Molecular Laboratory of National Animal Health Diagnostic and Investigation Center, Sebeta, Oromia, Ethiopia
E-mail: delesa_damenaa@yahoo.com

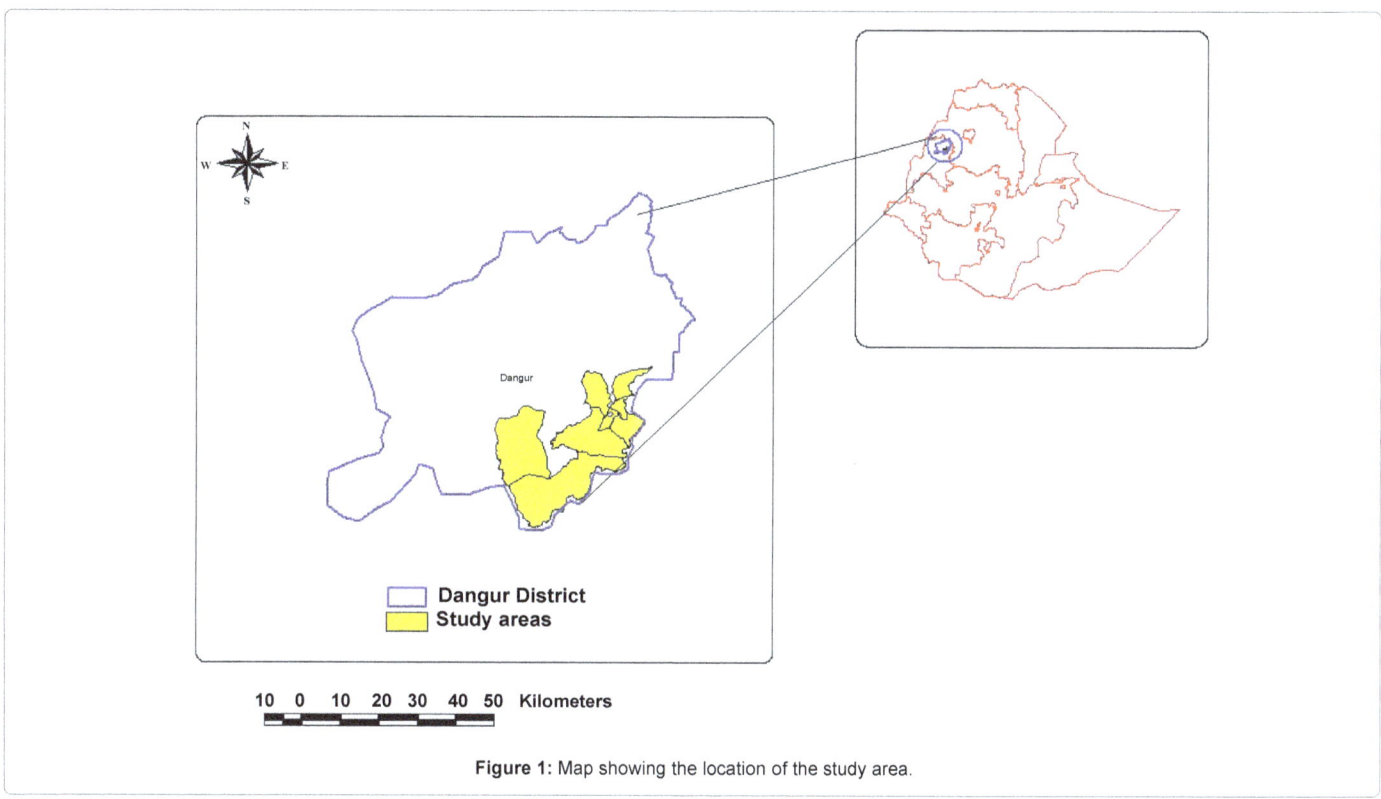

Figure 1: Map showing the location of the study area.

area are: Arundodonax, Arundinariaalina, Strykinosspynosa, Acacia abyssinica, Ficussycomonus, Prunusafricana and Piliostigmathonningi trees together with wooded grasslands. The main crop types cultivated in this area are teff, sesame, maize, peanut and sorghum. The commonly found wild animals are buffalos, antelopes, monkeys, leopard, lion, hyena and elephants [11].

Study animals

The study population constituted of indigenous zebu cattle managed under smallholder mixed crop-livestock farming system. The animals are kept under traditional extensive husbandry system with communal grazing and watering points [11]. Animal population of the district consists of 23,610 cattle, 7,945 sheep, 17,201 goats, 18 horses, 63 mules, 6194 donkeys and 43,448 poultry [11].

Sampling and sample size determination

A cross-sectional study design was conducted in dry season (November 2011-March 2012) to estimate the prevalence of trypanosomosis in cattle in the area. The study sites (kebeles) were selected based on their accessibility to transport. Sample size allocation was done based on the cattle population of the respective kebeles. Cattle owners were informed one day a head of sample collection to gather their animals at one place and simple random sampling technique was employed to select the study animals from the population. The sample size required was calculated at 50% prevalence with level of precision at 5% and 95% confidence interval using the formula described by Thrusfield [12]. As the actual prevalence was unknown, 50% was used to produce the largest sample size possible. Hence, a total of 384 animals were needed to be sampled. However, 543 animals were sampled to increase the precision of the study. Age, sex and body condition score of the studied animals were recorded during sampling. The age was estimated by means of their dentition [13]. The

body condition status of selected animals was assessed and ranked as good, medium and poor [14].

Parasitological and hematological data

Blood samples were collected from superficial ear veins using sterilized lancet and heparinized micro-haematocrit capillary tubes. Immediately after blood collection, the tubes were sealed on one side with Cristaseal (Hawksley Ltd, Lancing, UK). The capillary tube was then transferred to a hematocrit centrifuge and spun for 5 min at 1200 revolutions per minute. The centrifuged capillary tube was measured on a hematocrit reader to estimate the Packed Cell Volume (PCV) as an indicator of anaemia. Then, the capillary tube was cut using a diamond tipped pen 1 mm below the buffy coat to include the uppermost layers of the red blood cells. The content of the capillary tube was expressed on to slide, homogenized onto a clean glass slide and covered with a 22 × 22 mm cover slip. The slide was examined using the 40 × objective for the movement of parasites [15]. Then Packed Cell Volume (PCV) was calculated using micro-haematocrit reader. For the purpose of species identification, thin blood smears were made and fixed with methanol for 3 minutes, stained with Giemsa stain for 30 minutes and examined under a microscope using the oil immersion 100 x objectives [16].

Entomological data

A total of 78 monopyramidal traps including 16, 20, 15, 6 and 21 were deployed in the riverside and wooded grassland areas of Kitili, Burji, Gublak, Ipupuwa and Beles 2 kebeles, respectively. The density and species of tsetse flies were assessed using odour-baited monopyramidal traps deployed at 200-250 m intervals. The odour baits used contained acetone, octanol and cow urine with appropriate apertures in order to release the necessary amounts of attractants. After 48 hours of trapping, the trap cage was collected [17]. The species and sex of the captured flies were identified based on morphological characteristics [18]. The apparent density of tsetse flies was determined based on the daily mean number of flies captured in baited traps and recorded as fly per trap per day (F/T/D) [19].

Data analysis

Raw data were entered into a Microsoft Excel spreadsheet and descriptive statistics were used to summarize the data. STATA* version 11.0 statistical software programs were used to analyze the data. The point prevalence was calculated for all data as the number of infected individuals divided by the number of individuals examined and multiplied by 100. The association between the prevalence of trypanosome infection and risk factors were assessed by chi-square test (χ^2), whereas the two sample student's t-test was used to assess the difference in mean PCV between trypanosome positive and negative animals. The test result was considered significant when the calculated p-value was less than 0.05 at 95% confidence interval.

Results

Parasitological results

A total of 543 animals were sampled including 123, 129, 70, 119 and 102 from Kitili, Burgi, Gublak, Ipupuwa and Beles 2 kebeles, respectively. Out of these, 46 (8.5%) were infected with trypanosomes. The majority (95.5%) of trypanosome species identified was *T. congolense* and the remaining 4.5% was *T. vivax*. Statistically different variation was observed in the infection status among different sites (Table 1, p=0.01). The prevalence of trypanosome in different age groups was 7.6%, 8.7% and 6.7% in young, adult and old animals respectively (Table 2). The prevalence of trypanosomosis was not significantly different among age and sex groups. Of the 543 cattle examined, 97 (17.9%), 247 (45.5%) and 199 (36.7%) were in poor, medium and good body conditions, respectively. Higher proportion (18.3%) of cattle ranked as having poor body conditions were significantly more infected compared to those ranked as medium (8.1%) and good (4%) body conditions (Table 3, p=0.001).

The mean PCV value of the parasitemic animals (22.6%) was lower compared to the mean PCV value of aparastemic animals (26.9%) as indicated in Table 4. There was a statistically significant difference in mean PCV among parasitemic and aparasitemic animals (p=0.02). Besides, a total of 528 tsetse flies were caught (Table 5). The majorities

Kebele	No. of animals examined	Prevalence N (%)	95% CI
Kitili	123	12 (9.8)	5.1-16.4
Burgi	129	19 (14.7)	9.1-22
Gublak	70	9 (12.9)	6-23
Ipupuwa	119	3 (2.5)	0.5-7
Beles 2	102	3 (2.9)	0.6-8
Overall prevalence	543	46 (8.5)	6.3-11.1

Table 1: Prevalence of trypanosomes in different sites (Kebeles) in eastern part of Dangur district.

Variables		Number examined	Prevalence (%)	95% CI
Sex	Male	302	9.9	6.8-13.88
	Female	241	6.6	3.8-10.56
Age group	Young (<1 years)	150	7.6	5.5-12.75
	Adult (1-3 years)	200	8.7	5.9-13.50
	Old (>3 years)	193	6.7	3.9-10.87

Table 2: Prevalence of trypanosomosis in association with sex and age groups in eastern part of Dangur district.

Body condition	No. of animals examined	Prevalence N (%)	95% CI
Good	199	8 (4)	1.8-7.8
Medium	247	20 (8.1)	5-12
Poor	97	18 (18.6)	11.4-27.7
Total	543 46 (8.5)		6.3-11.1

Table 3: Relationship between infection and body condition of cattle in eastern part of Dangur district.

Infection status	No. of animals examined	Mean PCV (%)	t-test	P-value
Aparasitemic	497	27.0	6.4	0.00001
Parasitemic	46	22.6		

Table 4: Association between trypanosome infection and PCV value of cattle in eastern part of Dangur district.

Kebele	Altitude (masl)	Number of traps	*G. m. submorsitans* Male	Female	*G. tachinoides* Male	Female	Total	F/T/D
Kitili	1228	16	3	7	26	28	64	2
Burji	1316	20	43	60	27	30	160	4
Gublak	1300	15	4	6	27	23	60	2
Ipupuwa	1240	6	17	9	6	4	36	3
Beles 2	1245	21	0	0	123	85	208	4.95
Total	_	78	67	82	209	170	528	3.38

Table 5: Species and sex of tsetse flies caught in 5 kebeles of eastern part of Dangur district.

(71.8%) of the flies were *G. tachinoides* and the remaining were *G. m. submorsitans*.

Discussion

In this study, the overall prevalence of bovine trypanosomosis was 8.5% (95% CI=6.3-11.1). Similar findings were reported from different parts of Ethiopia. Earlier studies indicated the prevalence of bovine trypanososmosis ranging from 8.6 to 9% and from 6.6 to 11.3% in southwestern and north western parts of the country respectively [20-25].

However, our finding was higher than previous reports from districts in southern part of Ethiopia that showed the diseases prevalence ranging from 4.2 to 4.4% [26,27]. In these districts tsetse control has been carried out by the southern tsetse and trypanosomosis control project for many years which significantly reduced the prevalence. On the other hand, the current finding is lower than other reports of earlier studies in Ethiopia where the prevalence ranging from 17.3% to 28.1% were reported [28-30]. These variations could be attributed to seasonal differences during sampling periods and methods employed for the studies. The present study showed that the majority (95.5%) of the infections is caused by *T. congolense* and the remaining 5% is caused by *T. vivax*. The predominance of *T. congolense* in tsetse infested areas of Ethiopia has been reported by many authors. In Southwest Ethiopia, Abebe and Jobre reported an infection rate of 58%, 31.2% and 3.5% for *T. congolense, T. brucei* and *T. Vivax*, respectively [10]. Another study in south western Ethiopia recorded an infection rate of 37% for *T. congolense* [31]. The present finding is also supported by earlier works done in which 82.4% *T. congolense* and 5.9% *T. vivax* infections in Arbaminch, southern Ethiopia has been reported [26]. The predominance of *T. congolense* infection in cattle may be due to the high number of serodems of *T. congolense* as compared to *T. vivax* and the development of better immune response to *T. vivax* by the infected animal [9].

The trypanosome infection in male animals is slightly higher than in the female animals, but the variation was not statistically significant (p=0.21); showing that both male and female cattle were equally susceptible to trypanosomosis infection. This is in line with previous studies in Ethiopia [22,23].

There was a significant difference in trypanosome prevalence between the study kebeles (p=0.001). The high prevalence of the disease in Burji might have been attributed to the presence of relatively more suitable habitats (denser grassland and bush coverage) for the vectors compared to other areas. However in Beles 2 lower disease prevalence was observed despite a dense tsetse fly population. This could be attributed to the proximity of this Kebele to a veterinary clinic where the community has more easily access to animal health care compared to other areas. Treating animals with prophylactic drugs against the disease minimizes the prevalence of trypanosomosis in high tsetse fly population densities [32].

This study also showed that there is strong association between the body condition of cattle and trypanosome infection. The occurrence of infection was 4%, 8.1% and 18.6% in cattle with good, medium and poor body conditions, respectively. Thus, the majority of the infected animals manifest poor body conditions because of the effect of the disease. However, poor body condition could also be the consequence of other pathogens and nutritional stress [33]. The finding agrees with the reports of earlier studies in Ethiopia [21,28]. In this study, strong associations existed between the mean PCV value of the animals and occurrence of parasitaemia. The mean PCV value of aparastaemic (27.0%) was significantly higher than that of parastaemic animals (22.6%). The lower mean PCV value in parasitaemic animals than that of aparasitaemic ones was well recorded in previous studies in Ethiopia [34,35]. Another study conducted in southwestern Ethiopia indicated that in an increase in PCV value, the proportion of positivity decreases and hence mean PCV is a good indicator for the health status of the herd in endemic areas [36]. As anaemia is the classical sign of the disease pathogenicity [16], the low PCV in parasitaemic animals could have contributed in reducing the mean PCV of the cattle.

The 8.5% overall prevalence of bovine trypanosomosis recorded in this study might not fully express the true extent of the disease burden because of the very low sensitivity and high variability of the parasite detection methods. Even though relatively high in acute state of infection, the sensitivity of buffy coat technique decreases over the course of the infection and becomes very low in chronic state of the disease [37]. A study conducted in Zambia also indicated that the buffy coat method fails to detect 66% of the infected animals [38]. However; the authors suggested that, the PCV-value of an individual animal is a good indicator of the presence of a trypanosomal infection. Therefore, the apparent parasitological prevalence of trypanosomosis is a little or much lower than the true parasitological prevalence in endemic areas. Hence, in endemic areas, it is necessary to complement the parasitological detection methods with PCR/RFLP and other sensitive molecular techniques to better understand the epidemiology of trypanosomosis and institute appropriate interventions.

The entomological survey revealed that tsetse fly species in the study area are G. m. submorsitans and G. tachinoides. In the study area, there is a typical habitat pattern for riverine species (G. tachinoides) along the rivers surrounded by savannah habitats suitable for G. m. submorsitans. Both of the identified fly species in the present study are among the five Glossina species recorded in Ethiopia [8]. The overall apparent density of tsetse flies was 3.38 F/T/D. Earlier studies in the western part of the country, reported the apparent density of Glossina species ranging from 0.3 to 24.4 F/T/D [26,39,40]. Such wide variations could have been resulted from differences in season and density of vegetation cover and types of traps deployed, type and volume of odour attractants utilized during the studies. The low density of tsetse in the study area may have been due to the expansion of settlements and farmlands in the area. It may also be explained by the migration of the game as a result of climate and habitat changes [9]. The relative abundance of G. tachinoides (71.8%) than G. m. submorsitans (28.2%) might have been due to ability of this species to adapt to unsuitable habitats. Riverine flies appear to be largely unaffected by human population density and can even adapt to human-made environments [41].

Conclusion

In conclusion, T. congolense is the predominant species of trypanosome in the study area although T. vivax was also present. Tsetse fly species caught in the study area were G. m. submorsitans and G. tachinoides. This study also indicated that infection with trypanosomosis negatively affects the body condition and PCV profile of animals. Taken together, tsetse borne trypanosomosis is posing a considerable threat to cattle production in Dangur district, western Ethiopia. Therefore, it is imperative to extend and strengthen the national tsetse and trypanosomosis control scheme in tsetse infested areas in Ethiopia to minimize the burden of the disease.

Competing Interests

The authors have declared that no competing interests exist.

Acknowledgements

The authors are grateful to National Tsetse and Trypanosomosis Investigation and Control Center funding and facilitating the fieldwork.

References

1. Taylor KA (1998) Immune responses of cattle to African trypanosomes: protective or pathogenic? Int J Parasitol 28: 219-240.

2. Uilenberg G (1998) A field guide for diagnosis, treatment and prevention of African animal trypanosomosis. Food and Agricultural Organization, Rome, pp: 43-135.

3. Singla LD, Aulakh GS, Juyal PD, Singh J (2004) Bovine trypanosomosis in Punjab, India. Proceeding of The 11th International Conference of the Association of Institutions for Tropical Veterinary Medicine and 16th Veterinary Association Malaysia Congress, 23-27 August 2004, Petaling Jaya, Malaysia, pp: 283-285.

4. d'Ieteren GD, Authié E, Wissocq N, Murray M (1998) Trypanotolerance, an option for sustainable livestock production in areas at risk from trypanosomosis. Rev Sci Tech 17: 154-175.

5. Bourn D, Reid R, Rogers D, Snow B, Wint W (2001) Environmental change and the autonomous control of tsetse and trypanosomosis in sub-Saharan Africa: case histories from Ethiopia, Gambia, Kenya, Nigeria and Zimbabwe. p: 175.

6. Aulakh GS, Singla LD, Singh J (2005) Bovine trypanosomosis due to *Trypanosoma evansi*: clinical, haematobiochemical and therapeutic studies. In: New Horizons in Animal Sciences. Sobti RC, Sharma VL (eds.), Vishal Publishing and Co., Jalandhar, India, pp: 137-144.

7. Radostits OM, Gay C, Constable PD (2007) Veterinary Medicine: A text book of diseases of cattle, horses, sheep, pigs and goats. 10th edn. Elsevier, London. pp: 1531-1540.

8. Keno M (2005) The current situation of tsetse and trypanosomiasis in Ethiopia. Ministry of Agriculture and Rural development, Veterinary service department, in proceedings of the 28th meeting of International Scientific Council for Trypanosomiasis Research and Control (ISCTRC), Addis Ababa, Ethiopia.

9. Leak SGA (1999) Tsetse biology and ecology: their role in the epidemiology and control of trypanosomiasis. Tydskr S Afr vet Ver 70: 172-176.

10. Abebe G, Jobre Y (1996) Trypanosomosis: A threat to cattle production in Ethiopia. Rev Med Vet 147: 897-902.

11. ARDODW (2011) Agricultural and Rural Development Office of Dangur District Annual Report. pp: 25-28.

12. Thrusfield M (2005) Veterinary Epidemiology. 3rd edn. Blackwell Science, Oxford, p: 233.

13. Pasquini C, Spurgeon T, Pasquini S (2003) Anatomy of domestic animals: Systemic and regional approach. 10th edn. Sudz Publishing, USA, p: 255.

14. Nicholson MG, Butterworth MH (1986) A guide to condition scoring of Zebu cattle. International Livestock Center for Africa (ILCA), Addis Ababa, Ethiopia.

15. Paris J, Murray M, McOdimba F (1982) A comparative evaluation of the parasitological techniques currently available for the diagnosis of African trypanosomiasis in cattle. Acta Trop 39: 307-316.

16. Murray M, Murray PK, McIntyre WI (1977) An improved parasitological technique for the diagnosis of African trypanosomiasis. Trans R Soc Trop Med Hyg 71: 325-326.

17. Bekele J (2004) Evaluation of Deltamethrin applications in the control of tsetse and trypanosomosis in the southern rift valley areas of Ethiopia. Vet Parasitol 168: 177-184.

18. Food and Agriculture Organization (2009) Key for the identification of adults of the species of Glossina. Collection of entomological baseline data for tsetse area-wide integrated pest management programmes. Chapter 5, Food and Agriculture Organization of The United Nations, Rome.

19. Leak SGA, Woume KA, Colardeue C, Duffera W, Feron A, et al. (1987) Determination of tsetse challenge and its relationship with trypanosomosis prevalence in trypanotolerant livestock at sites of the African trypanotolerant livestock network. The African Trypanotolerant Livestock Network, Nairobi, Kenya, pp: 43-52.

20. Tafese W, Melaku A, Fentahun T (2012) Prevalence of bovine trypanosomosis and its vectors in two districts of East Wollega Zone, Ethiopia. Onderstepoort J Vet Res 79: E1-4.

21. Bekele M, Nasir M (2011) Prevalence and host related risk factors of bovine trypanosomosis in Hawa-gelan district, West Wellega zone, Western Ethiopia. Afr J Agri Res 6: 5055-5060.

22. Dagnachew S, Shibeshi S (2011) Prevalence and vector distributions of bovine trypanosomosisin control (Sibu Sire) and noncontrol (Guto Gida) districts bordering Upper Anger valley of East Wollega zone, Western Ethiopia. Ethiop Vet J 15: 77-86.

23. Mihret A, Mamo G (2007) Bovine trypanosomosis in three districts of East Gojjam Zone bordering the Blue Nile River in Ethiopia. J Infect Dev Ctries 1: 321-325.

24. Cherenet T, Sanl RA, Panandam JM, Nadzr S, Spcybroeck N, et al. (2004) Seasonal prevalence of bovine trypanosomosis in a tsetse-infested zone and a tsetse-free zone of the Amhara Region, north-west Ethiopia. Onderstepoort J Vet Res 71: 307-312.

25. Dagnachew S, Girma H, Abebe G (2011) A cross-sectional study on bovine trypanosomosis in Jawi district of Amhara Region, Northwest Ethiopia. Ethiop Vet J 15: 69-78.

26. Teka W, Terefe D, Wondimu A (2012) Prevalence study of bovine trypanosomosis and tsetse density in selected villages of Arbaminch, Ethiopia. J Vet Med Anim Health 4: 36-41.

27. Tadesse A, Tsegaye B (2010) Bovine trypanosomosis and its vectors in two districts of Bench Maji zone, South Western Ethiopia. Trop Anim Health Prod 42: 1757-1762.

28. Ali D, Bitew M (2011) Epidemiological study on bovine trypanosomiasis in Mao-komo special district Benishangul-Gumuz regional State, Western Ethiopia. Glob Vet 6: 402-408.

29. Zeleke G (2011) Preliminary survey on tsetse flies and trypanosomosis at grazing fields and villages in and around the Nech Sar National Park, Southern Ethiopia. Ethiop Vet J 15: 59-67.

30. Mulaw S, Addis M, Fromsa A (2011) Study on the prevalence of major trypanosomes affecting bovine in tsetse infested Asosa district of Benishangul Gumuz Regional State, Western Ethiopia. Glob Vet 7: 330-336.

31. Rowlands GJ, Mulatu W, Authié E, d'Ieteren GD, Leak SG (1993) Epidemiology of bovine trypanosomiasis in the Ghibe valley, southwest Ethiopia. 2. Factors associated with variations in trypanosome prevalence, incidence of new infections and prevalence of recurrent infections. Acta Trop 53: 135-150.

32. Kahn CM, Line S (2005) The Merck Veterinary Manual. 9th edition. Wiley Publishers, USA, pp: 18-35.

33. Pereckiene A, Kaziūnaite V, Vysniauskas A, Petkevicius S, Malakauskas A, et al. (2007) A comparison of modifications of the McMaster method for the enumeration of Ascaris suum eggs in pig faecal samples. Vet Parasitol 149: 111-116.

34. Afework Y (1998) Field investigation on the appearance of drug resistant population of trypanosomes in Metekel district, Northwest Ethiopia. MSc Thesis, Addis Ababa University and FreieUniverstat Berlin, Faculty of Veterinary Medicine, Ethiopia.

35. Tewelde N (2001) Study on the occurrence of drug resistant trypanosomes in cattle in the Farming in Tsetse Control Areas (FITCA) project in Western Ethiopia. MSc Thesis, Addis Ababa University, Faculty of Veterinary Medicine, Debre-Zeit, Ethiopia.

36. Rowlands GJ, Leak SG, Peregrine AS, Nagda SM, Mulatu W, et al. (2001) The incidence of new and the prevalence and persistence of recurrent trypanosome infections in cattle in southwest Ethiopia exposed to a high challenge with drug-resistant parasites. Acta Trop 79: 149-163.

37. Office of International Epizootes (2012) Trypanosomosis (tsetse-transmitted) Manual of diagnostic tests and vaccines for terrestrial animals. Paris, France.

38. Marcotty T, Simukoko H, Berkvens D, Vercruysse J, Praet N, et al. (2008) Evaluating the use of packed cell volume as an indicator of trypanosomal infections in cattle in eastern Zambia. Prev Vet Med 87: 288-300.

39. Regassa F, Abebe G (2009) Current epidemiological situation of bovine trypanosomosis in Limu Shay tsetse controlled area of upper Didessa valley. Ethiop Vet J 13: 19-33.

40. Tilahun G, Balcha F, Kassa T, Birrie H, Gemechu T (1999) Tsetse and trypanosomiasis plot trial at Pawe settlement area, Tana Bales valley, Metekel zone, North-Western Ethiopia. Proceedings of the 13th Annual Conference of the Ethiopian Veterinary Association, Addis Ababa, Ethiopia.

41. Jordan AM (1986) Trypanosomiasis control and African rural development. Longman, London, UK.

38

Bovine Mastitis: Prevalence and Associated Risk Factors in Alage ATVET College Dairy Farm, Southern Ethiopia

Muluken Tuke[1], Dawit Kassaye[2], Yimer Muktar[2]*, Tsegaye Negese[3] and Kifle Nigusu[3]

[1]Asella City Administration Livestock Development and Fishery Office, Asella, Ethiopia
[2]College of Veterinary Medicine, Haramaya University, P.O. Box 138, Dire Dawa, Ethiopia
[3]Hirna Regional Laboratory, P.O. Box 36, Hirna, Ethiopia

Abstract

Purposive cross-sectional types of study was carried out to determine the prevalence of mastitis in lactating dairy cows, and assess the associated risk factors in Alage agricultural technical vocational and training (ATVET) college dairy farm. The study was carried out in 138 dairy cows based on data collection, regular farm visit, clinical examination, and California mastitis test (CMT). In the present study, in general the prevalence of mastitis was 94 (68.11%) and (46.37%) at cow and quarter level respectively. The prevalence of clinical and subclinical mastitis was (16.67% and 51.44%), subclinical (5.25% and 41.12%) at cow and quarter level respectively. In this study prevalence of mastitis was considerably correlated with breed, parity and production status (milk yield per lactation period) ($p<0.05$). However, stage of lactation and age of the cow was not statistically significant in this study. Taking into consideration the different huge losses that could be incurred by both clinical and subclinical mastitis, regular checkup for the exposure of subclinical mastitis and appropriate treatment of the clinical cases should be practiced and also attention should be paid for further detailed investigation and control measure of cases.

Keywords: Alage ATVET college; Bovine mastitis; Prevalence; Southern Ethiopia

Introduction

The world human population is expected to increase from time to time and it will be expected that 7.2 million in the year 2010 the majority of the boost will be in tropical developing countries, where there will be migration from rural areas to urban centers which may led to shift in the pattern of food production, marketing and consumptions [1]. The dairy market is more preferred than meat production and where milk production, provides a regular income generation for the producers since it has easy access to the market. The dairy activity is labor intensive and it creates considerable employment opportunities during production processing and in the marketing area [2].

The proportion of livestock in Ethiopia remained the largest figure in any Africa until recent times but levels of production are one of the lowest. Factors for the poor productivity of livestock in Ethiopia include; disease, poor nutrition, unimproved genotypes, inappropriate managements, socio-economic and institutional constraints [3]. On the other hand, milk production from these animals is not sufficient to the need of the population in the country. Many constraints are faced by increasing the demand for milk and dairy products in the country is huge and the consequential opportunities for the smallholders farming are large. However, low animal output, inappropriate technologies, insufficient research and extension support, poor infrastructure and unfavorable external factors have contributed to the low performance of the dairy cows in general, and of the dairy industry and the products in particular [3]. Only a few modern dairy farms are operational in Ethiopia and most of the milk products come from conventional dairy farm [4].

Mastitis as a disease is the most common and costly production diseases affecting the dairy cattle business worldwide [5]. It is a disease of many mammalian species, at least, 137 infectious causes of bovine mastitis are known to date and in large animal, the commonest pathogens are *S. aureus*, *S. agalactiae*, and other *Streptococcus* species and *Coliforms* [6]. It may also be associated with many other microorganisms including *Actinomyces pyogens*, *Pseudomonas aeruginosa*, *Nocardia asteroids*, *Clostridium perfinges* and other like *Mycobacterium*, *Mycoplasma*, *Pasteurella* and *Prototheca* species and Yeasts [7]. The majority of the cases are caused by only a few common bacterial pathogens namely *Staphylococcus* species, *Streptococcus*, *Coliforms* and *Actinomyces pyogens* [8,9]. Most of the above mentioned microorganisms are usually found in and around the cows environ thus the dairy animals without doubt can got *via* the udder and easily contracted the disease [10]. In Ethiopia, mastitis has got less emphasis as disease, particularly the subclinical form of mastitis mainly caused by *S. aureus* [11,12].

In Ethiopia, most of the previous studies were focused in Addis Ababa and it's surrounding the capital of the country and fails to represent the incidence of mastitis under different management and ecological situation. Moreover, the subclinical mastitis, has received very little consideration in many of the previous studies. Therefore, the objective of this study was to determine the prevalence of mastitis in lactating dairy cows, and assess the assumed risk factors from milk samples of mastitic cows.

Materials and Methods

Study area and period

The study was conducted from November 2014 to April 2015 in Alage ATVET college dairy farm, Southern Ethiopia. The college is

*Corresponding author: Yimer Muktar, College of Veterinary Medicine, Haramaya University, P.O. Box 138, Dire Dawa, Ethiopia
Email: yimermktr21@gmail.com

situated at 217 km Southwest of Addis Ababa. Its absolute location is about a longitude of 38°30' East and latitude of 7°30' North. The area covers 4200 hectares of land with an altitude of 1600 meters above sea level. This is characterized by mild subtropical weather with minimum and maximum temperature ranging from 11°C to 29°C. The area experiences bimodal rainfall distribution with an annual average of 700-900 mm. The three defined Seasons based on rainfall distribution are; short rainy season (March to April); long rainy season (June to September) and long dry season (October to January). The dominant soil type is black clay soil (vertisol) with sand slit clay with PH of 7.9 [13].

Study population

The target population was lactating cattle comprising of 34 Local Borena and 104 Holstein Friesian (HF) breeds with a total of 138 dairy cows. In the study area, the dairy cows managed intensively were kept in exclusive stalls and given with extra diets together with hay and natural grazing pasture.

Study design

A purposive cross-sectional type of study was carried out on lactating dairy cows of Alage ATVET college. The study dairy farm was selected purposively based on accessibility and willingness of dairy farm owner i.e. the Alage ATVET college to determine the occurrence of bovine mastitis and a total of 138 lactating dairy cows were sampled based on none probability sampling method. Semi structured questionnaire was prepared and information regarding cow attributes and farm attributes were collected. The age, breed, lactation stage, and production status were recorded from farm record documents, farm owners and milkers. The study animals were categorized into the different age, parity groups, and production status according to Quinn. Cows were grouped into three lactation stage groups that are up to less than 4 months (Early), 5-7 months (Middle) and over 8 months (Late) lactation stage according to Quinn [10].

Sample size determination

The sample size was determined using the formula given by Thrusfield [14] by assuming the expected prevalence to be 10% while the statistical confidence level was 95%. Accordingly, the sample size of lactating cows was determined to be 138.

$$n = \frac{1.96^2 \left(P_{exp}\left(1 - P_{exp}\right)\right)}{d^2}$$

Where: n=required sample size

P_{exp}=expected prevalence

d=desired absolute precision

Study methodology

California mastitis test (CMT): The CMT was carried out to detect the occurrence of subclinical mastitis. It was conducted in each quarter milk sample immediately after collection. A drop of milk, nearly 2 ml from each quarter was placed in each of the four wells of

the CMT paddle and an equal amount of the CMT reagent was applied to each cup. A gentle circular movement was applied to the mixture, in a horizontal plane for seconds. Clinical mastitis was diagnosed on the basis of visible or palpable sign of inflammation together with a change in consistency and color of milk secreted. On the other hand, CMT was applied to all samples for screening of sub clinical mastitis according to the reaction obtained the results were classified as negative (no gel formation), trace 1,2,3 reaction in which one and above results are considered positive [10]. Cows were considered positive for CMT when at least one quarter turned out to be positive for CMT. A herd was considered positive for CMT when at least one cow in a herd was tested positive with CMT.

Data management and analysis

All the information collected throughout the study period was entered into Microsoft Excel data sheet and then statistical analysis was done by SPSS Version 20 statistical software. The variations between different factors were analyzed using chi-square (χ^2) test. A P-value<0.05 was considered to be statistically significant.

Results

From the total of 138 lactating cows examined using CMT screening the overall prevalence of mastitis was 68.1% and 48.8% at cow and quarter level respectively where 16.67% and 51.4%, cows were found with clinical and subclinical mastitis, respectively. Out of the 552 quarters examined, (41.12%) quarters were found to be positive for subclinical mastitis and (5.25%) for clinical mastitis (Table 1).

In this study 17.64% clinical and 23.52% sub clinical and 17.30% clinical and 61.53% sub clinical prevalence at cow base and 5.46% clinical and 10.93% subclinical and 5.80% clinical and 53.03% subclinical prevalence at quarter base were observed from local borena and exotic breeds respectively (Table 2).

Prevalence of mastitis associated to assumed factors was determined by the total animal examined to positive cows. Breed, parity, and production status showed significant variation on the occurrence of bovine mastitis (p<0.05). Exotic HF cows had prevalence of 61.51%. A higher prevalence (100%) was recorded in cow calved more than 6 times followed by cow calved 5-6 times (77.77%) as compared to cows calved 2, and 3-4 times and cows that gave more production had (>450 liters) higher prevalence (100%) of mastitis (Table 3).

Discussion

The result of current study showed that an overall prevalence of mastitis was 68.11%. The finding was similar with Nibret et al. [15], Mekonnen et al. [16] and Tesfaheywet and Gerema, [17], who reported prevalence of 60.9%, 62.9%, and 64.3% respectively, and comparable with the result of 71% around Holeta town [18], 59.1% in Borana [19],56.5% in Batu and its surrounding [11,20], 56.16% in West Algeria [21], and 50.03% in the districts of North Showa and Borana zones of pastoral area [22]. However, the current study is different from the result of 75.22% in Jimma town [23], 74.3% in Addis Ababa area [24], 53.25% in Dire Dawa town [25], 52.78% in and around Sebeta [26],

Types of mastitis	Total examined cows	Total number affected cows (%)	Total examined quarter	Total number affected (%)
Clinical	138	23 (16.67)	552	29 (5.25)
Subclinical	138	71 (51.44)	552	227 (41.12)
Total	138	94 (68.11)	552	256 (46.37)

Table 1: The overall prevalence of mastitis at cow and quarter levels.

Level	Types of Mastitis	Local borana (n=34)	Exotics (n=104)
		Prevalence, N (%)	Prevalence, N (%)
Cow level	Clinical	6 (17.64)	18 (17.30)
	Subclinical	8 (23.52)	64 (61.53)
Quarter level	Clinical	7 (5.46)	23 (5.80)
	Subclinical	14 (10.93)	210 (53.03)

Table 2: Prevalence of mastitis in local Borana and exotic breed at cow base and quarter level.

Risk factor	Examined animal	positive animals	Prevalence (%)	χ^2	p value
Age					
3-5 years	91	42	46.15	6.59	0.086
6-8 years	23	11	47.82		
9-11years	15	9	60.0		
>11years	9	8	88.88		
Breed					
Local Borana	34	6	17.64	19.74	0.001
Exotic HF	104	64	61.51		
Parity					
Calved up to 2	92	42	45.65	9. 034	0.029
Calved 3-4 times	28	13	46.42		
Calved 5-6 times	9	7	77.77		
Calved>6	4	4	100.0		
Stage of lactation					
Early	55	25	45.45	5.406	0.067
Mid	42	18	42.85		
Late	41	27	65.85		
Production status					
<150 liter	45	13	28.88	15.537	0.001
150-300 liter	67	41	61.19		
300-450 liter	22	12	54.54		
>450 liter	4	4	100.0		

Keys: HF: Holstein Friesian; MY/LP: Milk Yield/Lactation Period

Table 3: The prevalence of both clinical and subclinical mastitis in milking cows based on assumed risk factors.

46.7% in Adama town [27], 44.1% around Holeta areas [28], 32.6% in and around Gondar [15], 28.2% in Bahir Dar and its surroundings [29], and 34.9% in Southern Ethiopia [30]. The variation in these studies could be due to the disparity in the breed, management system, and the epidemiological status [31].

The present study also confirmed that prevalence of 16.67% for clinical mastitis that was similar with the repot of 19.6% in Addis Ababa [24], and 16.11% in and around Sebeta [26] and comparable to the reports of 9.09% in Dire Dawa town [25], 10.0% in Adama town [27], 10.3% at Asella [32], 10.3% around Holeta town [28], and 11.9% in Bahir Dar and its surroundings [29] and 10.7% Eastern harrarghe zone [17] and 9.5% in North Showa and Borana zones of pastoral area [22]. However, the result of the current study was much higher than the findings of 0.93% in and around Gondar [15], 5.3% in Batu and its surroundings [20] and lower than the reports of 22.4% around Holeta town [18], Animals, pathogen, and environment were the most important determining factors which influence the occurrence of clinical mastitis that could contribute for variation in the prevalence of mastitis [31].

The present study also confirmed that prevalence of subclinical mastitis was 51.44% this result was in line with the result of 51.8% in Eastern harrarghe zone [17] and also in close harmony with the result of 55.1% in Addis Ababa [24], 55.8% in Asella [19], 44.6% around Holeta town. The finding of the present study was comparable with earlier findings such as the findings of 40.6% in Batu and its surroundings [20],

40.7% in North showa and Borana zones of pastoral area [22], 33.8% around Holeta areas [28]. However lower than the finding of 36.67% in and around Sebeta [26], 31.67% in and around Gondar [15], and 23.0% in Bahir Dar and its environments [29]. The prevalence of subclinical mastitis varies in dairy cows this might be due environmental factors that play an important role in the occurrence of the disease [31].

The current finding confirmed that lower prevalence of clinical mastitis compared with the subclinical mastitis. Other studies also shared similar observations [17,22-24,33,34]. This could be attributed to the indistinguishable and silent character of subclinical mastitis in most of the time that gives little concentration by the farms and veterinary professionals during treatment unlike that of the clinical mastitis which have given more emphasis in the treatment and control efforts of the disease [17,28,35].

The prevalence of mastitis with regard to lactation stage was studied and the result showed an increase in early and late stages of lactation with a prevalence rate of 45.45% and 65.85%, respectively. This observation was similar with the previous result of Nesru [36], Mungube et al. [37], and Biffa et al. [30] in Ethiopia. The former two authors reported a high prevalence of subclinical mastitis for cows in the late stage of lactation while the late two reported higher prevalence in the early stage of lactation this is associated with most new infection occurs in the first two month of lactation especially the environmental infection probably due to stress and following weakening of immunity. In the late lactation stage the chance of the cow picking up the infection would be high and this result in an increase in prevalence of mastitis in early and late stage of lactation [38].

The higher prevalence of mastitis observed in exotic breed lactating cows (61.51%) than local borana breed (17.64%) was considerably associated with variation in certain physiological and anatomical characteristics between the breeds. This is similar with Lakew et al. [32] who found significant difference between crosses and local Arsi breed and Biffa et al. [30] found a significant difference between local zebu, Holstein Friesian, and Jersey breeds. Exotic breed cows have been found more vulnerable to mastitis due to the position of teat, udder, and anatomy of teat canal. Differences in the genetic structure of teat canal sphincter muscle, keratin in the teat canal or shape of teat end where pointed end are prone to injury which induces infection. [31].

The study showed that there were significant statistical associations ($p<0.05$) the prevalence of mastitis with the parity number of animals, cows with many numbers of calves were with higher prevalence of mastitis and the risk of subclinical mastitis increases with increasing parity number in this study agrees with the finding of Busato and Schallibaum [39] and Bitew et al. [29]; Girma [28]; Nibret et al. [15] who found that the risk of clinical and subclinical mastitis increase significantly with increasing parity number of the cow. The higher prevalence in cows at three and above calved could be due to increase ease of penetration of the teat duct by pathogens and accumulated previous infection [7]. It is postulated that younger animal is less susceptible; through a more effective host defense mechanism. Older cows, especially after four calving are more prone to mastitis [40].

The study showed that there were significant statistical associations ($p<0.05$) between the different production status of the cow. Prevalence of mastitis was higher in high yielding cows than that produce low milk yield per lactation period. Radostits et al. [7] stated that high yielding cows are more susceptible to mastitis than low yielding. This could be due to the ease with which injuries are sustained in large udders so that foci for the entrance of pathogens are created, and stress associated with a high milk yield may upset the defense system of the cow. It has been shown that genotype favorable for milk yield are more susceptible to mastitis [41]. The long-term selection pressure for milk production may have had a negative effect on polymorphism of gene linked to major histocompatibility complex (Bola) in dairy breeds [42,43]. Once inside teat cistern pathogens encounter a group of nonspecific bacteriostatic and bactericidal factors. When these fail, phagocytic cell aided by Immunoglobulins are called into action. Variation among cows has been observed in most of mechanisms, apportion of which is attributable to heredity [41].

Conclusions

The finding of this study confirmed that a total prevalence of 68.11%, which could indicate that mastitis, was the main important health constraints of dairy cows in the study farm which decreases the output of dairy business and thus which urges the need of serious concentration for the disease. Occurrence of subclinical mastitis was more prevalent in the study farm (51.44%) which might indicate dairy farm owners, managers and veterinary professionals give due attention for clinical mastitis than subclinical infection which gives very little emphasis for the status of the subclinical mastitis. Furthermore, regular testing for the detection of subclinical mastitis and proper treatment of the clinical cases together with the appropriate treatment of cows during dry and lactation period should be practiced.

References

1. Sire C, Seinfeld H, Goenewold T (1996) World livestock system. Current status, issue and trends. Animal production and health paper, No: 127, FAO, Rome pp: 81.

2. World Bank technical paper (1991) Dairy development in Sub Sahara Africa: A study of issues and options. Africa technical department series Washington DC, the World Bank.

3. Williams TO, Derosa A, Badiance O (1995) Macroeconomic, International trade and sect oral economic policies in livestock development: A with particular reference to low income countries ILRI, Addis Ababa Ethiopia, pp. 45-68.

4. Asfaw W (1997) Livestock development policy in Ethiopia In: CTA, OAU/IBAR, Ministry of agriculture and cooperatives, Swaziland (editors). Livestock development policies in eastern and southern Africa paper presented in a seminar held in Mbabane, Swaziland, 28 July-August 1997.

5. Seegers H, Fourichon C, Beaudeau F (2003) Production effects related to mastitis and mastitis economics in dairy cattle herds. Vet Res 34: 475-491.

6. Sumathi BR, Veeregowda BM, Mitha RA (2008) Prevalence and anti biogram profile of bacterial isolates from clinical bovine mastitis. Vet World 1: 237-338.

7. Radostits OM, Gay CC, Hinch, KW (2002) Mastitis Veterinary Medicine. A text book of disease of cattle, sheep, pigs, goats and horses 9th (ed). WB Saunders, London, UK, pp. 603-700.

8. Dupreeze JH (2000) Bovine mastitis therapy and why it fails. J S Afr Vet Assoc 71: 201-208.

9. Quinn PJ, Carter ME, Markey B, Carter GR (2004) Clinical Veterinary Microbiology. Mosby Publishing, London, UK, pp. 43-55.

10. Quinn PJ, Carter, ME, Markley B, carter GR (2002) Clinical Veterinary microbiology. Wolf publishing, London, UK, pp. 405-420.

11. Bishi AB (1998) Cross-sectional and longitudinal prospective study of Bovine clinical, sub clinical mastitis in peri urban and urban dairy production system in Addis Ababa region. MSc Thesis Addis Ababa University, Faculty of Veterinary Medicine, Debre-Zeit, Ethiopia.

12. Mekonnen H, Workinesh S, Baylyegne M, Moges A, Tadele K (2005) Antimicrobial susceptibility profile of mastitis isolate from cow in three major Ethiopian dairies. Revue Med Vet 150: 391-394.

13. CSA (2008) Federal Democratic Republic of Ethiopia. Central statistical Agency, Agricultural sample survey report on livestock and livestock characteristics. Volume II, Addis Ababa Ethiopia.

14. Thrusfield M (2005) Veterinary Epidemiology. Blackwell science Ltd, Oxford, UK.

15. Nibret M, Yilikal A, Kelay B (2011) A cross sectional study on the prevalence of sub clinical mastitis and associated risk factors in and around Gondar, Northern Ethiopia. Int J Anim Vet Adv 3: 455-459.

16. Mekonnen L, Tesfu K, Azage T (2012) Clinically manifested major health problem of cross breed dairy herds in urban and peri-urban production system in central highlands of Ethiopia. Trop Anim Health Prod 33: 85-93.

17. Tesfaheywet Z, Gerema A (2017) Prevalence and Bacterial Isolates of Mastitis in Dairy Farms in Selected Districts of Eastern Harrarghe Zone, Eastern Ethiopia. J Vet Med: ID 6498618, 7 pages.

18. Mekibib B, Furgasa M, Abunna F, Megersa B, Regassa A (2010) Bovine mastitis: prevalence, risk factors and major pathogens in dairy farms of Holeta town, central Ethiopia. Vet World 3: 397-403.

19. Bedane A, Kasim G, Yohannis T, Habtamu T, Asseged B, et al. (2012) Study on prevalence and risk factors of bovine mastitis in Borana pastoral and agro-pastoral settings of Yabello District, Borana Zone, Southern Ethiopia. American-Eurasian J Agricult Environ Sci 12: 1274-1281.

20. Bedacha BW, Mengistu HT (2011) Study on prevalence of mastitis and its associated risk factors in lactating dairy cows in Batu and its environments, Ethiopia. Global Veterinaria 7: 632-637.

21. Benhamed N, Moulay M, Aggad H, Henni JE, Kihal M (2011) Prevalence of mastitis infection and identification of causing bacteria in cattle in the oran region West Algeria. J Anim Vet Adv 10: 3002-3005.

22. Dinaol B, Yimer M, Adem H, Nateneal T, Tadesse K, et al. (2016) Prevalence, Isolation of Bacteria and Risk Factors of Mastitis of Dairy Cattle in Selected

Zones of Oromia Regional States, Ethiopia. Global J Med Res: C Microbiol Pathol 16: 39-45.

23. Sori T, Hussien J, Bitew M, (2011) Prevalence and susceptibility assay of *Staphylococcus aureus* isolated from bovine mastitis in dairy farms of Jimma town, South West Ethiopia. J Anim Vet Adv 10: 745-749.

24. Zeryehun T, Aya T, Bayecha R (2013) Study on prevalence, bacterial pathogens and associated risk factors of bovine mastitis in small holder dairy farms in and around Addis Ababa, Ethiopia. J Anim Plant Sci 23: 50-55.

25. Biniam T, Rediet T, Yonus A (2015) Prevalence and potential risk factors of bovine mastitis in selected dairy farms of Dire Dawa Town, Eastern Ethiopia. Appl J Hygiene 4: 06-11.

26. Sori H, Zerihun A, Abdicho S (2005) Dairy cattle mastitis in and around Sebeta, Ethiopia. Int J Appl Res Vet Med 3: 332-338.

27. Abera M, Demie B, Aragaw K, Regassa F, Regassa A (2010) Isolation and identification of Staphylococcus aureus from bovine mastitic milk and their drug resistance patterns in Adama Town, Ethiopia. J Vet Med Anim Health 2: 29-34.

28. Girma D (2010) Study on prevalence of dairy cows around Holeta Areas, West Shewa Zone of Oromia Region, Ethiopia. Global Veternaria 5: 318-323.

29. Bitew M, Tafere A, Tolossa T (2010) Study on bovine mastitis in dairy farms of Bahir Dar and its environments. J Vet Anim Adv 9: 2912-2917.

30. Biffa D, Debela E, Beyene F (2005) Prevalence and risk factors of Mastitis in lactating dairy cow in southern Ethiopia. Int J Appl Res Vet Med 3: 189-198.

31. Radostits OM, Gay KW, Hinchcliff C, Constable PD (2007) Mastitis: in Veterinary Medicine: A Text Book of Disease of Cattle, Sheep, Pigs, Goats, and Horses (10th ed). Bailliere Tindall, London, UK, pp. 674-762,

32. Lakew M, Tolosa T, Tigre W (2009) Prevalence and major bacterial causes of bovine mastitis in Asella, South Eastern Ethiopia. Trop Anim Health Prod 41: 1525-1530.

33. Workineh S, Bayleyegn M, Mekonnen H, Potgieter LN (2002) Prevalence and aetiology of Mastitis in cows from two major Ethiopian dairies. Trop Anim Health Prod 34: 19-25.

34. Dego OK, Tareke F (200) Bovine mastitis in selected areas of southern Ethiopia. Trop Anim Health Prod 35: 197-205.

35. Karimuribo ED, Fitzpatrick JL, Bell CE (2006) Clinical and subclinical mastitis in smallholder dairy farms in Tanzania: risk, intervention and knowledge transfer. Prev Vet Med 74: 84-98.

36. Nesru H (1999) A cross sectional and longitudinal study of bovine mastitis in urban and peri urban dairy system in the Addis Ababa region. MSc. Thesis. Free University Berlin and Addis Ababa University, Ethiopia.

37. Mungube EO, Tenhagen BA, Regassa F, kyule MN, Shiferaw Y, et al. (2005) Reduced milk production in udder quarters with sub clinical mastitis and associated economic losses in cross bred dairy cows in Ethiopia. Trop Anim Health Prod 37: 1573-7438.

38. Schalm DW, Carroll EJ, Jain C (1971) Bovine Mastitis. Lea and Fibiger, Philadelphia, Pa, USA.

39. Busato A, Trachsel P, Schalibaum M, Blum JW (2000) Udder health and Risk factor for sub clinical mastitis in organic dairy farm in Switzerland. Prev Vet Med 44: 205-220.

40. Dullin AM, Paape MJ, Nickerson SC (1988) Comparison of phagocytosis and chemiluminescence's by blood and mammary gland neutrophils from multi parous cows. Am J Vet Res 49: 172-177.

41. Shook GE (1989) Selection for disease resistance. J Dairy Sci 72: 1349-1362.

42. Lewin H (1989) Disease resistance and immune response genes in cattle: Strategies for their detection. J Dairy Sci 72: 1334-1348.

43. Lipman LJ (1995) *Escherichia coli and Staphylococcus aurius mastitis*: Epidemiology and pathogenesis. PhD Thesis, University Utrecht, Netherlands.

39

Rapid Detection of Type 2 Porcine Reproductive and Respiratory Syndrome Virus by a Duplex Reverse Transcription Insulated Isothermal PCR on a Field-Deployable System

Hung-Chih Kuo[1], Dan-Yuan Lo[1], Chiu-Lin Chen[1], Chien-Hsien Lee[2], Yu-Han Shen[2], Yung-Long Tsai[2], Pei-Yu Alison Lee[2]* and Hsiao-Feng Grace Chang[2]

[1]Yunlin-Chiayi-Tainan of Animal Disease Diagnostic Center, College of Veterinary Medicine, National Chiayi University, Chiayi, Taiwan

[2]GeneReach Biotech, Taichung, Taiwan

Abstract

Porcine reproductive and respiratory syndrome virus (PRRSV) is an important porcine pathogen globally. Reverse transcription-polymerase chain reaction (RT-PCR) for PRRSV detection is an important tool for disease management and control. Clinical sensitivity of RT-PCR for PRRSV detection is compromised to a certain degree by the high genetic diversity in the PRRSV genome. A duplex RT-insulated isothermal PCR (RT-iiPCR) for the North America lineage of PRRSV (PRRSV-NA) has been developed by targeting both ORF6 and ORF7 to increase test inclusivity. In this study, its limit of detection 95% was determined to be about 5 genome equivalents per reaction by testing a serial dilution of in-vitro transcribed RNA. The PRRSV-NA duplex RT-iiPCR was compared with an ORF7 real-time RT-PCR (rRT-PCR) published previously for the evaluation of analytical and clinical performance. Both tests did not react with seven common swine pathogens. The two methods had similar detection endpoints for viral RNA of two PRRSV-NA isolates. Further tests with 187 swine samples showed that 14 of the 90 rRT-PCR-negative and 2 of the 97 rRT-PCR-positive samples were positive and negative by the duplex RT-iiPCR, respectively. The two methods had 91.44% agreement (95% confidential interval: 87.26 - 95.62%, κ=0.83). Repeat testing could not resolve 13 of the discrepant samples (all negative by rRT-PCR and positive by RT-iiPCR). Further RT-nested PCR analysis and DNA sequencing analysis of the ORF7 region supported that the target RNA was present in these samples. Therefore, the PRRSV-NA duplex RT-iiPCR appeared to have higher clinical sensitivity than the reference rRT-PCR. Working on a field-deployable device, the PRRSV-NA duplex RT-iiPCR has potential to serve as a fast and sensitive tool for PRRSV detection at points of need.

Keywords: PRRSV; Reverser transcription-insulated isothermal PCR; RT-iiPCR; Molecular detection; Field-deployable; Point of need

Introduction

Infection of porcine reproductive and respiratory syndrome virus (PRRSV) can lead to decreased pork production, and the costs for disease management were estimated $664 million annually in the USA in 2011 [1,2]. PRRSV, a member of genus Arterivirus, family Arteriviridae, is an enveloped virus containing a positive single-stranded RNA of approximately 15 kb, which encodes 11 open reading frames (ORFs). ORF1a and ORF1b encode the nonstructural proteins, Nsp1α, Nsp1β, and Nsp2 to -12 [3]; ORF2 to ORF7 encode the structural proteins, GP2, E, GP3, GP4, GP5, M, and N [4]. PRRSV evolves rapidly and is divided into two genotypes sharing only about 60% nucleotide identity: the type 1 European lineage (PRRSV-EU, prototype the Lelystad strain) and the type 2 North American lineage (PRRSV-NA, prototype the VR-2332 strain) [5-8]. PRRSV-NA is prevalent in North America, South America, and Asia; and has also been found in Europe in recent years [8-12].

PRRSV can infect pigs of all ages. Its clinical symptoms include mild to severe respiratory syndromes in nursery-grown pigs, and reproductive failures characterized by infertility, late fetal mummification, abortions, stillbirths, and/or weak piglets [9,13]. Most importantly, PRRSV infection has been associated with the complicated porcine respiratory disease complexes [13]. Although various modified-live and inactivated vaccines are commercially available in many countries, their protection efficacy was limited to infection by PRRSV strains closely related to the vaccine strain, making the control of PRRS difficult [9,14]. Therefore, adoption of strict biosecurity measures to help avoid or reduce the introduction and transmission of PRRSV plays an important role in the control and eradication of PRRSV; sensitive and specific detection of the etiological agent is crucial to these measures [15,16].

Several methods, including serological tests, virus isolation, and reverse transcription polymerase chain reaction (RT-PCR), are available for to help follow the status of PRRSV infection. The immunoassays, such as ELISA tests, for PRRSV-specific antibody have been commonly used to follow the immunization status of the pigs. Detection of the PRRSV by virus isolation is time-consuming and requires specific facility, technician, and cell line; furthermore, not all PRRSVs can be isolated. With high sensitivity and specificity, the RT-PCR methodology has been accepted for PRRSV detection recently [9]. The RT-PCR assays for PRRSV detection reported so far were designed to target either the ORF6 or ORF7 gene [17-22], the regions found to be the most conserved among the available PRRSV sequences [23].

*Corresponding author: Pei-Yu Alison Lee, GeneReach Biotech, Keyuan Second Road, Central Taiwan Science Park, Taichung, Taiwan
E-mail: peiyu329@genereachbiotech.com

Nevertheless, PRRSV mutates quickly and has a high degree of genetic diversity [24]. False-negative results in RT-PCR tests due to sequence variations in the primer and probe target areas have been reported. Consequently, the inclusion of more than one PRRSV RT-PCR test was recommended by OIE for PRRSV detection [9,25].

A duplex RT-insulated isothermal PCR (RT-iiPCR) was developed recently for PRRSV-NA (POCKIT™ PRRSV-NA Reagent Set, GeneReach Biotech, Taichung, Taiwan) to increase the strain coverage for PRRSV detection by RT-PCR. It was designed to target two of the most conserved regions found in the ORF6 and ORF7 genes in the PRRSV genome [23]. Furthermore, in iiPCR, natural liquid convection established in a capillary tube can cycle the reaction components sequentially through different temperature zones to achieve the 3 stages (denaturation, annealing, and extension) of PCR [26-28]. Consequently, the annealing step is not done at a fixed temperature in iiPCR, allowing primers and probes to bind to sequences with minor mismatches [29]. Clinical performance of various iiPCR for various bacterial and viral pathogens in companion animals, livestock animals, and aquaculture animals, food safety, and health care has been demonstrated to be comparable to that of the reference nested PCR, real-time PCR, and/or virus isolation method [28,30-41]. In several cases, clinical sensitivity slightly higher than that of the reference real-time PCR methods was observed for targets with notable sequence variations; clinical specificity can be maintained by careful design of the primer and probe [36,42-44].

Additionally, the iiPCR works on a field-deployable device, the POCKIT™ Nucleic Acid Analyzer (POCKIT™; GeneReach, Taichung, Taiwan), which is compact (28 × 25 × 8.5 cm, W × D × H) and lightweight (2.1 kg). Automatically interpreted results are generated within one hour. The regent is ready in a lyophilized format and minimal steps are involved in reaction assembly. Essentially, the iiPCR method is ready in a format for point-of-need applications to facilitate efficient biosecurity management and timely disease control.

In this study, analytical and clinical performance of the PRRSV-NA duplex RT-iiPCR on the POCKIT™ device was evaluated and compared to a previously published rRT-PCR which was also routinely used in a diagnostic laboratory.

Materials and Methods

Microorganisms and clinical samples

One PRRSV Taiwan isolate (CH18-2) and a VR-2332-derived PRRSV-NA vaccine (Ingelvac PRRS® MLV, Boehringer Ingelheim Vetmedica, Saint Joseph, MO, USA) were used in the sensitivity comparison study. Sequencing analysis showed that CH18-2 was closely related to the previously reported PRRSV-NA MD001 strain found in Taiwan (data no shown); it was grouped into the lineage 3 of PRRSV based on its ORF5 sequence (maximum-likelihood analysis [Tamura-Nei model] with bootstrap analysis of 1000 replicates). The exclusivity test panel included PRRSV-EU (AMERVAC® PRRS, Laboratorios Hipra S.A., Amer, Spain), porcine circovirus type 2 (PCV2; Circovac®, Merial, Lyon, France), Japanese encephalitis virus (JEV; SUIGEN® Swine Japanese Encephalitis Live Virus Vaccine-at Strain, SBC Virbac Biotech, Kaohsiung City, Taiwan), pseudorabies virus (PRV; SUIGEN® Swine Pseudorabies Gene Deleted Live Vaccine, SBC Virbac Biotech), classic swine fever virus (CSFV; Dried Lapinized Hog Cholera Vaccine, Animal Health Research Institute, Council of Agriculture, New Taipei City, Taiwan), porcine parvovirus (PPV; PORCILIS® PARVO, MSD Animal Health, Kenilworth, NJ, USA), and *Mycoplasma*

hyopneumoniae (Ingelvac MycoFLEX®, Boehringer Ingelheim Vetmedica, Saint Joseph, MO, USA). The clinical performance studies included 130 serum samples from diseased pigs and 57 postmortem lung tissues from animals with respiratory symptoms collected for surveillance or diagnostic purposes in Taiwan in 2016.

In vitro transcription

A linearized plasmid template containing the consensus sequences of ORF6 (nt 14285 - 14809, GenBank accession number KP89034) and ORF7 (nt 1 - 372, GenBank accession number JX046380) downstream of a T7-promoter was synthesized (Shanghai Generay Biotech, Shanghai, China). The consensus sequences were derived from alignment analyses of 792 ORF6 and 1168 ORF7 sequences. From this plasmid, an artificial ORF6/ORF7 RNA was produced by *in vitro* transcription (IVT) by using the MEGAscript® T7 Kit (Thermo Fisher Scientific, Carlsbad, CA). RNA concentrations were calculated from OD260 readings measured by a NanoDrop 2000 spectrophotometer (Thermo Fisher Scientific, Wilmington, DE) according to the following formula:

$$\text{No. of RNA molecules / } \mu l = \frac{\text{Avogadro number}\left(6.022 \times 10^{23}\right) \times \text{RNA concentration}\left(g / \mu l\right)}{\left(\text{RNA molecular weight}\left(g\right)\right)}$$

The RNA was aliquoted and stored at –80°C until use; dilutions were made in 40 ng/μl of yeast tRNA.

Nucleic extraction

Nucleic acid extraction was performed with the taco™ DNA/RNA Extraction Kit (GeneReach Biotech) on taco™ mini Nucleic Acid Automatic Extraction System (taco™ mini; Gene Reach Biotech) according to the manufacturer's instructions. For the lung tissue, 80 mg was homogenized in 500 μL phosphate-buffered saline in a taco™ Prep (GeneReach Biotech) and centrifuged at 12,000 x g for 5 min. After the wells of the extraction plate were filled with the designated buffers, 200 μL of the serum or the supernatant from homogenized lung tissues were loaded to the first well of the extraction plate. The plate was subsequently loaded into a taco™ mini device for automatic nucleic acid extraction. The nucleic acids were eluted individually in 200 μL Eluting Buffer, transferred to fresh tubes, and stored at -70°C for later use.

RRSV duplex RT-iiPCR

The PRRSV-NA duplex RT-iiPCR (POCKIT™ PRRSV Detection Kit) targeted both the ORF6 and ORF7 genes of PRRSV-NA; their amplicons were detected by the 550-nm and 520-nm channels, respectively, in the POCKIT™ device. Briefly, the lyophilized reagent was reconstituted with 50 μL Premix Buffer B and mixed with 5 μL nucleic acid extract. Subsequently, 50 μL of the final mixture were transferred to an R-tube™ (GeneReach Biotech) which was loaded into a POCKIT™ device. Qualitative results were generated by the built-in algorithm and shown on the display screen within 1 hour. Samples generating positive signals from either ORF6 or ORF7 marker were considered PRRSV positive.

PRRSV real-time RT-PCR

The reference PRRSV-NA rRT-PCR (Table 1) [17,45] was routinely used as a tool to facilitate PRRSV diagnosis at the Animal Disease Diagnostic Center, National Chiayi University. It targeted the ORF7 gene. The 25-μL reaction contained 1x PCR Reaction Buffer (BioMi, Taichung, Taiwan), 0.5 mM dNTP, 0.25 μM forward primer, 0.5 μM reverse primer, 0.2 μM probe, 0.3 μM ROX, 60 units of MMLV reverse transcriptase (BioMi), 2 units of Taq polymerase (BioMi), and 2 µL of sample nucleic acids. The reaction was performed on an Applied Biosystems® Step One Plus™ system (Thermo Fisher Scientific) at 42°C for 30 min followed by 40 cycles of 93°C for 15 s and 60°C for 1 min. A representative standard curve of the rRT-PCR analyses with a serial dilution of the ORF6/ORF7 IVT RNA had a linearity range between 10^2 and 10^6 copies with a slope of -3.21 (correlation coefficient, 0.99; y-intercept, 39.78; data not shown). All results that had a recorded threshold cycle (Ct) value were considered PRRSV positive.

PRRSV ORF7 RT-nested PCR and sequencing analysis

To amplifying the target region of the PRRSV-NA rRT-PCR, a degenerate RT-nested PCR (Table 1) was designed and optimized to target the highly conserved sequences found in the 212 sequences of PRRSV-NA available in the GenBank database. Briefly, the 10-µL solution containing the sample and 1 µM random primers was heated to 80°C for 10 min and cooled immediately on ice. Next, the 20-µL RT reaction containing 1 × Reaction Buffer, 0.5 mM dNTP, 200 units of MMLV reverse transcriptase (Thermo Fisher Scientific), and 10 µL of the pretreated template was incubated at 37°C for 1 hour, 42°C for 30 min, and 94°C for 5 min. For both steps in the nested PCR, the 20-µL reaction contained 1x PCR Reaction Buffer (BioMi), 0.125 mM dNTP, 0.25 µM each of the forward and reverse primers, 2 units of Taq polymerase (BioMi), and 2 µL sample. The first PCR (n-f1 and n-r1 primers, Table 1) was performed with the following program: 95°C for 30 s; 30 cycles of 95°C for 20 s, 61°C for 20 s, and 72°C for 40 s; and 72°C for 5 min. The program for the second PCR (n-f2 and n-r2 primers, Table 1) was 95°C for 30 s; 30 cycles of 95°C for 20 s, 56°C for 20 s, and 72°C for 40 s; and 72°C for 5 min. The PCR products of the expected size were verified on a 2% agarose gel stained with ethidium bromide and sent to Genomics (Taipei, Taiwan) for DNA sequencing analysis. Phylogenetic trees were constructed by using the maximum-likelihood method by the MEGA 5 software [46].

Statistical analysis

Limit of detection 95% (LOD95%) of a reaction was determined by probit analysis at 95% confidence interval by SPSS v14 (SPSS, Chicago, IL, USA). The 2 x 2 contingency tables were analyzed by kappa statistic using SPSS to determine the inter-rater agreement.

Results

Analytical sensitivity of the PRRSV-NA duplex RT-iiPCR

To assess the analytical sensitivity of the PRRSV-NA duplex RT-iiPCR, a serial dilution of the ORF6/ORF7 IVT RNA was tested. The detection rates of the 100- (10/10), 50- (20/20), 20- (20/20), and 10-copy (20/20) reactions were 100%; those of the 5-, 1-, and 0-copy ones were 95% (19/20), 25% (5/20), and 0% (0/24), respectively. Probit regression analysis determined that the LOD95% of the reaction was about 5 genome equivalents per reaction.

The analytical sensitivity of the PRRSV-NA duplex RT-iiPCR for PRRSV RNA was compared to that of the reference PRRSV-NA rRT-PCR [17,45] using serial dilutions of the nucleic acid extracts of a Taiwan isolate (CH18-2) and a VR-2332-derived vaccine. The 100% endpoints of the duplex RT-iiPCR and the rRT-PCR were at the 10^{-5} and 10^{-4} dilution, respectively, with both samples (Table 2), demonstrating that the RT-iiPCR and the rRT-PCR had similar sensitivity for the viral RNA of the PRRSV isolates.

Analytical specificity of PRRSV-NA duplex RT-iiPCR

Analytical specificity of the PRRSV-NA duplex RT-iiPCR was verified with a PRRSV-EU strain, and CSFV, PCV2, PRV, PPR, JEV, and *M. hyopneumoniae*, whose infection also causes respiratory symptoms, production failure, and/or gross lesion in the lungs on infected animals. The PRRSV-NA duplex RT-iiPCR did not detect any of these pathogens.

Clinical performance of the PRRSV-NA duplex RT-iiPCR

The PRRSV-NA duplex RT-iiPCR was compared with the reference rRT-PCR to evaluate its clinical performance for the detection of PRRSV in swine samples. Totally, 130 sera and 57 lung tissues collected in Taiwan in 2016 were tested by the two methods in parallel. Among them, 97 were positive and 90 negative by the rRT-PCR; 109 were positive and 78 negative by the duplex RT-iiPCR (Tables S1 and 3a). Two of the 97 rRT-PCR-positive samples were negative by the RT-iiPCR; notably, 14 of the 90 rRT-PCR negative samples were positive by the duplex RT-iiPCR. Based on these results, the agreement between the two assays was 91.44% (95% confidential interval: 87.26% - 95.62%; κ=0.83). Repeating tests by the two tests were performed to help resolve the discrepancy. Three of the samples (S29, S77, and S81) were positive by both methods (rRT-PCR, 1/5[Ct=38.78], 2/5 [Ct=39.90, 38.54], and 2/5 [Ct=37.96, 37.55], respectively; duplex RT-iiPCR, 3/5, 2/5, and 2/5, respectively); the other 13 specimens still showed discordant results after repeat testing (Table S2).

RT-nested PCR and sequencing analysis of the discrepant samples

An RT-nested PCR was established to amplify the target region of the rRT-PCR in ORF7 from the 13 samples. The results of the RT-nested PCR can help resolve the discrepancies between the results of the rRT-PCR and RT-iiPCR methods, and the amplicons obtained, if any, were subjected to further sequencing analysis. Mutations at the primer/probe binding sites can lead to false-negative results in PCR assays [9,25]. RT-nested PCR products of the expected size and ORF7 sequences (nt 2-350, Figure 1) were obtained from all 13 samples, supporting that the samples were PRRSV positive. Sequencing analysis revealed that 1-3 mismatches were found in the forward primer, 1-2 mismatches in the probe, and 0-1 mismatches in the reverse primer sequences of the rRT-PCR assay. The phylogenetic tree generated from

Reaction	Name	Nucleotide sequence (5' - 3')	position*
rRT-PCR	PRRSVf2	GGGGAATGGCCAGYCAGTCAA	14927 - 14947
	PRRSVr2	GCCAGRGGAAAATGKGGCTTCTC	15061 - 15039
	US probe	FAM-CTGGGYARGATYATCGCCCAGCA-BHQ1	14964 - 14986
RT-nested PCR	n-f1	GGCCCCTGCCCACCAC	14704 - 14719
	n-r1	GGCARACTRAACTCCACAGYGTAACT	15208 - 15183
	n-f2	ACCACGTYGAAAGTGCCG	14715 - 14732
	n-r2	AACTCCACAGTGTAACTTATYCTCCC	15199 - 15174

*Nucleotide position is based on the sequence of the VR-2322 strain (GenBank accession no. U87392.3)
Table 1: Sequences of primers and probe used in the PRRSV-NA rRT-PCR and RT-nested PCR.

these nucleotide sequences suggested that the 13 PRRSV samples all belonged to the PRRSV-NA lineage (data not shown).

Discussion and Conclusion

Among the tools recommended by OIE for the detection of PRRSV (virus isolation, immunoassay, RT-PCR) [9], the PCR methodology is gaining momentum in recent years. However, testing with multiple PCR methods has been recommended to help mitigate the risks of false-negative results due to the high genetic variations found in the viral genome. The PRRSV-NA duplex RT-iiPCR was designed to amplify two of the most conserved regions found in the PRRSV-NA sequences available in the GenBank database, i.e., in ORF6 and ORF7 genes, to help boost the detection inclusivity/sensitivity of the reaction for PRRSV-NA. Notably, 13 of the 90 rRT-PCR-negative samples reacted positively in the duplex RT-iiPCR test (Table S2). The positive RT-nested PCR results and sequencing analyses of these samples provided evidences for the presence of PRRSV RNA in the samples. After integrating the results of all tests, 111 PRRSV-positive samples were found; all were positive by the duplex RT-iiPCR and 13 of them were negative by the rRT-PCR (Tables 3b), implying that the duplex RT-iiPCR had higher clinical sensitivity (inclusivity) than the reference rRT-PCR. The fact that the annealing step was not carried out at a specific temperature may have also allowed the reaction to tolerate sequence mismatches to some extent in iiPCR.

Although the reference rRT-PCR contained degenerate primers and probes to be inclusive for as many strains of PRRSV as possible [17], significant numbers of mutations in the forward primer (1-3

mismatches) and/or probe binding sites (1 - 2 mismatches) were found in the 13 rRT-PCR false-negative samples. Similarly, mutations at the primer/probe binding sites caused by genetic variations led to the false-negative results in certain PRRSV real-time PCR assays [9,25]. Sequence mismatches could have decreased the binding efficiency between the oligonucleotides and the target sequences (Figure 1), leading to reduction in the melting temperatures (Tm) and negative effects on the annealing step. For 12 of the 13 discrepant samples, substantial Tm reductions (~15-30°C) between the probe of the rRT-PCR and the target sequences were suggested by bioinformatics analysis (75 mM monovalent ion and 3 mM Mg^{2+}; OLIGO 7 software; Molecular Biology Insights, Colorado Springs, CO, USA) [49]); for the one (L2) with minor probe Tm reduction (~8°C), significant Tm reductions in both primers were predicted. One base-pair mismatch in the probe biding site had substantial influence on the sensitivity of different real-time PCR tests for influenza virus and swine hepatitis E virus [47,48].

Information of the PRRSV infection status is important for PRRSV control and elimination [15]. However, issues such as time-consuming procedures, carry-over contamination, and/or expensive equipment and special technicians have limited the application of conventional RT-PCR at points of need. The sensitive and specific iiPCR/POCKITTM system described herein is a practical tool for settings with limited resources. The device can be powered on a rechargeable or car battery; the lyophilized reagent can be shipped without a cold chain and stored for up to two years in a refrigerator. Its protocols, involving only a couple of assembly steps, can be accomplished by any

Strain	Dilution Factor	rRT-PCR (Ct)			duplex RT-iiPCR		
		test 1	test 2	test 3	test 1	test 2	test 3
VR2332-derived vaccine	10^2	29.54	29.74	29.69	+	+	+
	10^3	31.97	32.51	32.31	+	+	+
	10^4	**36**	**37.01**	**35.56**	+	+	+
	10^5	-	-	-	+	+	+
	10^6	-	-	-	+	-	-
Taiwan CH18-2 isolate	10^2	29.5	29.11	29.09	+	+	+
	10^3	32.85	33.01	32.57	+	+	+
	10^4	**37.13**	**35.42**	**38.74**	+	+	+
	10^5	-	39.65	-	+	+	+
	10^6	-	-	-	-	-	+

Table 2: Detection limit of the PRRSV-NA duplex RT-iiPCR: comparison with the rRT-PCR.

(a) Variables		rRT-PCR		Total
		+	-	
Duplex	+	95	14	109
RT-iiPCR	-	2	76	78
Total		97	90	187
(b) Variables		rRT-PCR		Total
		+	-	
Duplex	+	98	13	111
RT-iiPCR	-	0	76	76
Total		98	89	187

Table 3: A 2 × 2 contingency between the rRT-PCR and duplex RT-iiPCR for PRRSV-NA detection in swine samples.

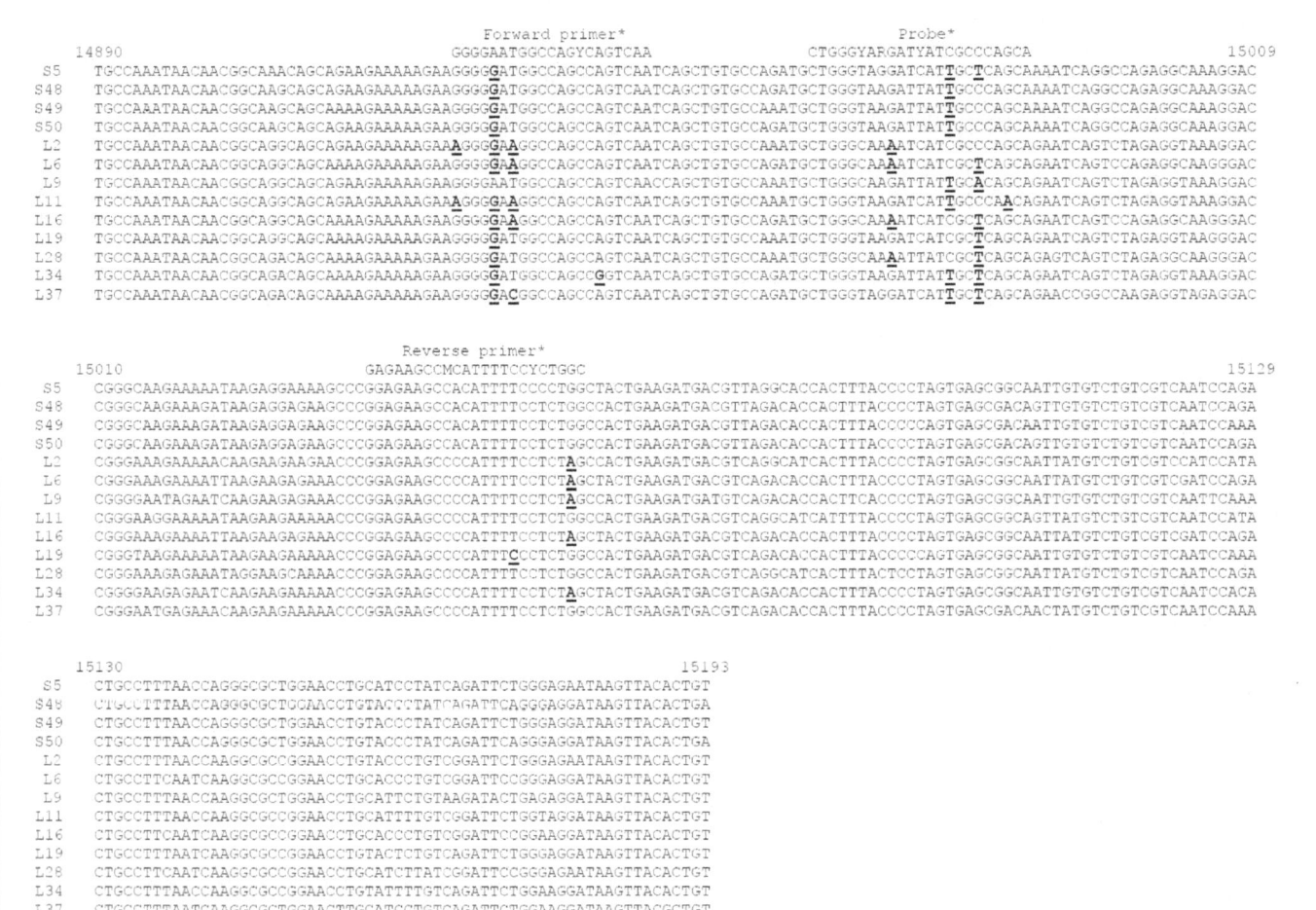

Figure 1: Sequence alignment of the *ORF7* region of the 13 rRT-PCR-negative/ duplex RT-iiPCR-positive samples. Nucleotide positions were based on the sequence of the PRRSV-NA VR-2332 strain (GanBank accession no. U87392). *, rRT-PCR primer and probe sequences; bold and underlined, nucleotide different from that of the primer or probe sequence.

users with basic training. Implemented in a closed system, the system has relatively low risks of amplicon cross-contamination. The relatively inexpensive system can be performed at locations close to or at the pen side, reducing the turn-around time to facilitate timely implementation of the measures for the control and management of PRRSV infection.

A nucleic acid extraction step before PCR is generally required to remove the reaction inhibitors from the sample matrix [49]. A field-deployable automatic nucleic acid extraction method, namely taco™ mini, is available to help reduce the labor costs and increase the performance consistency of the procedure. This device can also be operated on rechargeable car battery. The protocol combining the taco™ mini with the POCKIT™ device can generate qualitative test results within 2 hours with minimal hands-on time.

With great analytical sensitivity and specificity, the PRRSV-NA duplex RT-iiPCR was shown to have higher clinical sensitivity than the reference rRT-PCR. Working on the field-deployable taco™ mini/ POCKIT™ system in a rapid and user-friendly manner, this test can provide timely information on the status of PRRSV infection to facilitate efficient biosecurity and disease management in the swine industry.

References

1. Lunney JK, Benfield DA, Rowland RR (2010) Porcine reproductive and respiratory syndrome virus: an update on an emerging and re-emerging viral disease of swine. Virus Res 1: 1-6.

2. Holtkamp DJ, Kliebenstein JB, Neumann E, Zimmerman JJ, Rotto H, et al. (2013) Assessment of the economic impact of porcine reproductive and respiratory syndrome virus on United States pork producers. J Swine Health Prod 2: 72-84.

3. Ropp SL, Wees CEM, Fang Y, Nelson EA, Rossow KD, et al. (2004) Characterization of emerging European-like porcine reproductive and respiratory syndrome virus isolates in the United States. J Virol 7: 3684-3703.

4. Stadejek T, Oleksiewicz M, Potapchuk D, Podgorska K (2006) Porcine reproductive and respiratory syndrome virus strains of exceptional diversity in eastern Europe support the definition of new genetic subtypes. J Gen Virol 7: 1835-1841.

5. Allende R, Lewis T, Lu Z, Rock D, Kutish G, et al. (1999) North American and European porcine reproductive and respiratory syndrome viruses differ in non-structural protein coding regions. J Gen Virol 2: 307-315.

6. Nelsen CJ, Murtaugh MP, Faaberg KS (1999) Porcine reproductive and respiratory syndrome virus comparison: divergent evolution on two continents. J Virol 1: 270-280.

7. Forsberg R (2005) Divergence time of porcine reproductive and respiratory syndrome virus subtypes. Mol Biol Evol 11: 2131-2134.

8. Brar MS, Shi M, Murtaugh MP, Leung FCC (2015) Evolutionary diversification of type 2 porcine reproductive and respiratory syndrome virus. J Gen Virol 7:

1570-1580.

9. OIE (2015) Porcine reproductive and respiratory syndrome: Manual of diagnostic tests and vaccines for terrestrial animals.(7), World Organisation for Animal Health (OIE), Paris, France.

10. Shi M, Lam TTY, Hon CC, Murtaugh MP, Davies PR, et al. (2010) Phylogeny-based evolutionary, demographical, and geographical dissection of North American type 2 porcine reproductive and respiratory syndrome viruses. J Virol 17: 8700-8711.

11. Shi M, Lam TTY, Hon CC, Hui RKH, Faaberg KS, et al. (2010) Molecular epidemiology of PRRSV: A phylogenetic perspective. Virus Res 1: 7-17.

12. Stadejek T, Stankevicius A, Murtaugh MP, Oleksiewicz MB (2013) Molecular evolution of PRRSV in Europe: Current state of play. Vet Microbiol 1: 21-28.

13. Lunney JK, Fang Y, Ladinig A, Chen N, Li Y, et al. (2016) Porcine Reproductive and Respiratory Syndrome Virus (PRRSV): Pathogenesis and interaction with the immune system. Annu Rev Anim Biosci 4: 129-154.

14. Chand RJ, Trible BR, Rowland RR (2012) Pathogenesis of porcine reproductive and respiratory syndrome virus. Curr Opin Virol 3: 256-263.

15. Rowland R, Morrison R (2012) Challenges and opportunities for the control and elimination of porcine reproductive and respiratory syndrome virus. Transbound Emerg Dis s1: 55-59.

16. Corzo CA, Mondaca E, Wayne S, Torremorell M, Dee S, et al. (2010) Control and elimination of porcine reproductive and respiratory syndrome virus. Virus Res 1: 185-192.

17. Lurchachaiwong W, Payungporn S, Srisatidnarakul U, Mungkundar C, Theamboonlers A, et al. (2008) Rapid detection and strain identification of porcine reproductive and respiratory syndrome virus (PRRSV) by real-time RT-PCR. Lett Appl Microbiol 1: 55-60.

18. Lin CN, Lin WH, Hung LN, Wang SY, Chiou MT (2013) Comparison of viremia of type II porcine reproductive and respiratory syndrome virus in naturally infected pigs by zip nucleic acid probe-based real-time PCR. BMC Vet Res 1: 181-182.

19. Chang CY, Deng MC, Wang FI, Tsai HJ, Yang CH, et al. (2014) The application of a duplex reverse transcription real-time PCR for the surveillance of porcine reproductive and respiratory syndrome virus and porcine circovirus type 2. J Virol Methods 201: 13-19.

20. Egli C, Thür B, Liu L, Hofmann MA (2001) Quantitative TaqMan® RT-PCR for the detection and differentiation of European and North American strains of porcine reproductive and respiratory syndrome virus. J Virol Methods 1: 63-75.

21. Kleiboeker SB, Schommer SK, Lee SM, Watkins S, Chittick W, et al. (2005) Simultaneous detection of North American and European porcine reproductive and respiratory syndrome virus using real-time quantitative reverse transcriptase–PCR. J Vet Diagn Invest 2: 165-170.

22. Revilla-Fernández S, Wallner B, Truschner K, Benczak A, Brem G, et al. (2005) The use of endogenous and exogenous reference RNAs for qualitative and quantitative detection of PRRSV in porcine semen. J Virol Methods 1: 21-30.

23. Stevenson G, Torremorell M (2012) Porcine reproductive and respiratory syndrome virus (porcine Arterivirus): Diseases of swine. (10thedn). Blackwell, Ames, IA, USA.

24. Murtaugh MP, Stadejek T, Abrahante JE, Lam TT, Leung FCC (2010) The ever-expanding diversity of porcine reproductive and respiratory syndrome virus. Virus Res 1: 18-30.

25. Wernike K, Bonilauri P, Dauber M, Errington J, Le Blanc N, et al. (2012) Porcine reproductive and respiratory syndrome virus: Interlaboratory ring trial to evaluate real-time reverse transcription polymerase chain reaction detection methods. J Vet Diagn Invest 24: 855-866.

26. Chang HFG, Tsai YL, Tsai CF, Lin CK, Lee PY, et al. (2012) A thermally baffled device for highly stabilized convective PCR. Biotechnol J 5: 662-666.

27. Tsai YL, Wang HT, Chang HF, Tsai CF, Lin CK, et al. (2012) Development of TaqMan probe-based insulated isothermal PCR (iiPCR) for sensitive and specific on-site pathogen detection. PLoS ONE 9: e45278.

28. Tsai YL, Wang HC, Lo CF, Tang-Nelson K, Lightner D, et al. (2014) Validation of a commercial insulated isothermal PCR-based POCKIT™ test for rapid and easy detection of white spot syndrome virus infection in Litopenaeus vannamei.

PLoS ONE 3: e90545.

29. Krishnan M, Ugaz VM, Burns MA (2002) PCR in a Rayleigh-Benard convection cell. Science 5594: 793.

30. Tsen HY, Shih CM, Teng PH, Chen HY, Lin CW, et al. (2013) Detection of Salmonella in chicken meat by insulated isothermal PCR. J Food Prot 8: 1322-1329.

31. Balasuriya UB, Lee PY, Tiwari A, Skillman A, Nam B, et al. (2014) Rapid detection of equine influenza virus H3N8 subtype by insulated isothermal RT-PCR (iiRT-PCR) assay using the POCKIT™ Nucleic Acid Analyzer. J Virol Methods 207: 66-72.

32. Wilkes RP, Tsai YL, Lee PY, Lee FC, Chang HF, et al. (2014) Rapid and sensitive detection of canine distemper virus by one-tube reverse transcription-insulated isothermal polymerase chain reaction. BMC Vet Res 10: 213.

33. Wilkes RP, Kania SA, Tsai YL, Lee PY, Chang HH, et al. (2015) Rapid and sensitive detection of feline immunodeficiency virus using an insulated isothermal PCR-based assay with a point-of-need PCR detection platform. J Vet Diagn Invest 4: 510-515.

34. Wilkes RP, Lee PY, Tsai YL, Tsai CF, Chang HH, et al. (2015) An insulated isothermal PCR method on a field-deployable device for rapid and sensitive detection of canine parvovirus type 2 at points of need. J Virol Methods 220: 35-38.

35. Lung O, Pasick J, Fisher M, Buchanan C, Erickson A, et al. (2015) Insulated isothermal reverse transcriptase PCR (iiRT-PCR) for rapid and sensitive detection of classical swine fever virus. Transbound Emerg Dis 63: e395-402.

36. Ambagala A, Pahari S, Fisher M, Lee PA, Pasick J, et al. (2015) A rapid field-deployable reverse transcription-insulated isothermal polymerase chain reaction assay for sensitive and specific detection of bluetongue virus. Transbound Emerg Dis doi: 10.1111/tbed.12388.

37. Tung H-Y, Wang SH, Chiang YC, Tsai MS (2016) Rapid screening of roundup ready soybean in food samples by a hand-held PCR device. Food Sci Biotechnol 4: 1101-1107.

38. Lin YH, Lin YJ, Chang TD, Hong LL, Chen TY, et al. (2016) Development of a TaqMan probe-based insulated isothermal polymerase chain reaction (iiPCR) assay for detection of Fusarium oxysporum f. sp. cubense Race 4. PLoS ONE 7: e0159681.

39. Chua KH, Lee PC, Chai HC (2016) Development of insulated isothermal PCR for rapid on-site malaria detection. Malaria J 1: 1.

40. Ambagala A, Fisher M, Goolia M, Nfon C, Furukawa-Stoffer T, et al. (2016) Field-deployable reverse transcription-insulated isothermal PCR (RT-iiPCR) assay for rapid and sensitive detection of foot-and-mouth disease virus. Transbound Emerg Dis doi: 10.1111/tbed.12554.

41. Zhang J, Tsai YL, Lee PYA, Chen Q, Zhang Y, et al. (2016) Evaluation of two singleplex reverse transcription-Insulated isothermal PCR tests and a duplex real-time RT-PCR test for the detection of porcine epidemic diarrhea virus and porcine deltacoronavirus. J Virol Methods 234: 34-42.

42. Soltan MA, Tsai YL, Lee PA, Tsai CF, Chang HG, et al. (2016) Comparison of electron microscopy, ELISA, real time RT-PCR and insulated isothermal RT-PCR for the detection of Rotavirus group A (RVA) in feces of different animal species. J Virol Methods 235: 99-104.

43. Wilkes RP, Kania S, Tsai YL, Lee PY, Chang HH, et al. (2015) Rapid and sensitive detection of feline immunodeficiency virus using an insulated isothermal polymerase chain reaction-based assay with a point-of-need PCR detection platform. J Vet Diagn Invest 27: 510-515.

44. Drigo M, Franzo G, Belfanti I, Martini M, Mondin A, et al. (2014) Validation and comparison of different end point and real time RT-PCR assays for detection and genotyping of porcine reproductive and respiratory syndrome virus. J Virol Methods 201: 79-85.

45. Tamura K, Peterson D, Peterson N, Stecher G, Nei M, et al. (2011) MEGA5: Molecular evolutionary genetics analysis using maximum likelihood, evolutionary distance, and maximum parsimony methods. Mol Biol Evol 10: 2731-2739.

46. Klungthong C, Chinnawirotpisan P, Hussem K, Phonpakobsin T, Manasatienkij W, et al. (2010) The impact of primer and probe-template mismatches on the sensitivity of pandemic influenza A/H1N1/2009 virus detection by real-time RT-PCR. J Clin Virol 2: 91-95.

47. Gerber PF, Xiao CT, Cao D, Meng XJ, Opriessnig T (2014) Comparison of real-

time reverse transcriptase PCR assays for detection of swine hepatitis E virus in fecal samples. J Clin Microbiol 4: 1045-1051.

48. Rychlik W (2007) OLIGO 7 primer analysis software. Methods Mol Biol 402: 35-60.

49. Schrader C, Schielke A, Ellerbroek L, Johne R (2012) PCR inhibitors - Occurrence, properties and removal. J Appl Microbiol 5: 1014-1026.

40

Study on the Prevalence of Endoparasites in Small Holder Dairy Farm in and around Harar Town, Oromia Regional State, Eastern Ethiopia

Lamessa Keno[1], Birhanu Abera[2*], Diriba Lemma[2], Eyob Eticha[2] and Guluma Assefa[1]
[1]East Shoa Zone Livestock and Fishery Resource Office, Adama, Ethiopia
[2]Asella Regional Veterinary Laboratory, PO Box 212, Asella, Ethiopia

Abstract

A cross- sectional study of prevalence of Gastro-intestinal helminthiasis of small holder dairy cows was carried out from December 2007 to April 2008 with an attempt to determine the prevalence in Harar town and its surrounding, Eastern Ethiopia. Amongst the 287 coprological analysis or quantitative faecal analysis on dairy cows were performed with an overall prevalence rate 139 (48.4%) by using coprological examination. Coprological examination (Direct, Floatation, sedimentation and Mc Master Techniques) were the methods followed to study the prevalence of GI - parasitic infestation. An overall GI-parasitic infestation of 48.4% was found in this study. The result also revealed that nematodes Strongyles (38.4%) and Trichuris (8.4%), paraphistomum (13.9%) and Coccidia (10.5%) in that order. The helminth eggs present were identified in general terms as strongyloid eggs, since relevant nematode genera produce eggs that are similar in appearance and cannot be discriminated easily, except for eggs of Nematodirus, Strongyloides and Trichuris. In view of the prevalence of hazardous parasitic gastro intestinal parasites with a potential of entailing serious direct and indirect losses, and accompanying in these small holder dairy cows deserve attention and pertinent action to see they are controlled because high economic importance deserving due attention in helminth control programs in the study area.

Keywords: Small holder; Dairy cow; Prevalence; Helminthiasis; Harar; Eastern Ethiopia

Introduction

The growing demand for the meat and milk in developing world, changing function of livestock and changing consumers perspectives are the major driving forces in the global livestock sector during the next two decades [1].

The Ethiopian dairy system can be paraphrased by the statement that "though there is huge livestock population with high potential for milk and dairy production and there are ever more people tend to drink milk and consume more dairy products yet milk production is still too low in the country to satisfy the needs which is hampered by bucketful of paradoxes, hopes and heartbreaks". The Ethiopian livestock population is the highest in African continent and there has been efforts exerted to develop the sector, but the outcomes are insignificant (the paradox) [2].

Helminth infection, especially subclinical gastrointestinal nematode infections are among the major health problems limiting the productivity in dairy animals [3]. Economic losses are caused by gastrointestinal parasites in a variety of ways. The losses can be through lowered fertility, reduced work capacity, involuntary culling, a reduction in food intake and reduced weight gain, lower milk production, treatment costs and mortality in heavily parasitized animals [4].

Infectious diseases especially gastrointestinal parasites and exo-parasites are considered as the major diseases of cattle in the study area. Helminth parasite infections in cattle are of the major importance in many agro ecological zones and are a primary factor in the reduction of productivity. This is further aggravated in small holder dairy farmers due to the limited availability of land and feed resources. Year round utilization of communal grazing and watering places shared livestock kept by smallholder are a major source of infection. The prevention and control of helminth parasites is not based on disease epidemiology rather is targeted at sick individual [5].

Gastrointestinal parasite infection is one of the major causes of wastage and decreased productivity exerting their effect through mortality, morbidity, decreased growth rate, weight loss in young growing calves and late maturity of slaughter stock, reduced milk and meat production and working capacity of the animal mainly in developing countries [6]. These effects largely relates to specific damage caused by the parasites including villous atrophy at the site of gastrointestinal nematode attachment and liver trauma resulting from the presence of migratory liver fluke [7]. Indirect effects have also been described, including altered feed intake, digest flow rate, nutrient absorption and liver metabolic activity, endocrine status and immunological response [8].

A number of helminths species are known to infect cattle worldwide. The most important ones include nema-todes like Strongyle species (Haemonchus, Ostartagia, Trichostrongylus, Cooperia) and trematodes of economic importance Fasciola species (Fasciola hepatica and Fasciola gigantica) and Paraphistomum species (Paraphistomum cervei), while cestodes like Monezia species (Monezia benideni and Monezia expanza) could also be important constraints in animal production [9].

Small holders or pastoralist may not easily detect the effects of internal parasites on their animals, because of generally sub-clinical or chronic nature of the nematode infections [10,11]. Thus the subclinical parasite infections are responsible for significant economic loss, because

*Corresponding author: Birhanu Abera, Asella Regional Veterinary Laboratory, PO Box 212, Asella, Ethiopia
E-mail: birhanuabera27@yahoo.com

once clinical disease is noticed in a group of animal productivity has already occurred [12,13].

Parasitic gastro enteritis is very important causes of production losses including the direct effect of severe clinical signs such as anemia, associated edema, diarrhea and anorexia [14]. The investigation and identification of the prevalence and to know the burden of gastro-intestinal parasites are very important to give veterinary care and to get expected product from dairy cattle. Therefore the objective of this study was to know prevalence of endoparasites and to identify species of parasites in the area based on coprological examination.

Study Materials and Methods

Description of the study area

A cross sectional study was carried out from December 2007 to April 2008 in Harar town and its surrounding (capital of eastern Hararghe region). Harar is situated 526 km east of Addis Ababa altitudes ranges from 1300 to 2200 m and total coverage of the area is 343.2 km². Mean annual temperate and rainfall ranger between 19.2°C - 20°C and 67.1-804.7 mm respectively according to Harar agricultural office report. This area has a mid-tropical weather (woyna dega) and highland temperate climate (Dega) accounting respectively 76% and 24% of the climate. Agriculture is the main occupation of the population of the area. The agricultural activities are mainly mixed type with cattle, sheep, goats, rearing and crop production undertaken side by side. According to the information obtained from the veterinary section of Harar agricultural office report 1998/1999 [15], the total livestock population of this region was estimated at 36,098 cattle, 19,973 goats, 6,067 sheep, 6,487 equines and 34,525 poultry. The major annual crops include sorghum, wheat, maize and chat. The major types of soil in the area supporting the crops and the flora of the area are chromic cambisols 7%, chromic luvisols 48%, chromic vertisols 1%, eutric nitosols 3% and vertic luvisols 41% type of soils.

Study animals

The study was conducted on small holder dairy farm in and around Harar town on 287 dairy cattle (253 female and 34 male). All the cattle found in each farms during the study period were subjects of the study.

Study design

A cross sectional survey was made on small holder dairy farm animals during the study period to investigate the prevalence of endoparasites through examination. Regular visits were made to the area for faecal sample collection. After a through collection of faecal sample and the sample was undertaken some examination.

Coprological examination

In field faecal samples were collected from study animals, directly from rectum and was transported to laboratory and examined. Three laboratory techniques were employed: Faecal samples were directly taken from the rectum and transported to laboratory for examination through direct smear, floatation, sedimentation and McMaster techniques.

Direct smear: A few drops of water plus an equivalent amount of faecal are mixed on a microscopic slide. Tilting the slide then allows the lighter eggs to flow away from the heavier debris, a coverslip is placed on the fluid and the preparation is then examined microscopically. It is possible to detect most eggs or larvae by this method, but due to

the small amount of faeces used it may only detect relatively heavy infection [16].

Floatation method: The basis of any floatation method is that when worm eggs are suspended in a liquid with a specific gravity higher than that of the eggs, the latter will float up to the surface. Nematode and cestode eggs float in a liquid with a specific gravity of between 1.1 and 1.2, trematode eggs, which are much heavier, require a specific gravity of 1.3 to 1.35. The floatation solution used for nematode and cestode ova are mainly based on Nacl or sometimes MgSO₄. A saturated solution of these is prepared and stored for a few days and the specific gravity checked prior to usage.

Sedimentation method: From collected samples for each case 3 gms of faeces was measured and put in to a mortar. Then 42 ml of ZnSO₄ (zinc sulfate) solution as floating medium was added and crusher thoroughly with a pistle. The suspension then allowed passing through a mesh sieve in to a beaker and the one left was discarded. After gentle shaking, the suspension was poured in to conical centrifuge tube and centrifuged at 1500 rpm for 3 minutes. After decanting the supernatant, the sediment was agitated till thick homogeneous fluid is obtained at the bottom of the tube and then filled equal amount of water to previous level. The content of the tube was mixed thoroughly with thumb over the open end of the tube. And then using a pasture pipette a 0.15 ml fluid is taken from the suspension and placed on a microscope slide covered with cover slip. Then examined under low power objective [11].

McMaster method: This quantitative technique is used where it is desirable to count the number of eggs or larvae per gram of faeces. An abbreviated version of this techniques is to homogenize the 3 gm of faeces in 42 ml of salt solution, sieve, and pipette the filtrate directly in to the mc master slide. Finally number of eggs observed was registered and the total egg from two chamber and then multiply by 50 to get the total number of eggs per gram of faeces [16].

Data Management and Analysis

The data collected from the study area were coded and analyzed by using SPSS version 20. The prevalence was calculated by dividing the number of animals harboring a given parasite by the total number of animals examined. Percentage to measure the prevalence of helminth and chi-square and t-test to measure association between prevalence of the helminth and the breeds, age, sex, lactation condition and body conditions of animals were employed. Variation of prevalence among or between age group, sex group and techniques was analyzed by chi-square (X^2) test. Confidence interval was held at 95% and $p<0.05$ was set for significance level.

Results

Out of 287 dairy cattle examined in smallholder farms during the study period, using faecal sample qualitative examination, 139 (48.4%) were detected to positive for internal parasites. Hence, the prevalence of internal parasites among age, sex and techniques of small holder dairy cows in and around Harar town shown in Tables 1-5 respectively. There were no statistically significant differences ($p>0.05$) in infection rates between female and male, young and adult. Both sexes and age groups are equally susceptible and exposed to the parasite.

Discussion

During the study period in the study area, nine farms had been visited. The managemental supplementation given to the animal to the

Number of farms	Address	Number of animals examined
1	Kebele 13	30
2	Kebele 16	60
3	Kebele 16	30
4	Aretagna	23
5	Amaressa	31
6	Amaressa	30
7	Kebele 17	24
8	Kebele 18	14
9	Abirabata	45
	Total	287

Table 1A: Indicates the number of animal examined, address and number of farms.

Age	Total examined	No. of positive	Prevalence (%)
<2	1	0	0
3 ≤ 4	19	2	10.5
>4	267	41	15.4
Total	**287**	**43**	**15**
Sex			
F	253	124	15.4
M	34	15	11.8
Total	**287**	**139**	**15**
Techniques			
Direct smear	85	40	47.1
Floatation	106	59	55.7
Sedimentation	96	40	41.7
Total	**287**	**139**	**48.4**

Table 1B: The overall prevalence of helminthosis examined in the study area.

Age	Total examined	no. of positive	Prevalence (%)	X²	p-value
<2	1	0	0		
3 ≤ 4	19	2	10.5	0.5016	0.778
>4	267	41	15.4		
Total	287	43	15		
Sex					
F	253	39	15.4	0.3135	0.576
M	34	4	11.8		
Total	287	43	15		
Techniques					
Direct smear	t85	6	7.1		
Floatation	106	18	17		
Sedimentation	96	0	0		
Total	287	24	8.4		

Table 2: Prevalence of *Strongyle* eggs in small holder dairy cow by age, sex and techniques.

animal in the all farm is almost similar. Regarding to housing system, among the type of housing system, the all farms are loose type from opening type of housing system and closed type of housing system in which its ground surface was concrete. In relation to feeding system, concentrate, Roughages and feed residue like residues of wheat from Harar brewery always supplied to the all age groups. Besides the health aspects, mastitis is the most core point of diseases that commonly affect lactating animals. Such serious condition may be due to low milking management in the farms. Regarding noninfectious disease, bloat is commonly affect farms. The animals are dewormed twice annually.

Based on the result of this study livestock diseases and their consequences have severe impact on the small holder farmer's livelihood directly or indirectly. The direct cause of disease is mortality of animals and the indirect effects include low out put such as meat, milk and

draft power. Animal diseases have also been indicated as public health hazard which is the same with the current study [17].

Endo parasite is a wide spread ruminants health problems and cause significant economic loss to the livestock in Ethiopia. Lemma et al. [18] have reported that water logged and poorly drained areas with acidic soils in the highlands are often endemic areas for parasites.

Cross sectional study showed that *Strongyle, Coccidia, Trichuris* and *Paramphistomum* are the most internal parasites commonly affect

Age	Total examined	no. of positive	Prevalence (%)	X²	p-value
<2	1	0	0		
3 ≤ 4	19	3	15.8	0.7279	0.695
>4	267	27	10.1		
Total	287	30	10.5		
Sex					
F	253	28	11.1	0.8608	0.354
M	34	2	5.9		
Total	287	30	10.5		
Techniques					
Direct smear	85	6	7.1		
Floatation	106	18	17		
Sedimentation	96	0	0		
Total	287	24	8.4		

Table 3: Prevalence of coccidian oocyst in small holder dairy cow by age, sex and techniques.

Age	Total examined	No. of positive	Prevalence (%)	X²	p-value
<2	1	0	0		
3 ≤ 4	19	0	0	1.9698	0.373
>4	267	24	9		
Total	287	24	8.4		
Sex					
F	253	24	9.5	3.5347	0.060
M	34	0	0		
Total	287	24	8.4		
Techniques					
Direct smear	85	6	7.1		
Floatation	106	18	17		
Sedimentation	96	0	0		
Total	287	24	8.4		

Table 4: Prevalence of *Trichuris* eggs in small holder dairy cows by age, sex and techniques.

Age	Total examined	No. of positive	Prevalence (%)	X²	p-value
<2	1	0	0		
3 ≤ 4	19	4	21.1	1.0098	0.604
>4	267	36	13.5		
Total	287	40	13.9		
Sex					
F	253	31	12.3	5.0510	0.025
M	34	9	26.4		
Total	287	40	13.9		
Techniques					
Direct smear	85	2	2.4		
Floatation	106	0	0		
Sedimentation	96	38	39.6		
Total	287	40	13.9		

Table 5: Prevalence of *Paramphistomum* eggs in small holder dairy cows by age, sex and techniques.

the animals. Irrespective of their prevalence *Strongyle* is the most prevalent parasites affect the animal in the study area while *Trichuris* is the least one. The prevalence rates of the above parasitic infection are 15%, 10.5%, 8.4% and 13.9% in *Strongyle*, *Coccidia*, *Trichuris* and *Paramphistomum* respectively.

The present study is conducted with the aim of identifying GI-helminth and their prevalence on dairy cows. Coprological examination was performed on 287 dairy cows and the overall prevalence of GI-parasites was found to be 48.4% which comparable to the report on dairy cow by Derib [19] in Bahir-Dar and its surrounding which is 50%. The higher prevalence was also reported by Etsehiwot [20] to be 82.8% in Holeta and its surroundings and by Zerfu [21] to be 81% in Assela and its surroundings. The prevalence difference in different study area could have resulted from difference in management system, topography, deworming practices, and climatic condition that favors the survival of infective stage of the parasite and intermediate hosts.

There was no statistically significant difference (p>0.05) in prevalence between females (15.4%) and males (11.8%). This shows that sex seems have no effect on the prevalence and both sexes are equally susceptible and exposed to the disease. In this study, no significant variation in prevalence of internal parasites in dairy cow of different age groups, calves percentage is zero, young's (10.5%) and adults (15.4%) were observed statistically (p>0.05). This indicates that age groups do not matter for the presence or prevalence of internal parasites in dairy cows and hence both age groups are equally susceptible to the diseases as well.

According to the current study result which indicated the prevalent helminth egg with respect to their 139(48.4%) were infested by internal parasites genera like *Strongyle* (15%). *Coccidia* (10.5%), *Trichuris* (8.4%) and *Paramphistomum* (13.9%). In this result, the *Strongyle* species were highly prevalent than other parasite genera. This result lower when compare with Adame [22] who reported *strongyles* (23.4%), *Coccidia* (2.6%), *Paramphistomum* (33.3%) prevalence in dairy cow in cheffa dairy farm. The prevalence difference among the genera of helminth in different study area indicates that the topography and climatic condition of each study area vary from one another in supporting infectivity of different parasite and development of their intermediate hosts.

Conclusion and Recommendations

The present study conducted on small holder dairy farm on endoparasites from December up to end of April for five months in and around Harar town of Oromia regional state, Eastern Ethiopia. This study showed that an internal parasite in small holder dairy cow is one of the most prevalent diseases in the area affecting the well-being of the animals. However, the attention given to disease so far was not satisfactory in that there were perhaps little or no attempts made to study the epidemiology of the disease. Hence, to get clear epidemiological picture of the disease, comprehensive study should be launched in the area where small holder dairy cows are abundant and practically participating in agricultural practices and play significant role in this sector.

Even though, small holder dairy farms are paramount important animals in the farming system of the country, the existing livestock extension package programmed of region, saying little out the management and health aspects of small holder daily cows. Based on the aforementioned conclusion, the following recommendations are indicated: significance of these parasites should not be underestimated as they reduce the growth, productivity, reproductive potential of animals; Strategic treatment with appropriate, effective and broad spectrum anathematic should be practiced at the beginning and after the end of rainy seasons. Such treatment regime is targeted to get rid-off the parasites burden of the host animals and minimize pasture contamination by dropping faecal output; the government should formulate an appropriate policy regarding small holder dairy cow's management and health aspects and this should be hold in the livestock extension package programmed; the field veterinarians and stock owners should be aware of the importance and burden of the parasitic disease in small holder dairy farm; this study did not consider the breeds of animals, management and feeding systems, seasonal helminth dynamics, and identification of parasite to species level. Therefore, future detailed works should be undertaken.

Competing Interest

The authors declare that they have no competing interest.

Acknowledgements

Authors would like to thank the faculty of veterinary medicine of Haramaya University support of this work and dairy farm owners for their cooperation.

References

1. World Bank (2001) Livestock Development Report, World Bank, Washington DC, USA.

2. Felleke G, Woldearegay M, Haile G (2009) SNV Ethiopia. Dairy Policy Inventory of Ethiopia, pp: 5-14.

3. Johannes C, Johan H, Georg VSM, Pierre D, Jozef V (2009) Gastrointestinal nematode infections in adult dairy cattle: Impact on production, diagnosis and control. Veterinary Parasitology 164: 70-79.

4. McLeod RS (1995) Costs of major parasites to the Australian livestock industries. International Journal for Parasitology 25: 1363-1367.

5. Alekaw L (2000) Distribution of ticks and tick born diseases at Metekel branch, Ethiopia. J Ethiop Vet Assoc 4: 40-60.

6. Newman RL (1995) Recommendation to Minimize Selection for Anthelminthic Resistance in Nematode Control Program. CSIRO Division of Animal Health, pp: 161-169.

7. Murray M, Rushton B (1997) The Pathology of Fasciolosis and the Effect of Large Doses of GIT Nematodes on the Histology and Biochemistry of the Small Intestine of Lambs. Int J Parasitol 3: 349-361.

8. Hansen J, Perry B (1994) The Epidemiology, Diagnosis and Control of Helminth Parasites of Ruminants. A handbook. ILRAD, Nairobi, Kenya.

9. Onah DN, Nawa Y (2000) Mucosal Immunity Against Parasitic Gastrointestinal Nematodes. Korean J Parasitol 38: 209-236.

10. Soulsby ESW (1982) Helminths, Arthropods and Protozoa of Domesticated Animals. 7th edn. Bailliere Tindall, London; lea and Febiger, Philadelphia, pp: 212-258.

11. Urquhart GM, Armour J, Duncan JL, Dunn AM, Jennings FW (1996) Veterinary Parasitology. 2nd edn. Blackwell Science, United Kingdom, p: 307.

12. Kaplan RM (2006) Update on parasite control in small ruminants 2006: addressing the challenges posed by multiple-drug resistant worms. Proc Am Assoc Bovine Pract, Saint Paul, Minnesota 39: 1-16.

13. Tibbo M, Aragaw K, Philipsson J, Malmfors B, Nasholm A, et al. (2005) Economics of sub-clinical helminthosis control through anthelmintics and supplementation in Menz and Awassi-Menz crossbred sheep in Ethiopia. 56th Annual Meeting of the EAAP, pp: 5-8.

14. Ploeger HW, Kloosterman DC, Borge Steede FH, Eysken M (1990) Effect of Natural occurring Nemotod infection in the 1st and 2nd grazing season on the growth of second year grazing cattle. Veterinary Parasitology 36: 57-70.

15. Harar Agricultural Office (1999) Harar agricultural office annual report of the 1998/1999 fiscal year.

16. Urquhart GMJ, Armour JL, Duncan AM, Dunn FW, Jennings J (1987) Department of Veterinary Parasitology. 2nd edn. Blackwell science, United Kingdom, p: 22.

17. Assegid W (2000) Constraints to live stock and its products in Ethiopia: Policy implications. DVM Thesis, Faculty of Veterinary Medicine, Addis Ababa University, Debre-Zeit, Ethiopia, p: 52.

18. Lemma B, Gabre-Ab F, Tedla S (1985) Studies on fascioliasis in four selected sites in Ethiopia. Veterinary parasitology 18: 29-37.

19. Derib Y (2005) The Study on Endoparasite of Dairy Cattle in Bahir-Dar and its Surrounding. DVM Thesis, FVM, AAU, Debre Zeit, Ethiopia.

20. Etsehiwot W (2004) Study on bovine gastrointestinal helminthes in dairy cows in around Holetta. DVM Thesis, Debre Zeit, Ethiopia.

21. Zerfu M (1991) The Study on the Prevalence of Gastro-Intestinal Helminthes of Cattle in Chilalo Awraja Arsi Administrative Region. DVM Thesis, Debre Zeit, Ethiopia.

22. Adame Z (1985) Importance of helmintaisis in the cheffa dairy farm. DVM Thesis, FVM, AAU, Ethiopia, p: 2.

41

Major Causes of Liver Condemenation and its Economic Significance in Small Ruminanats Slaughtered at Luna Export Abattoir, East Shoa Zone, Centeral Ethiopia

Elias Gezahegn[1]*, Birhanu Abera[2], Dinku Assefa[3] and Hussen Yunus[4]

[1]Bale Zone Pastoral Area Development Office, Ethiopia
[2]Asella Regional Veterinary Laboratory, Ethiopia
[3]Yem Special District Livestock Development and Fishery Office, Ethiopia
[4]Bale Zone Livestock Development and Fishery Office, Ethiopia

Abstract

A study was conducted from December, 2014 to April 2015 to identify the major causes of liver condemnation and its economic significance in small ruminants slaughtered at Luna Export Abattoir, Ethiopia. By considering age, origin and species as a risk factors major abnormalities encountered were identified and considered accordingly. A simple random sampling was used where 384 each sheep and goats were sampled with a total of 768 animals and postmortem examinations was applied on liver. Out of 768 sheep and goats slaughtered 67.7% of liver revealed total condemnation. The major cause of these liver condemnations are due to *Cysticercus tenuicullosis* (11.5%), Calcification (20.31%), Cloudiness (20.57%), Cirrhosis (5.08%), Hepatitis (5.9%), Fatty degeneration (2.99%), *Steilesia hepatica* (3.65%), Adhesion (7.42%), and Hydatidosis (0.13%). Except in *C. tenuicollis*, calcification and cloudiness (p<0.05) which has a significance difference were observed between sheep and goats, insignificance difference (p>0.05) were recorded between sheep and goats in other lesions. Concerning the origin of the animal significance difference (p<0.05) in cloudy lesion were observed on sheep originated from Somali, GammuGoffa and Awash but insignificant difference observed in another lesion. Similarly, significance difference were observed in *C tenuicollis*, Calcification, and fatty degeneration (p<0.05), among goats originated from Borena, Afar and Wollo and insignificance difference was observed in other lesions. Regarding age and species in other lesions different rates of prevalence were recorded in the current study. Moreover, from total condemnation rate of liver, economic loss of 335,000.00 USD per annum was estimated. Due to such small ruminant health problems and these pathological lesions results in significance economic loss in small ruminants, continuous surveillance and strategically prevention and control of these abnormalities shall be implemented in these animals.

Keywords: Liver; Condemnation; International market; Economic; Abattoir; Small ruminant

Introduction

The total number of Sheep and goats in Ethiopia is estimated to be nearly 48 million. Sheep and goats are widely adapted to different climates and are found in all production systems [1], They generate cash income from export of meat, edible organs, skins and live animals. There is also a high domestic meat demand from these animals, particularly during religious festivals [2], Hence, an increase in small ruminant's production could contribute to the attainment of food self-sufficiency in the country, particularly in response to the protein requirement for the growing human population as well as to enhance the export earnings [3].

Even though this sub-sector contributes much to the national economy, its development is hampered by various constraints. These include endemic animal diseases, poor nutrition, poor husbandry, poor infrastructure and shortage of trained labor and lack of government policies [4], Each year a significant loss result from, death of animals, inferior weight gain, condemnation of edible organs and carcass at slaughter. This production loss to the livestock industry is, estimated at more than 900 million USD annually [5].

The 2009/10 annual report of the veterinary services [6], indicated that out of 1,261,886 animals slaughtered at all export abattoirs during the year 2009/10; 379,517 liver, 336,536 lungs; 13,722 kidneys; and 5,809 heart were condemned. The organs which were found affected with disease and abnormalities were mostly liver and lung and they accounted for 49.1% and 43.5% respectively of the total rejections [6].

In view of this proper evaluation of economic loss due to major causes of liver condemnation in sheep and goats at abattoir surveillance is needed which of great relevance.

Therefore, the objective of this study was-

• To determine the major causes of liver condemnation in small ruminants slaughtered at Luna Export Abattoir.

• To estimate the magnitude of direct Economic loss incurred due to condemned liver.

Materials and Methods

Study area

The study was conducted from December 2014 to April 2015 in the private owned Luna export abattoir, Modjo town, central Ethiopia. It has a latitude and longitude of 8°N 39°E with an elevation between 1788

*Corresponding author: Elias Gezahegn, Bale Zone Pastoral Area Development Office, Ethiopia, E-mail: eluccaa@gmail.com

and 1825 m. a. s. l. [7], The Luna export slaughter house was established in 2003 and located in Modjo town with 50,000 square meters of area. This is one of the abattoirs which export meat to Saudi Arabia, Turkey, Egypt and United Arab Emirates

Study populations

Study populations are apparently healthy of sheep and goats, slaughtered at Luna Export Abattoir, Modjo town. The origins of slaughtered animals are from different areas of the country such as, Borena, Afar, Somali, Wollo, Eastern Hararghe and the Southern part of the country. The study conducted in the Luna Export abattoir indicates that most of the animals are comes from pastoral and semi-pastoral areas, which are preferred breeds.

Study design and sampling method

The cross-sectional abattoir survey was conducted on slaughtered sheep and goats to determine the major causes of liver condemnation. A simple random sampling method is employed and the study animals were randomly selected and recorded tagged and followed up throughout the whole slaughtering process. The required sample size of the study for both species of animals was determined by the formula given in [8], 50% expected prevalence with 95% of Confidence interval and at 5% desired precision.

Thrus field formula = $n = \dfrac{1.96^2 \left(P_{exp} \left(1 - P_{exp} \right) \right)}{d^2}$

Where n=Required sample size

Pexp=Expected prevalence

d²=Desired absolute precision

Hence, the required sample sizes for each species were = 384 and 768 samples were used for both species.

Abattoir survey

Postmortem inspection: Post-mortem examination involved visual inspection, palpation and making systemic incision of liver to look for the presences of cysts, adult parasites, and other abnormalities. Pathological lesions were differentiated and judged based on FAO guidelines on meat inspection for developing countries [9].

Economic loss assessment: The direct Economic losses incurred due to liver condemnation were, estimated by using the formula indicated below [10].

EL=[S_{SR} X OC_{Li} X R_{Li}]

Where **EL**=Estimated annual economic loss due to liver Condemnation.

S_{SR}=Annual shoats slaughter rate of the abattoir

OC_{Li}=Average cost of liver /cost of rejected liver

R_{Li}=Rejection rate of liver.

So, to calculate the above formula the following data is considered.

• The annual slaughter rate of the abattoir

• The average retail market of the liver.

• The rejection rate of the liver will be required.

Data management and analysis: Data generated from postmortem inspection was recorded in the Microsoft Excel 2007 program. Descriptive statistics was used to determine the variation between condemnation rates of the liver in relation to, the origin of the animal and age groups were evaluated by person's chi-square (X^2) and percentage. The significance among and/or between rejection rates of specific organs in age groups, origins and species of animals were evaluated using p-value where it is significance if ($p \geq 0.05$).

Results

Postmortem examination

As shown in Tables 1 and 2, from all examined animals, the major causes for liver condemnations are cloudiness (20.57%), calcification, (20.31%), *C. tenuicollis*, (11.46%) and adhesion (7.42%) are the major causes for rejection of the liver from international market and also miscellaneous factors are a principal causes for liver condemnations. Generally, these causes of the liver found to be high in goats than in sheep with a high significance ($p \geq 0.05$) in first three abnormalities.

Among the origin of animals, although insignificance difference was observed in all abnormalities but cloudiness has a significance (p<0.05) in sheep, and *C. tenuicollis*, calcification and fatty degeneration has (p<0.05) in goats (Table 3).

With regard to age group except cirrhosis in sheep P-value (p<0.05), and *C. tenuicollis*, and miscellaneous abnormalities in goat P-value (p<0.05), but all other liver abnormalities observed in current study shows insignificance difference between considered age groups (Table 4).

Economic loss assessment

The annual direct economic loss incurred due to condemned liver as a result of pathological, parasitological and other abnormalities at abattoir were estimated from international market of the abattoir estimated to be 3,685,000 ETB (Ethiopian Birr) or 184,250 USD (United States Dollar) in present study. The cost analysis guidance was as shown in Table 5 below. The liver of sheep and goats are similar and weighs 500-700 gram [11].

Discussion

In this study from 768 samples taken from both sheep and goats 520(67.7%) samples were found positive for one or more lesion

Origin	Number of animals examined				
	Sheep	No	Goat	No
	Somali	218	Borena	202
	GamuGofa	87	Afar	164
	Awash	79	Wollo	18
Total		384	Total	384
Age	Young	101	Young	214
	Adult	283	Adult	170
Total		384	Total	384

Table 1: Random sample distributions in relative to Species, origin and age.

which is 245(31.9%) and 275(35.8%) positive samples from sheep and goats respectively rejected. Major causes of liver condemnations from international market were found to be Cloudiness (20.57%), Calcification (14.58%), *C. tenuicollis* (16.67%), Adhesion (7.42%), Cirrhosis (5.47%) and Hepatitis (5.99%) found to be the major causes of liver condemnations in the abattoir. From both species of animals goats were mostly affected and responsible for high rejection rate of the liver, which has a statistical significance value (p<0.005). This is due to the feeding habit of the animals in which sheep are grazers, whereas goats feed substantial amount of browse and mostly exposed to toxic plants especially of from low land areas, which resists the dry periods [12], results damage to the liver.

From the sheep samples, drawn from different origins cloudiness is more in sheep brought from Somali origin, and has a significance value (P<0.05). It is probably due to the fact that vegetative coverage of the arid and semi arid weather conditions, plants that are found there can resist drought and are mostly toxic plants and ingestion of these

plant leaves resulting cloudy degeneration of the liver, responsible for rejection because of aesthetic value and hazard to public Gracey et al. [13], suggests the same reason.

In this study, hydatidosis has low prevalence only (0.26%) and (0.00%) in sheep and goats respectively as the same as Getachew and Mesfin and Mekonnen [14], also reported that 0% of hydatidosis of goats in Hawassa and Luna export abattoir respectively. This is probably due to that low population of dogs, which is the definitive host in the pastoral and semi-pastoral areas, which decrease the contact between dogs with sheep and goats. On the other hand, the difference between the prevalence of sheep (1) and goat (0) hydatidosis is due to feeding habit of goats that are mostly browsers Kusiluka and Kambarage, Abdella [15], reported that from 1476 samples of sheep and goats from three abattoirs (Hashim, Elfora and Luna) reported that all recovered cysts except three (2 sheep and 1 goat located in the liver) were located in lungs in both sheep and goats. In addition, [16], reported that hydatid cysts were more frequently observed in the lungs than livers of small ruminants.

Major Causes	Out of 768 Total Prevalence No. (%)	Species Prevalence			
		Sheep (384) No. (%)	Goat (384) No. (%)	x^2	P-value
C. tenuicollis	88(11.46)	24(6.25)	64(16.67)	20.5348	0.000
Calcification	156(20.31)	100(26.04)	56(14.58)	15.5737	0.000
Cloudiness	158(20.57)	67(17.45)	91(23.70)	4.5898	0.032
Cirrhosis	39(5.08)	18(4.69)	21(5.47)	0.2431	0.622
Hepatitis	45(5.86)	22(5.73)	23(5.99)	0.0236	0.878
Fatty. Degeneration	23(2.99)	9(2.34)	14(3.65)	1.1205	0.290
S. hepatica	28(3.65)	11(2.86)	17(4.43)	1.3344	0.248
Adhesion	57(7.42)	24(6.25)	33(8.59)	1.5350	0.215
Hydatid cyst	1(0.13)	1(0.26)	0(0.00)	1.0013	0.317
Others	35(4.56)	13(3.39)	22(5.73)	2.4248	0.119
Total	630(82.03)	289(75.26)	341(88.8)		

Table 2: Distributions of major causes of liver condemnations in small ruminants.

Species	No. examined	Origin	*C. tenuicollis*(%)	Calcification n(%)	Cloudiness n(%)	Cirrhosis n(%)	Hepatitisn(%)	Fatty Degenerationn(%)	*S. hepatica* n(%)	Hydatid Cyst n(%)	Adhesion n(%)	Simultaneous causes n(%)
Sheep	210	Somali	15(6.88)	63(28.90)	37(16.9)	11(5.05)	12(5.50)	8(3.67)	3(1.38)	1(0.46)	16(7.34)	3(1.38)
	89	GG	5(5.75)	20(22.9)	7(8.05)	3(3.45)	6(6.90)	4(4.60)	2(2.30)	0(0.00)	8(9.20)	5(5.75)
	79	Awash	4(5.06)	17(21.52)	23(29.11)	4(5.06)	4(5.06)	2(2.53)	6(7.59)	0(0.00)	0(0.00)	5(6.33)
Total	384		24(6.25)	100(26.04)	67(17.45)	18(4.69)	22(5.73)	14(3.65)	11(2.86)	1(0.26)	24(6.25)	13(3.39)
		x^2	0.37	2.18	12.83	0.39	0.30	0.50	8.19	0.7635	6.99	6.27
		P-value	0.83	0.34	0.002	0.82	0.86	0.78	0.017	0.683	0.030	0.044
Goat	202	Borena	24(11.88)	16(7.92)	46(22.77)	11(5.45)	10(4.95)	3(1.49)	12(5.94)	0(0.00)	12(5.94)	11(5.45)
	264	Afar	35(21.34)	29(17.68)	40(24.39)	8(4.88)	11(6.71)	4(2.44)	4(2.44)	0(0.00)	18(10.9)	9(5.49)
	18	Wollo	5(27.78)	11(61.11)	5(27.78)	2(11.11)	2(11.11)	2(11.11)	2(11.11)	0(0.00)	3(16.67)	2(11.11)
Total	384		64(30.5)	56(28.90)	91(24.98)	21(7.15)	23(5.01)	9(5.01)	18(6.5)	0(0.00)	33(11.2)	22(7.35)
		x^2	7.5112	39.7445	0.3049	1.2194	1.3759	6.7022	5.6101	-	4.4880	1.0131
		P-value	0.023	0.000	0.85	0.544	0.503	0.035	0.061	-	0.106	0.603

Table 3: Summary of the rejection rate of liver condemnations based on Origin of the sheep and goats.

Species	No. examined	Age	C. tenuicoillisn(%)	Calcification n(%)	Cloudiness n(%)	Cirrhosis n(%)	Hepatitis n(%)	Fatty Degeneration n(%)	S. hepatica n(%)	Adhesion n(%)	Hydatid cyst n(%)	Simultaneous causesn(%)
Sheep	101	Young	6(5.94)	25(24.7)	24(23.7)	10(9.90)	7(6.9)	2(1.98)	5(4.95)	6(5.94)	0(0.00)	6(5.94)
	283	Adult	18(6.36)	75(26.5)	43(15.1)	8(2.83)	15(5.3)	12(4.24)	6(2.12)	18(6.36)	1(0.35)	7(2.47)
Total	384		24(6.25)	100(26.0)	67(17.4)	18(4.69)	22(5.7)	14(3.65)	11(2.86)	24(6.25)	1(0.26)	13(3.3)
		X²	0.0224	0.1183	3.7937	8.3374	0.3663	1.0823	2.1430	0.3578	0.0224	2.7356
		P-value	0.881	0.731	0.051	0.004	0.545	0.298	0.143	0.550	0.881	0.098
Goat	214	Young	25(11.6)	28(13.0)	54(25.2)	9(4.21)	16(7.4)	3(1.40)	8(3.74)	16(7.48)	0(0.00)	7(3.27)
	170	Adult	39(22.9)	28(16.4)	37(21.7)	12(7.06)	7(4.1)	6(3.53)	9(5.29)	17(10.00)	0(0.00)	15(8.8)
Total	384		64(16.6)	56(14.5)	91(23.70)	21(5.47)	23(5.9)	9(2.34)	17(4.43)	33(8.59)	0(0.00)	22(5.7)
		X²	8.6469	0.8722	0.6305	1.4919	1.8983	1.8736	0.5420	0.7679	-	5.4080
		P-value	0.003	0.350	0.427	0.222	0.168	0.171	0.462	0.381	-	0.020

Table 4: Summary of rejection rate of liver condemnations in Sheep and Goats based on age.

Species	Annual slaughtering rate of shoats	Frequency of Positives No (%)	Rejection rate (%)	Average cost of liver from market
Sheep		245	63.8	
Goats	250,000	275	71.6	2 USD/Kg
Total		520	67.7	

Table 5: Liver rejection rate in small ruminant and related economic loss.

Though *C. tenuicollis* and *S. hepatica* do not have public health importance, they considered as an important cause of economic loss in the meat industry since liver harboring them, are rejected for aesthetic reasons. Similarly, Jibat [17-20], reported that out of 2688 animals examined one-tenth of the total condemned livers were due to mechanical damage that was caused by faulty practices during evisceration. However, in this study liver condemnations due to mechanical damage are low in Luna Export Abattoir, which is due to experienced personnel and good slaughtering operations.

Losses from liver condemnation were assumed to occur since hepatic pathology is associated to infection that might have public health and aesthetic value [16]. The current study disclosed that from 768 samples taken from both sheep's and goats 520 liver samples of sheep and goats liver rejected from international market, with an estimated annual economic loss of 3,685,000.00 ETB or 335,000.00 USD per annum.

Conclusion and Recommendations

Several diseases are the major concern to small ruminant farming as it causes extensive financial waste because of direct and indirect economic losses. In general pathological conditions and parasitic diseases were the major causes of financial loss through liver condemnations at Luna Export Abattoir, which may also reflect the same scenario in other slaughter houses in Ethiopia. To mitigate the economic and public health impacts of diseases of small ruminants, proper disposal of offal, prohibition of backyard slaughter of small ruminants, construction of slaughterhouses, better disease control strategies, enhancing animal welfare, adequate training of abattoir personnel on the slaughtering operation and regular deworming of dogs are recommended. Furthermore, Small ruminants ranching at pastoral areas where the shoat population is vast should be put into practice for the purpose of export market and the total (true) economic impact of the diseases of small ruminants at depth should be investigated. Since most cases of liver condemnation was found to be Cloudiness and Calcification caused by ingestion of toxic plants which are found in arid and semi arid areas further investigation is required to isolate them for many purposes. From public health and live stock disease control point of view, abattoir surveillance of these abnormalities were found to be important to take control measures.

Acknowledgements

The authors would like to thank the Luna Export abattoir for their unreserved cooperation and facilities that they provided for this study.

Conflict of Interest

The authors declare that they have no conflict of interest.

References

1. Adane H, Girma A (2008) Economic significance of Sheep and Goats. Sheep and Goats Production Handbook for Ethiopia. Alemu Y, Merkel RC (eds.), Ethiopia Sheep and Goat Productivity Improvement Program, pp: 2-3.

2. FAO (2010) Food and Agricultural Organization of the United Nation statistical year book.

3. Teferi M (2000) An epidemiological study on given pasteurellosis in Arsi, south east Ethiopia.

4. Jobre Y, Lobago F, Tiruneh R, Abebe G, Dorchies PH (1996) Hydatidosis in three selected regions in Ethiopia. An assessment trial on its prevalence on economic and public health importance. Rev Med Vet. pp: 797-804.

5. MOA (2009/10) Ministry of Agriculture: Animal and Plant Health Regulatory Directorate, Ethiopia. Animal Health Year Book, Inspection and Quarantine Services. p: 28.

6. EMPDA (1984) Educational Material and Distribution Agency. Atlas for secondary High school of Ethiopia. Kindergarten and Formula Curriculum division. Social Science Panel. Ministry of Education, Macmillan Publisher.

7. Thrusfield M (2005) Surveys. In: veterinary epidemiology, 3rd edn. Blackwell Science Ltd, London, pp: 228-246.

8. AO (1994) Manual on Meat Inspection for Developing Countries. Food and Agriculture Organization (FAO), Rome, Italy.

9. Ogurinade A, Ogurinade BI (1980) Economic importance of Fasciolosis in Nigeria. Trop Anim Health Prod. pp: 155-159.

10. Wilson WG (2005) Wilson's Practical Meat Inspection. 7th edn, Revised from the original text Practical Meat Inspection by Andrew Wilson. Blackwell Publishing, p: 52.

11. Zewde S, Lidetu D (2006) Sheep and Goat Flock Health.A Hand Book of Sheep and Goats Productivity Improvement Program (ESGIP). p: 213.

12. Gracey JF, Collins OS, Huey RJ (1999) Meat Hygiene. 10th edn. London. Bailliere Tindall, pp: 223-260.

13. Mesfin G, Mekonnen A (2014) Causes of Liver and Lung Condemnation among Apparently Healthy Slaughtered Sheep and Goats at Luna Abattoir, Modjo, Ethiopia. Middle-East J Scient Res 21: 2346-2351.

14. Kusiluka L, Kambarage D (1996) A hand book of Diseases of small ruminants in Sub-saharan Africa. Diseases caused by Helminthes. Overseas Development administration. Animal Health Program, pp: 8-9.

15. Budke CM, Deplazes P, Torgerson PR (2006) Global Socio Economic impact of cystic echinocccosis. Emerg Infec Dis. 12: 296-302.

16. Jibat TB (2006) Causes of organ and carcass condemnation in small ruminants slaughtered at HELMEX Abattoir, Debrezeit. Faculty of Veterinary Medicine, Addis Ababa University, DVM Thesis, pp: 1-2.

17. ILCA (1993) International livestock center for Africa. A Hand book of African livestock statistics. Addis Ababa, Ethiopia.

18. LMA (2001) Livestock Marketing in Ethiopia: A review of structure, performance and development initiatives. Socio-economics and Policy Research Working, p: 52.

19. Radostits OM, Blood DC, Gay CC, Hinchllif FW (2007) Disease of the liver and pancreas: Veterinary Medicine. 9 edn. ELBS, Baiviere Tindall, London, UK, pp: 313-332.

20. Debrezeit, Addis Ababa University, DVM Thesis, p: 32.

42

Major Cause of Organ and Carcass Condemnation in Apparently Healthy Small Ruminant Slaughtered at Addis Ababa Abattoir Enterprise, Ethiopia

Dinku Assefa[1], Elias Gezaheng[2], Birhanu Abera[3]*, Eyob Eticha[3], Diriba Lemma[3] and Tekle Hailemariam[4]

[1]*Yem Special District Livestock and Fishery Resource Office, SNNPRS, Ethiopia*

[2]*Bale Zone Pastoral Area Development Office, Bale Robe, Ethiopia*

[3]*Asella Regional Veterinary Laboratory, Asella, Ethiopia*

[4]*Kembata Tembaro District Livestock and Fishery Resource Office, SNNPRS, Ethiopia*

Abstract

Study was conducted from November 2008 to March 2009 to determine the major causes of organ and carcass condemnation and associated annual magnitude of financial loss at Addis Ababa abattoir enterprise. Out of 1052 examined sheep and goats 459 (43.6%) livers, 307 (29.18%) lungs, 130 (12.36%) Hearts, 108 (20.27%) kidney and 28 (2.66%) carcass were condemned. The major causes of condemnation were parasite 52.24%, cirrhosis (11.2%), hepatitis (9.2%) and mechanical damage (8.12%) for liver; pneumonia (32.2%), emphysema (19.5%) and hydatidosis (15.9%) for lung; pericarditis (43.07%), calcification (17.7), Abscess (5.4%), *Cysticercus ovis* (8.4%) and other (25.4%) for heart; nephritis (30.5%) for kidneys, abscess (50%), bruising (29%) and other causes for carcasses. Rate of condemnation due to hydatidosis was higher in the lungs (4.3% in sheep and 5.0% in goats) than in the liver (3.3% in sheep and 3.4% in goats) significant higher rate of liver, lung, heart, kidney and carcass condemnation were not observed between age groups (p>0.05), but significantly higher rate of organ and carcass condemnation were observed with in sex group of sheep (P<0.05). However significant difference in the rate of organ and carcasses condemned were not observed by species of the animals (p>0.05). Total annual loss due to organ and carcass condemnation was estimated one million Ethiopian Birr (90909.09 USD). Result of the present work warrant immediate need for the prevention of causes of organ and carcass condemnation and pathological abnormalities through development of and animal health delivery, enforcement of slaughter policy, education of sheep and goat traders, and training of slaughter house personnel on standard slaughter operations.

Keywords: Abattoir; Addis Ababa; Carcass; Condemnation; Financial loss; Goats; Organ; Sheep

Introduction

Ethiopia, with over 42 million head, has the third largest number of sheep and goat among African nations and rank eighth in the world [1]. Small ruminant (sheep and goats) are among economically important livestock in Ethiopia. There are about 25.5 million sheep and 22.78 million goats [2]. They contribute a quarter of domestic meat consumption, about half of the domestic wool requirements about 40% of fresh skin and 92% of the value of semi-processed skin and hide export trade it is estimated that 1,078.000 sheep and 1.128.000 goats are used in Ethiopia for domestic consumption annually.

Many important livestock diseases that inflict major socio - economic losses in Ethiopia occur every year. Annual disease losses amount to 8-10%, 14-16% and 11-13% of cattle, sheep and goats populations respectively. It is estimated that some 700 Million Birr (1 US$=9.2) is lost annually due to helminthes (internal parasite) infestation of domestic animals. Besides affecting the quantity and quality of livestock products, the prevalence of infectious and economically important animal disease in Ethiopia excludes the country from profitable international markets; there by greatly reducing the country's foreign exchange earnings poor husbandry practice and inadequate veterinary services are of the major factors favoring the expansion of livestock diseases [1].

However, each year a significant loss result from death of animals, inferior weight gain, condemnation of edible organs and carcass at slaughter house. This production loss to the livestock industry is estimated at more than 900 million USD annually [3]. A recent study conducted at HELMEX abattoir, Debre Zeit, Ethiopia indicate the annual direct financial loss form international and domestic markets

due to organ and carcass condemnations from different pathological lesions was estimated at 2.7 million Ethiopian Birr (312,655 USD) annually. This total loss could be partitioned in to the loss incurred due to disease which amounted to 187,868.6 USD and the rest, 124,686.4 USD, was due to human factors either as a result of mishandling of animals during transport to the slaughter house or due to faulty slaughter operations in the abattoir [4].

As the meat are the main sources of protein to human being, it should be clean and free from diseases of particular importance to the public such as tuberculosis and cysticercosis. Meat is also condemned at slaughter house to break the chain of some zoonoses which are not transmitted to man directly via meat like hydatidosis and other important diseases of animals such as fasciolosis [5,6].

Yet meat is also condemned from human consumption because of aesthetic values caused by diseases and mechanical damage during slaughtering operation procedures [7]. A report of the prevalence of

***Corresponding author:** Birhanu Abera, Asella Regional Veterinary Laboratory, Asella, Ethiopia, E-mail: birhanuabera27@yahoo.com

Echinococcus granulosis (adult stage of the hydatid cyst) in dogs indicated 25.45% [8]. The presence of hydatidasis was also reported in man in the south–west Ethiopia. Hydatidosis is maintained as a major zoonotic disease in the country because small ruminants are mainly slaughtered at the backyard for home consumption without any veterinary inspection, the absence of rigorous and enforced meat inspection legislation and long standing habit of feeding offal to dogs. The presence of large number of stray dogs throughout the country exacerbates the problem. However, there is no information describing the causes and associated magnitude of organs and carcass condemnation in slaughtered sheep and goat at Addis Ababa Abattoir Enterprise. Determination of the causes and magnitude of organ and carcass condemnation in these animals using abattoir surveillance by considering associated risk factors for evaluation of associated economic loss are needed where economic realities often determine the type and scope of preventive measures to be used. Therefore the objectives of this study were; to determine the major causes of organ and carcass condemnation in apparently healthy sheep and goat slaughtered and to estimate the associated magnitude of economic loss at Addis Ababa Abattoir enterprise.

Materials and Methods

Study area

The study was conducted at Addis Ababa Abattoir Enterprise, Ethiopia, from December 2008 to April 2009. Where cattle, small ruminant and swine are slaughtered. The average annual slaughtered animals where 36,000 sheep and 18,000 goat according to animal report of the abattoir of LMA, 2009 [9]. The obtained beef, mutton, lamb, goat meat and edible organs like liver, lung, heart and kidney, was distributed to the customers. Addis Ababa is the capital city and administrative center for the Federal Democratic Republic of Ethiopia. Geographically, the area is located with in an altitude of about 2,400 m above sea level and receives a mean annual rainfall of season 18000 mm in bimodal with average minimum and maximum temperatures are 10.7°C and 25.6°C respectively [10].

Study animals

A total of 1052 animals comprising (600 sheep and 452 goats) where randomly selected and identified by species, age, and sex during ante mortem inspection. The animals were originating from different areas of the country (Arsi, Bale, Afar, Shoa, Ogaden, Wollo, Omo, Jimma, and Borena) representing different agro ecological zones (highland, semi arid and arid). It was impossible to track back the origin of each animal as they were being mixed before they arrive at the abattoirs. Animals were transported to the abattoir using vehicles and on foot. Age grouping in to young for goats less than 1 year and sheep less than 1.25 years while adult for goat more that 1 year and sheep more than 1.25 years [11]. Random sample size distributions were as shown in Table 1 below.

Abattoir survey

Detailed meat inspection procedure were applied and examination

Species	Sex				Total (%)
	Male		Female		
	Young (%)	Adult (%)	Young (%)	Adult (%)	
Sheep	159 (38.4)	255 (61.6)	34 (18.3)	152 (81.7)	600 (100)
Goats	111 (29.5)	265 (70.5)	17 (22.4)	59 (77.6)	452 (100)
Total	270 (25.6)	520 (49.4)	51 (4.9)	211(19.6)	1052 (100)

Table 1: Number of animals examined.

were done after evisceration, the liver, lung, heart, kidney and carcass were thoroughly examined by visual inspection, palpation and systematic incisions for the presence of gross pathological lesions and parasite were differentiated and judged based on guidelines on meat inspection for developing countries [7].

Study design

Cross sectional study by abattoir survey were conducted for the determination of major causes of organ and carcass condemnation in apparently healthy sheep and goat slaughtered at Addis Ababa Abattoir Enterprises by post mortem examination.

Data management and statistical analysis

Data collected during study period were entered in to Excel spreadsheet (Microsoft Excel 2007). Descriptive statistics were used to determine major cause of organ and carcass condemnation rate by using percentage. Association of the risk factors were calculated with consideration of age, sex, species and abnormalities were evaluated by person's chi-square (x^2) and differences were regarded statistically significant if P-values were less than 0.05.

Assessment of economical losses

To evaluate the economic losses, only the direct monetary losses due to rejection of liver, lung, heart, kidney and carcass were considered. The analysis was based on annual slaughter capacity of the abattoir considering market demand, average market price on domestic markets, and rejection rates of specific organs and carcasses. The annual slaughter rates were estimated from retrospective slaughter data recorded in the past three years. Financial losses were then computed mathematically by adapting the formula of Ogunrinade 1980 for liver [12].

EL srx * coy * Roz

Where

EL - Estimated annual economic loss due to organs and carcass condemnation from domestic market.

Srx - Annual sheep /goat slaughter rates of the abattoir.

Coy - Average cost of each sheep/goat liver /lung/Heart/Kidney/carcass.

Roz - Condemnation rates of sheep /goat liver /bung/Kidney/Heart/ carcass.

Results

Post mortem examination

Out of 1052 small ruminant examined during the study period, 459 (43.6%), 307 (29.18%), 130(12.36%), 108 (10.27%) and 28 (2.66%) of all liver, lungs, hearts, kidney and carcasses, respectively, were condemned, respectively from gross abnormalities as unfit for human consumption (Table 2). The most frequently condemned organ was liver followed by the lungs. Significant difference in the rate of organs and carcasses condemned were not observed by species of animals and pathological abnormalities (P>0.05).

Percentage of condemnations of Liver (43.2%), Lung (27.83%), Heart (11.67%), Kidney (12.33%) and Carcass (2.5%) in sheep like wise (44.25%) (30.1%) (13.27%) (17.5%) and (2.88%) were condemned in respective organ and carcass of goats. Regarding age insignificance was observed (Table 2) between both sexes in both study species (P>0.05).

Risk factors		Number of Examined	Liver (%)	Lung (%)	Heart (%)	Kidney (%)	Carcass (%)
Sheep	Male Female	414 186	167(40.34) 92(49.46)	103(24.88) 64(34.41)	42(10.14) 28(15.05)	44(10.63) 30(16.13)	- -
	X^2			4.3551	5.8022	3.009	3.5920	6.0488
	P-value			0.037	0.016	0.083	0.058	0.014
	Young Adult	193 407	2.1509 0.142	2.2654 0.132	0.9166 0.338	1.0219 0.312	2.5009 0.114
	X^2			2.1509	2.2654	0.9166	1.0219	2.5009
	P-value			0.142	0.132	0.338	0.312	0.114
Total		600	259(43.17)	167(27.8)	70(11.67)	74(12.3)	15(2.5)
Goat	Male Female	376 76	156(41.49) 37(48.68)	113(03.05) 27(35.53)	48(12.77) 12(15.79)	25(6.65) 9(11.84)	12(3.19) 1(1.32)
	X^2			1.3376	0.8858	0.5020	2.4510	0.7963
	P-value			0.247	0.347	0.479	0.117	0.372
	Young	129	63(49.2)	37(28.9)	12(9.4)	11(8.6)	2(1.56)
	Adult	323	137(42.3)	103(31.8)	48(14.8)	23(7.1)	11(3.4)
	X^2			3.1022	0.3569	2.3584	0.2948	1.1031
	P-value			0.078	0.550	0.125	0.587	0.294
Total		452	200(44.25)	140(30.1)	60(13.3)	34(17.5)	13(3.0)
Overall		1052	459(43.63)	307(29.2)	130(12.4)	108(10.3)	28(2.66)

Table 2: Total condemnations of organ and carcass Rate (%).

The frequency of liver condemnation was statistically significant difference was not observed in sheep (259/600, 43.17) and goats (193/452,42.70) (p>0.05), but frequency of kidney condemnation, statically significant difference was not observed in condemnation of rates of lung, heath, kidney and carcass between the two species of animals (p>0.05). In sheep, significantly higher (p<0.05) rate of condemnation of liver, lung and carcasses were observed in the female than male, but there was significant difference were observed in sex of goats (p.0.05). No age difference was observed in the organs and carcass condemnation rates in sheep and goat (P>0.05) (Table 3).

In sheep age difference was observed in liver cirrhosis (0.00% in young and 8.84 in the adult) (p=0.000), Stilesia *hepatica* (6.74% in young and 3.19% in the adult) (p=0.47) and mechanical damage (4.15% in young and 1.47% in the adult) (p=0.043). In goat there was no statistically significant age difference between young and adult age categories (Table 3) concerning the cause of liver condemnation, except mechanical damage caused significant loss of liver in young (13.28%) than in adult (1.55%) p=0.000).

Pneumonia was the major causes of lung rejection with a rate of 32.14% (99/308) followed by emphysema (19.48%, 60/308) (Table 4). There was no statistically significant difference between sheep (117/600, 29.5%) and goats (131/452, 28.98%) (p>0.05); however, statistically significant difference was observed (p<0.05) between the young and adult age groups of both species in the frequency of lung condemnation from any causes, except statistically high significant difference observed in adult sheep in case of emphysema (7.86%) than in goat 95.57%) (p=0.012).

Significant difference between the sex groups in sheep and goats, with relation to specific causes was not observed (p>0.05), except calcification causes significant lung condemnation in Male sheep (3.62%) than in female sheep (1.6%) (P=0.007 (Table 4); Frequency and percentage of organ and carcass condemnation by sex (0.5%). Rate of condemnations due to hydatidosis was higher in the lung (4.33% in

sheep and 5.09% in goats) than in the liver (3% in sheep and 3.54% in goats) (Table 4).

Out of a total of 130 hearts condemned, pericarditis contributed 43.08% (56/130) followed by other unidentified causes (24.62%) calcification (17.6%), *Cysticercus ovis* (8.4%) and abscess (5.38%) (Table 5). No statistically significant difference was observed between the two species (p.0.05) in heart condemnation rate. In both species no statistically significant difference within age and sex categories regarding the causes of heart condemnation rare (Table 5).

Renal problems were observed in 108 pairs (10.27%) of the total kidneys examined (Table 6). Nephritis accounting for 30.56% (33/108) was the major pathological lesion. There was no statistically significant difference between the age, groups and sex groups (p>0.05) However nephritis caused higher rate of kidney condemnation in female goats (5.34%) than in male sheep (2.41%) (p=0.018).

The major pathological conditions for carcass rejection from human consumption were Abscess accounting for 50% (24/28), bruising 28.57% (8/28) and poor body condition (21.43% 6/28) (Table 6) and other causes.

Fasciolosis caused statistically higher liver condemnations (Table 7) in sheep (11.67%) than in goats (7.3%) (P=0.018), hepatitis was found to be a major cause of liver condemnation in goats (5.31%) than in sheep (2.83%) (p=0.017), Mechanical damage has caused statistically higher rate of liver condemnation in goat (4.87%) than in sheep (2.33%) (p=0.025). In sheep, there was no statistically significant difference between male and female sex categories except for *Fasciola* species where it was significantly higher in the female sheep (15.59%) than in the males (9.90%) (p=0.045). In goat, there was no statistically significant difference between male and female categories regarding the cause of liver condemnation.

Assessment of direct economic loss

The annual direct financial loss from domestic markets due to

Abnormality	Frequency and percentage of condemnation (%)									
	Sheep (n=600)					Goat (n=452)				
	Young (n=193)	Adult (n=407)	Totat	X^2	p-value	Young n (129)	Adult n (323)	Total n (452)	X^2	p-value
Fasciola	18(9.3)	52(12.7)	70(11.7)	1.5120	0.219	7(5.4)	26(8.03	33(7.3)	0.9373	0.333
Cirrhosis	0(0.0)	36(8.8)	36(6.0)	18.161	0.00	2(1.5)	11(3.4)	13(2.9)	1.1358	0.287
Hepatitis	7(3.6)	10(2.4)	17(2.8)	0.6509	0.420	7(5.4)	17(5.3)	24(5.3)	0.0049	0.944
Stilesia hepatica	13(6.7)	13(3.2)	26(4.3)	3.9612	.047	6(4.6)	12(3.7)	18(4)	0.2112	0.646
Cysticercus tenicollis	10(5.2)	15(3.7)	25(4.2)	1.6829	0.431	5(3.9)	19(5.9)	24(5.3)	0.7381	0.390
Calcification	1(0.52)	17(4.2)	18(3.0)	9.4133	0.052	2(1.5)	13(4.0)	15(3.3)	1.0436	0.903
Mechanical damage	8(4.2)	6(1.5)	14	4.0981	0.043	17(13.2)	5(1.55)	22(4.9)	26.929	0.000
Hydatid cyst	4(2.1)	16(3.03)	20(3.4)	1.4112	0.703	4(3.1)	12(3.7)	16(3.5)	1.4742	0.831
Abscess	1(0.5)	11(2.7)	12(2.0)	9.0083	0.109	4(3.0)	11(3.4)	15(3.3)	2.8925	0.576
Other	6(3.0)	8(1.9)	14(2.3)			4(3.1)	6(1.8)	10(2.2)		

Table 3: Cause of Liver condemnation by age.

Abnormality	Frequency and percentage of condemnation (%)									
	Sheep(n=600)					Goat(n=452)				
	Male% (n=414)	Female%(n=186)	Total% (n=600)	X^2	p-value	Male%(n=376)	Female% (n=76)	Total% (n=452)	X^2	p-value
Pneumonia	37(8.8)	21(11.3)	58(9.7)	0.8138	0.367	36(9.6)	5(6.6)	41(9.1)	0.6878	0.407
Emphysema	22(5.3)	15(8.1)	37(6.2)	1.6780	0.195	16(4.3)	7(9.2)	23(5.1)	3.2142	0.073
Hydatid cyst	14(3.4)	12(6.45)	26(4.3)	3.7714	0.287	19(5.05)	4(5.3)	23(5.1)	1.4742	0.831
Abscess	3(0.7)	2(1.1)	5(0.83)	12.2601	0.031	3(0.8)	1(1.3)	4(0.9)	2.8925	0.576
Calcification	15(3.6)	3(1.6)	18(3.0)	14.2503	0.007	16(4.3)	3(3.95)	19(4.2)	1.0436	0.903
Other	13(3.14)	20(10.75)	33(5.5)			14(3.7)	7(5.2)	21(4.6)		
Overall	104(25.12)	73(39.24)	177(29.5)			104(27.65)	27(53.52)	131(28.98)		

Table 4: Frequency and percentage of condemnation Lung.

Abnormality	Frequency and distribution of lesions												
	Sheep and goat (n=1052)			Sheep(n=600)					Goats (n=452)				
	Sheep n=600	Goat n=452	Total n=1052	Young n=193	Adult n=407	Total n=600	X^2	p-value	Youngn=129	Adult n=323	Total	X^2	p
Pericarditis	31(5.1)	25 (5.5)	56(5.3)	11(5.7)	20(4.9)	31(5.7)	0.1649	0.685	6(4.6)	19(5.8)	25(5.5)	0.2674	0.605
Calcification	12(2)	11(2.4)	23(2.2)	2(1)	10(2.4)	12(2)	9.4133	0.042	2(1.5)	9(2.8)	11(2.4)	4.0024	0.406
Abscess	5(0.8)	2(0.4)	7(0.6)	1(0.5)	4(0.9)	5(0.8)	9.0083	0.109	0.00	2(0.6)	2(0.4)		
Cysticercus ovis	7(1.2)	4(0.8)	11(1.1)	2(1)	5(1.5)	7(1.6)	0.5032	0.438	1(0.7)	3(0.9)	4(0.8)	0.0248	0.875
Other	15(2.5)	18(3.8)	33(3.4)	2(1)	13(3.9)	15			2(1.5)	16(2.4)	18(3.4)		
overall	70(11.6)	60(13.2)	130(12.3)	18(9.3)	42(10.3)	70(11.6)			11(8.5)	49(15.2)	60(13.2)		

Table 5: Frequency and percentage lesions causing heart condemnation.

organ and carcass condemnation at Addis Ababa abattoir enterprise was estimated at 998,430.8 Ethiopian Birr. This total loss could be due to diseases and human factors either as a result of mishandling animals during transports to the slaughterhouse or due to faulty slaughter operations in the abattoir.

Risk factors		Number of examined	Calcification	Abscess	Pneumonia	Emphysema	Bruise	Nephritis	Pericarditis	Hydronephrosis	Hepatitis	Cirrhosis	Mechanical damage	Calculi	Others
Species	Sex														
sheep	Male	414	32(7.7)	15(3.6)	37(8.9)	22(5.3)	3(0.7)	12(2.9)	18(4.3)	7(1.6)	13(3.4)	21(5.0)	11(2.6)	4(0.9)	31(7.4)
	Female	186	25(13.4)	17(9.1)	21(11.3)	15(8.1)	-	9(4.9)	13(6.9)	4(2.2)	4(2.2)	15(8.1)	3(1.6)	4(2.1)	20(10.7)
	Total	600	57(9.5)	32(5.3)	58(9.6)	37(6.2)	3(0.5)	21(3.5)	31(5.1)	11(1.8)	17(2.8)	36(6.0)	14(2.3)	8(1.3)	51(5.1)
	X^2	23.82	11.5541	12.260	0.8138	1.6780	1.354	1.403	1.8275	0.150	0.4565	2.0371	0.6139	1.3684	1.3684
	P-value	0.000	0.021	0.031	0.367	0.159	0.244	0.232	0.176	0.698	0.499	0.153	0.433	0.242	1.3684
Goat	Male	376	40(10.6)	21(5.6)	36(9.5)	16(4.3)	4(1.1)	7(1.8)	21(5.6)	1(0.2)	17(4.5)	9(2.4)	18(5.3)	4(1.1)	
	female	76	10(13.2)	5(6.6)	5(6.6)	7(9.1)	1(1.3)	5(6.6)	4(5.2)	2(2.6)	7(9.2)	4(5.3)	4(5.3)	-	
	Total	452	50(11.1)	26(5.7)	41(9.1)	23(5.1)	5(1.1)	12(2.6)	25(5.5)	3(0.6)	24(5.8)	13(2.8)	22(4.8)	4(0.8)	
	X^2	1.056	1.0436	2.8925	0.6878	3.2142	0.367	5.4436	0.0125	5.366	2.7650	1.8636	0.0309	0.8157	
	P-value	0.304	0.903	0.576	0.407	0.073	0.848	0.020	0.911	0.021	0.096	0.172	0.860	0.366	

Pathological lesions (%)

Table 6: Pathological cause organ and carcass condemnation.

Discussion

The present study revealed that parasite and poor management practices are the major causes of organ and carcass condemnations. Parasitic causes like *Fasciola* species, *Hydatid cyst*, *Stilesia hepatica* and *Cysticercus tenuicollis* were found to be the major parasitic conditions responsible for organ condemnation. Even it impossible to draw back the origin of animal the frequency occurrence of pathological abnormalities show that parasitic disease of sheep and goats are widely distributed through to out the country. The major managemental practice that rendered organ and carcasses unfit for human consumption were faulty evisceration and bruising of carcass mainly brought about by mishandling of animals during transportation to the slaughter houses. Pneumonia was the major cause of lung condemnation in both species. It is observed that animals transported on foot long distance suffer from transportation stress and lack of feed and water. Those which were transported on open trucks are over crowed. Furthermore, animals are suffocated at the lairages and there was short resting time before slaughter for the animals to recover from physical stresses. Those conditions were causes of pneumonia and emphysema an observed at a higher case of incidence in this study. This indicates also violations of animal welfare stretching from farm to slaughter houses. The higher rate of occurrence of pneumonic lungs and poor meat quality are related to mishandling.

Liver condemnations are generally associated with infections of public health importance and for aesthetic reasons [13]. More than half of liver were condemned due to parasites; the rate of livers condemned in this study was relatively higher than a report in Debre Zeit HELMEX abattoir by Ejeta et al. [14] where 9.7% was recorded and a report in Kenya [15]. Mungube et al. have also reported frequency of liver condemnation due to *Fasciola* in goats at a rate of 6.6% which is lower than present finding 7.3%. The higher rate of fasciolosis observed in sheep in comparison with goat could be due to their feeding behavior where sheep are usually grazers and goat tend to be more of browsers making them less exposed to parasites. Mungube et al. have also reported cumulative incidence of liver condemnation due to *Stilesia hepatica* at 28% and 22% in sheep and goats respectively, which is higher than the result obtained in this study (4.33% and 3.98% in sheep and goats, respectively) and also Ejeta et al. reported higher incidence rate of liver condemnation due to *Stilesia hepatica* at 9.5% and 12.1% in sheep and goats, respectively. Ejeta et al. have also reported cumulative incidence of liver condemnation due to *Cysticercus tenuicollis* at 5.2% and 8.3% in sheep and goats, respectively, which is higher than the result obtained in this study (4.33% and 5.31% in sheep and goat, respectively) [14]. The epidemiology of *S. hepatica* and *C. tenuicollis* was not well established in sheep and goats; hence, it may be difficult to explain why significantly more livers were condemned in goats than in sheep. However Bekele et al. have reported a prevalence rate of 37.1% *C. tenuicollis* in sheep slaughtered at Addis Ababa Abattoir which higher than the present report in sheep (4.2%) [16]. This may be due to increase the health services in the conditions in the country. One-tenth of the total condemned livers were due to mechanical damage that was caused by faulty practices during evisceration. Higher frequency of mechanical damage was observed in young animals than adults which might be related to the difficulty associated with the removal of liver from the thoracic cavity.

The presence of small ruminant hydatidosis at slaughter house has been documented in Ethiopia. Bekele et al. reported a prevalence rate of 16.4% in sheep which is higher than the finding in this study [16]. Similarly Jobre et al. reported prevalence rate of 11% and 6% from

Risk factors			PARASITOLOGICAL LESIONS				
Species	Age	No. of Examined animal	Fasciola n (%)	Stilesia hepatica n (%)	Cysticercus tenicollis n (%)	Hydatid cyst n (%)	Cysticercus ovis n (%)
Sheep	Young	193	18(9.33)	6(3.11)	11(5.69)	10(5.18	2(1.04)
	Adult	407	52(12.78)	20(4.91)	15(3.69)	40(9.83)	5(1.23)
	Total	600	70(11.67)	26(4.33)	26(4.33)	50(8.33)	7(1.17)
	X^2		1.512o	1.0291	2.2057		0.0420
	P-value		0.219	0.310	0.332		0.838
Goat	Young	129	7(5.43)	6(4.65)	5(3.88)	7(5.43)	1(0.78)
	Adult	323	26(8.05)	12(3.72)	19(5.88)	28(8.67)	3(0.93)
	Total	452	33(7.30)	18(3.98)	24(5.31)	35(7.74)	4(0.88)
	X^2		0.9373	0.2112	0.7381		0.0248
	P-value		0.333	0.646	0.390		0.875
Overall		1052					

Table 7: Parasitological causes of organ condemnation.

south Omo and Debre Zeit slaughter houses, respectively in sheep and goats which is similar with the present finding (8% and 9.78% in sheep and goat, respectively) [8].

In present finding, hydatid cysts were more frequently observed in lungs than liver of sheep and goats. Additionally similar findings were reported also reported by different authors [17-19]. However, the most common site for hydatid cyst was the liver followed by the lungs in the Middle East [20].

Bruising caused more than one-fourth of all carcasses condemned. Bruising occurs due to use of rough vehicles and beating of animals during transportation. Bruising also caused by excessive uses of sticks while driving to the abattoir, mishandling of animals during loading and unloading, improper transport vehicle where responsible causes at slaughter. Bruising could be also a result of in the slaughter houses when animals struggle during slaughter as stunning of small ruminants was not practiced at Addis Ababa abattoir in particularly and in other abattoir in Ethiopia in general [21]. It has been suggested that bruising during transportation is the major sources of economic loss in Africa and Asia [22].

Abscess, calcification, cirrhosis, nephritis and pericarditis important causes for the condemnation of edible organs like liver, heart and kidney [23]. Ojo reported similar cases in Nigeria and was able to isolate bacteria with public health significance. Salmonella serotypes 14.5% of mutton samples examined from various super markets in Addis Ababa reported [14].

Though *Cysrticercus tenuicollis, Cysticercus ovis* and *Stilesia hepatica* do not have public health importance, they are considered as important causes of economic loss, since viscera harboring them are rejected for economic loss and aesthetic reasons. The threat these parasites pose to small ruminant's meat industry in Ethiopia is evident due to the present situation of improper disposal of offal at abattoirs and backyard slaughter. The presence of freely roaming/living stray dogs on grazing land together with live stock and the deep rooted habit of feeding dogs with offal are important risk factors. This may lead to perpetuation of the life cycle between intermediate hosts (ruminants) and the final host dogs for *C. ovis, C. tenuicollis* and hydatidosis.

The financial loss in the abattoir is considered high. However, realization of the total (true) economic loss from organ and carcass condemnation is difficult and complex. The indirect losses from mortality at the lairage and public health implication were not included in the analysis in this study. Thus, the total economic loss attributable to diseases of small ruminants and hence, abattoir wastage could be

much higher. The economic analysis of livestock disease in Ethiopia is scarce and inadequate because of lack of information on the prevalence and partly by the complexity of the analysis. Ngategize et al. reported a financial loss associated with liver condemnation due to ovine fasciolosis alone in the central highlands of Ethiopia amounting to be 2-3 million Ethiopian Birr (460.000 USD) [24]. Similarly Jobre et al. have estimated a total annual loss of 1.3 million Ethiopian Birr (260.000 USD) resulting from offal condemnation and carcass weight loss [8].

Conclusion and Recommendations

Slaughter houses provide excellent opportunities for detecting disease of both economic and public health importance. Government and other programs in Africa can use abattoirs as a source of data to assist in monitoring diseases, provide feedback to producer, to produce whole some products and to protect the public from zoonotic hazards. The present survey report indicates that parasitic disease, other pathological conditions, mechanical damage evisceration and bruising were the major cause of organ and carcass condemnation and financial loss through organ at Addis Ababa abattoir enterprise, which may also reflect the same scenario in other slaughter houses in Ethiopia. To mitigate the economic and public health impacts of diseases of small ruminants, proper disposal of offal, prohibition of backyard slaughter of small ruminants and construction of slaughter houses, better disease control strategies, adequate training of abattoir personnel on the slaughtering operation and regular deworming of stray and home dogs and Education of small ruminant traders how to transport the livestock from farm to markets recommendations are forwarded.

Competing Interest

The authors declare that they have no competing interest.

Acknowledgements

Authors I would like to thank the entire staff members of Addis Ababa abattoir enterprise and administrative office for their cooperation and support of this work.

References

1. Alemu Y, Merkel RC (2008) Sheep and Goat Production Handbook for Ethiopia: Ethiopia Sheep and Goat Productivity Improvement Program /ESGPIP/, Ministry of Agriculture and Rural Development, pp: 15-53.

2. CSA (2016) Federal Democratic Republic of Ethiopia Central Statistical Agency Agricultural Sample Survey 2015/16 Volume II Report on livestock and livestock characteristics. Statistical Bulletin, p: 532.

3. Jacob L (1979) Seminar for Animal Health Officials. Minster of Agriculture and Settlement, Animals and Fisheries Authority, Addis Ababa, Ethiopia.

4. Jibat T, Ejeta G, Asfaw Y, Wudie A (2008) Causes of Abattori condemnation in apparently healthy slaughtered sheep and Goats at HELMEX (Hashim Nurs' Ethiopian Livestock and Meat Export) abattoir at Debre Zeit, Ethiopia. Revue Med Vet. 5: 305-311.

5. Arbabi M, Hooshyr H (2006) Survey of Regions might have accounted for variation of the Echinococcosis and Hydatidosis in Kashan Region, Prevalence in different areas of a country Central Iran. Iran J Public Health 35: 75-81.

6. Fufa A, Loma A, Bekele M, Alemayehu R (2010) Bovine fasciolosis: coprological, abattoir survey and its economic impact due to liver condemnation at Sodo Municipal abattoir, Southern Ethiopia. Trop Anim Health Prod. 42: 289-292.

7. Herenda D, Chambers PG, Ettriqui A, Senevirat Nap, da Silva TJP (1994) Manual on meat inspection for developing countries, Food and Agricultural Organization of the united nations (FAO), Rome, Italy.

8. Jobre Y, Lobago F, Tiruneh R, Abebe G, Dorchies PH (1996) Hydatidosis in three Selection Region in Ethiopia: An Assessment Trial on its Prevalence, Economic and Public Health Importance. Revue med Vet. 147: 797-804.

9. LMA (2009) Brief baseline information on Ethiopian livestock resources base and its trade, livestock Marketing Authority, Addis Ababa, Ethiopia.

10. NMA (2011) National Meteorology Service Agency. Addis Ababa, Ethiopia.

11. Steele M (1996) Goats: The tropical Agriculturist. Macmillan Education Ltd, CTA Publishing, London, pp: 79-83.

12. Ogunrinade A, Ogunrinade BI (1980) Economic importance of bovine fasiolosis in Nigeria. Trop Anim Prod. 12: 155-160.

13. Edwards DS, Johnston AM, Mead GC (1997) Meat Inspection and Overview of Present Practice and Future Trends. Vet J. 154: 135-147.

14. Ejeta G, Molla B, Alemayehu D, Muckle A (2008) Salmonella serotypes isolated from minced beef, mutton and pork in Addis Ababa Ethiopia. Revue Med Vet. 155: 547-551.

15. Mungube EO, Bauni SM, Tenhagen BA, Wamael W, Nyinyi JM, et al. (2006) The prevalence and econmic significance of Fasciola gigantica and stelesia hepatica in slaughtered animals in semi-arid costal Kenya. Trop Anim Hlth Prod. 38: 475-483.

16. Bekele T, Mukassa ME, Kasali OB (1988) The prevalence of cysticercosis and Hydatidosis in Ethiopian sheep. Vet Parasitol. 28: 267-270.

17. Khan AH, El–Buni AA, Ali MY (2001) Fertility of the Cyst of Echinococcus Granulosus in Domestic Herbiivorse from Benghazi, Libya, and the Ractivityof Antigens Produced from them. Ann Trop Med Parasitol. 95: 337-342.

18. Dalimai A, Motamedi GH, Hosseini M, Mohammadian B, Malaki H, et al. (2002) Echinococcosis/hydatidosis in western Iran. Vet Parasitol. 105: 161-171.

19. Daryani A, Alaei R, Arab R, Sharif M, Dehghan MH, et al. (2007) The Prevalence, Intensity and Viability of Hdatidcysts in Slaughtered Animals in the Ardavil Province Northwest Iran. J Helminthol. 81: 13-17.

20. Kamhawi S, Hijjawi N, Abu-Ghazaleh A, Abbas M (1996) Pevalence of Hydatid Cyst in Livestock from Five Regions in Jorda. Ann Trop Med Hyg. 147: 797-804.

21. Gracey JF, Collins OS, Hueyr J (1999) Meat hygiene. Tenth Edition, Baillier Tindall, London Philadelphia, Toronto, pp 223-260.

22. Mitchell JR, Slough CAB (1980) Guide to Meat inspection in the Tropics, Common Wealth Bureau of Animal Health, UK.

23. Ojo SA (1996) Survey of Pathological Conditions in Slaughtred Goats at Zaria Slaughter houses. In: Lebbie SHB, Kagwini E (eds). Small Ruminant Research and Development in Africa. Proceeding of the Third Biennial conference of the African small ruminant Research network, UICC, Kampala, Uganda, 5-9 December 1994, International Livestock Research Institute (ILIRI), Nairobi, Kenya.

24. Ngategize PK, Bekele T, Tilahun G (1993) Financial Losses caused by Ovine Fasciolosis in the Ethiopian Highlands. Trop Anim Health Prod. 25: 155-161.

43

Absence of Rabies and Rabies-Related Lyssaviruses in Some Wild Animal Species in Enugu State, Nigeria

Lynda O Obodoechi[1]*, Chidi O Anyaoha[1], Nnenna E Ibezim[1], Majesty E Alukagberie[1], Chika I Nwosuh[3], John A Nwanta[1] and Chukwunyere O Nwosu[2]

[1]Veterinary Public Health and Preventive Medicine, University of Nigeria, Nsukka, Nigeria
[2]Veterinary Parasitology and Entomology, University of Nigeria, Nsukka, Nigeria
[3]National Veterinary Research Institute, Vom, Plateau State, Nigeria

Abstract

This study investigated the presence of rabies and rabies-related lyssaviruses in the brain, liver and spleen of some wild animal species (rodents, shrews and civet cats) slaughtered for human consumption in Enugu State, Southeastern Nigeria. Attempts were made to establish possible exposure potential of humans to rabies and rabies-related lyssaviruses through handling, processing, selling, buying and consumption of these wild animals and establish the species of the viral isolates if any. A total of four hundred and eighty four 329) wild animals were sampled for rabies and rabies-related lyssaviruses using florescent antibody technique (FAT), cell culture test for the isolation and Reverse Transcriptase Polymerase Chain Reaction (RT-PCR) for detection of lyssavirus nucleic acid. The animals sampled include eighty nine land squirrels (*Xerus erythropus*), seventy African giant rats (*Cricetomysgambians*), one hundred and one black rats eighty bush rats (*Rattus fuscipes*), seventy two shrews and seventy civet cats (*Civetticitis civetta*). The animals were collected fresh from hunters or markets, restaurants and bars where they are slaughtered and consumed as delicacy in the study area. There was no lyssavirus isolated from the three hundred and forty rodent samples (brain, liver, spleen) examined. Similarly, there was no lyssavirus isolated from the seventy civet cat samples (liver, spleen, brain). And samples (liver, spleen, brain) from seventy two shrews. The results of this study suggest that rodents and civet cats slaughtered for human consumption in Enugu State, Nigeria are free of rabies and rabies-related lyssaviruses. Therefore, there is no exposure potential to rabies or rabies-related lyssaviruses in those involved in the hunting, handling, processing, selling, buying and consumption of bush meat of these animal species. Also, the shrews and some other rodents such as black rats (*Rattus rattus*) were noted to be free of rabies and rabies-related lyssaviruses in the study area.

Keywords: Rabies; Rabies-related; Lyssaviruses; Rodents; Shrews; Civetcats

Introduction

The ecological persistence of pathogenic viruses has been the focus of many studies [1-3]. Nigeria occupies a strategic position wherever the history of lyssavirus is recounted [4]. This is because three species have been reported in the country. Lyssaviruses are negative stranded RNA viruses belonging to the family Rhabdoviridae [5]. Lyssaviruses are persistent and emerging infectious agents that cause disease in a range of domesticated and wild animal species including man [6]. The wild species reported to have been infected include foxes, ferrets, raccoons, bats, and several species of rodents [7]. Among the domesticated species, dogs and cats are mainly affected by the lyssaviruses but dogs have been established as the predominant vector of rabies in Nigeria [8-10]. Lyssavirus genus includes 11 recognized species [11]. The species type, Rabies virus (RABV) is distributed worldwide among carnivores and bats. Lagos bat virus (LBV) circulates among pteropid bats in sub-Saharan Africa with infrequent spill over into other mammals [12]. Mokola virus (MOKV) has been isolated in sub-Saharan Africa from shrews, domestic cats, dogs, rodents and humans [13,14]. Whereas rabies is probably the most important and definitive viral zoonosis world wide, Mokola virus infection has to date been reported from the African continent only [13]. Mokola virus was originally isolated in 1968 from pooled viscera of 3 insectivorous shrews (*Crocidura* spp.) from Mokola district of Ibadan, Nigeria [15]. It has been isolated twice from human beings from Nigeria in 1972 and since then there is no evidence of further isolation [16]. Rabies is one of the most important and widespread zoonotic diseases and it is with the exception of a few countries, a truly global dilemma [17-19]. Although dog is the predominant vector of

rabies in Nigeria [9], rabies has been reported in wildlife species (lynx, civet cats, monkeys, insectivorous bats, chimpanzee, lion, hyrax) [20-23]. In the USA, Canada, and Western Europe, where canine rabies has been controlled, dogs are responsible for very few cases of the disease. Rather, human rabies develops from bites of wild animals (especially bats, squirrels, rats, raccoons, skunks, and foxes) or occur in travelers bitten by dogs elsewhere in the world [24]. Mokola virus has been detected in Shrews and wild rodents but not bats, and its reservoir host is still uncertain [14]. In Nigeria, rabies cases still abound in spite of the yearly massive anti rabies vaccination, there may be thus an alternative reservoir for the virus. The overwhelming mortality associated with rabies infection makes it one of the most feared diseases of humans and animals. Dogs are the major animal reservoirs in the developing regions, wild life maintains cycle of infection even in developed countries and new viral aetiologic agents continue to emerge [25]. The domestic dog, *Canis familaris*, is recognized as the reservoir for classical rabies virus and the straw-coloured fruit bat for Lagos bat virus. The reservoir for

---

*Corresponding author: Lynda O Obodoechi, Veterinary Public Health and Preventive Medicine, University of Nigeria, Nsukka, Nigeria
E-mail: onyinye.obodoechi@unn.edu.ng

Mokola virus remains unidentified but shrews could be the reservoir [4]. The human cases of Mokola virus infection have demonstrated its zoonotic potential [16,26] but a natural reservoir is yet to be identified [27]. The fact that all cases of Mokola virus infection in South Africa, as well as all but one from domestic animals from other countries in Africa [28-31] have been confined to cats, strongly suggests that the reservoir is to be found among their prey (shrews and rodents) as the virus has been isolated from them [15,32-34]. Mokola virus was last isolated in Nigeria in 1972 and since then, no further isolation has been done. Monitoring of animals especially the bush-meat in Africa has revealed that zoonotic viruses frequently spill over into the human populations that hunt, or manage the animals; which have provided significant insights into origins, geographic distributions, temperate limitations, and emergence potential of several important human pathogens [35]. In Enugu state, there is increase in wild life meat consumption with an increase in the population of people who hunt. Consequently, the rate of contacts between the indigenes and wild life is increased which could pose a very big risk should these animals be reservoirs of the viruses. It is against this background that this study was carried out to find out if lyssaviruses would be isolated from these animal species for a better understanding of the epidemiologic situation, circulation pattern and public health significance in order to establish control strategy in Enugu State in particular and Nigeria in general.

Study Design

The study was a one year cross- sectional study. This was achieved through collection of shrews civet cats and rodents from markets, bushes, restaurants and bars for viral isolation and identification from brain tissues and visceral organs (spleen and liver) using FAT, tissue cell culture in mouse neuroblastoma cell line (MNA) and RT-PCR.

Sample collection

Purposive sampling method was adopted for sample collection from markets where fresh rodents and wild cats exist and bars and restaurants where their meat are sold as delicacy for human consumption. However, some of the rodents and shrews were collected directly from hunters from purposively selected bushes where the wild animals reside.

A total of four hundred and eighty four animals were collected for lyssaviruses screening. The animals included were 89 land squirrels (*Xerus erythropus*), 70 African giant rats(*Cricetomysgambians*), 101 black rats *Rattus rattus* 80 bush rats (*Rattus fuscipes*), 72 shrews (*Cocidura spp*) and seventy Civet cats (*Civetticitis civetta*) were used for the study. The samples were stored at -20°C until analysis.

Detection of rabies and rabies- related lyssaviruses was done using FAT and RT-PCR while isolation was done on mouse neuroblastoma cell line (MNA) as described by Zanoni et al. [36].

Direct Fluorescent Antibody Technique (DFA)

Glass slides were properly degreased and labeled accordingly. A known positive sample normally challenge virus strain (positive control) and a normal 3-week-old mice brain (negative control) were used as controls. Thin impression smears of the negative control, positive control and test brain samples were made on the centre of the properly labeled glass slides.

The smears were air-dried at room temperature and fixed in cold acetone contained in coplin jar for thirty minutes at -20°C. The slides were air-dried for thirty minutes at room temperature and the smears encircled with wax pencil. 150 µl of the diluted aliquot of the FITC anti-

rabies monoclonal globulin conjugate made by Fujirebio Diagnostics Inc. Malvern, PA, USA that detects the four African lyssaviruses (Rabies virus, Lagos bat virus, Mokola virus and Duvenhage virus) was added to cover the smears within the encircled areas of the slides in the moist chamber and incubated at 37°C for 30 minutes. Afterwards, the slides were properly washed in phosphate buffered saline (pH 8.5) for 30 minutes to remove the unbound DFA reagent in the smears. The slides were allowed to air-dry at room temperature. Two drops of 50% buffered glycerol mounting medium was added and cover slips were mounted and the slides were viewed under florescent microscope. The test impression and the positive and negative control impressions stained with FDI FITC anti- rabies monoclonal globulin were examined with a fluorescence microscope. A test impression was scored as positive when brilliant apple-green fluorescence was observed. The test is valid when brilliant apple-green fluorescence was observed in the positive control, but no apple- green fluorescence was seen in the negative control. A test impression was negative when no apple-green fluorescence was observed.

Tissue cell culture in mouse neuroblastoma cell line (MNA)

This procedure involved the isolation and culture of all lyssavirus from a homogenate of a suspect test specimen in mouse neuroblastoma cells (MNA) (ATCC HB-12317) from America Type Culture Collection Center, USA. Ten percent homogenate of the brain and pooled visceral organs (spleen and liver) were separately made using Phosphate buffered saline of pH 7.2 and antibiotic (a combination of Penicillin, streptomycin and Fungizone). This was clarified by centrifugation for 10 minutes at 10,000 g in a cold centrifuge and filtered using 0.45 µ Millipore filter. Using 96 well cell culture plates 100 µl of each sample was inoculated in quadruplet into 80% confluent MNA cells in DMEM (Dulbecco's Modified Eagle's Medium) without sodium pyruvate but with 10% fetal calf serum and 1.5 gm/liter of sodium carbonate and incubated for four days at 37°C with 5% CO_2. The medium was harvested separately, labeled and stored at -20°C while the plates were fixed in 80% cold acetone for 30 mins, washed and stained with fluorescent labeled antirabies conjugate. Positive samples showed bright 'apple' green fluorescence inclusions generally in the peri-nuclear area cells. A negative sample had no fluorescence and appeared dull green or red/green.

Reverse Transcriptase Polymerase Chain Reaction (RT-PCR)

RNA extraction: Total Viral RNA was extracted from pooled sample of the brain, spleen and liver using TRIzol® reagent (invitrogen™, U.S.A). The spleen and liver were included because previous isolates of Mokola virus were from pooled viscera organs.

Approximately 300 µl of the sample was homogenized in 1000 µl of TRIzol Reagent and vortex mixed and incubated at room temperature (RT) for 5 minutes allowing for complete dissociation of the nucleoprotein complex. Two hundred microlitres of chloroform was added to the homogenate, vortex mixed and kept for 5 minutes at RT and then centrifuged at 14000 g for 10 minutes to separate the phases. Five hundred microlitres of the aqueous phase was transferred to a fresh sterile Eppendorf tube and 200 µl of 75% ethanol was added and 500 µl of isopropanol (SIGMA U.S.A) was added gently mixed and kept at RT for 10 minutes to enhance precipitation of the RNA. The RNA pellet was recovered by centrifugation at 14000 g for 10 minutes, washed with 1000 µl of 75% ethanol and air-dried. The RNA pellet was then solubilized in 50 µl of RNA suspension solution (DEPC treated water) (Thermo Scientific, USA) in heating block (Thermo Scientific, USA). The solubilized RNA was stored at -20°C.

Reverse Transcription (RT): Approximately 2 µl of the total RNA was heat-natured and annealed with messenger sense primers JW12 and Lys001 at 65°C for 2 minutes and cooled on ice for 1 minute. This was immediately followed by reverse transcription performed at 37°C for 60 minutes in a 0.5 µl reaction containing 200 units of Murine Moloney Leukemia Virus Reverse Transcriptase (M-MLV, USB™), 20 units of RNasin® ribonuclease inhibitor (promega), 4.0 of dNTP mixture, 2.0 of DTT and 2.0 reverse transcriptase reaction buffers. At the end of the reverse transcription reaction, the cDNA mixture was inactivated at 85°C for 5 minutes, 37°C for 20 minutes then stored at -20°C (Plate 1).

Polymerase Chain Reaction (PCR): In brief, a 50 µlreaction mixture containing 2 µl of the cDNA, 0.5 µlof the Takara Taq DNA polymerase (Takara Biotechnology, Japan), 4 µl of 10 mM DNTP mixture, 4 µl each of 10 pmol Lys001 and 550B, 0.5 µl of 10X Taq polymerase reaction buffer and made up to 50 µl with nuclease free water. The amplification was carried out with an ABI 9700 thermocycler with an initial denaturation at 94°C for one minute, followed by 40 cycles of (94°C for 30 seconds, 37°C for 30 seconds and 72°C for 90 seconds) and a final extension at 72°C for 10 minutes. The amplified DNA products were visualized under UV transillumination after electrophoresis through 1% ethidium bromide stained agarose gels (Labnet, power station 300) with a 100 bp DNA ladder as the molecular weight maker (Promega).

Results

Out of the three hundred and forty brains of rodents, seventy two shrews and 70 brains of civet cats sampled and examined on florescent antibody test, none (0%) was positive for rabies or rabies-related lyssaviruses nor isolated on mouse neuroblastoma cell line (MNA). In addition, out of the total 329 pooled brain, liver and spleen, there was no rabies or rabies-related lyssavirus nucleic acid detected on RT-PCR test techniques. On the other hand, the positive control samples remained positive while the negative controls were also negative for all the test techniques used.

Discussion

In the present study, a total of three hundred and forty samples made up of brain, liver and spleen homogenates of rodents (89 squirrels, *Xerus erythropus*; 80 bush rats, *Rattus fuscipes*; and 70 African giant rats *Cricetomys gambianus* and 101 black rats, *Rattus rattus* were analyzed for the presence of rabies and rabies-related viruses. The brain, spleen and liver of these animal species were examined using FAT, RT-PCR and tissue cell culture in mouse neuroblastoma cell line (MNA) for viral isolation. Although, the FAT has been recommended by the OIE and WHO, and used worldwide for the diagnoses of rabies [8], it failed to detect any lyssavirus antigen in the present study because none of the samples had lyssavirus antigen. However, in spite of the FAT being the most common, rapid and sensitive diagnostic test for rabies, other supplementary diagnostic methods are employed when a questionable FAT result is obtained in order to arrive at a definite conclusion.

Consequently, several molecular biology-based diagnostic methods which target the nucleic acids of the causative agents have been employed for such further confirmatory tests. Accordingly, diagnostic methods based on RT-PCR have been confirmed to be useful and sensitive in detecting viruses that cause lyssaviral diseases [24]. In the present study, no lyssavirus nucleic acid was detected using the RT-PCR.

Virus isolation in cell culture is fast and results can be given in 24-48 hours. The cell lines most suitable for virus isolation are of neural origin and the most commonly used cell line is the murine neuroblastoma cell line Neuro-2a. Other cell lines which are used but may not be as sensitive as Neuro-2a include chicken embryo-related (CER) and baby hamster kidney (BHK 21) cells. In this research, we were not able to isolate any rabies nor rabies- related lyssaviruses using MNA cell line since there was no growth of any virus. The 0% prevalence of rabies and rabies-related lyssavirus in the animal species sampled suggests that there may not be lyssavirus in these animal species in the study area. Inspite of isolations of rabies virus in wildlife, the role of wildlife in the

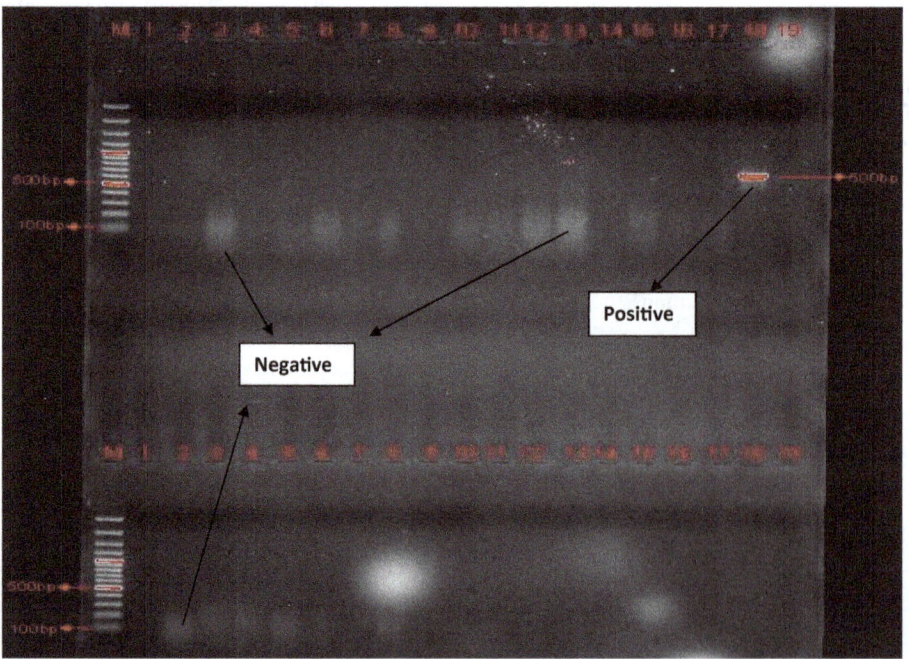

Plate 1: Annotated picture of the RT-PCR result showing all samples to be negative except for the positive control trapped at 500 bp.

transmission of rabies in Nigeria is still not clearly defined. Bougler and Hardy failed to isolate rabies virus from the brains and salivary glands of 1,913 rats collected in Lagos [37]. The present findings agree with the recommendations of the CDC that bites from squirrels and rats do not call for post exposure prophylaxis as they rarely carry rabies [38]. According to CDC, squirrels and rats may get rabies, but their chances of contracting it are slim to none. In order for these animals to get rabies, they would have to hang around with animals that are common carriers. However, this does not usually happen because many of the animals that would carry rabies (dogs, cats, foxes) are arch enemies of rodents which, ordinarily, would avoid them. In addition, squirrels are so quick at evasion and with 180 degree vision; the chances of them being bitten by rabid animal are very remote [39].

According to CDC, rats almost never carry rabies and are not considered a serious rabies risk. Rabies transmission in rats is extremely rare, not because rats have dry bites but because they almost never carry rabies, presumably because rats do not survive the attack of a rabid animals like raccoons, skunks, foxes, cats or dogs. Most animals that carry rabies, if they get hold of rats and squirrel would more likely kill them and thus would end the possibility of such rats and squirrels carrying and transmitting the disease. This therefore reaffirms the public health community's general assumption that rodents, with the exception of large-bodied species, carry little risk of transmitting RABV [40]. The findings of this study is also in harmony with Winkler, who stated that although rodents may become infected with rabies, there is actually little or no naturally occurring rodent rabies [41]. This however, does not rule out rodents as factor in rabies epidemiology in Nigeria. First, there is belief that a bite from a rodent, the ground squirrel (*Xerus erythropus*) results in madness and death one to six months after the bite and with Mokola virus been isolated from shrews. Reports of Oboegbulem and Garba showed that in Nigeria, only 1 rat was positive for rabies between 1991 and 2005 [9,42]. Similarly, the findings of this study (0% prevalence) is lower than the prevalence of 0.04% recorded in rats in Poland (WHO), 1% in rats in Isreal and 4.7% in rats in Norway [8,24,25]. Rodents represented less than 1% of all species tested for rabies in the United States of America, and virtually all of those tested and found rabid were large species such as woodchucks (*Marmota monax*) and beavers (*Castor canadensis*) [39,43]. Winkler reviewed rabies in rats over 18 years period (1953 to 1970) and reported that only 39 rats were found rabid in the United States of America; only 11 rabid rats were rabid between 1953 and 1955 while during the three year period of 1968-1970, only 2 rats were rabid [41]. The result of this study does not agree with the work done by some authors in Nigeria and other countries, who have implicated rodents in the maintenance of RABV but critical data to support these contentions are elusive [23,44,45].

The present study recorded 0% prevalence of rabies and rabies-related lyssaviruses in shrews. Mokola virus was first isolated from shrews (*Cocidura spp*) in 1968 [46]. Since the initial isolation was from the visceral organs, pooled samples of the brain, spleen and liver were equally analyzed using mouse neuroblastoma cell line (MNA) and there was no viral growth. This suggests that there may not be rabies or rabies-related lyssaviruses in the animals sampled in the study area. The 0% prevalence of Mokola virus recorded in shrews in this study agrees with Kantakamalakul who investigated five hundred rodents and shrews for rabies virus using direct immunoflorescnce and reported 0% prevalence [47]. Kgaladi et al. after his survey on Moklola virus (1968-2012) reported that although, the first isolates of Mokola virus were from Nigeria and other Congo basin countries, all reports over the past 20 years have been from Southern Africa [27].

The results obtained from this study showed 0% prevalence of rabies and rabies–related lyssaviruses in civet cats since we were not able to isolate any virus suggesting that rabies and rabies-related lyssaviruses do not exist in the civet cats sampled in the study area. Civet cats are nocturnal in habit and rarely found during the day. Dogs which are the main reservoir of rabies in Nigeria often move around during the day, thus reducing the chances of interaction between civet cats and dogs [9]. However, this result is not in harmony with the works of Kasali who reported a case of rabies in a wild cat in Jos, Nigeria and Ogunkoya who reported a prevalence of 21.4% in 22 civet cats screened in Bauchi State, Nigeria [20,23]. Furthermore, Umoh and Belino incriminated civet cats as wild life reservoirs of rabies in Nigeria [48].

The 0% prevalence of rabies and rabies related lyssavirus observed in the wild animal species studied, agrees with the previous works done by researchers like Okoh who reported 0% prevalence of rabies in over 200 wild animals tested between the period 1923 and 1970 [44]. Furthermore, the National Veterinary Research Institute (NVRI) Vom, Nigeria diagnosed 538 cases of rabies between 1970 and 1978 with 504 (94%) of the cases in dogs and the rest in domestic cats. This therefore conforms to previous reports that wild life rabies is not given prominence in some countries like Nigeria were dogs are the major reservoirs of rabies [7,9,49].

Conclusion

In conclusion, the 0% prevalence of rabies and rabies-related lyssaviruses observed in the rodents shrews and civet cats examined in Enugu State, Nigeria suggests that lyssaviruses may not exist in these animal species in the study area at the time of the study. It further suggests that these animal species may not be important in the epidemiology of lyssaviruses in the study area.

References

1. Bartlett MS (1960) The critical community size for measles in the United States. J Royal Statistical Soc 123: 37-44.

2. Black FL (1966) Measles endemicity in insular populations: Critical Community six and its evolutionary implications. J Theor Biol 11: 207-211.

3. Anderson RM, May RM (1991) Infectious disease of humans. New York: Oxford University Press.

4. Dzikwi AA, Garkida AD, Umoh JU (2011) World Rabies Day: Efforts Towards Rabies Awareness in Zaria, Nigeria. Nigerian Vet J 32: 133-136.

5. Tordo N, Kouknetzoff A (1993) The rabies virus genome: An overview. Onderstepoort J Vet Res 60: 263-269.

6. Okoh AEJ (2007) Rabies in Nigeria: Issues and Challenges. 6th Inaugural lecture, University of Agriculture Makurdi, 26th September, 2007. pp. 1-2.

7. Bishop GC, Durrhicim, Kloeck PE, Godlonton JP, Bingham J, et al. (2003) Rabies: Guide for the Medical, Veterinary and allied Professions. I edition. Government Printer Pretoria.

8. World Health Organization (1992) WHO Expert Committee on Rabies Technical Report Series No. 824, Geneva.

9. Oboegbulem SI (1994) Rabies in man and animals. 1st edition. Fidelity Publishers Enugu pp. 5-15, 238.

10. Cleaveland S, Kaare M, Knobel D, Laurenson MK (2006) Canine vaccination-providing broader benefits for disease control. Vet Microbiol 117: 43-50.

11. Kuzmin IV, Mayer AE, Niezgoda M, Markotter W, Agwanda B, et al. (2010) Shimoni bat virus, a new representative of the Lyssavirus genus. Virus Res 149: 197-210.

12. Markotter W, Kuzmin I, Rupprecht CE, Nel LH (2008a) Phylogeny of Lagos bat virus: challenges for lyssavirus taxonomy. Virus Res 135: 10-21.

13. Nel L, Jacobs J, Jafta J, Von Teichman B, Bingham J (2000) New cases of Mokola virus infection in South Africa: a genotypic comparison of Southern

African virus isolates. Virus Genes 20: 103-106.

14. Sabeta CT, Markotter W, Mohale DK, Shumba W, Wandeler AI, et al. (2007) Mokola virus in domestic mammals, South Africa. Emerg Infect Dis 13: 1371-1373.

15. Shope RE, Murphy FA, Harrison AK, Causey OR, Kemp GE, et al. (1970) Two African viruses serologically and morphologically related to rabies virus. J Virol 6: 690-692.

16. Familusi JB, Moore DL (1972) Isolation of a rabies related virus from the cerebrospinal fluid of a child with aseptic meningitis. African J Med Sci 3: 93-96.

17. Blancou J (1988) Epizootiology of rabies: Eurasia and Africa. In: Rabies. Campell JB & Chalton KM (eds.) Kluwer Academic publishers, Boston, 243-265.

18. World Health Organisation (1989) WHO expert committee on Rabies: WHO Technical Report, WHO. Geneva.

19. World Health Organisation (1991) WHO expert Committee on Rabies: WHO Technical Report, WHO. Geneva

20. Kasali OB (1977) Rabies in a civet cat (virtacirtta); case report. Vet Rec 100: 291.

21. Okoh AEJ (1986a) Dog ecology with reference to surveillance of rabies and characterization of rabies virus isolates in Plateau State, Nigeria. Ahmadu Bello University, Zaria.

22. Enurah LU, Ocholi RA, Adenryi KO, Ekwonu MC (1988) Rabies in civet cat in Jos Zoo, Nigeria. Br Vet J 144: 515-516.

23. Ogunkoya AB (2008) Review of rabies and problems of rabies in Nigeria. Proceedings of the National Conference/Workshop on Rabies, IDR-ABU, Zaria, Nigeria.

24. Smith JS (1996) New aspects of rabies with emphasis on epidemiology, diagnosis, and prevention of the disease in the United States. Clin Microbiol Rev 9: 166-176.

25. Rupprecht CE, Willoughby R, Slate D (2006) Current and future trends in the prevention, treatment and control of Rabies. Expert Rev Anti Infect Ther 4: 1021-1036.

26. Warrell MJ, Warrell DA (2004) Rabies and other lyssavirus diseases. Lancet 363: 959-969.

27. Kgaladi J, Wright N, Coertse J, Markotter W, Martson D (2013) Diversity and Epidemiology of Mokolavirus. PLoS Negl Trop Dis 7: e2511.

28. Foggin CM (1982) Atypical rabies virus in cats and a dog in Zimbabwe. Vet Rec 110: 338.

29. Foggin CM (1983) Mokola virus infection in cats and a dog in Zimbabwe. Vet Rec 113: 115.

30. Foggin CM (1988) Rabies and rabies-related viruses in Zimbabwe: Historical, virological and ecological aspects. PhD Theses, University of Zimbabwe, Harare.

31. Mebatsion T, Cox JH, Frost JW (1992) Isolation and characterization of 115 street rabies virus isolates from Ethiopia by using monoclonal antibodies: Identification of 2 isolates as Mokola and Lagos bat viruses. J Infect Dis 166: 972-977.

32. Kemp GE, Causey OR, Moore DRL, Odelola A, Fabiyi A (1972) Serological evidence of infection of dogs and man in Nigeria by lyssaviruses (family Rhabdoviridae). Trans R Soc Trop Med Hyg 21: 356-359.

33. Le Gonidec G, Rickenbach A, Robin T, Heme G (1978) Isolation of a strain of Mokola virus in Cameroon. Ann Microbiol 129A: 245-249.

34. Saluzzo JF, Rollin PE, Daugard C, Digoutte JP, Georges AJ, et al. (1984) First isolation of the Mokola virus from a rodent (Lophuromys sikapusi). Annalies de l'Institut Pasteur: Virology 135E: 57-66.

35. Wolfe ND, Heneioe W, Carr JK, Garcia AD, Shanmugam V, et al. (2007) Naturally acquired simian retrovirus infections in central African hunters. Lancet 363: 932-937.

36. Zanoni RG, Hornlimann B, Wandler AI (1990) Rabies tissue culture infection test as an alternative for mouse inoculation test. Altex 7: 15-23.

37. Bougler LR, Hardy J (1960) Rabies in Nigeria. West Africa Med J 9: 233-234

38. Centers for Disease Control and Prevention (1969) Wild rats and Disease.

39. Centers for Disease Control and Prevention (2011) Rabies and pet risk.

40. Real LA, Childs JE (2005) Spatial-temporal dynamics of rabies in ecological communities. Collinge 12: 170-186.

41. Winkler WG (1973) Rabies in the United States, 1951-1970. J Infect Dis 125: 674-675.

42. Garba A (2011) What you must know about Rabies. 1st edn. Sanies Press Jos Nigeria.

43. World Health Organisation (1998) WHO World survey of Rabies. Report Series No. 34, Geneva.

44. Okoh AEJ (1986b) Investigation of possible rabies reservoirs in rodents in Nigeria. Int J Zoonoses 13: 1-5.

45. Summa ME, Carrieri ML, Favoretto SR, Chamelet EI (1987) Rabies in the state of Sao Paulo: the rodents question. Rev Inst Med Trop S Paulo 29: 53-58.

46. Kantakamalakul W, Siritantikorn S, Thongcharoen P, Singchai C, Puthavalthana P (2003) Prevalence of rabies virus and Hantaan virus infections in commensal rodents and shrews trapped in Bankok. J Med Assoc Thai 86: 1008-1014.

47. Shope RE (1978) Rabies in viral infections of Humans: Epidemiology and control. pp: 351-363.

48. Umoh JU, Belino ED (1070) Rabies in Nigeria A historical review: Int J Zoonoses 6: 41-48.

49. Fooks AR, Brookes SM, Johnson N, McElhinney LM, Hutson AM (2003a) Epidemiol Infect 131: 1029-1039.

Permissions

List of Contributors

Arup Sen and Abu Torab
Department of Microbiology and Veterinary Public Health, Chittagong Veterinary and Animal Sciences University, Chittagong, Khulshi, Bangladesh

Abdus Salam SM, Bhubon Halder and Alauddin MD
Faculty of Veterinary Medicine (FVM), Chittagong Veterinary and Animal Sciences University, Chittagong, Khulshi, Bangladesh

Chala Bedasa and Mekdes Getachow
College of Agriculture and Veterinary Medicine, Jimma University, Jimma, Ethiopia

Ararsa Duguma
College of Veterinary Medicine, Haramaya University, PO Box 138, Diredawa, Ethiopia

Shubisa Abera
Yabello Regional Veterinary Laboratory, Yabello, Ethiopia

Teroj Abdulrehman Muhamed
Department of Medicine and Surgery, College of Veterinary Medicine, University of Duhok, Iraq

Lokman T Omer Al-barwary
Department of Pathology and Microbiology, College of Veterinary Medicine, University of Duhok, Iraq

Bonaparte A, Heo J and Murtaugh RJ
VCA All Care Animal Referral Center, 18440 Amistad Street, Fountain Valley, CA 92708, USA

Dhaliwal RS
Silicon Valley Veterinary Specialists, 7160 Santa Teresa Boulevard, San Jose, CA 95139, USA

Lawal JR and Ibrahim UI
Department of Veterinary Medicine, University of Maiduguri, Nigeria

El-Yuguda AD
Animal Virus Research Laboratory, Department of Veterinary Microbiology and Parasitology, University of Maiduguri, Nigeria

Christopher T Cornelison, Blake Cherney, Kyle T Gabriel, Courtney K Barlament and Sidney A Crow Jr
Applied and Environmental Microbiology, Georgia State University, Atlanta, GA, USA

Desalegn Deferes
Lemu Bilbilo District Livestock and Fisheries Resource and Development Office, Arsi, Ethiopia

Minda Asfaw Geresu
School of Agriculture, Animal and Range Sciences Course Team, Madda Walabu University, Bale-Robe, Ethiopia

Pinar Can, Murat Caliskan, Irem Gul Sancak and Omer Besalti
Department of Surgery, Faculty of Veterinary Medicine, Ankara University, Ankara, Turkey

Sevil Atalay Vural and Arda Selin Coskan
Department of Pathology, Faculty of Veterinary Medicine, Ankara University, Ankara, Turkey

Cisel Yazgan
Department of Radiology, Faculty of Medicine, Hacettepe University, Ankara, Turkey

Wondwossen Belay, Daniel Teshome and Abebaw Abiye
School of Veterinary Medicine, Wollo University, Amhara, Ethiopia

Kumela Lelisa
National Institute for Control and Eradication of Tsetse Fly and Trypanosomosis, Addis Ababa, Ethiopia

Adem Abdela
College of Veterinary Medicine, Haramaya University, Dire Dawa, Ethiopia

Delesa Damena
National Animal Health Diagnostic and Investigation Center, Sebeta, Ethiopia

Dinaol Belina, Abdurahman Giri, Shimelis Meng-istu and Amare Eshetu
College of Veterinary Medicine, Haramaya University, PO Box 138, Dire Dawa, Ethiopia

Azeem Riaz M, Aslam A, Rehman M and Yaqub T
Department of Pathology, University of Veterinary and Animal Sciences, Lahore, Pakistan

Christopher Jacob Kasanga and Gerald Misinzo
Department of Veterinary Microbiology and Parasitology, Sokoine University of Agriculture, Chuo Kikuu, Morogoro, Tanzania

Tebogo Kgotlele
Department of Veterinary Microbiology and Parasitology, Sokoine University of Agriculture, Chuo Kikuu, Morogoro, Tanzania
Molecular Biology Section, Botswana National Veterinary Laboratory, Gaborone, Botswana

Emeli Torsson
Department of Veterinary Microbiology and Parasitology, Sokoine University of Agriculture, Chuo Kikuu, Morogoro, Tanzania
Department of Biomedical Sciences and Veterinary Public Health, Swedish University of Agricultural Sciences, SE-750 07 Uppsala, Sweden

Jonas Johansson Wensman
Department of Veterinary Microbiology and Parasitology, Sokoine University of Agriculture, Chuo Kikuu, Morogoro, Tanzania
Department of Clinical Sciences, Swedish University of Agricultural Sciences, SE-750 07 Uppsala, Sweden

Robert P Lavan
Outcomes Research, Animal Health Center for Observational and Real-World Evidence, Merck & Co. Inc., Kenilworth, NJ 07033, USA

Robert Armstrong
Animal Health Global Marketing, Merck & Co. Inc., Madison, NJ 07940, USA

Dorothy Normile
Animal Health Technical Services, Merck & Co. Inc., Madison, NJ 07940, USA

Dongmu Zhang and Kaan Tunceli
Center for Observational and Real-World Evidence, Merck & Co. Inc., Kenilworth, NJ 07033, USA

Ezeddin Adem
Metema Woreda Office of Agriculture and Rural Development, Metema, Gondar, Ethiopia

Tewodros Alemneh
Woreta City Office of Agriculture and Environmental Protection, S/Gondar, Woreta, Ethiopia

Qianrong Wu, Lee L Schulz
Department of Economics, Iowa State University, Ames, Iowa, USA

Glynn T Tonsor
Department of Agricultural Economics, Kansas State University, Manhattan, Kansas, USA

Julia M Smith
Department of Animal and Veterinary Sciences, The University of Vermont, Burlington, Vermont, USA

Mohamed Kedir
National Tsetse and Trypanosomosis Investigation and Control Center, Bedele, Ethiopia

Kumela Lelisa
National Institute for Control and Eradication of Tsetse Fly and Trypanosomosis, Ethiopia

Delesa Damena
National Animal Health Diagnostic and Investigation Center, Sebeta, Ethiopia

Amare Eshetu, Tilahun Ayele, Shimelis Mengistu, and Dinaol Belina
College of Veterinary Medicine, Haramaya University, PO Box-138, Dire Dawa, Ethiopia

Tolosa Shane and Teshome Gunse
Arsi Zone Livestock and Fisheries Development Office, Ethiopia

Fanos Tadesse Woldemariyam
College Veterinary Medicine and Agriculture, Addis Ababa University, Ethiopia

Eyob Eticha, Diriba Lemma and Birhanu Abera
Asella Regional Veterinary Laboratory, PO Box 212, Asella, Ethiopia

Hani Selemon
Arsi University School of Agricultural and Environmental Science, Asella, Ethiopia

Nesradin Yune and Nejash Abdela
School of Veterinary Medicine, College of Agriculture and Veterinary Medicine, Jimma University, PO Box 307, Jimma, Ethiopia

Solomon Abreham, Merry Hailu and Ali Worku
Veterinary Drugs and Feed Administration Control Authority, Addis Ababa, Ethiopia

Solomon Tsegaye
College of Agriculture, Woldia University, Woldia, Ethiopia

Tagesu Abdisa and Tolera Tagesu
Jimma University College of Agriculture and Veterinary Medicine, Jimma, Ethiopia

Nesradin Yune and Nejash Abdela
School of Veterinary Medicine, College of Agriculture and Veterinary Medicine, Jimma University, Jimma, Ethiopia

Wolde Akalu Biruk
Ministry of Agriculture and Rural Development, Ethiopia

Kassahun Tessema, Hussen Bedu and Mebrat Ejo
Department of Biomedical Sciences, Faculty of Veterinary Medicine, University of Gondar, Gondar, Ethiopia

Adem Hiko
Department of Veterinary Epidemiology, Microbiology and Public Health, College of Veterinary Medicine, Haramaya University, Haramaya, Ethiopia

Abdeljelil Ghram
Laboratory of Epidemiology and Veterinary Microbiology, Pasteur Institute of Tunis, University Tunis El Manar, 13 Place Pasteur, Tunis- Belvedere, Tunisia

Rim Aouini and Nacira Laamiri
Laboratory of Epidemiology and Veterinary Microbiology, Pasteur Institute of Tunis, University Tunis El Manar, 13 Place Pasteur, Tunis- Belvedere, Tunisia
Faculty of Sciences Bizerte, University of Carthage, Zarzouna Bizerte, Tunisia

Javid Sadraie and Ehsan Shariat Bahadory
Medical University of Tarbiat Modaress, Tehran, Iran

Fanos Tadesse Woldemariyam
College of Veterinary Medicine and Agriculture, Addis Ababa University, Addis Ababa, Ethiopia

Yidnekachew Tadesse
Horo Guduru Zone Livestock and Fisheries Office, Ethiopia

Iyasu Angani Dereja and Dagnachew Hailemichael
Animal Products, Veterinary Drug and Feed Quality Assessment Center, Addis Ababa, Ethiopia

Zirintunda G, Etiang P , Akullo J and Ekou J
Department of Animal Production and Management, Faculty of Agriculture and Animal Sciences, Busitema University, Soroti, Uganda

Omadang L, Mawadri P
Department of Animal Production and Management, Faculty of Agriculture and Animal Sciences, Busitema University, Soroti, Uganda
National Livestock Resources Research Institute, National Agricultural Research Organization, Tororo, Uganda

Demelash Mekonnen, Amare Eshetu and Tesfaheywet Zeryehun
College of Veterinary Medicine, Haramaya University, PO Box 301, Dire Dawa, Ethiopia

Sena Meskela
Akaki Woreda Livestock and Fisheries Development, Ethiopia

Abebaw Gashaw
College of Agriculture and Veterinary Medicine, Jimma University, Ethiopia

Ebisa Mezgabu, Eyob Hirpa and Lama Yimer
School of Veterinary Medicine, Wollega University College of Medical and Health Science, PO Box 395, Nekemte, Ethiopia

Dasselegn Begna
Holeta Research Institute, Bee Research Center, Holota, Ethiopia

Abdisa Bayan
Gudeya Bila Veterinary Clinic, Ethiopia

Misganu Chali
Haru District Jeto Veterinary Clinic, Ethiopia

Anmaw Shite, Bemrew Admassu, and Yosef Malede
Faculty of Veterinary Medicine, Unit of Biomedical Sciences, University of Gondar, PO Box: 196, Gondar, Ethiopia

Tadesse Guadu
Faculty of Veterinary Medicine, Department of Veterinary Epidemiology and Public Health, University of Gondar, PO Box: 196, Gondar, Ethiopia

Tesfaye Belachew
Assela Regional Animal Health Diagnostic Laboratory, Assela, Oromiya, Ethiopia

Endalu Mulatu
Mettu University, Bedelle College of Agriculture and Forestry, Mettu, Oromia, Ethiopia

Kumela Lelisa
National Institute for Control and Eradication of Tsetse and Trypanosomosis, Addis Ababa, Ethiopia

Delesa Damena
National Animal Health Diagnostic and Investigation Center, Sebeta, Oromia, Ethiopia

Muluken Tuke
Asella City Administration Livestock Development and Fishery Office, Asella, Ethiopia

Dawit Kassaye and Yimer Muktar
College of Veterinary Medicine, Haramaya University, P.O. Box 138, Dire Dawa, Ethiopia

Tsegaye Negese and Kifle Nigusu
Hirna Regional Laboratory, P.O. Box 36, Hirna, Ethiopia

Hung-Chih Kuo, Dan-Yuan Lo and Chiu-Lin Chen
Yunlin-Chiayi-Tainan of Animal Disease Diagnostic Center, College of Veterinary Medicine, National Chiayi University, Chiayi, Taiwan

Chien-Hsien Lee, Yu-Han Shen, Yung-Long Tsai, Pei-Yu Alison Lee and Hsiao-Feng Grace Chang
GeneReach Biotech, Taichung, Taiwan

Lamessa Keno and Guluma Assefa
East Shoa Zone Livestock and Fishery Resource Office, Adama, Ethiopia

Birhanu Abera, Diriba Lemma, Eyob Eticha
Asella Regional Veterinary Laboratory, PO Box 212, Asella, Ethiopia

Elias Gezahegn
Bale Zone Pastoral Area Development Office, Ethiopia

Birhanu Abera
Asella Regional Veterinary Laboratory, Ethiopia

Dinku Assefa
Yem Special District Livestock Development and Fishery Office, Ethiopia

Hussen Yunus
Bale Zone Livestock Development and Fishery Office, Ethiopia

Dinku Assefa
Yem Special District Livestock and Fishery Resource Office, SNNPRS, Ethiopia

Elias Gezaheng
Bale Zone Pastoral Area Development Office, Bale Robe, Ethiopia

Birhanu Abera, Eyob Eticha and Diriba Lemma
Asella Regional Veterinary Laboratory, Asella, Ethiopia

Tekle Hailemariam
Kembata Tembaro District Livestock and Fishery Resource Office, SNNPRS, Ethiopia

Lynda O Obodoechi, Chidi O Anyaoha, Nnenna E Ibezim, Majesty E Alukagberie and John A Nwanta
Veterinary Public Health and Preventive Medicine, University of Nigeria, Nsukka, Nigeria

Chukwunyere O Nwosu
Veterinary Parasitology and Entomology, University of Nigeria, Nsukka, Nigeria

Chika I Nwosuh
National Veterinary Research Institute, Vom, Plateau State, Nigeria

Index

www.ingramcontent.com/pod-product-compliance
Lightning Source LLC
Chambersburg PA
CBHW080411190526
45161CB00003B/206

* 9 7 8 1 6 4 1 1 6 0 9 4 0 *